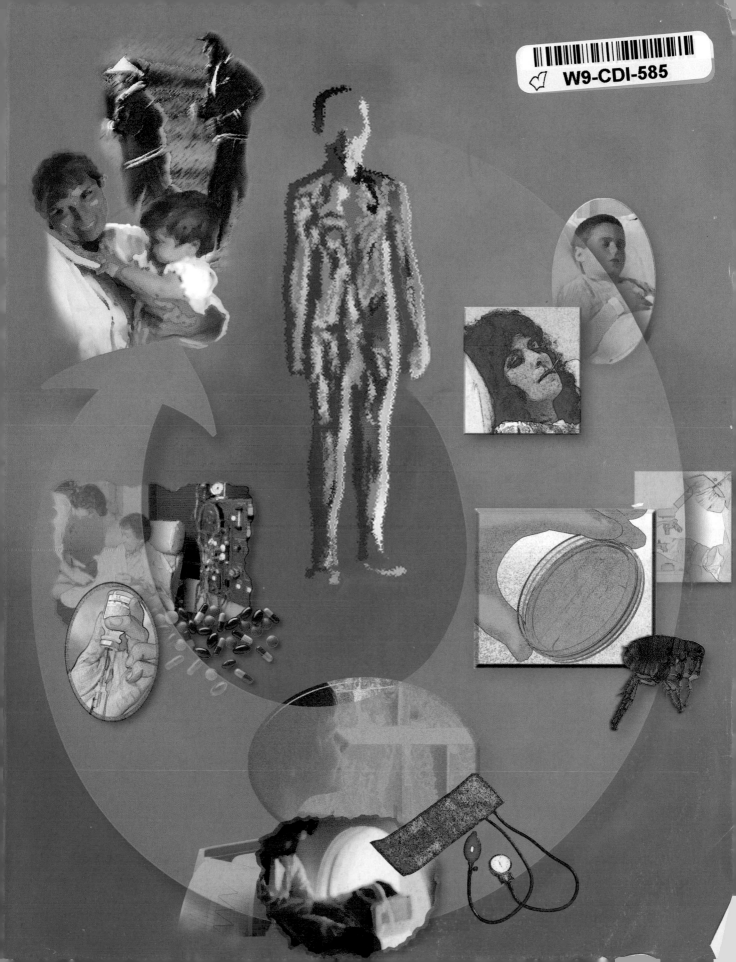

Essentials of Human Diseases and Conditions

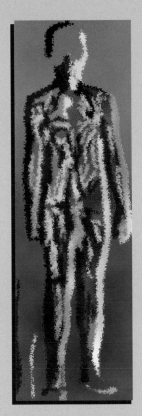

Essentials of Human Diseases and Conditions

Second Edition

MARGARET SCHELL FRAZIER, RN, CMA, BS
formerly
Department Chair, Health and Human Services Division
Program Chair, Medical Assisting Program
Ivy Tech State College, Northeast
Fort Wayne, Indiana

JEANETTE WIST DRZYMKOWSKI, RN, BS
formerly
Associate Faculty
Ivy Tech State College, Northeast
Fort Wayne, Indiana

SANDRA J. DOTY, RN, ADN
Contributing author

W.B. SAUNDERS COMPANY
An Imprint of Elsevier Science
Philadelphia   London   New York   St. Louis   Sydney   Toronto

W.B. SAUNDERS COMPANY
An Imprint of Elsevier Science

The Curtis Center
Independence Square West
Philadelphia, Pennsylvania 19106

Editor-in-Chief: Andrew Allen
Senior Acquisitions Editor: Adrianne Williams
Senior Developmental Editor: Helaine Barron
Project Manager: Evelyn Adler
Senior Production Manager: Pete Faber
Illustration Specialist: Margaret Shaw
Book Designer: Nicholas Rook

Library of Congress Cataloging-in-Publication Data

Frazier, Margaret Schell.
    Essentials of human diseases and conditions / Margaret Schell Frazier,
Jeanette W. Drzymkowski; Sandra J. Doty, contributing author.—2nd ed.

        p. cm.

Includes index.

ISBN 0–7216–8475–0

    1. Diseases.   2. Internal medicine.   3. Pathology. I. Drzymkowski, Jeanette
    W. II. Doty, Sandra J. III. Title.

[DNLM: 1. Pathology.   2. Disease. QZ 140 F848e 2000]

RC46.F79 2000

616–dc21   99–057048

ESSENTIALS OF HUMAN DISEASES AND CONDITIONS   ISBN 0–7216–8475–0

Printed in China

Last digit is the print number: 9   8   7   6   5   4

To Dave, you are my love and my strength.
To our children, Mark, Mischelle, Mary, and Margaret Ann (Pegi),
you are our hope and dreams.
To our grandchildren, Matthew, Michael, Mitchell, Andrew, and those yet to be born,
you are our joy.
To the memory of Dad and Mom, Alfred O. and Emma Margaret Schell,
you were my motivation.
And, finally, to
Maverick Luther Musser,
January 10, 1998 to August 18, 1999,
Chapter 2 is for you and about you.
You came into this world too early and left it too early.
You were a blessing in our lives.
Your heart lives on in another as you will forever live on in our hearts.
Love, Grandma Margie

Dedicated with love and gratitude to
Frank
and to the Wist-Drzymkowski generation, Michael, Mark, Gregory, and Wanda;
their spouses, Annemarie, Michele, and Steven;
our grandchildren,
Kristina, Justin, Michael Matthew, Christian, Brandy, Kevin Francis, and Billy;
to Daniel, never to be forgotten;
proudly to my parents, Wanda and Ed Wist,
in the year of their 60th wedding anniversary.
Jeanette

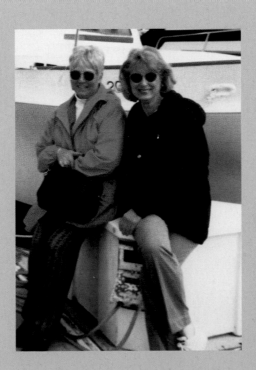

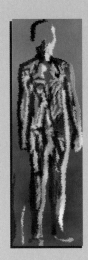

Preface

Essentials of Human Diseases and Conditions is a user-friendly textbook intended to promote a stimulating and enjoyable learning experience for students as well as providing an invaluable teaching tool for instructors. This encyclopedic but simplified textbook includes comprehensive information about hundreds of diseases and conditions. Supplementary facts highlighted throughout the text offer additional clarification of information.

Because disease conditions are universally experienced, there is a natural curiosity about and interest in understanding them. Written by experienced nurses, who are educators of para-professionals, this book attempts to condense and simplify current medical information on the more common clinical disorders encountered in the health field. Students in the field of medical assisting, medical transcription, insurance coding, or other allied health programs, who have had a prior introduction to basic anatomy and physiology of the human body and medical terminology, will find this system of learning orderly, concise, and easy to comprehend. The sheer magnitude of the body of knowledge represented in this field would overwhelm any beginning student if it was not streamlined into a logical format.

Each chapter is introduced with a brief review of the normal function of the specific body system discussed in that chapter and reinforced with clear illustrations. Important pathologic mechanisms are explained and illustrated as well. Each disease entity is presented in a format that discusses the nature of the disease in symptoms experienced by the patient and signs detected by the physician, etiologic factors, diagnosis, and treatment options. This format also considers the inherent progression of a patient's scenario: (1) the individual reports symptoms to a health care provider, usually in a clinical setting; (2) abnormal signs of a clinical disorder may be elicited during the physical examination and/or subsequent diagnostic testing; and (3) an appropriate treatment option is initiated and monitored for results.

Additional features included in each chapter are a chapter outline, which introduces the topics discussed in that chapter and indicates how topics are arranged, and learning objectives, which inform both the student and the instructor about the goals that should be achieved after studying the chapter. Key terms are also featured in chapter openers. Each key term has the phonetic spelling of that term next to it so that students know the correct pronunciation and become comfortable with the use of these medical expressions in oral discussion. These key terms are considered common words or phrases that medical personnel are likely to encounter in the specific specialty. A summary at the end of each chapter gives an overview of the material discussed. The review challenge contains study questions at the completion of the text material. Bolded words found in the chapters are defined in the glossary for the purpose of review or clarification of meaning. Some bolded words may appear in the key terms list.

The authors have kept before them the advantages to the student in better understanding clinical disorders. These include (1) great professional gain when one comprehends the effects that a disease has on a person, (2) increased communication skills with the entire health care team, and (3) personal education that has many practical applications.

Preface

The information presented in this book represents research into the mainstream of medical knowledge and its application in clinical practice. In the actual practice of the dynamic art and science of medicine, great variations and opposing views result in either more conservative or more aggressive concepts. The material presented in this text should not take the place of individualized consultation with medical experts.

Margaret Schell Frazier, RN, CMA, BS
Jeanette Wist Drzymkowski, RN, BS

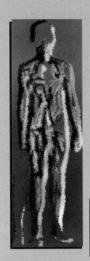

Acknowledgments

We extend our gratitude to and acknowledge our professional reviewers and those who provided guidance, assistance, encouragement, and support in the development and the revision of the second edition of this book.

The expertise of the following professionals assures the readers that the information presented in this book was reviewed for its accuracy. We thank them for taking the time to critique the material: Jacqueline L. Akey, MD, Gilbert H. Bierman, MD, Donald A. Bollheimer, MD, Dean D. Dauscher, MD, Thomas V. Doty, DDS, Sheema Farooqui, MD, Margaret Ann Frazier, MSEd, Alan R. Gilbert, MD, Thomas Hayhurst, MD, Steven M. Jones, MD, Craig T. Marks, MD, Michael F. O'Hear, PhD, and Alan W. Sidel, MD. Special thanks to the following professionals who so patiently answered our numerous questions as we revised the manuscript. Tai Min Chen, MD; Toni Cruse, CMA, ASCP, PBT; Dean D. Dauscher, MD; Margaret Ann Frazier, MSEd; Mary Sue Frazier, MSEd; Debra Green, CMA; Jodie Inskeep, RN, ASN; Mischelle Frazier Musser, RN, ASN; David P. Schlueter, MD; and Kimberly Weaver, RN, ASN.

To Adrianne Williams, Senior Acquisitions Editor, thank you for your vision in this second edition; to Helaine Barron, Senior Developmental Editor, once again we had the privilege of working with you. Thanks for coordinating our efforts, keeping us on track, and being our main communication link; to Evelyn Adler, Project Manager, thanks for all your help and troubleshooting; to Mickie Hall, thanks for your skillful achievement as our copy editor; to Nicholas Rook, our designer, for your artistic design of the cover and interior; and to Peter Faber, our production manager, for your astute scrutiny.

To Maverick Luther Musser and his family. Thank you for teaching us about the joy and value of life by displaying courage and strength during the 19 months Maverick blessed our lives. Also thanks for making us aware of the technology available to very premature neonates. The situations you faced enlightened us to the challenges and possible conditions resulting from premature birth.

Finally, to each other. We shared joys and sorrows, laughter and tears, and still accomplished this revision long distance thanks to the Internet. Modern technology and friendships are wonderful.

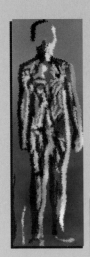

Contents

Contents

Contents

ENRICHMENTS

Essentials of
Human
Diseases and
Conditions

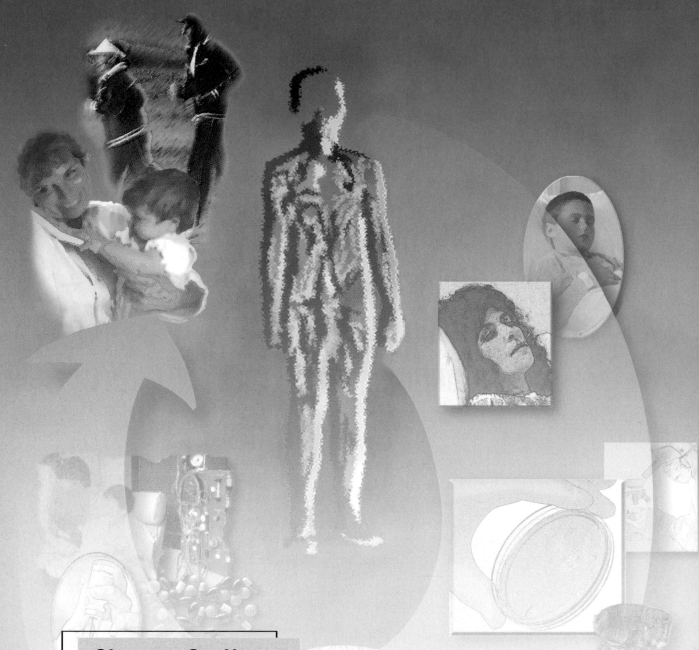

Chapter Outline

Mechanisms of Disease, Diagnosis, and Treatment

Learning Objectives

After studying Chapter 1, you should be able to:

1. Explain how a pathologic condition impacts the homeostasis of the body.
2. Describe the difference between
   Signs and symptoms of disease
   Acute and chronic disease
   Benign and malignant neoplasms
3. Identify the predisposing factors of disease.
4. Describe the ways in which pathogens may cause disease.
5. Track the essential steps in diagnosis of disease.
6. List the prevention guidelines for cancer.
7. Explain the inflammation response to disease.
8. Describe the hospice concept of care.
9. Name two ways an individual can practice positive health behavior.
10. Describe (a) the physiology of pain, (b) how pain may be treated, and (c) what is meant by referred pain.
11. Define the holistic approach to medical care.
12. Describe examples of alternative medical therapies.

Key Terms

allergen	(**AL**–ler–jen)	hospice	(**HAUS**–pis)
anaphylaxis	(**an**–ah–fih–**LAK**–sis)	ischemia	(is–**KEY**–me–ah)
antigen	(**AN**–tih–jen)	karyotype	(**KARE**–ee–o–type)
asymptomatic	(**a**–sim–toh–**MAH**–tik)	metastasis	(meh–**TAS**–tah–sis)
auscultation	(**aws**–kel–**TAY**–shun)	mutation	(meu–**TAY**–shun)
cachexia	(kah–**KEX**–e–ah)	nociceptor	(**no**–see–**SEHP**-tor)
carcinogenic	(**kar**–sih–no–**JEN**–ik)	oncogene	(**AHN**–ko–jeen)
chromosome	(**KRO**–mo–sohm)	pathogenesis	(**path**–o–**JEN**–eh–sis)
genotype	(**JEN**–o–type)	phagocytic	(**fag**–o–**SIT**–ik)
homeostasis	(**ho**–me–o–**STA**–sis)	somatoform	(so–**MAT**–o–form)

Pathology at First Glance

Pathology, the scientific study of disease, is the objective description of the traits, causes, and effects of abnormal conditions. Pathologic conditions involve measurable changes in normal structure and function that threaten the internal stability, or **homeostasis,** of the body.

In human disease, the negative characteristics, or departures from normal status, are described subjectively by patients as symptoms. Signs, or abnormal objective findings, are the evidence of disease found by physical examination and diagnostic testing. Signs of disease frequently correlate with the symptoms. In other instances, the signs of disease may be noted in an **asymptomatic** patient, as in the discovery of a painless tumor or the finding of an abnormal blood pressure reading in a person with undiagnosed essential hypertension. A defined collection of signs and symptoms that characterize a disorder or condition is termed a syndrome.

The development of disease occurs in stages, described as the **pathogenesis.** In the course of infection, for instance, the pathogenesis may include an incubation period, a period of fullblown symptoms, and then remission or convalescence. The pathogenesis of a disease varies with the individual patient, the causative factors, and medical intervention.

Diseases frequently are described as acute or chronic. Acute refers to an abrupt onset of more or less severe symptoms that run a brief course (usually shorter than 6 months) and then resolve or, in some cases, result in death. When a disease develops slowly, or is intermittent, and lasts longer than 6 months, it is described as chronic. Additionally, persons who have continuous pain as part of chronic syndromes often experience depression.

Mechanisms of Disease

Human disease, a universal occurrence, has varied manifestations, any of which threatens a person's ability to adapt to internal and external stressors and to maintain a state of well-being.

Systemic health, or internal equilibrium, is preserved by numerous body organs and structures that work in concert to meet specific cellular needs. Any disruption of the body's equilibrium produces degenerative changes at the cellular level that may produce signs and symptoms of disease. Major disruptions in the body's cellular equilibrium that threaten homeostasis include fluid and electrolyte imbalance and excessive acidity or alkalinity.

Elements involved either directly or indirectly in pathogenesis include predisposing factors, genetic diseases, infection, inflammation and repair, neoplasms, physical trauma, chemical agents, malnutrition, immune disorders, aging, psychological factors, and mental disorders.

PREDISPOSING FACTORS

Predisposing factors, also called risk factors, make a person or group more vulnerable to disease. Although the recognition of risk factors may be significant in prevention, diagnosis, and prognosis, it does not precisely predict the occurrence of disease, nor does the absence of predisposing factors necessarily protect against the development of disease. A person may be susceptible to one or more risk factors that overlap or occur in combination, to a greater or lesser degree. Predisposing factors include age, sex, lifestyle, environment, and heredity.

Age. From complications during pregnancy and the postpartum period to maladies associated with aging, there exist increased risks of diseases intrinsic to one's stage in the human life cycle.

Sex. Certain diseases are more common in women (e.g., multiple sclerosis and osteoporosis) and other disorders are more frequent in men (e.g., gout and Parkinson's disease).

Lifestyle. Occupation, habits, or one's manner of living can have negative cumulative effects that impose threats to health. Some known risk factors associated with lifestyle may be controlled in favor of promoting health instead of predisposing to disease; examples include smoking, excessive drinking of alcohol, poor nutrition, lack of exercise, and certain psychological stressors.

Environment. Pollution of air and water is considered a major risk factor for illnesses such as cancer and pulmonary disease. Poor living conditions, excessive noise, chronic psychological stress, and a geographic location conducive to disease also are environmental risk factors.

Heredity. Genetic predisposition (inheritance) currently is considered a major risk factor.

Family histories of coronary disease, cancer, and renal disease are known hereditary risk factors. Hereditary factors in disease that appear regularly in generations are likely to affect males and females equally. Hereditary or genetic diseases frequently originate from the combined effects of inheritance and environmental factors. Examples are mental illness, cancer, hypertension, heart disease, and diabetes. Some evidence shows that smoking, a sedentary lifestyle, and a diet high in saturated fat, combined with a positive family history, compound a person's risk for heart disease. Schizophrenia may result from a combination of genetic predisposition and numerous psychological and sociocultural causes.

PREVENTIVE HEALTH CARE

Preventive health care places emphasis on strategies for prevention of disease. There currently is statistical evidence that positive personal health behavior, in conjunction with prophylactic medical services, may reduce the mortality rate in certain diseases, such as cardiovascular disease. Identification of risk factors and specific screening tests allow individuals the opportunity to modify their lifestyles, and use medical measures to help prevent the onset of disease or at least minimize complications. For example, a fatty diet may contribute to the risk of cancer or coronary heart disease. Smoking is known to contribute to one in six deaths in the United

States. Many injuries are preventable by: (1) improved safety measures in occupational machinery and automobiles; (2) protective labeling and packaging of consumable food, drugs, and toxic products; and (3) general public safety education. Family violence is a serious and growing epidemic in the United States, resulting in psychological stress and physical trauma. In many cases, early intervention may be preventive. Legal, social, and medical authorities can be instrumental in identifying and protecting those caught in the cycle of domestic violence before the onset of serious medical consequences.

GENETIC DISEASES

Every cell in the body is coded with genetic information arranged on 23 pairs of chromosomes, half inherited from one parent and half from the other parent. Each cell in an individual's body contains the same chromosomes and genetic code (genotype). A **karyotype** is an ordered arrangement of photographs of a full chromosome set (Fig. 1–1). Genes, the basic units of heredity, are small stretches of a DNA (deoxyribonucleic acid) molecule, situated at a particular site on a chromosome. A gene is termed X linked when it is located on an X chromosome.

Genetic diseases are (1) produced by an abnormality in, or a mutation of, the genetic code in a single gene; (2) caused by several abnormal genes (producing so-called polygenic diseases);

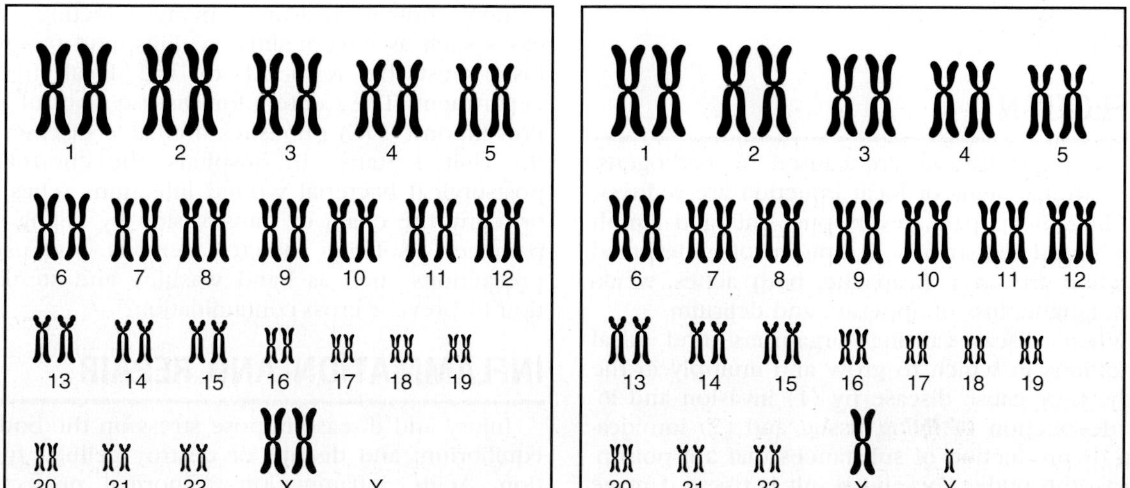

Figure 1–1

Examples of karyotypes. *A,* Normal female (46,XX). *B,* Normal male (46,XY). (From Damjanov I: Pathology for the Health-Related Professions. Philadelphia: WB Saunders, 1996.)

or (3) caused by the abnormal presence or absence of an entire chromosome or alteration in the structure of chromosomes. Harmful genetic **mutations,** or changes in the genetic code, passed from one generation to the next may occur spontaneously or be caused by agents known to disrupt the normal sequence of DNA units. Agents (called mutagens) that can damage DNA include certain chemicals, radiation, and viruses. The mutant gene may produce an abnormal protein that causes a disease, or it may fail to produce a normal cellular function. Hereditary diseases may be congenital or may not appear until later in life. Many genetic diseases are compatible with life, and some are not.

The following examples of genetic abnormalities are discussed in this book:

Huntington's chorea
Down syndrome
Hemophilia
Klinefelter's syndrome
Polycystic kidney
Dwarfism
Albinism
Hyperopia
Hemolytic anemia
Cystic fibrosis
Epilepsy
Hirschsprung's disease
Phenylketonuria
Turner's syndrome
Hemolytic disease of newborn
Cleft palate
Myopia

INFECTION

Infectious diseases are caused by pathogens. The cardinal signs of local infection are redness, swelling, heat, pain, fever, pus, enlarged lymph glands, and red streaks. Symptoms of widespread infection are fever, headache, body aches, weakness, fatigue, loss of appetite, and delirium.

When disease-causing organisms find ideal conditions in which to grow and multiply in the body, they cause disease by (1) invasion and local destruction of living tissue and (2) intoxication or production of substances that are poisonous to the body. The end result is tissue damage that has the potential for producing systemic involvement.

The sources of infection can be endogenous (originating within the body) or exogenous (originating outside the body). Modes of transmission of pathogenic organisms are direct or indirect physical contact, inhalation or droplet nuclei, ingestion of contaminated food or water, or inoculation by an insect or animal. Pathogenic agents include bacteria, viruses, fungi, and protozoa (Table 1-1).

A communicable or contagious disease can be transmitted directly from one person to another. Carriers are asymptomatic persons or animals that harbor in their bodies pathogens that can be transferred to others.

The body's natural defense systems against infection include (1) natural mechanical and chemical barriers, such as the skin, the cilia, body pH, and normal body flora; (2) the inflammatory response; and (3) the immune response. When these mechanisms of defense fail to contain or eliminate infection, appropriate and prompt medical intervention is required to treat the host and to control transmission of the infectious disease. This is accomplished by first isolating and identifying the organism by laboratory testing. Subsequently, appropriate antimicrobial therapy using antibiotic (antibacterial), antifungal, antiparasitic, or antiviral agents can begin. Analgesics for pain and antipyretic agents for fever, as well as other comfort measures, are dispensed. Adequate fluid intake, infection control measures, and rest are important for management.

Fundamental to preventing the spread of certain infections are isolation of the infected individual when necessary, implementation of immunization programs, and rudimentary public health teaching. To facilitate early intervention and infection control measures, many infectious diseases such as encephalitis, syphilis, and tuberculosis must be reported to the local health department. The Centers for Disease Control and Prevention (CDC) publishes notifiable diseases in the United States. In hospitals, the control of postsurgical bacterial wound infections relies on breaking the chain of transmission by killing the pathogen, isolating infected persons, and using precautions such as hand washing and sterilization to prevent cross-contamination.

INFLAMMATION AND REPAIR

Injury and disease impose stress on the body's equilibrium and disrupt or destroy cellular function. Acute inflammation, a normal protective physiologic response to tissue injury and disease, is accompanied by redness, heat, swelling, pain, and loss of function. Widespread inflammation is marked by systemic symptoms, such as fever, malaise, and loss of appetite. Blood testing may reveal an elevated white blood cell count or an

TABLE 1–1 ➤ Common Pathogens and Some Infections or Diseases That They Produce

ORGANISM	RESERVOIR	INFECTION OR DISEASE
Bacteria		
Escherichia coli (E. coli)	Colon, manure	Enteritis, mild to severe
Staphylococcus aureus	Skin, hair, anterior nares	Wound infection, pneumonia, food poisoning, cellulitis
Streptococcus (beta-hemolytic group A) organisms	Oropharynx, skin, perianal area	"Strep throat," rheumatic fever, scarlet fever, impetigo
Streptococcus (beta-hemolytic group B) organisms	Adult genitalia	Urinary tract infection, wound infection, endometritis
Mycobacterium tuberculosis	Lungs	Tuberculosis
Neisseria gonorrhoeae	Genitourinary tract, rectum, mouth, eye	Gonorrhea, pelvic inflammatory disease, infectious arthritis, conjunctivitis
Rickettsia rickettsii	Wood tick	Rocky Mountain spotted fever
Staphylococcus epidermidis	Skin	Wound infection, bacteremia
Viruses		
Hepatitis A virus	Feces, blood, urine	Hepatitis A (infectious hepatitis)
Hepatitis B virus	Feces, blood, all body fluids and excretions	Hepatitis B (serum hepatitis)
Herpes simplex virus	Lesions of mouth, skin, blood, excretions	Cold sores, aseptic meningitis, sexually transmitted disease
Human immunodeficiency virus (HIV)	Blood, semen, vaginal secretions (also isolated in saliva, tears, urine, breast milk, but not proven to be sources of transmission)	Acquired immunodeficiency syndrome (AIDS)
Hantavirus	Deer mouse urine, feces, and saliva	Upper respiratory infection (URI) to lower respiratory infection (LRI) to adult respiratory distress syndrome (ARDS)
Fungi		
Aspergillus organisms	Soil, dust	Aspergillosis
Candida albicans	Mouth, skin, colon, genital tract	Thrush, dermatitis
Protozoa		
Plasmodium falciparum	Mosquito	Malaria

From Potter P, Perry A: Fundamentals of Nursing: Concepts, Process, and Practice, 3rd ed. St Louis: Mosby-Year Book, 1993. Used with permission.

elevated erythrocyte sedimentation rate (ESR). The intensity of inflammation depends on the cause, the area of the body involved, and the physical condition of the person. An inflammatory response is considered a nonspecific immune response. Infection with pathogens, the effects of toxins, physical trauma, **ischemia**, and **necrosis** are some conditions that induce the inflammatory response.

Acute inflammation, an exudative response, attempts to wall off, destroy, and digest bacteria and dead or foreign tissue. Vascular changes allow fluid to leak into the site, with the release of chemicals that permit **phagocytic** activity by white blood cells. The process prevents the spread of infection with the help of antibodies and other chemicals released by cells with more specific immune activity. After the mechanisms of inflammation have contained the insult and

"cleaned up" a damaged area, repair and replacement of tissue can begin (Fig. 1–2). A normal inflammatory response can be inhibited by immune disorders, chronic illness, or the use of certain medications, especially long-term steroid therapy.

When an inflammatory response is chronic or too intense, damage can result in the affected tissue, inhibiting the healing process. Diseases with a component of chronic inflammation include arthritis, asthma, and eczema.

NEOPLASMS

A **neoplasm** (tumor) is a new growth of cells that proliferate without a purpose. Tumors result when cells begin growing rapidly and independently at the expense of the healthy organism. Neoplasms are classified as either benign or malignant and according to the tissue of origin (Tables 1–2 and 1–3).

Benign tumors develop slowly and can arise from any connective tissue. They tend to remain encapsulated and do not infiltrate surrounding tissue. When examined microscopically, benign tumor cells are well differentiated; they resemble the tissue of origin. Because tumors take up space, complications can result from compression of tissue by the lesion or obstruction of organs. Benign tumors rarely recur after surgical removal.

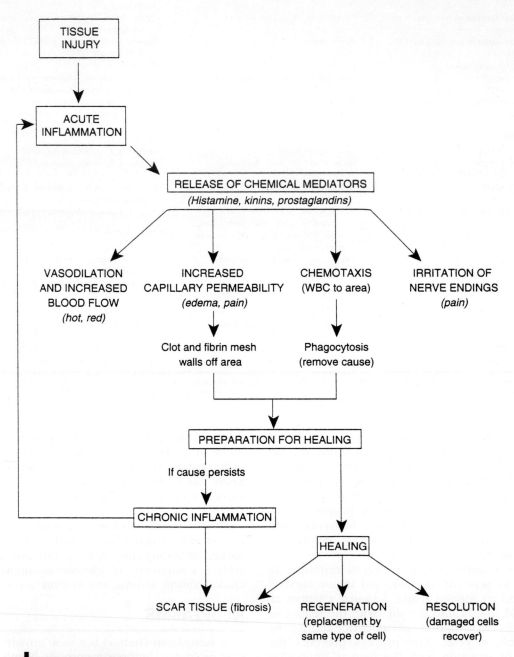

Figure 1–2

The course of inflammation and healing. (From Gould BE: Pathophysiology for the Health-Related Professions. Philadelphia: WB Saunders, 1997.)

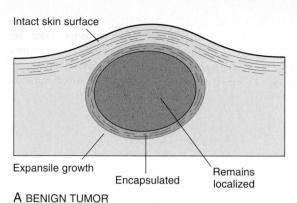

Intact skin surface

Expansile growth

Encapsulated

Remains localized

A BENIGN TUMOR

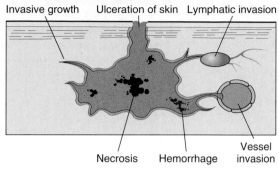

Invasive growth   Ulceration of skin   Lymphatic invasion

Necrosis   Hemorrhage   Vessel invasion

B MALIGNANT TUMOR

Gross appearance of benign *(A)* and malignant *(B)* tumors.

Malignant, or cancerous, tumors can represent a serious threat to the life and well-being of a person. The tumors consist of invasive cells that multiply excessively and can infiltrate other tissues. They tend to bleed, ulcerate, and become infected. Cancer cells are variable in appearance and disorderly (anaplastic), with irreversible changes in structure; they are usually poorly differentiated and do not resemble the tissue of origin. A major characteristic of cancerous cells is **metastasis,** which is the capacity to spread from the original site of tumor to distant sites in the body. The metastatic process results when cancer cells spread through the blood and lymph system, causing secondary tumors or seeding tumors in adjacent body cavities. If the spread is not controlled, the effects on the body can be **cachexia** and death.

Cancer is actually many different diseases with numerous causes. Cancer may be caused by both external exposure to **carcinogens** (chemicals, radiation, and viruses) and internal factors (hormones, immune conditions, and inherited mutations). Ten years or longer may pass between exposures or mutations and the onset of detectable cancer. Cancer can develop in anyone, but the frequency increases with age. Figure 1–3 shows the leading sites of cancer incidence and death.

Recommendations to decrease the risk of cancer encompass guidelines and appropriate screening tests for early detection and treatment. Primary prevention guidelines include:

• A low-fat, high-fiber diet rich in fruits and vegetables for vitamin A and E;
• Elimination of active and passive exposure to cigarette smoke;

TABLE 1–2 ➤ Comparison of Benign and Malignant Tumors

CHARACTERISTICS	BENIGN	MALIGNANT
Mode of growth	Relatively slow growth by expansion; encapsulated; cells adhere to each other	Rapid growth; invades surrounding tissue by infiltration
Cells under microscopic examination	Resemble tissue of origin; well differentiated; appear normal	Do not resemble tissue of origin; vary in size and shape; abnormal appearance and function
Spread	Remains localized	Metastasis; cancer cells carried by blood and lymphatics to one or more other locations; secondary tumors occur
Other properties	No tissue destruction; not prone to hemorrhage; may be smooth and freely movable	Ulceration and/or necrosis; prone to hemorrhage; irregular and less movable
Recurrence	Rare after excision	A common characteristic
Pathogenesis	Symptoms related to location with obstruction and/or compression of surrounding tissue or organs; usually not life threatening unless inaccessible	Cachexia; pain; fatal if not controlled

TABLE 1–3 ➤ Classification of Neoplasms by Tissue of Origin		
TISSUE OF ORIGIN	**BENIGN**	**MALIGNANT**
Connective tissue		Sarcoma
Embryonic fibrous tissue	Myxoma	Myxosarcoma
Fibrous tissue	Fibroma	Fibrosarcoma
Adipose tissue	Lipoma	Liposarcoma
Cartilage	Chondroma	Chondrosarcoma
Bone	Osteoma	Osteogenic sarcoma
Epithelium		Carcinoma
Skin and mucous membrane	Papilloma	Squamous cell carcinoma
Glands		Basal cell carcinoma
		Transitional cell carcinoma
	Adenoma	Adenocarcinoma
	Cystadenoma	Cystadenocarcinoma
Pigmented cells (melanocytes)	Nevus	Malignant melanoma
Endothelium		Endothelioma
Blood vessels	Hemangioma	Hemangioendothelioma
		Hemangiosarcoma
		Kaposi's sarcoma
Lymph vessels	Lymphangioma	Lymphangiosarcoma
		Lymphangioendothelioma
Bone marrow		Multiple myeloma
		Ewing's sarcoma
		Leukemia
Lymphoid tissue		Malignant lymphoma
		Lymphosarcoma
		Reticulum cell sarcoma
Muscle tissue		
Smooth muscle	Leiomyoma	Leiomyosarcoma
Striated muscle	Rhabdomyoma	Rhabdomyosarcoma
Nerve tissue		
Nerve fibers and sheaths	Neuroma	Neurogenic sarcoma
	Neurinoma	
	(Neurilemoma)	
	Neurofibroma	(Neurofibrosarcoma)
Ganglion cells	Ganglioneuroma	Neuroblastoma
Glial cells	Glioma	Glioblastoma
Meninges	Meningioma	Malignant meningioma
Gonads	Dermoid cyst	Embryonal carcinoma
		Embryonal sarcoma
		Teratocarcinoma

From Black JM, Matassarin-Jacobs E: Medical-Surgical Nursing, 5/E. Philadelphia, WB Saunders, 1997, p 550.

- Limitation of skin exposure to sunlight;
- Avoidance of heavy use of alcohol;
- Avoidance of excessive exposure to radiation and radon;
- Careful evaluation for estrogen replacement therapy (ERT);
- Avoidance of chemical agents known to be carcinogenic; and
- Increased physical activity.

Cancer detection employs general and specific techniques of physical examination, medical history-taking, and laboratory screening tests.

Screening examinations can detect cancers of the breast, rectum, colon, prostate, cervix, testis, tongue, mouth, and skin early, when treatment is more likely to succeed. These cancers account for approximately half of all new cancer cases.

Tumor cells produce and secrete substances called tumor markers. Screening tests for elevation of blood serum levels of tumor markers, when considered with other diagnostic data, are shown to have clinical value (1) in the diagnosis of cancer and (2) to evaluate response to therapy. For example, in primary and metastatic

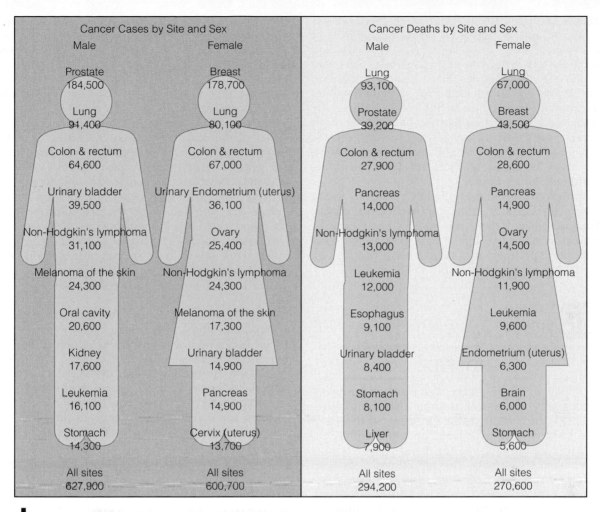

Figure 1–3

Leading sites of new cancer cases and deaths—1998 estimates, excluding basal and squamous cell skin cancer and in situ carcinomas except urinary bladder. (Reprinted by permission of the American Cancer Society, Inc. Cancer Facts and Figures—1998.)

prostate cancer, elevated prostate-specific antigen (PSA) may be found.

If cancer is suspected, additional diagnostic investigation is achieved with high-technology imaging techniques and most decisively by **biopsy** of the lesion. After a diagnosis of cancer is made, it is further defined by grading (assessing the degree of change in the appearance of tumor cells) and staging (determining the extent of spread of the tumor and regional lymph node involvement). The staging and grading of tumors is a guide for the physician in determining the course of treatment and the prognosis.

The goal of treatment of cancer is to eradicate every cancer cell in the body. This is attempted through surgery, radiation, radioactive substances, chemicals, hormones, and immunotherapy. These measures frequently are used in combination not only to cure but also to promote comfort, by shrinking tumor mass and relieving pain. Currently, approximately 4 of 10 patients who are diagnosed with cancer are alive 5 years after the diagnosis.

Advances in radiation and chemotherapy have diminished the need for radical surgery. Both radiation and most useful anticancer drugs have significant side effects that require constant surveillance and management. Pain management at every stage is a major concern for patients and includes generous use of various analgesics and noninvasive techniques that promote relaxation and distraction. Immunotherapy, although still investigative, may be most effective during early stages of cancer when used in combination with other modalities. Terminally ill persons can be referred to hospice care for compassionate, holistic case management. See the Enrichment describing hospice care.

Research into cancer therapy points to useful information about new approaches to cancer treatment that show promise. One theory is based on starving a tumor by inhibiting its blood supply. Experimental studies have shown that in-

hibiting the growth of new blood vessels (angiogenesis), which feed the tumor, causes the tumor to shrink. Since 1994, two angiogenesis inhibitors, angiostatin and endostatin, have had positive results in mice. Humans are scheduled to begin receiving experimental treatments with angiogenesis inhibitors.

Certain forms of cancer are inherited; thus, much of the current research is focused on cancer at its genetic roots. Scientists are investigating genetic switches that cause healthy cells to become disorderly. It has been observed that broken genes can send cells into spirals of cancerous growth. Herceptin, recently approved by the Food and Drug Administration (FDA), seems to disable cancer cells that are fueled by a bad gene. This new drug, specific for certain advanced aggressive types of breast cancer, bypasses healthy cells, reducing distressing side effects.

Since 1990, another experimental method of therapeutic intervention, gene therapy, has been used. Replacing or augmenting a defective human gene potentially mends the basis of the disease state. Inherited genetic diseases are logical targets for gene therapy; cystic fibrosis is one example. Indications for gene therapy are malignancies associated with mutations in **oncogenes.** Certain criteria are necessary for any gene therapy to be efficacious.

Specific types of cancer are discussed in subsequent chapters of this book.

PHYSICAL TRAUMA AND CHEMICAL AGENTS

Physical trauma is the major cause of death in children and young adults. Common mechanisms of acute injury are falls; motor vehicle accidents, including those involving pedestrians; physical abuse; penetrating injuries; drowning; and burns. Emergency management begins with triage to determine the priorities of care. Persons who sustain trauma require precise assessment and management to prevent infection, to minimize the insult to the body tissues, to combat shock and hemorrhage, and to restore homeostasis.

Chemical agents or irritants that are potentially injurious include pollutants, poisons, drugs, preservatives, cosmetics, and dyes. Extreme heat or cold, radiation, electrical shock, and insect and snake bites are other instruments of injury to the body.

See Chapter 15 for a discussion of specific types of trauma.

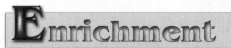

HOSPICE

The word hospice describes a unique concept of care developed to help patients and their families deal with life-threatening illness. Hospice philosophy of care includes a compassionate staff pledged to respect the patient's choice for care, providing comfort, dignity, and privacy. The focus is comfort and supportive care for the family unit during the illness and bereavement period. Financial assessment determines eligibility for financial assistance if needed.

The philosophy of hospice affirms life and neither hastens nor postpones death. Dying is recognized as a normal process, even when it is the result of disease. Through appropriate care and the promotion of a caring community sensitive to their needs, patients and families may be free to attain a degree of mental and spiritual preparation for death that is satisfactory to them. The hospice team and services may include a physician, a registered nurse available day and night, a social worker, a home health aide as needed, a chaplain as needed, volunteers, therapists, and a pharmacist.

Hospice provides a full range of care in a variety of settings, such as the hospice care center, home care, and respite care.

MALNUTRITION

Disorders of nutrition, as discussed in Chapter 8, may be the result of a deficient diet or disease conditions that do not allow the body to break down, absorb, or use food. An example of a severe deficiency disease is protein-calorie malnutrition (kwashiorkor), the starvation associated with famine. Other nutritional disorders include iron deficiency, anemia, obesity, and hypervitaminoses.

IMMUNE DISORDERS

The immune system is a complex network of specialized cells and organs that has evolved to defend the body against attacks by foreign organisms. Immune disorders are the result of a breakdown in the body's defense system that may generate (1) hypersensitivity (allergy), (2) autoimmune diseases, or (3) immunodeficiency disorders.

Allergic disease is a hypersensitivity of the body to a substance (**allergen**) ordinarily considered harmless. Common allergens include inhalants (dust, molds, and fungi), foods, drugs, chemicals, and physical agents (heat, cold, and radiation). Initial exposure to an allergen, which acts as **antigen** (a substance that causes the allergic response), stimulates the production of immunoglobulin E (IgE) antibodies, and the person thus is sensitized. Subsequent exposures trigger the allergic response, which is an antigen-antibody reaction causing the release of histamine and other chemicals (Fig. 1-4). The chemicals cause a variety of persistent and bothersome symptoms, including nasal congestion, sneezing, coughing, wheezing, itching, burning, swelling, and diarrhea. Common allergic conditions include seasonal allergic rhinitis (hay fever), allergic sinusitis, bronchial asthma, urticaria (hives), eczema, and food, drug, or venom allergy. These conditions may range from mild and self-limiting to severe and life threatening.

When the offending allergens can be identified, they are eliminated from the diet or the environment. Symptomatic treatment includes the use of antihistamines, bronchial dilators, and corticosteroids. Desensitization with a series of injections may be recommended to build immunity to some antigens. Severe systemic manifestations of allergic responses include **anaphylaxis,** serum sickness, arthralgia, and **status asthmaticus.** For example, anaphylactic shock, the result of a severe systemic allergic reaction, calls for emergency lifesaving intervention.

Autoimmune diseases represent a large group of disorders marked by an inappropriate or excessive response of the body's defense system that allows the immune system to become self-destructive. Normally, the immune system is able to distinguish self-antigens, which are harmless, from foreign antigens, which present a threat to the body. In autoimmune diseases, antibodies are formed against self-antigens mistaken as foreign. Why the body becomes confused or what triggers an autoimmune response remains a mystery. Many serious diseases appear to have a strong autoimmune component. Examples are glomerulonephritis (see Chapter 11), Hashimoto's disease (see Chapter 4), and rheumatoid arthritis (see Chapter 3).

Immunodeficiency disorders result from a depressed or absent immune response. Causative factors can be primary, manifested by a characteristic decrease in the number of T cells and B cells, leaving the body in a weakened state; the body has difficulty in defending itself against infection and tumors. Immunodeficiency also may be secondary to disease or infection or may be the result of damage to the immune system from drugs, radiation, or surgery. Acquired immunodeficiency disease (AIDS), a prominent example of an immunodeficiency state, is caused by infection with a virus.

Chapter 3 discusses specific diseases of the immune system.

AGING

Because of the gradual diminishment of body functions, the aging process, although not considered a disease in itself, is a risk factor for the onset of many health problems. For this reason, a yearly physical examination with specific screening tests is recommended after age 50 years. Screening examinations include determination of blood cholesterol levels for **hyperlipidemia, electrocardiogram** (ECG) for heart disease, rectal examination for bowel cancer and prostate enlargement, blood pressure check for hypertension, Pap (Papanicolaou) smear for cervical cancer, mammogram for breast cancer, and urinalysis for possible diabetes and renal disease. Other common concerns in older persons are substance abuse, overmedication, loss of mental acuity, depression, and nutritional problems.

PSYCHOLOGICAL FACTORS

The constant interaction between mind and body potentially affects a person's state of well-

12

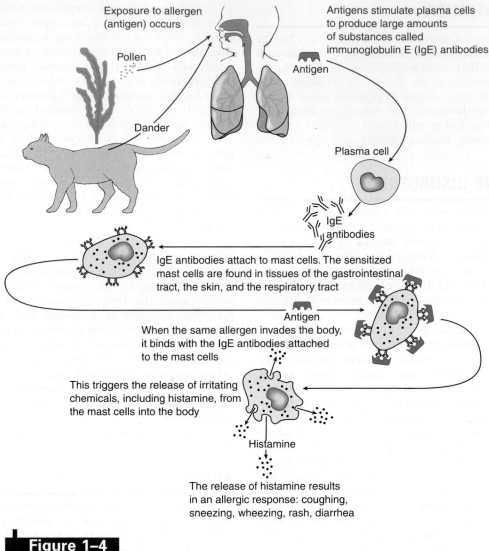

Exposure to allergen
(antigen) occurs

Pollen

Dander

Antigens stimulate plasma cells
to produce large amounts
of substances called
immunoglobulin E (IgE) antibodies

Antigen

Plasma cell

IgE
antibodies

IgE antibodies attach to mast cells. The sensitized
mast cells are found in tissues of the gastrointestinal
tract, the skin, and the respiratory tract

Antigen

When the same allergen invades the body,
it binds with the IgE antibodies attached
to the mast cells

This triggers the release of irritating
chemicals, including histamine, from
the mast cells into the body

Histamine

The release of histamine results
in an allergic response: coughing,
sneezing, wheezing, rash, diarrhea

Figure 1–4

Mechanisms of allergic reaction.

ness or illness. When a person seeks medical attention, assessment of mental status is intertwined with physical evaluation. Psychological evaluation encompasses the observation of behavior, appearance, mood, communication, judgment, and thought processes. Because people react differently to disease, or the threat of illness, a treatment plan must be tailored to meet their psychological needs. Preservation of self-esteem is of great importance.

Illness can disrupt activity and change the patient's life and affect the family as well. In the face of disease, the person experiences an altered body image and emotional and social changes that are best understood in terms of past personal experience and perception. For example, when the patient was a child, did illness elicit empathy and a "chicken soup" approach or was illness met with aversion and a "tough it out" attitude?

Chronic disease is a stressor that can affect a person's self-esteem and behavior. Fear, helplessness, and lack of control are typical feelings. A patient passes through stages of anxiety, shock, denial, anger, withdrawal, and depression. If these stages are sustained without the person's coming to acceptance of the disease, the patient may acquire psychological disturbances.

PAIN

All of us experience pain at some time in our lives. What is pain, how do we describe pain, how do we interpret pain, what are the types of pain, why are tolerance levels different, and why do we have pain? The answers to these questions are necessary to develop an understanding of pain and how the health-care provider can be involved in the relief of pain.

Pain is described in many ways. It can be an uncomfortable sensation, hurting, an unpleasant experience, distress, strong discomfort, suffering, agony, physiologic, or psychological. Pain can be referred, acute, chronic, transient, or intractable. It also can be classified as superficial, deep, or visceral. Pain is subjective and individualized and is perceived only by the individual experiencing it. Pain is a necessary entity in life. The physiology of pain involves the stimulation of specialized nerve endings called **nociceptors.** These pain receptors are found on free sensory nerve endings in the superficial portions of the skin, in some tissues of internal or visceral organs, in joint capsules, in the periosteum of bones, surrounding the walls of blood vessels, and in certain deep tissue. Pain often is a signal of injury or tissue damage and as such is a protective mechanism that makes us aware of the insult to the tissue. It is a signal to locate and eliminate or reduce the source of tissue damage. However, pain can occur in the absence of injury. Pain also may be a part of the normal healing process as a reply to the inflammatory response.

Pain interpretation as to its intensity is subjective depending on many factors. The individual's perception and response to pain may be based on cultural values, past experiences, religious beliefs and background, emotional support, anxiety, education, and the particular situation. Stress can alter both perception and response to pain. Threatening situations can cause individuals to lack pain perception until they have escaped the danger of the threat. The cerebral cortex is responsible for the interpretation of pain and therefore must be functioning at normal capacity. Superficial pain is described as being located on the body surface. Deep pain refers to pain that usually is correlated with muscles, joints, or tendons. Visceral pain is attributed to internal organs.

Pain is not always reported accurately. Many of the internal organs are poorly supplied with nociceptors, and therefore the tissue insults in these organs are not always reported as such. The free nerve endings have large receptive fields, consequently making it difficult to determine the true source of the pain stimuli. Additionally, neurons from certain organs may travel a parallel pathway along the spinal cord to the brain, resulting in referred pain. Generally, the referred pain follows a **dermatome** that is supplied by the same spinal nerve as the nerve that has been stimulated by the insult, causing the pain to be projected to the body surface. For example, the patient experiencing myocardial ischemia or angina describes the pain as chest pain radiating to the left arm. Likewise, the nervous tissue of the brain has no pain receptors; nevertheless, headaches are commonly reported. Often the pain is caused by pressure on the blood vessel walls or pressure on the meninges. Tissue insult or inflammation to the gallbladder often results in pain referred to the right scapular region (Fig. 1–5).

Pain may be classified as acute, chronic, transient, or intractable. Acute pain usually has a sudden onset and is severe in intensity. It also usually is of short duration. Individuals with acute pain have a tendency to guard the painful area; may exhibit distractive behavior, such as crying or moaning; are restless, anxious, or listless; and may have altered thought processes. Blood pressure and pulse often increase whereas respiratory rates may increase or decrease. Occasionally, sudden onset of very severe pain may cause vascular collapse and a resulting state of shock. Facial movements may indicate a grimace, and the skin may become diaphoretic. Acute pain, such as the pain experienced from myocardial infarction, postoperatively after surgical intervention, from severe trauma, and during terminal illness can be treated with narcotics or opioid-related drugs. Chronic pain is usually less severe and has a duration of longer than 6 months. Pain from inflammatory conditions such as arthritis and bursitis is considered chronic. Patients with chronic pain often exhibit weight loss or gain, insomnia or altered sleep patterns, anorexia, inability to continue normal activities, and guarded movements. Psychosocial relationships may be altered. Chronic pain often is treated with acetaminophen, antiprostaglandins, steroids, or anti-inflammatory agents such as nonsteroidal anti-inflammatory drugs (NSAIDs). Chronic intractable pain, usually generated by nerve damage, is debilitating and can cause depression. Transient pain comes and goes, usually has a brief duration, and often is not significant.

As previously mentioned, pain relief can be achieved by the use of analgesic drugs including narcotics and non-narcotic agents. Other meth-

13

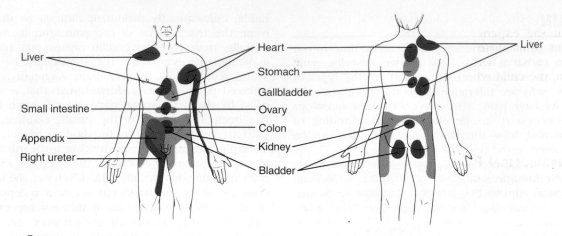

Figure 1–5

Referred pain, anterior and posterior views. (From Miller-Keane Encyclopedia and Dictionary of Medicine, Nursing, & Allied Health, 5th ed. Philadelphia: WB Saunders, 1992.)

ods include massage of the painful area to increase the blood flow to and from the area and to increase the flow of lymph from the area. Acupuncture, a very ancient form, is thought to cause pain relief by the needles used to stimulate nerves deep in the tissue, thus arousing the pituitary gland and other parts of the brain to release endorphins, the brain's own natural opioids. Endorphins reduce the perception of pain while the stimulus remains. Transcutaneous electrical nerve stimulation (TENS) uses electrical impulses to the nerve endings intending to block nerve transmission to the brain. (Some insurance companies consider TENS and electrical stimulation for pain relief experimental and will not provide reimbursement for this procedure.)

Pain is the result of tissue insult from noxious (harmful) stimuli, including heat and cold, pressure, chemicals, electrical shock, and trauma. Pain receptors respond to three types of stimuli: (1) temperature extremes, (2) mechanical damage, and (3) dissolved chemicals, including potassium, acids, histamines, acetylcholine, bradykinin, and prostaglandins. A very strong stimulus may excite all three types, creating a burning-type sensation. Additional causes of painful stimuli include hypoxia and ischemia to the tissues and muscle spasms.

Pain may be described in several ways by the individual experiencing it. Dull and aching is often the way that overuse of the musculoskeletal system is described. Burning-type pain along a nerve route is often an indication of peripheral nerve insult. Patients use the term cramping to characterize abdominal–visceral type pain. Head pain or pain along a blood vessel commonly is described as throbbing. Other descriptions include shooting, stabbing, stinging, dull, and, referring to thermal, burning. When concerned about how the pain is affecting them, patients may use terms such as frightening, sickening, tiring, discomforting, intense, unbearable, mild, excruciating, and vicious to categorize the pain.

Pain impulses travel from the nerve ending through the spinal cord to the thalamus, where they then proceed to the sensory cortex. Adaptation to painful stimuli does not occur because the receptors continue to respond while the stimulus remains, stopping only after the tissue damage has ended.

Pain is necessary for survival. It is a warning signal that tissue damage is occurring. Without pain, the individual would have no idea that something was going wrong in the body. An example is the person who has broken a bone in the leg and continues to walk until the bone protrudes through the skin, creating awareness of a fracture. Another example is the person whose coronary vessels are narrowing but who feels no anginal pain with increased activity. He or she continues the activity, unaware of the ischemia and permanent damage being done while the vessels completely occlude. The probable outcome is death. An additional example is the woman with an ectopic pregnancy. She is not cognizant that the pregnancy growing inside the fallopian tube has caused the tube to rupture until she experiences vaginal bleeding. At that point, immediate surgical intervention may be able to save her life. Continuing in the same vein, the child who touches an object that is hot will withdraw his or her hand, thus preventing additional tissue damage. Although most of us find pain to be an unpleasant experience, it is an essential part of our survival.

Psychological Pain

Psychological or emotional pain is as real as physical pain to the person experiencing it. This type of pain also can be acute, chronic, transient, or intractable.

Acute psychological pain often is triggered by a catastrophic event, such as the death of a loved one, severe trauma, extreme loss, brutal or cruel incidents, and abusive situations. Coping or defense mechanisms are called into play but are not always effective in helping the individual deal with the extreme stress of the situation. The reaction to the acute stressor may be immediate or it may be delayed. This pain may be described as feelings of despair, anger, helplessness, rage, depression, and hopelessness. Thought processes and sleep patterns may be disrupted. The individual may cry or may exhibit signs of withdrawal. Often, they become nonfunctional in a normal environment or they may function unaware of their surroundings. Diagnoses for these situations include major depression, post-traumatic stress disorder, and a variety of anxiety disorders. Should the individual present with these manifestations, intervention is indicated in the form of counseling, drug therapy, or both.

Chronic psychological pain usually has a more subtle and insidious onset. Often the individual is unaware of the changes taking place in personality and functioning. This type of pain also is very real, but with the gradual onset, adaptive behavior and defense or coping mechanisms come into play, assisting the individual to continue in a fairly normal fashion. Over a period of time, family, friends, coworkers, and even the individuals themselves notice personality and functional changes taking place. As in acute emotional pain, thought processes and sleep patterns are altered along with eating habits. The individual may experience anorexia or overeating, with corresponding weight loss or gain. A change in appearance may take place as caring about appearance becomes less significant. Posture takes on a slumping attitude, and energy diminishes. Often sadness is expressed with tears and crying whereas laughter and humor are experi-enced on a less frequent basis. Depression, de-layed reaction to post-traumatic stress, seasonal affective disorder, situational involvement or lack of involvement, loss, and the grieving process all are responsible for chronic emotional pain. Inter-vention in the form of counseling and drug ther-apy is helpful to relieve this pain.

Transient emotional pain, like transient physi-cal pain, is of very short duration and often re-solves itself as the situation modifies.

Intractable psychological pain is a true emer-gency. The individual finds him- or herself in a hopeless situation and with very few coping mechanisms on which to rely. When intractable psychological pain is brought to the attention of the health-care provider, immediate intervention should be initiated. If left to their own resources, these individuals react to the hopelessness of the situation either with violent behavior or with at-tempted, and many times successful, suicide.

Health-care providers must recognize the im-portance of an awareness of the depth and signif-icance of psychological pain and assist the pa-tient in receiving appropriate treatment. Chapter 14 discusses mental health disorders in more de-tail. An awareness of how any of us may be touched by psychological pain and events caus-ing such pain is necessary to provide the best care possible to our patients. It also serves to make the community more aware of the inci-dence of mental disorders and remove the stigma from mental illness.

MENTAL DISORDERS

Generally, mental disorders are described as clinically significant behavioral or psychological syndromes that are associated with psychic pain, a distressing symptom, or impairment of func-tion. Although sometimes cloaked in mystery, their common occurrence and their potential for disability dictate the same ardent handling as for any sickness. Chapter 14 addresses mental disor-ders, including grief response, dementia, mood disorders, and **somatoform** disorders.

Diagnosis

When a person seeks medical attention with symptoms and/or signs of disease, the clinician begins an orderly series of steps to investigate the cause and make a diagnosis (Figure 1–6). Establishing a diagnosis is a decision-making process in which data collected from the medical history, physical examination, and diagnostic tests are analyzed, integrated, and interpreted. A diagnosis provides a logical basis for treatment and prognosis.

The importance of the patient's medical history as the primary source of data cannot be overstated because it provides vital clues and background for the rest of the assessment. During the patient interview, medical information, such as predisposing factors or pre-existing conditions, is skillfully noted. Other relevant information ascertained, such as the existence of drug allergy and current therapy, can be the foundation for an individualized treatment plan. Finally, the clinician focuses questions on the onset and nature of the present illness.

Next, a methodical physical examination of the patient from head to toe (a systems review) is done to detect the physical signs of disease. Assessment skills used to evaluate health status are inspection (observation and measurement, including vital signs), **auscultation** (trained listening), palpation (investigation by sense of touch), and percussion (tapping that produces vibration and sound). Information gathered then is measured against norms or standards.

The final source of assessment data is a wide variety of appropriate diagnostic studies and laboratory tests. These include microscopic examination and chemical analysis. Although diagnostic testing is considered important as scientific measurement, laboratory data are not interpreted apart from other clinical data gathered from the history and physical examination. In the process of deciding or confirming the identification of a

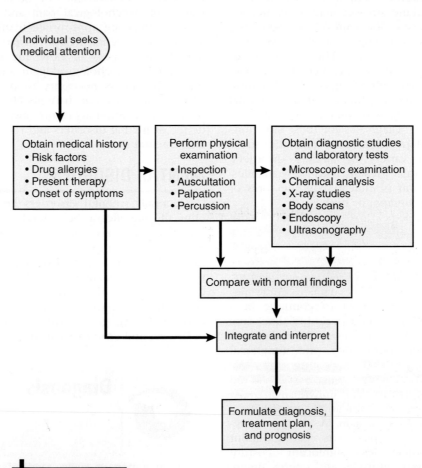

Figure 1–6

Essential steps in diagnosis.

disease, the results of diagnostic studies are integrated with the medical history and physical examination findings. In fact, physicians currently have computer systems that help to analyze large numbers of patient records to quantify probabilities and to devise an orderly approach to diagnosis (a decision tree). As a result, the physician is reminded of a full range of possible diagnoses for a given set of symptoms and signs; in other words, the physician is aided in making a differential diagnosis especially when two or more diseases resemble one another.

Laboratory tests, particularly biochemical profiles obtained by testing blood and urine, are used routinely to screen for imbalances or to detect early signs of disease. They also are used to monitor the effectiveness of therapeutic medications and other medical treatment (Table 1–4).

TABLE 1–4 ➤ Common Laboratory and Diagnostic Tests

BLOOD ANALYSIS

Complete Blood Count (CBC): Evaluation of cellular components of the blood. Includes red blood cell count, red blood cell indices, white blood cell count, white blood cell differential, hemoglobin, hematocrit, and platelet count. Sometimes referred to as hemogram. Often the differential must be ordered specifically as CBC with differential.

Hemoglobin (Hgb): Measurement of the oxygen-carrying pigment of the red blood cells.

Hematocrit (HCT): Measurement of the percentage of red blood cells in a volume of whole blood.

Chemistries: Normal chemistry profiles may contain blood serum levels for albumin, alkaline phosphatase, aspartate aminotransferase, bilirubin, calcium, creatinine, lactate dehydrogenase, phosphorus, total protein, urea nitrogen, and uric acid.

Thyroid Function Tests: Thyroid thyroxine (T4), triiodothyronine (T3), and thyroid-stimulating hormone (TSH).

Lipid Profile: Total cholesterol, triglycerides, high-density lipoprotein (HDL) cholesterol, low-density lipoprotein (LDL) cholesterol.

Electrolytes (lytes): Blood serum test for chloride, potassium, sodium, and carbon dioxide.

Clotting and Coagulation Studies: Partial thromboplastin time (PTT), prothrombin time (PT), platelet (thrombocyte) count, bleeding times.

Erythrocyte Sedimentation Rate (ESR): The rate at which red blood cells (erythrocytes) fall out of well-mixed whole blood to the bottom of the test tube.

Glucose Tolerance Test (GTT): Fasting blood glucose (FBS) levels.

Toxicology Studies, Drug screens.

Drug Levels: Digoxin, digitoxin, theophylline, lidocaine, lithium, and various drugs for therapeutic and/or toxic levels.

Arterial Blood Gas (ABG) Analysis: Measurement of dissolved oxygen and carbon dioxide in arterial blood. Also measures pH and O_2 saturation of the arterial blood.

Cardiac Enzymes: Creatine kinase (CK), CK isoenzymes, lactate dehydrogenase (LD), lactate dehydrogenase isoenzymes, aspartate aminotransferase (ASL, SGOT), alanine aminotransferase (ALT, SGPT)

URINE STUDIES

Urinalysis (UA): A screening test using a urine specimen that gives a picture of the patient's overall state of health and the state of the urinary tract. Measurements include pH and specific gravity of the urine, presence of ketones, protein, sugars, bilirubin, urobilinogen. Color and odor are noted, as is the presence of abnormal blood cells, casts, bacteria, other cells, and crystals.

Culture and Sensitivity (C & S) of Urine: *Culture:* Sample of urine specimen is placed in/on culture medium to see whether microbial growth occurs. If growth occurs, identification of the pathogenic microbe is determined. *Sensitivity:* A portion of the specimen is placed on a sensitivity disk (which has been impregnated with specific antibiotics) to determine which antibiotic the pathogen is resistant or to which it will be responsive.

CARDIOLOGY TESTS

Electrocardiogram (ECG, EKG): A record of the electrical activity of the myocardium used to diagnose ischemia, arrhythmias, conduction difficulties, activity of cardiac medications.

Echocardiogram: An ultrasound examination of the cardiac structure to define the size, shape, thickness, position, and movements of the cardiac structures, including valves, walls, and chambers.

Holter Monitor: A miniature electrocardiograph that records the electrical activity of the heart for an extended period of time, usually 24 to 48 hours. The patient records all activities during the time period for the examiner to correlate activity with cardiac abnormalities.

Thallium Scan: A scan to indicate myocardial profusion and the location and extent of myocardial ischemia and/or infarction and to predict the possible prognosis of the cardiac condition.

MUGA Scan: A scan that assesses the function of the left ventricle and identifies abnormalities of the myocardial walls.

Stress Testing, Treadmill, Exercise Tolerance Testing: An assessment of cardiac function during moderate exercise after a 12-lead electrocardiogram.

Pulse Oximeter: An instrument (spectrophotometer) that provides a noninvasive measurement of the O_2 saturation of the arterial blood.

Cardiac Catheterization: Fluoroscopic visualization of right or left side of heart by passing a catheter into right or left chamber and injecting dye. Angiograms consist of the catheter being passed into the coronary vessels where the dye is injected and fluoroscopic images are recorded.

(continued on the following page)

TABLE 1–4 ➤ Common Laboratory and Diagnostic Tests *(continued)*

IMAGING STUDIES

X-rays: Visualization of internal organs and structures by electromagnetic radiation. Radiographs of bone; the abdomen; the chest; paranasal sinuses; and kidneys, ureters, and bladder (KUB) and mammograms do not require contrast medium. Contrast medium is used to distinguish soft tissue and some organs such as the gallbladder, esophagus, stomach, and small and large intestines.

Magnetic Resonance Imaging (MRI): Uses a magnetic field instead of radiation to visualize internal tissues. It is possible to view tissue and organs in a three-dimensional manner with MRI. Helpful in determining blood flow to tissues and organs, in studying condition of blood vessels, in detecting tumors, in differentiating healthy and diseased tissues, and in detecting sites of infection. The patient is not exposed to ionizing radiation during MRI.

Computed Tomography (CT) Scans: A radiographic technique using a scanner system that can provide images of the internal structure of tissue and organs both geographically and characteristically.

Fluoroscopy: A real-time imaging process that provides continuous visualization of the area undergoing radiography. Still films and video recordings are made of the process for more extensive examination. Used in procedures and to study the functioning of tissues and organs.

Sonograms, Ultrasound, Echogram: A beam of sound waves is projected into target tissues or organs, resulting in a bouncing back of the wave off the target structure. An outline of the structure is produced and recorded on film or videotape for examination.

Myelogram: An imaging examination of the spinal cord and spinal nerve roots. Contrast medium (dye) and/or air are injected into the subarachnoid space and recorded on radiographic film and videotape. Fluoroscopy generally is used in this procedure.

STOOL ANALYSIS

Guaiac Tests: For occult blood.
Ova and Parasite Tests

SPUTUM ANALYSIS

Sputum Studies: Microscopic studies of sputum, including culture and sensitivity, acid-fast bacteria culture and stain, Gram stain, and cytology studies.

ENDOSCOPY TESTS

Endoscopy: Visual inspection of internal organs and/or cavities of the body using appropriate scope.
Gastroscopy: Visualization of the stomach by a gastroscope.
Colonoscopy: Visualization of the colon with a colonoscope.
Sigmoidoscopy: Visualization of the sigmoid portion of the colon and the rectum with a sigmoidoscope.
Proctoscopy: Visualization of the rectum with a proctoscope.
Cystoscopy: Visualization of the structures of the urinary tract with a cystoscope.
Bronchoscopy: Visualization of the trachea and bronchi with a bronchoscope.

PULMONARY FUNCTION STUDIES

Peak Flow: The patient blows into a flowmeter to determine the volume of an expiratory effort.
Spirometry: A measurement of lung capacity, volume, and flow rates by a spirometer.
Methacholine Challenge: A test for asthma in which measurement of lung volumes is taken before and after the inhalation of methacholine, a bronchial constrictor.
Pulmonary Function
Tidal Volume, Expiratory Reserve Volume, Residual Volume, Inspiratory Reserve Volume

MISCELLANEOUS TESTS

Culture and Sensitivity (C & S): *Culture:* Sample of specimen is placed in/on culture medium to see whether microbial growth occurs. If growth occurs, identification of the pathogenic microbe is determined. *Sensitivity:* A portion of the specimen is placed on a sensitivity disk (which has been impregnated with specific antibiotics) to determine which antibiotic the pathogen is resistant or to which it will be responsive. The specimen could be blood, stool, urine, sputum, any discharge fluid, or from a wound.

Bone Marrow Studies: Aspiration of bone marrow by needle from the sternum, posterior or superior iliac spine, or the anterior iliac crest for diagnosis of neoplasms, metastasis, and blood disorders.

Immune and Immunoglobulin Studies: Studies of the functioning or nonfunctioning of the patient's immune system.
Serologic Testing: Analysis of blood specimens for antigen–antibody reactions. Used to detect bacterial infections, including syphilis, Lyme disease, chlamydia, and streptococcal infections; antibodies from viral sources including infectious mononucleosis, rubella, hepatitis, rabies, HIV, herpes, and cytomegalovirus; antibodies from fungal sources such histoplasmosis and candida; and antibodies from the parasitic source, toxoplasmosis.
Biopsies: The excision of tissue from the living body, followed by microscopic examination, for purpose of exact diagnosis.

Lumbar Punctures (LP): A surgical procedure to withdraw spinal fluid for analysis.
Electroencephalogram (EEG): A recording of the electrical activity of the cerebral cortex of the brain.
Electromyelogram (EMG): An electrodiagnostics assessment and recording of the activity of the skeletal muscles.
Gastric Analysis: Used in the diagnosis of pernicious anemia and peptic ulcers.
Pregnancy Tests: Human chorionic gonadotropin (HCG–UCG). Used in diagnosis of pregnancy, abortion, ectopic pregnancy, and uterine pathology.
Gram Stain: Used to identify gram-positive or gram-negative microorganism of infectious process.

TABLE 1–4 ➤ **Common Laboratory and Diagnostic Tests** *(continued)*

SCREENING

Hepatic Screening: Liver function tests–Liver profile: Usually includes alanine aminotransferase, alkaline phosphatase, aspartate aminotransferase, bilirubin, and gamma-glutamyl transpeptidase.

Tuberculosis (TB) Screening: *Mantoux:* An intradermal injection of tuberculin is done usually on the inner aspect of the lower arm. Localized thickening of the skin in the area, along with redness, indicates the presence of active or dormant tuberculosis. Positive reaction requires further investigation, usually including a chest radiograph.

Prostatic-Specific Antigen (PSA): A serum blood test to determine the level of PSA. Increased levels may indicate benign prostatic hypertrophy, prostate cancer, inflammatory conditions of the prostate. This is a screening test that should be followed by a digital rectal examination of the prostate gland to determine any abnormalities. Often additional diagnostic studies are indicated.

Pap (Papanicolaou) Smear: A cytologic examination of cells that have been scraped or aspirated from the cervix and cervical os. A screen test is done annually, especially before any female hormones are prescribed.

Mammograms: A radiographic examination of the breast tissue. A screen test is done on an annual basis for women older than 40 years of age to detect the presence of breast disease. This screening also should be accompanied by a manual examination of the breast tissue by a physician. Monthly breast self-examinations are recommended.

These are many of the common diagnostic procedures that may be ordered and performed. Many more diagnostic procedures may be used in the process of arriving at the patient's diagnosis and prognosis. More diagnostic tests and procedures are discussed, along with the corresponding disease or condition, in subsequent chapters.

Refer to Appendix I for additional information regarding normal and abnormal values and indications for tests.

Treatment

After the initial assessment is completed and a diagnosis is established, appropriate medical intervention is implemented. The plan of treatment is directly related to an identified expected outcome. The goal may be specifically to cure, to control symptoms, or to be supportive, or it may be a combination of these. Therapeutic elements of a conventional medical care plan may be used conservatively or aggressively and include one or more of the following: preventive measures, therapeutic procedures, administration of medications, surgery, physical therapy, diet modification, psychotherapy, patient education, and follow-up care.

After a medical treatment plan is implemented, it is evaluated and modified as needed. The current trend is to involve patients directly in the choices of treatment and to emphasize their responsibility to make choices that promote their recovery. A team approach to medical treatment, involving the patient, medical personnel, family, and community support systems, is optimum for complicated cases.

The concept of holistic medicine is comprehensive care that focuses on the needs of the whole person (Figure 1-7). The physical and psy-

chological well-being of the individual are dependent on each other. A mind-and-body interaction has been established to compel the health-care provider to consider the patient as a whole person. Rather than narrowly defining a disease in terms of physical pathologic changes, the patient's social, emotional, intellectual, and spiritual components also are considered. Individualized care is important when personality, environment, and lifestyle are factored into identifying the needs of a sick person. The holistic practitioner must recognize the uniqueness of the patient and consider the needs, aspirations, perception, comprehension, and insight of the patient. The illness or event should be looked on as an emergence of a dysfunction of the entire or whole person and not an isolated dimension. Love, humor, hope, and enthusiasm can become part of the healing process, whereas feelings of hostility, fear, anger, grief, rage, shame, and greed fuel the illness process. The absence of illness does not necessarily indicate optimal health. Holistic care encourages the patient to consciously pursue the highest expressions of being, including those of spirit, mind, emotion, environment, socialization, and physical being. An emphasis on the patient's active participation in the recovery process is essential to this system of care. Although integrating all the needs of a patient is compatible with traditional comprehensive treatment plans, holistic medicine also may connote a variety of nontraditional methods of treatment, which may be empirical or experimental.

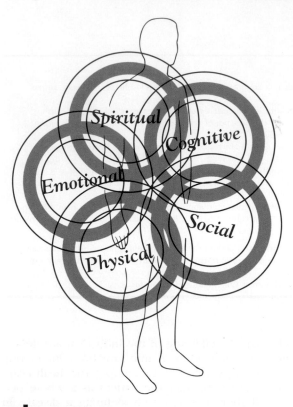

Figure 1–7

Human beings from a holistic viewpoint. The expanding and receding circles represent the dynamic interaction of the physical, social, emotional, spiritual, and cognitive needs that constitute humanness. (From Luckmann J, Sorensen K: Medical–Surgical Nursing: A Pathophysiologic Approach. Philadelphia: WB Saunders, 1987.)

ALTERNATIVE MEDICINE

Many patients and practitioners are accepting safe alternative medicine as an adjunct therapy to traditional medicine. Some of the therapies are osteopathy, chiropractic, massage, reflexology, aromatherapy, herbs, diet and nutrition, acupuncture, acupressure, shiatsu, magnetic therapy, hypnosis, relaxation, Reiki, energy movement, and music therapy.

Osteopathy is probably the most widely accepted form of alternative medicine. In the United States, osteopathic physicians (Doctors of Osteopathy, DOs) are trained medical doctors with emphasis on the stimulation of the body's natural process to provide healing and well-being. In addition to traditional medical and surgi-

cal concepts, osteopathic physicians use manipulation techniques to realign body structure, restoring balance and promoting healing.

Chiropractic medicine relies on the concept of the body's nervous system as a basis for health and that undue pressure on or an insult to the nervous system may result in pain and disease. Emphasis is placed on correct alignment of the spinal vertebrae, and many chiropractic adjustments involve manipulation of the spine.

Massage, although not a new concept, is just beginning to be recognized by the U.S. medical community as an alternative therapy or type of medicine. Using the Eastern approach along with Swedish concepts, massage encourages the drainage of the lymphatic system and increases the circulation to the tissues.

Reflexology, a form of massage, directs its efforts to massage primarily of the feet and sometimes of the hands. The theory is that the body is divided into zones and that these zones are reflected in specific areas of the feet or hands. Manipulation of these areas is expected to cause a therapeutic effect on the organ or system represented in that zone.

Aromatherapy uses essential oils to promote wellness for stress relief and for healing. Although using the olfactory system (Fig. 1–8) by inhalation, the oils also are absorbed through the skin and transported to the various body tissues and systems by the circulatory system. The essential oils are diluted and then used for massage or placed in a steam inhaler for inspiration. Some of the more common essential oils used in aromatherapy are chamomile, clary, sage, clove, eucalyptus, geranium, ginger, lavender, orange, peppermint, rosemary, sage, tea tree, and ylang ylang. Often aromatherapists mix the oils to meet the needs of their clients.

Herbs have been used in medicine for many centuries, with ancient Egyptians the first known culture to record lists of herbs. Sometimes called natural medicines, herbs are being substituted for pharmaceutical products. Common herbal products include *Ginkgo biloba,* garlic, saw palmetto, ginseng, passion flower, angelica, chamomile, fennel, lavender, peppermint, rosemary, sage, Saint John's wort, valerian, and yarrow. Herbs may be purchased in a pharmacy or herbal drug store, or by mail. Herbal remedies are professed to treat allergies, arthritis, gastrointestinal (GI) problems, headaches, hypertension or hypotension, insomnia, urinary problems, menstrual or menopausal symptoms, and skin diseases. Many of these products do not have FDA approval and may even damage health if taken unwarily.

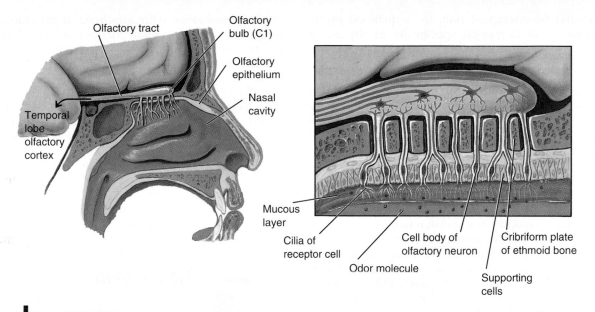

Olfactory tract

Olfactory bulb (C1)

Olfactory epithelium

Nasal cavity

Temporal lobe olfactory cortex

Mucous layer

Cilia of receptor cell

Odor molecule

Cell body of olfactory neuron

Supporting cells

Cribriform plate of ethmoid bone

Figure 1–8

Structure of the olfactory receptors. (From Applegate EJ: The Anatomy and Physiology Learning System: Textbook. Philadelphia: WB Saunders, 1995.)

Diet and nutrition therapy is not a new concept; however, many are following special diets and addressing nutritional needs, hoping to eliminate toxins from the body and allow it to function at optimum level. Diet therapy may include fat-free, low saturated fat, low-sugar, high-protein, low-carbohydrate, vegetarian, no or low-caffeine, and seafood diets. Vitamin and mineral supplements often are added to the daily routine. Vitamins and minerals may be toxic in megadoses. Check with a physician or pharmacist before starting any nutritional supplement regimen.

Acupuncture, an Asian therapy using meridians, attempts to adjust the body's energy (chi [chee]) flow by inserting needles into acupuncture points. After insertion, the needles are manipulated by twirling or by a gentle pumping action. Recent advances in techniques use electrical or laser stimulation. Acupuncture should be attempted only by professionals trained in the art.

Acupressure, similar to acupuncture, involves the manipulation of acupoints by means of finger pressure. There is an attempt to balance the flow of energy along the meridians to promote healthy functioning of internal organs. Acupressure often is incorporated into massage as a method of muscle relaxation and stress reduction.

Shiatsu (she-AT-sue), a form of therapy from Japan that is similar to acupressure, usually is performed on a mat on the floor. The client remains clothed, and the pressure is applied to the acupoints and along the meridians by fingertips, knuckles, elbows, knees, or even the feet.

Magnetic therapy, a relatively new concept in the United States, is not approved by the FDA. However, it is used extensively in veterinary medicine, especially equine, and in Europe and the United Kingdom, magnetic therapy has been accepted for use in humans as well. Although the theory has not been proved according to FDA standards, it is believed that magnets increase circulation to the area, thereby increasing oxygen (O_2) and nutrients while transporting away the waste products of metabolism and the inflammatory process. It also is postulated that the magnetic field interferes with the conduction of the sensory nerves by preventing the movement of the sodium (Na) and potassium (K) ions in and out of the nerve cell, thereby reducing the conduction capability of the sensory nerve. Advocates of this therapy state that magnets are useful in muscle and nerve pain, inflammation, and migraines.

Hypnosis and hypnotherapy only have been accepted means of psychological therapy for approximately the past 40 years. The therapist places the patient or client in a trance-like state, often resembling sleep. In this trance, the subject follows acceptable suggestions. Often relaxation and pain relief can be achieved. This therapy

www.bach

should be attempted only by a qualified practitioner who is trained specifically in the art of hypnosis.

Relaxation frequently can be in the form of self-hypnosis. Many forms of relaxation techniques are available to the individual. Physical relaxation usually is a starting point for the subject with psychological relaxation often following. Relaxation is used to treat stress-related physical and emotional problems, pain, anxiety, asthma, arthritis, depression, panic attacks, and hypertension. Many forms of relaxation include a repetition of action, images, or sounds to passively erase everyday thoughts from the mind.

Reiki (ray-KEE) is a transference of healing energy from the practitioner to the client. Usually the practitioner starts at the head of the client either by touching the head or moving the hands close to the head into the aura. Other parts of the body then are touched by the hands, or the hands move into the aura space. Healing energy then is transferred to the client. The intention of this therapy is the promotion of physical, emotional, and spiritual well-being.

The practitioner using energy movement perceives shortages in the energy field of the client and attempts to balance the energies with interaction. Energy from a "higher power" is transferred through the practitioner to the client, thus not exhausting the practitioner's energy supply. This noninvasive approach uses energy balancing to effect significant changes in the physical, emotional, and spiritual well-being of the client.

Music therapy, often a healing influence, recognizes the involvement of vibrations, rhythms, and sound in the well-being of individuals. Relaxation can be achieved by listening to music by composers of the Baroque period, such as Bach.

Music is used along with anesthesia or pain medication for mood elevation, for its calming effect, and for sedation to lessen muscle tension and to alleviate fear and anxiety. Trained and qualified music therapists design the therapy to fit the client's needs.

Homeopathy, polarity therapy, rolfing, tai chi (tie-chee), iridology, naturopathy, hydrotherapy, and Ayurveda are some of the additional forms of alternative medicine. Although any of these forms may be a form of alternative medicine, the patient and practitioner should check with the physician before attempting to involve them in the course of treatment. When used, they should be considered as adjunct treatment and not necessarily proven medical treatment.

Conclusion

Human pathologic processes involve complex mechanisms that can be weighed separately as elements of the disease process but that ultimately converge into the total picture of how and why an individual is sick and what is required as a remedy.

It is worth the effort to strive to understand the nature and impact of human disease on the person and humankind. One can expect to find great personal and professional satisfaction in knowing the nature, signs, symptoms, causes, and treatment of the pathologic conditions that alter or seriously threaten health. This knowledge also fosters insight into the scenario imposed by diseases and compassion for the people affected by them.

Summary

Pathologic conditions involve measurable changes in the normal stability, or homeostasis, of the body. These changes elicit symptoms described by the patient, and signs demonstrated by abnormal physical and laboratory findings. Assessment of the diagnostic data, systematically collected and analyzed, points to the nature and severity of disease.

A wide range of diagnostic tests are readily available to study, in detail, the components of blood and urine; results are compared with nor-

mal values. Specimens of body tissue or body fluids can be examined microscopically or cultured for microbial growth. Imaging studies allow visualization of internal organs and structures. Endoscopy allows direct examination of body organs or cavities. Electrical activity of the heart and brain can be measured. Analyzers and computers currently are more available, generating in-depth diagnostic data.

The complex mechanisms of disease include predisposing factors, genetics, infections associated with pathogens, and neoplasms both malignant and benign. Physical trauma, malnutrition, immune disorders (including allergies), and mental disorders are other factors. Ill health impacts the physical and psychological well-being of the person. Prevention and early detection introduce the element of control in certain threats to health.

Treatment modalities, although specific to the disease condition, may be directed to cure the disease, control symptoms, or be strictly supportive. The team approach to a medical treatment plan, with emphasis on individualized care, controls for optimal health and comfort of the patient. Proven and tested therapies are preferred in the mainstream of medical practice. Alternative medicine is finding acceptance by some as adjunct therapy. Examples of alternative medicine include osteopathy, chiropractic, the use of diet supplements and herbs, massage, and aromatherapy.

Pain, although universal, remains subjective and takes many forms. Physical or psychological pain can be acute, chronic, intractable, or transient. Relief of pain can be attained by many formulas, once the cause has been diagnosed and individual needs have been weighed.

Review Challenge

REVIEW QUESTIONS

1. How may the following predisposing factors make a person more vulnerable to disease?
   Age
   Sex
   Lifestyle
   Environment
   Heredity
2. Describe three ways that genetic diseases are caused.
3. Name three of the body's natural defense mechanisms.
4. How does acute inflammation protect against infection?
5. What is allergic disease? What are the symptoms, and how may they be treated?

6. What is the goal of cancer treatment, and what therapeutic measures may be used?
7. List the normal sequence of steps in formulating diagnosis.
8. What is the difference between benign and malignant tumors?
9. What is the emphasis in preventive health care?
10. Explain the importance of knowing the types of pain, the possible causes, and how it may be described by the patient.
11. What are the components of the holistic concept of medical care?
12. Discuss osteopathy as a form of alternative medicine.

RESOURCES

Cancer Information Service
Office of Cancer Communications
National Cancer Institute
Building 31, Room 10A24
9000 Rockville Pike, Bethesda, MD 20892
800-4-CANCER, 800-524-1234
http://www.nci.nih.gov/

Center for Health Promotion and Education
Centers for Disease Control and Prevention
Building 1 South, Room SSB249
1600 Clifton Road NE
Atlanta, GA 30333
404-329-3492
http://www.cdc.gov/

American Cancer Society Response Line
1599 Clifton Road NE

Atlanta, GA 30329
800-227-2345

American Academy of Allergy and Immunology
611 East Wells Street
Milwaukee, WI 53202

National Institute of Allergies and Infectious Diseases
9000 Rockville Pike
Building 31, Room 7A32
Bethesda, MD 20892
301-496-5717

National Council on Aging
600 Maryland Avenue SW
West Wing, Suite 100
Washington, DC 20024
800-424-9046
http://www.aoa.dhhs.gov/

Chapter Outline

DEVELOPMENTAL AND CONGENITAL DISORDERS

DEVELOPMENTAL CHARACTERISTICS
AND CONGENITAL ANOMALIES
DEVELOPMENTAL CHARACTERISTICS

Congenital Anomalies

METHODS OF PRENATAL DIAGNOSIS
PREMATURITY

Infant Respiratory Distress Syndrome
Bronchopulmonary Dysplasia
Retinopathy of Prematurity
Necrotizing Enterocolitis

DISEASES OF THE NERVOUS SYSTEM

Cerebral Palsy
Muscular Dystrophy
Spina Bifida
Meningocele
Myelomeningocele
Hydrocephalus
Anencephaly
*Cri du Chat Syndrome (Cat's Cry Syn-
  drome)*
Down Syndrome

CONGENITAL CARDIAC DEFECTS

Fetal Circulation
Acyanotic Defects
  Ventricular Septal Defect
  Patent Ductus Arteriosus
  Coarctation of the Aorta
  Atrial Septal Defect
Cyanotic Defects
  Tetralogy of Fallot
  Transposition of the Great Arteries

MUSCULOSKELETAL DISEASES

Clubfoot (Talipes Equinovarus)
Congenital Hip Dysplasia
Cleft Lip and Palate

GENITOURINARY DISEASES

Cryptorchidism (Undescended Testes)
Wilms' Tumor
Phimosis

DISEASES OF THE DIGESTIVE SYSTEM

Congenital Pyloric Stenosis
*Hirschsprung's Disease (Congenital
  Aganglionic Megacolon)*

METABOLIC DISORDERS

Cystic Fibrosis
Phenylketonuria

ENDOCRINE DISEASES

Klinefelter's Syndrome
Turner's Syndrome

CHILDHOOD DISEASES

INFECTIOUS DISEASES

Chickenpox (Varicella)
Diphtheria
Mumps (Epidemic Parotitis)
Pertussis (Whooping Cough)
Measles (Rubeola)
*Rubella (German Measles, Three-Day
  Measles)*
Tetanus
Influenza
Common Cold

RESPIRATORY DISEASES

Sudden Infant Death Syndrome
Croup
Epiglottiditis
Acute Tonsillitis
Adenoid Hyperplasia
Asthma

GASTROINTESTINAL DISORDERS

Infantile Colic
Helminth (Worm) Infestation
Diarrhea
Vomiting

BLOOD DISORDERS

Anemia
Leukemia
*Erythroblastosis Fetalis (Hemolytic
  Disease of the Newborn)*
Lead Poisoning

MISCELLANEOUS DISEASES

Reye's Syndrome
Fetal Alcohol Syndrome
Diaper Rash

CHAPTER 2

Developmental, Congenital, and Childhood Diseases and Disorders

Learning Objectives

After studying Chapter 2, you will be able to:

1. List the possible causes of congenital anomalies.
2. Discuss the purpose and procedure of amniocentesis.
3. Trace fetal circulation.
4. Describe the condition of prematurity and associated disorders: the causes and the treatment.
5. Distinguish between muscular dystrophy and cerebral palsy.
6. Describe patent ductus arteriosus.
7. Name and describe the most common congenital cyanotic cardiac defect.
8. List the major clinical manifestations of cystic fibrosis.
9. Distinguish between Klinefelter's syndrome and Turner's syndrome.
10. Describe the clinical condition of congenital rubella syndrome.
11. Discuss the treatment of asthma.
12. List the symptoms and signs of anemia; describe the pathology of leukemia.
13. Explain the etiology of erythroblastosis fetalis.
14. Name some warning signs of lead poisoning.
15. Describe the infant born with fetal alcohol syndrome.

Key Terms

acetabulum	(**ass**–eh–**TAB**–u–lum)	anencephalic	(**an**–en–seh–**FAL**–ik)
acyanotic	(a–**sigh**–ah–**NOT**–ik)	ataxic	(ah–**TACH**–sik)
adenosarcoma	(**ad**–eh–no–sar–**KO**–mah)	azoospermia	(azo–**SPIR**–me–a)
		bicornate	(bye–**KOR**–nate)
amniocentesis	(**am**–nee–o–sen–**TEE**–sis)	contracture	(kon–**TRACK**–chur)
		dysplasia	(dis–**PLAY**–zee–ah)

dystonia	(dis–**TOE**–nee–ah)	nevus	(**NEE**–vus)
dystrophy	(**DIS**–troe–fee)	pyelography	(**pye**–eh–**LOH**–grah–fee)
electromyography	(e–**LECK**–tro–my–**og**–ra–fee)	pylorus	(pye–**LOR**–us)
foramen ovale	(for–**A**–men o–**VAL**–a)	stenosis	(ste–**NO**–sis)
meconium	(meh–**KOH**–nee–um)	syncope	(**SIN**–koh–pee)
meninges	(men–**IN**–jeez)	tachypnea	(**tack**–ip–**NEE**–ah)
neonates	(**NEE**–o–nates)	trisomy	(**TRY**–so–me)

Developmental and Congenital Disorders

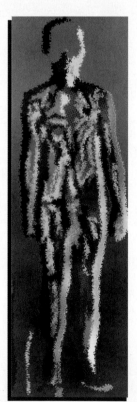

Developmental Characteristics and Congenital Anomalies

DEVELOPMENTAL CHARACTERISTICS

The developmental process commences with conception and progresses as a gradual modification of structure and characteristics of the individual. The embryonic period is considered the first 2 months of the gestational period, after which the developing human being is considered a fetus. At any point in this prenatal development, during the birth process (perinatal period) or during the neonatal and postnatal periods, a divergence from normal may evolve, generating a developmental dilemma. Causes of these dilemmas can be numerous or even unknown. Pregnant women are encouraged to refrain from smoking, consuming alcohol, and taking any form of medication without their physician's knowledge and consent and to avoid any situation that may expose the developing fetus to toxic substances. Table 2–1 lists information concerning specific stages of development during this important period of life.

CONGENITAL ANOMALIES

Congenital anomalies can be mental or physical with a wide range of severity, from the trivial to the fatal. They are present at birth or are detected later in infancy or childhood. The limbs or organs may be malformed, duplicated, or entirely absent. Sometimes organs fail to move to the correct place or fail to open or close at the right time. Anomalies tend to occur together.

END OF MONTH*	SIZE	DEVELOPMENTS DURING THE MONTH
1	6 mm	Arm and leg buds form; heart forms and starts beating; body systems begin to form
2	23–30 mm, 1 g	Head nearly as large as body; major brain regions present; ossification begins; arms and legs distinct; blood vessels form and cardiovascular system fully functional; liver large
3	75 mm, 10–45 g	Facial features present; nails develop on fingers and toes; can swallow and digest amniotic fluid; urine starts to form; fetus starts to move; heartbeat detected; external genitalia develop
4	140 mm, 60–200 g	Facial features well formed; hair appears on head; joints begin to form
5	190 mm, 250–450 g	Mother feels fetal movement; fetus covered with fine hair called lanugo hair; eyebrows visible; skin coated with vernix caseosa, a cheesy mixture of sebum and dead epidermal cells
6	220 mm, 500–800 g	Skin reddish because blood in the capillaries is visible; skin wrinkled because it lacks adipose in the subcutaneous tissue
7	260 mm, 900–1300 g	Eyes open; capable of survival but the mortality rate is high; scrotum develops; testes begin their descent
8	280–300 mm, 1400–2100 g	Testes descend into the scrotum; sense of taste is present
9	310–340 mm, 2200–2900 g	Reddish skin fades to pink; nails reach tips of fingers and toes or beyond
10	350–360 mm, 3000–3400 g	Skin smooth and plump because of adipose in subcutaneous tissue; lanugo hair shed; fetus usually turns to a head down position; full term

TABLE 2–1 ➤ Monthly Changes During Prenatal Development

* These are 4-week (28-day) months.
From Applegate EJ: The Anatomy and Physiology Learning System: Textbook. Philadelphia, WB Saunders, 1995, p. 423.

The cause of congenital defects may be genetic, nongenetic, or a combination of both. Nongenetic causes include infection in the mother, drugs taken by the mother, the age of the mother, radiographic examination made early in pregnancy, or injury to the pregnant woman or the fetus. The cause frequently is unknown; thus, measures of prevention usually have not been effective. However, prenatal care and advanced surgical techniques have improved greatly the management of anomalies that are compatible with life.

The emotional and physical challenges imposed on the parents of a special-needs child deserve optimal medical attention. A team approach is ideal, with medical assessment by physicians, appropriate therapeutic measures, family involvement, and participation in a parent support group.

METHODS OF PRENATAL DIAGNOSIS

The diagnosis of congenital anomalies in a fetus can be accomplished by obtaining a sample of fluid taken from the amniotic sac between the 15th and 18th week of pregnancy. The procedure, known as amniocentesis, allows the testing of the fluid and microscopic examination of the cells for abnormal substances or chromosomal abnormalities An example of an abnormal substance would be an elevated alpha-fetoprotein (AFP) level. Amniocentesis is not without risk to mother and baby. Abnormalities of the spine and skull may be discovered during ultrasound studies of the fetus.

A newer procedure called chorionic villus biopsy (CVB) can be done in the second month of pregnancy. The gynecologist, guided by ultrasound, introduces an instrument toward the placenta in the womb to obtain a tissue sample. The safety of this procedure has not been proved, and some data link this test to limb abnormalities.

Many, but not all, congenital disorders can be detected (Fig. 2–1).

PREMATURITY

SYMPTOMS AND SIGNS

The condition of prematurity is described as the birth of a low-weight, underdeveloped, and short-gestational infant and is considered the leading cause of death during the neonatal period. These high-risk infants are born with incomplete organ system development.

Premature babies may range in weight from 12 ounces to 5 pounds, 8 ounces. Their physical

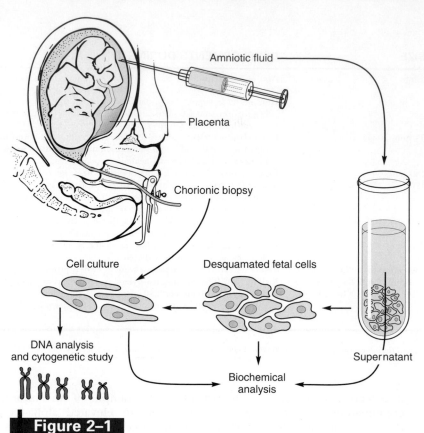

Figure 2–1

Methods of prenatal diagnosis. (From Damjanov I: Pathology for the Health-Related Professions. Philadelphia: WB Saunders, 1996.)

development is at various stages depending on the length of gestational time. The smaller of these infants has little subcutaneous fat, palms and soles with few creases, possible unde-scended testes in the male, and a prominent clit-oris in the female. Many of these very tiny and immature babies lack the ability to suck or swal-low or have weakened sucking or swallowing reflexes. The risk of infection is high because of an immature immune system.

ETIOLOGY

There are many reasons that these infants en-ter the world before reaching the traditionally accepted gestational age of 40 weeks and have very low birth weights. Causes of premature la-bor resulting in a premature infant may include an incompetent cervix, bicornate uterus, toxic conditions, maternal infection, trauma, premature rupture of the amniotic membranes, multiple ges-tation, intrauterine fetal growth retardation, and

other physical conditions of the mother, such as pregnancy-induced or chronic hypertension.

DIAGNOSIS

Diagnosis includes a gestational age of less than 37 weeks and a weight of less than 5 pounds, 8 ounces. Neonates diagnosed as small for gestational age (SGA) are not premature but are low-weight infants.

TREATMENT

Advances in technology have made survival of low-weight and short-gestation infants possible.

Treatment varies depending on the gestational age, weight, subsequent or present conditions, anomalies, and nutritional status. Intravenous (IV) fluids and **hyperalimentation** are necessary to encourage growth and development of the pre-mature infant. Airway management and pulmo-nary functioning are monitored very closely. Many of the smallest babies are intubated endotracheally, and respiration is maintained by mechanical ventilation. Pulse oximeters provide constant monitoring of the oxygen (O_2) saturation levels and heart rate. Body temperature is monitored closely and maintained at normal levels (Fig. 2–2).

Prognosis for these children is variable because of gestational age and weight as well as the occurrence of anomalies and developmental deficits. There are documented cases of 12-ounce and/or 22-week gestational babies surviving. They fall into the 1% of those born at that weight and gestational age. Being born before the normal prenatal development is complete, these children often have numerous problems to overcome (Fig. 2–3).

A primary concern is a cerebral bleed that may occur during the labor and delivery process or by handling after delivery. The cerebral bleed may result in the development of cerebral palsy or mental functioning deficiencies. Another major concern is underdevelopment of the pulmonary system, including the lung tissue and the airway. Some pulmonary conditions experienced by these infants include infant respiratory distress syndrome (IRDS), bronchopulmonary dysplasia (BPD), laryngomalacia, tracheomalacia, and bronchomalacia. Lack of body fat can impact the body temperature maintenance. Underdevelopment of the central nervous system (CNS) and the circulatory system may be responsible for hydrocephalus. Any stress or increased or high supplemental O_2 flow may be responsible for retinopathy of prematurity (ROP) and possible blindness. Necrotizing enterocolitis (NEC) is a danger in the digestive system because of the decreased tolerance of the alimentary tract. Atrial septal defect (ASD) and patent ductus arteriosus (PDA) often are present because the fetal circulatory system fails to mature.

Approximately 1% survive the birth process and the perinatal period. Improvements in technology are making it possible for more and more of these tiniest infants to survive (Fig. 2–4).

Prevention of prematurity includes good prenatal care, adequate nutrition, and addressing a pregnant patient's risk factors for premature labor.

Infant Respiratory Distress Syndrome

SYMPTOMS AND SIGNS

IRDS or **hyaline membrane** disease is similar to adult respiratory distress syndrome because

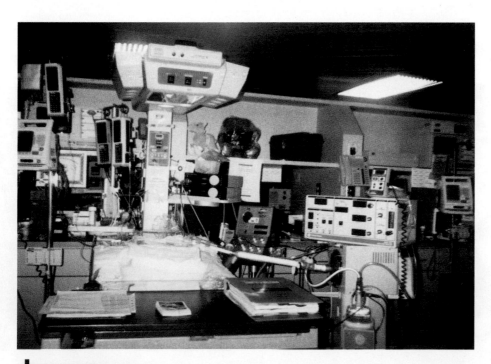

Figure 2–2
Technology in a neonatal intensive care unit. (Courtesy of David L. Frazier, 1999.)

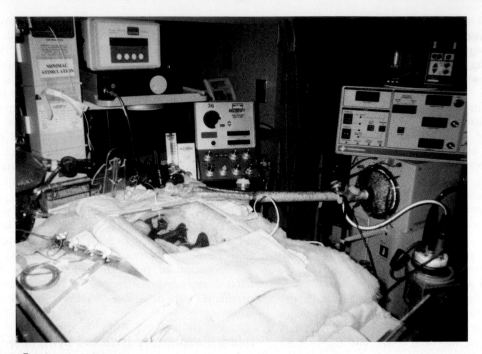

Figure 2–3

Four-day-old premature infant. Weight is 14.6 oz and gestational age is 22 weeks. (Courtesy of David L. Frazier, 1999.)

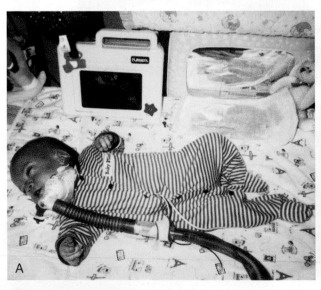 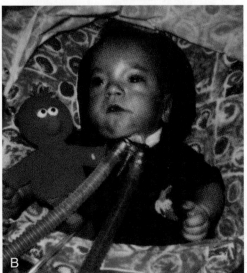

Figure 2–4

A, Same premature infant from Figure 2–3 at age 9 months, 11 lbs, 8 oz. *B,* Same infant at age 10 months, weight 13 lbs. (Courtesy of David L. Frazier, 1999.)

there is acute hypoxemia caused by infiltrates within the alveoli. Shortly after birth, the neonate exhibits signs of respiratory distress, including nasal flaring, grunting respirations, and sternal retractions. Blood gas studies indicate decreased oxygen tension and ineffective gas exchange. The infant becomes **cyanotic,** with mottled skin.

ETIOLOGY

The lungs of the neonate fail to contain the **surfactant** necessary to allow the alveoli to expand. The surfactant normally is produced relatively late in fetal life; consequently, premature infants are at risk. The outcome of this inability of the lungs to expand is inadequate surface area for proper gas exchange and a potentially fatal lack of oxygen in the blood.

DIAGNOSIS

The first indication of IRDS is increased respiratory efforts of the newborn plus a history of prematurity. Blood gas studies demonstrate the reduced potential for adequate gas exchange. Radiographic chest films indicate the presence of the infiltrate or hyaline membrane.

TREATMENT

Treatment consisting of the administration of carefully titrated supplemental oxygen, which usually is administered by mechanical ventilation and positive end-expiratory pressure (PEEP) is of primary importance. Drug therapy, including the aerosol infusion of an exogenous surfactant such as beractant (Survanta) or colfosceril palmitate (Exosurf) into the pulmonary tree by an endotracheal tube as soon as possible after birth, helps to provide an artificial surfactant, allowing the alveoli to expand. This treatment should begin within the first 48 hours of life.

Prognosis for these infants' survival has improved greatly because of a better understanding of the condition and advanced technology in drug and respiratory therapy. The incidence of IRDS, along with its treatment modalities, often predisposes premature infants to the development of bronchopulmonary dysplasia (BPD).

Prevention is the best treatment; therefore, if time permits, the mother is injected with a corticosteroid (betamethasone [Celestone Soluspan]) 12 hours before delivery in an attempt to mature the surfactant-synthesizing system.

Bronchopulmonary Dysplasia

SYMPTOMS AND SIGNS

BPD, a chronic lung disease, results after an insult to the neonate's lungs. This may be a sequela to IRDS, a lung infection, or extreme prematurity. The lungs are stiff, obstructed, and hard to ventilate.

The infant experiences periods of dyspnea, including **tachypnea,** wheezing, cyanosis, nasal flaring, and sternal retractions. O_2 **saturation** rates decrease, as does the heart rate. The infant may experience coughing and difficulty feeding. The babies appear to be working very hard to breathe. Wet or crackling sounds are heard on auscultation of the lungs with a stethoscope.

ETIOLOGY

BPD occurs in many premature infants after IRDS, mechanical ventilation with supplemental oxygen, and infection or pneumonia. The pressure and oxygen needed to maintain life-sustaining oxygen levels can damage soft and fragile lung tissue, causing overinflation or scarring.

DIAGNOSIS

Observation of the infant indicates early respiratory distress. Radiographs of the chest are abnormal, indicating alveolar damage, either scarring or overinflation, sometimes described as a "ground glass" appearance. Arterial blood gases (ABGs) indicate a problem. Oxygen levels in the lungs may be low and carbon dioxide (CO_2) levels high.

TREATMENT

The goal of treatment is replacement of the damaged alveoli. Children grow new alveoli until about 8 years of age. Infants who have BPD need to grow new alveoli to make up for those damaged by scarring. As this replacement happens, the severity of the condition lessens. Supportive treatment includes supplemental oxygen and adequate nutritional support. The types of medications used include diuretics, bronchodilators, including beta$_2$-agonists, anticholinergic drugs, and theophylline. Anti-inflammatory drugs such as steroids also may be helpful.

Supplemental O_2 therapy may be necessary for several weeks, occasionally for more than 1 year. This therapy usually is by nasal canula; however, if the infant has a tracheostomy, it may be delivered by a tracheostomy collar or by continuous positive airway pressure **(CPAP)**. O_2 saturation levels must be monitored with a pulse oximeter to maintain them at 90% or greater. The pulse oximeter also monitors heart rate. As the infant grows and matures, blood oxygen saturation levels may be maintained on room air, usually by the age of 1 year.

Diuretics help to reduce fluid accumulation in the lungs and lessen the incidence of pulmonary hypertension and right-sided heart failure. Bronchodilators are administered to reverse the narrowing of the bronchi from inflammation or bronchospasm, thus allowing more oxygen to reach the lung tissue. These drugs may be administered orally as syrups or by aerosol inhalation. The anti-inflammatory drug agents help to prevent the inflammatory process from becoming severe.

Adequate nutrition is necessary for the infant's growth and to meet the increased caloric demand with the workload of difficult breathing. High-calorie formulas are fed to the infant. The infant must be held with the head raised slightly and the formula given frequently in small amounts to prevent gastroesophageal reflux disease (GERD). Some infants are given medications to prevent GERD and medications such as antacids or histamine-2 blockers to reduce gastric acid. Emotional support should be given to the parents because this condition usually requires prolonged or frequent hospitalizations.

Prognosis is good with early and aggressive intervention, prudent monitoring, and maintenance of adequate oxygen saturation levels and heart rate. Resolution of the condition is slow, and improvement is gradual. Complications include pulmonary edema and hypertension, right-sided heart failure (cor pulmonale), respiratory infections, apnea, tracheomalacia, asthma, and gastrointestinal (GI) reflux and aspiration. These children are particularly susceptible to respiratory infections such as pneumonias, including respiratory syncytial virus (RSV), and they may experience poor growth or delayed development. Many of these children outgrow the condition, whereas others may be susceptible to respiratory distress for life. Apneic periods and low oxygen saturation levels for an extended period of time may cause hypoxia to the brain, which may result in developmental deficits. Some infants may not survive.

There is no way to prevent BPD at the present time; however, early weaning from mechanical respiratory support may decrease its incidence. Early and aggressive intervention and treatment may prevent complications and permanent conditions, even death, from occurring.

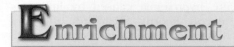

LARYNGOMALACIA, TRACHEOMALACIA, BRONCHOMALACIA

Laryngomalacia, tracheomalacia, and bronchomalacia all are forms of airway obstructive conditions. They can evolve as separate entities or can be a combination of two or even all three conditions. Although most frequently observed in the infant or young child, these conditions may be found in adults. The primary cause in all conditions is softened or underdeveloped cartilage, allowing the airway structure or structures to partially or completely collapse and compromise the airway. The infant with laryngomalacia exhibits respiratory stridor that is louder on inspiration. The infant with tracheomalacia also exhibits respiratory stridor; however, it is more pronounced on expiration. All these congenital conditions cause infants to experience dyspnea and possibly episodes of cyanosis. Oxygen saturation levels decrease and bradycardia may be experienced. Occasionally, infants may experience feeding difficulties. Diagnostic studies include chest x-ray, computed tomography (CT) and magnetic resonance imaging (MRI) scan, bronchoscopy, angiography, and echocardiography. Treatment is based on the underlying cause once it has been determined. Most of these children outgrow the disorders.

Retinopathy of Prematurity

SYMPTOMS AND SIGNS

ROP, or retrolental fibroplasia, is an abnormal growth of the blood vessels in the retinas of the infant's eyes. The condition occurs in the eyes of premature infants.

ROP occurs in infants born before 28 weeks of gestation is complete. There are no visible symptoms. Screening examinations are performed routinely on premature infants weighing less than 1500 g with a gestational age of less than 31 weeks. The entire retina is visualized to determine the stages of development of the blood vessels supplying it. These examinations first are performed when the infant is 4 to 6 weeks old.

ETIOLOGY

The vascularization of the retina begins at the back central part of the eye, growing out toward the edges. The blood vessels to the retina do not begin development until about the 28th week of gestation. In premature infants, this vascularization is not complete. Regardless of gestational age at birth, most ROP originates at 34 to 40 weeks after conception.

There are no specific risk factors identified for development of ROP. However, there is a group of risk factors that contribute to it. The more premature and low birth weight the infant, the greater the risk for developing ROP. High supplemental oxygen concentrations are responsible for many incidents of ROP. However, with close monitoring of oxygen saturation levels and appropriate adjustment and titration of oxygen concentration levels to the infant, the risk is reduced. Certain drugs, such as surfactant and indomethacin, administered to the neonate for treatment of immature lungs and PDA may increase the risk factor for the premature infant. Recently, intense artificial lighting in the nursery or crib has been considered a risk factor. Other risk factors cited include seizures, mechanical ventilation, anemia, blood transfusions, and multiple spells of apnea and bradycardia.

DIAGNOSIS

Diagnosis is made by an ophthalmologist using an indirect ophthalmoscope and scleral depression to visualize the retina. The lens and iris also are examined at this time.

TREATMENT

Most mild forms of ROP resolve on their own. Laser treatment to the area anterior to the vascular shunt eliminates abnormal vessels before their deposit of enough scar tissue to cause retinal detachment. Severe cases may require other procedures. Occasionally, the damage is so severe that blindness results.

There can be late complications of ROP that has resolved. These include crossed or wandering eyes (strabismus), "lazy eye" (amblyopia), nearsightedness (myopia), glaucoma, and late-onset retinal detachment. Many of these children may require corrective glasses.

There is no way to prevent ROP in the premature infant. Close monitoring and titration of oxygen concentrations have reduced the incidence of the condition. Neonatal intensive care units (NICUs) are currently protecting the premature infants' eyes from excessive exposure to artificial lighting. Attempts are made to reduce any stress factors to which the premature infant may be exposed. Screening examinations, staging, and appropriate intervention help to reduce the severity of the condition and hopefully prevent blindness.

Necrotizing Enterocolitis

NEC is an acute inflammatory process caused by ischemic necrosis of the mucosal lining of the small or large intestine, or both. It is a condition of premature infants or sick neonates that develops after birth, when the fragile intestinal tract of the premature or compromised newborn becomes active.

SYMPTOMS AND SIGNS

Feeding intolerance, abdominal distention, bile-colored emesis, diarrhea, blood in the stool, decreased or absent bowels sounds, lethargy, and body temperature instability a few days after birth are some of the initial symptoms exhibited by the preterm or low-weight infant. State of well-being diminishes as these infants experience respiratory problems to brief apneic periods, diminished urine output, hyperbilirubinemia, and erythema. The abdomen is tender to palpation.

ETIOLOGY

The etiology of NEC is unknown; however, it is thought to be a breakdown in normal defense systems of the GI tract, allowing the **normal flora** of the GI tract to invade the intestinal mucosa. This can happen when there is a shunting away of the blood from the GI tract, resulting in convulsive vasoconstriction of the mesenteric vessels and diminished blood supply, interfering with the normal production of protective mucus.

In addition to prematurity, factors that may predispose infants to NEC include hypovolemia, sepsis, umbilical catheters, exchange transfusions, and IRDS. Another factor is oral feeding of high-calorie concentrated formula.

DIAGNOSIS

Observation of the changes in the infant's feeding patterns, activity level, diminished body temperature maintenance, and respiratory difficulties, along with abdominal distention and tenderness, leads to further investigation. Complete blood count (CBC) indicates an elevated **white blood cell (WBC) count,** and guaiac test results of stool specimens for occult blood are positive.

Blood and stool cultures are done and may confirm the presence of bacteria. Radiographs of the intestine confirm the condition.

TREATMENT

Aggressive and immediate intervention is necessary if the infant is to survive. Feedings are stopped, making the infant's status NPO (nothing by mouth). A small tube is inserted into the stomach by way of the nose or mouth for decompression. Fluids are administered intravenously, as are antibiotics. Respiratory status and pH are monitored by ABGs. The infant's weight and intake and output are monitored closely, and fluid and electrolyte balance is maintained. Abdominal distention is monitored with frequent measurements of the abdomen by a tape measure. Radiographic monitoring of the intestinal tract also is done. Complications of intestinal perforation or peritonitis require surgical intervention with removal of the necrotic tissue. When necrosis is extensive, ileostomy or colostomy may be necessary until the infant grows, and closure with **anastomosis** can be performed.

Without immediate and aggressive intervention, many of these babies will die. NEC is a serious complication of prematurity, and some babies die even with aggressive treatment. Resection of a portion of the bowel can lead to an obstruction of the bowel or to malabsorption syndrome. Perforation can lead to sepsis and death.

Most of these babies are still in the hospital when NEC develops. Prudent nursing observations and reporting of any symptoms of NEC are essential. Because the infection can be spread from infant to infant, good hand-washing techniques must be followed. Breast milk appears to offer some immunity to this condition. An awareness of the high-risk infant is fundamental in the prevention and early intervention of this disease.

Diseases of the Nervous System

CEREBRAL PALSY

SYMPTOMS AND SIGNS

Cerebral palsy, the most common crippler of children, is a congenital, bilateral, nonprogressive paralysis that results from damage to the CNS. This syndrome primarily affects motor performance and might be noticed shortly after birth, when the infant has difficulty with sucking or swallowing. The muscles may be floppy or stiff, with diminished voluntary movement. When the infant is lifted from behind, the legs may be difficult to separate and the infant may cross his or her legs. There are three major types of cerebral palsy:

1. Spastic cerebral palsy is characterized by hyperactive reflexes or rapid muscle contractions. The older child manifests the scissor gait by walking on the toes and crossing one foot over the other. Approximately 70% of patients with cerebral palsy fall into this category.

2. Athetoid cerebral palsy is characterized by involuntary muscle movements, especially during times of stress, and decreased muscle tone. The child has difficulty with speech. Twenty percent of cases of cerebral palsy fall into this category.

3. Ataxic cerebral palsy is characterized by lack of control over voluntary movements, poor balance, and a wide gait.

A patient may exhibit signs of all three types in varying degrees from mild to severe. The symptoms tend to be more exaggerated as the child grows; however, they may be static (i.e., they neither get worse nor improve). Some persons have other related complications, including visual and auditory deficits, seizure activity, and mental retardation.

ETIOLOGY

Cerebral palsy usually stems from inadequate blood or oxygen supply to the brain during fetal development, during the birth process, or in early childhood until approximately 9 years of age. The syndrome is more common in premature infants and in male babies. Most insults to the brain occur from an interruption in the circulation of blood to the brain during labor and delivery or from infection or head trauma during the first month of life. It often is impossible to determine the exact cause of cerebral palsy.

DIAGNOSIS

Diagnosis is made from the clinical picture and neurologic examination findings. The child is examined to determine the degree of physical and mental impairment.

TREATMENT

There is no cure for cerebral palsy. In mild or severe cases, the goal of treatment is to minimize the handicap by providing every possible therapeutic measure to help the child reach his or her potential. This takes a team effort involving the family or caretaker and various medical specialists. Physical therapy, speech therapy, and special education may be required. Orthopedic intervention with casts, braces, and traction or surgery may be indicated. If the child experiences seizure activity, anticonvulsant agents are prescribed. Muscle relaxants help to reduce spastic muscle activity.

MUSCULAR DYSTROPHY

SYMPTOMS AND SIGNS

Muscular dystrophy (MD) is a progressive degeneration and weakening of the skeletal muscles. There are several types of the disease, but all are rare; the most common and well-known type is Duchenne's MD, which begins soon after birth or during early childhood, usually before the age of 5 years. Initially, it affects the muscles of the shoulders, the hips, and the thighs and calves of the legs, causing the characteristic waddling gait and toe walking. Affected muscles sometimes look larger than normal because fat replaces atrophied muscle. The child also may have lordosis or other spinal deformities. In addition, the child has difficulty with climbing stairs and running, tends to fall easily, and has difficulty with getting up. As the disease progresses, it involves all the muscles, causing crippling and immobility. **Contractures** typically develop, and the child becomes increasingly susceptible to serious pulmonary infections such as pneumonia. Frequently, children with Duchenne's MD also are impaired mentally.

ETIOLOGY

Duchenne's MD is the result of a genetic defect. As is the case for hemophilia and color blindness, the disease affects only males and generally is inherited through female carriers. In one third to one half of cases, there is no family history of MD. This means that the disease may be caused by a newly acquired mutation.

DIAGNOSIS

Characteristic symptoms along with family history of MD suggest the diagnosis. Muscle biopsy and **electromyography** confirm the diagnosis. Also, an elevated serum creatine kinase (CK) level is evident in the blood.

TREATMENT

There is no known successful treatment for Duchenne's MD. Physical therapy, exercise, surgery, and the use of orthopedic appliances can minimize deformities and preserve mobility.

The prognosis for a child with Duchenne's MD is poor. The child usually is confined to a wheelchair by the age of 9 to 12 years. Death usually occurs from cardiac or respiratory complications within 10 to 15 years of the onset of the disease.

SPINA BIFIDA

SYMPTOMS AND SIGNS

Spina bifida is a malformation of the spine in which the posterior portion of the bony canal containing the spinal cord (usually the lumbar region) is completely or partially lacking (Fig. 2–5). When this malformation exists without displacement of the cord or the meninges, it is known as spina bifida occulta and is asymptomatic. Other times, the only evidence of the neural tube defect is a dimpling, a tuft of hair, or a hemangioma over the site where the vertebrae have not completely fused.

ETIOLOGY

The etiology of this congenital anomaly is unknown, but it has been associated with exposure to ionizing radiation during early uterine life. The condition occurs when the neural tube fails to close in the early stages of fetal development. In spina bifida occulta, the posterior arches of the vertebrae, commonly in the lumbosacral area, fail to fuse; usually there is no spinal cord or spinal nerve involvement.

DIAGNOSIS

Maternal blood levels of AFP may be measured to detect possible neural tube defects. Diagnosis is made by prenatal ultrasonography or by postnatal physical examination, detection of neurologic symptoms, visual inspection of the spine, and radiographic studies. If the infant is asymptomatic, the condition may not be discovered unless it is sought.

TREATMENT

Spina bifida occulta usually requires no intervention other than prudent observation throughout the child's growth and development. Treatment depends on the degree of neurologic involvement. If the child becomes symptomatic with neurologic problems, surgical intervention to repair the deficit is necessary.

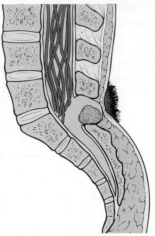 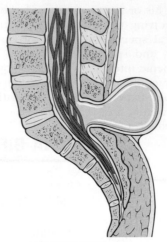 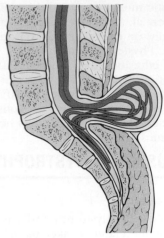

SPINA BIFIDA
Posterior vertebral arches have not
fused; there is no herniation of the
spinal cord or meninges

MENINGOCELE
External protruding sac
contains meninges and CSF

MYELOMENINGOCELE
External sac contains meninges,
CSF, and the spinal cord

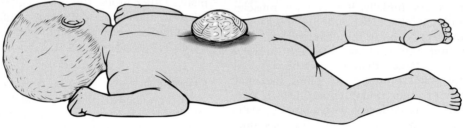

INFANT WITH MYELOMENINGOCELE

Figure 2–5

Congenital spinal cord defects.

MENINGOCELE

SYMPTOMS AND SIGNS

Meningocele is protrusion of the meninges through an opening in the spinal column, thus forming a sac that becomes filled with cerebrospinal fluid (CSF) (see Fig. 2-5). Because there is no nerve involvement, the infant usually has no neurologic problems. The skin over the area may be fragile, and rupture of the sac is a potential problem.

ETIOLOGY

As in spina bifida occulta, the posterior portion of the neural tube fails to close. The exact cause is not known. However, genetic and environmental factors may play a role.

DIAGNOSIS

Diagnosis is made by visual examination of the spinal area and verification of the presence of a sac. Radiographic studies of the spine confirm the clinical findings. The infant is assessed for hydrocephalus, which frequently is associated with neural tube defects.

TREATMENT

Treatment usually consists of surgical intervention to correct the deficit in the first 48 hours of life.

MYELOMENINGOCELE

SYMPTOMS AND SIGNS

Myelomeningocele (also known as spina bifida cystica) is a protrusion of a portion of the spinal cord and the meninges through a defect in the spinal column, usually in the lumbar region (see Fig. 2–5). Because spinal nerves or the spinal cord is present in this herniation, the infant exhibits neurologic symptoms. There may be musculoskeletal malformation, immobile joints, or paralysis of the lower extremities. Depending on the level of the anomaly, bowel or bladder control may be affected.

ETIOLOGY

As in spina bifida occulta and meningocele, the neural tube fails to close during fetal development. This allows the meninges and spinal nerves and the spinal cord to herniate through the opening of the posterior aspect of the spinal column. The etiology may include genetic factors; spinal cord defects are more frequent when prior offspring of the mother have had a similar defect.

DIAGNOSIS

Diagnosis is made by physical examination and imaging. Electromyography is employed to determine the extent of neurologic involvement. Surgical exploration verifies the severity of the disorder.

TREATMENT

Treatment is surgical intervention, usually within the first 24 hours of life, to prevent further deterioration of the involved nerves, infection, and rupture of the herniation. Additional procedures may be required as the child grows to correct any evolving problems. Children with myelomeningocele may have other anomalies, including hydrocephalus. Many of these children have no bowel or bladder control and may never be able to walk. A large number of these children die before the age of 2 years.

HYDROCEPHALUS

SYMPTOMS AND SIGNS

In hydrocephalus, the amount of CSF is increased greatly or there is blockage in its circulation, resulting in an abnormal enlargement of the head and characteristic pressure changes in the brain. The fontanelles begin to bulge, the sutures of the skull separate, and scalp veins become distended. The infant has a high-pitched cry, is irritable, and may have episodes of projectile vomiting. Eventually, there is a downward displacement of the eyes. Neurologic signs include abnormal muscle tone of the legs.

ETIOLOGY

In hydrocephalus, a large amount of CSF accumulates in the skull, causing increased intracranial pressure. An impairment of the circulation of the CSF in the ventricular circulation (obstructive hydrocephalus) may be caused by a lesion within the system or by a congenital structural defect. An impairment of the flow of the CSF in the subarachnoid space (communicating hydrocephalus) prevents the CSF from reaching the areas where normal reabsorption by the arachnoid villi occurs. This may be the result of intracranial hemorrhage from head trauma, a blood clot, prematurity, or infection (meningitis).

DIAGNOSIS

Diagnosis is made by the clinical picture, physical examination, and radiographic skull studies. CT and MRI scans demonstrate the condition.

TREATMENT

Treatment consists of surgical intervention to place a shunt in the ventricular or subarachnoid spaces to drain off the excessive CSF. Some catheters empty into the peritoneal cavity, whereas other shunt catheters empty into the right atrium of the heart (Fig. 2–6). One-way valves help to shunt the excessive CSF away from the cerebrospinal canal and to maintain a normal pressure. If left untreated, the increasing intracranial pressure of hydrocephalus causes mental retardation and eventually death.

ANENCEPHALY

SYMPTOMS AND SIGNS

The anencephalic fetus or neonate has no cranial vault and little cerebral tissue. Bones of the base of the skull and the orbits are present. Although most of these infants die before birth or during the birth process, a few survive for a short time.

ETIOLOGY

The etiology is essentially unknown, but this anomaly is characterized by failure of the neural tube at the cephalic (cranial) end to close completely during the second or third week of prenatal development. The occurrence of this defect tends to be familial; females are affected more frequently than males.

DIAGNOSIS

Diagnosis is made by ultrasonographic examination of the fetal head when blood tests of the

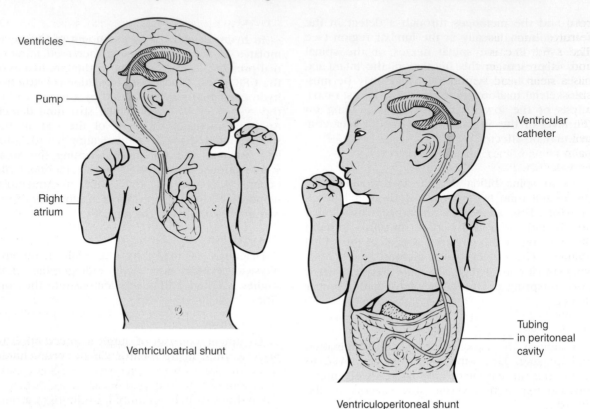

Ventricles

Pump

Right atrium

Ventriculoatrial shunt

Ventricular catheter

Tubing in peritoneal cavity

Ventriculoperitoneal shunt

Figure 2–6

Shunting procedures for hydrocephalus. Ventriculoperitoneal shunt is the preferred procedure.

mother indicate an elevated AFP level. The ultrasonogram shows symmetric absence of normal cranial bone structure and brain tissue.

TREATMENT

There is no effective treatment of this anomaly. Infants who survive the birth process die shortly afterward because many have numerous other neural tube anomalies not compatible with life.

CRI DU CHAT SYNDROME (CAT'S CRY SYNDROME)

SYMPTOMS AND SIGNS

Infants with cri du chat syndrome have an abnormally small head (microcephaly), with a deficiency of cerebral brain tissue, and mental retardation. Those who are born alive have a weak, cat-like cry. The orbits of the eyes are spaced far apart.

ETIOLOGY

Cri du chat syndrome, a hereditary condition, is the result of a chromosomal aberration caused by deletion of part of the short arm of chromosome 4 or 5 of the B group.

DIAGNOSIS

Diagnosis is made by the clinical picture of microcephaly and the characteristic cat-like cry of the infant. Confirmation is accomplished by a genetic study indicating the chromosomal defect.

TREATMENT

Treatment is supportive of body functions until the infant dies. Many fetuses with this chromosomal aberration die in utero.

DOWN SYNDROME

SYMPTOMS AND SIGNS

Down syndrome (formerly called mongolism) is a congenital form of mild to severe mental retardation accompanied by characteristic facial features and distinctive physical abnormalities. The syndrome is associated with heart defects and other congenital abnormalities. The infant has a small head with a flat back skull, a typical slant to the eyes, a flat nasal bridge, low-set ears, a protruding tongue, and small weak muscles (Fig. 2-7). The hands are short with stubby fingers and a deep horizontal crease across the palm (simian line). There is an exaggerated space between the big and little toes.

ETIOLOGY

Infants with Down syndrome have an extra chromosome on number 21 (trisomy 21). It occurs in 1 in 650 live births and more often in infants born to women older than 35 years of age (Fig. 2-8).

DIAGNOSIS

Infants with severe Down syndrome usually are identified at birth; milder forms are diagnosed later. The physical characteristics may be blatantly obvious. Findings on examination of the eyes may include the presence of small white dots on the iris. A **karyotype** showing the chromosomal abnormality can confirm the diagnosis.

TREATMENT

Care of the child with Down syndrome depends on the severity of the physical defects and the degree of mental impairment. There is no known cure. The treatment plan is individual and includes a multidimensional approach to maximize the development of motor and mental skills. Life expectancy has been improved through surgical correction of cardiac defects and antibiotic therapy for susceptibility to pulmonary disease. Some persons may be cared for in the home; others require residency at long-term care centers. Those who live long enough are known for their affectionate and placid personalities.

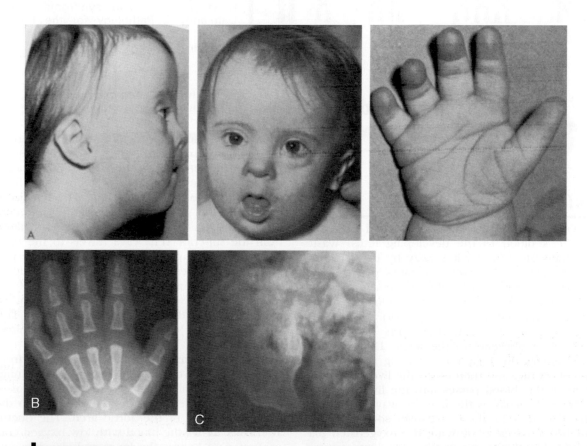

Figure 2–7

Child with Down syndrome. (From Jones KI: Recognizable Patterns of Human Malformation, 4th ed. Philadelphia: WB Saunders, 1988.)

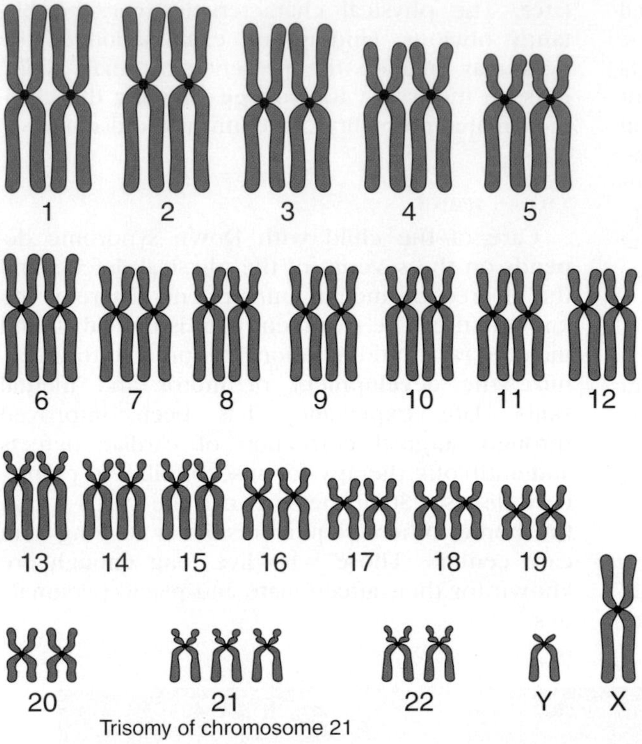

1 2 3 4 5

6 7 8 9 10 11 12

13 14 15 16 17 18 19

20 21 22 Y X

Trisomy of chromosome 21

Figure 2–8

Karyotype of Down syndrome. (From Damjanov I: Pathology for the Health-Related Professions. Philadelphia: WB Saunders, 1996.)

Congenital Cardiac Defects

FETAL CIRCULATION

Oxygen and nutrients are supplied from the mother's blood to the developing fetus. Waste products also are carried away by the maternal blood supply. The exchange takes place in the placental tissue. The umbilical vessels, two arteries and one vein, transport the blood between the placenta and the fetus (Fig. 2-9).

The umbilical vein transports oxygen-rich blood and nutrients to the fetus. The umbilical vein enters the fetal body passing through the umbilical ring and then on to the liver. Fifty percent of this blood passes into the liver, and the other 50% bypasses the liver by way of the ductus venosus. The ductus venosus soon joins the inferior vena cava, allowing the oxygenated placental blood to mix with the deoxygenated blood coming from the lower fetal body. This blood then travels to the right atrium through the vena cava.

Because of the nonfunctioning fetal lungs, this blood mostly bypasses the lungs. Most of the blood entering the right atrium by the inferior vena cava is shunted directly into the left atrium through the **foramen** ovale. There is a small valve on the left side of the atrial septum called the septum primum. This valve keeps blood from going back into the right atrium. The remaining fetal blood that has entered the right atrium containing a large amount of oxygen-poor blood from the superior vena cava travels to the right ventricle and into the pulmonary trunk. The pulmonary blood vessels have a high resistance to blood flow because of the collapsed state of the lungs, thus allowing only a small amount of blood to enter the pulmonary circulation. This small amount is enough to nourish the pulmonary tissue.

The blood that has been shunted away from the pulmonary circulation bypasses the lungs through the fetal vessel, the ductus arteriosus. This vessel connects the pulmonary trunk to the descending area of the aortic arch. The ductus arteriosus allows the blood with low oxygen concentration to bypass the lungs and also prevents it from entering the arteries leading to the brain.

The blood that has a high oxygen concentration and that has been shunted to the left atrium

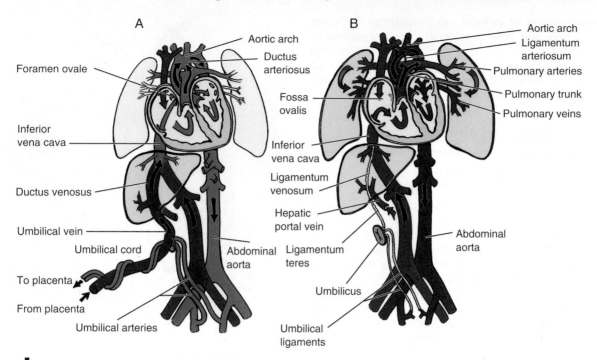

A

Aortic arch
Ductus arteriosus
Foramen ovale
Inferior vena cava
Ductus venosus
Umbilical vein
Umbilical cord
To placenta
From placenta
Umbilical arteries
Abdominal aorta

B

Aortic arch
Ligamentum arteriosum
Pulmonary arteries
Pulmonary trunk
Pulmonary veins
Fossa ovalis
Inferior vena cava
Ligamentum venosum
Hepatic portal vein
Ligamentum teres
Umbilicus
Umbilical ligaments
Abdominal aorta

Figure 2–9

Circulation patterns before and after birth. *A,* Fetal circulation. *B,* Circulation after birth. (From Applegate EJ: The Anatomy and Physiology Learning System: Textbook. Philadelphia: WB Saunders, 1995.)

by way of the foramen ovale mixes with the small amount of blood returning from the pulmonary circulation by way of the pulmonary veins. This blood flows into the left ventricle and then into the aorta. From the aorta, some travels to the coronary and the carotid arteries. A portion travels on through the descending aorta to other parts of the fetal tissue. The remaining blood travels into the umbilical arteries and back to the placenta for exchange of gases, nutrients, and waste.

After the birth process, the infant's respiratory effort, and the initial inflation of the lungs, the circulatory system undergoes important changes. The resistance to blood flow through the lungs is reduced because of the inflation of the tissue, allowing an increased blood flow from the pulmonary arteries. There now is an increased volume of blood flowing from the right atrium into the right ventricle and the pulmonary arteries. Additionally, the volume of blood flowing through the foramen ovale into the left atrium is reduced. The blood returning by way of the pulmonary veins from the lungs to the left atrium is increased in volume, causing an increase in the

pressure in the left atrium. Blood is forced against the septum primum because of decreased right atrial pressure and increased left atrial pressure, and the foramen ovale closes. If this does not happen, the infant has an ASD (discussed subsequently under congenital anomalies). The heart now is a two-sided pump.

With the lungs expanded and taking over the function of gas exchange, there no longer is a need for the ductus arteriosus to shunt blood from the pulmonary trunk to the descending aorta. Normally, the ductus arteriosus closes off in the first few days after birth. If it does not close, it is termed *patent,* a congenital birth defect, a PDA (discussed subsequently).

SYMPTOMS AND SIGNS

Congenital cardiac defects are developmental anomalies of the heart or the great vessels of the heart. They are present at birth, and the defects cause mild to fatal stress of the cardiac muscle. Signs and symptoms vary according to the nature of the anomaly, the severity of the defect, and its effect on the heart and the circulatory system. There can be more than one defect present, or a combination of defects can complicate the case. The common defects generally are categorized as follows: acyanotic, in which there is no mixing of deoxygenated and oxygenated blood, and cyanotic, in which mixing of oxygenated and deoxygenated blood occurs.

ACYANOTIC DEFECTS

Ventricular Septal Defect

The most common congenital cardiac disorder, ventricular septal defect, is an abnormal opening between the right and the left ventricle (Fig. 2–10). When the defect is small, there is little functional disease; when it is large, the results are serious. In this condition, a shunting of blood from the left to the right side of the heart is due to higher pressure in the left ventricle. A loud systolic **murmur** is heard during auscultation. Clinical features include failure to gain weight, restlessness, irritability, and increased heart rate and respirations.

42

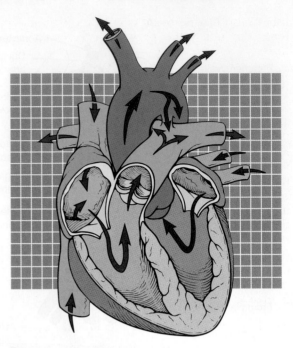

Figure 2–11

Patent ductus arteriosus. (Used with permission of Ross Products Division, Abbott Laboratories, from *Congenital Heart Abnormalities* [Clinical Education Aid no. 7], 1992.)

Patent Ductus Arteriosus

PDA results when the functional closure of the ductus fails to occur. During normal fetal circulation, the patent ductus short-circuits circulation to the lungs and directs blood from the pulmonary trunk to the aorta. If PDA still is present after birth, circulation of oxygen is compromised because this abnormal opening is a shunt that allows oxygenated blood to recirculate through the lungs (Fig. 2–11). PDA is detected during a physical examination when a classic "machinery" murmur is heard on auscultation and palpitation reveals a thrill. The infant's growth and development may be slowed, and various signs of heart failure may be present. Attempts at closure by drug therapy using an antiprostaglandin may be made. The other option is surgical closure of the ductus.

This condition is fairly common in premature infants and often is accompanied by ASD with failure of the foramen ovale to close.

Prognosis for these infants is dependent on the presence of other anomalies. Closure by either drug therapy or surgical intervention estab-

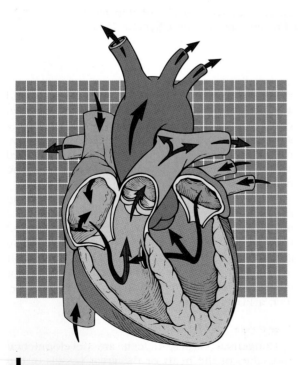

Figure 2–10

Ventricular septal defect. (Used with permission of Ross Products Division, Abbott Laboratories, from *Congenital Heart Abnormalities* [Clinical Education Aid no. 7], 1992.)

lishes a normal postnatal circulation path and affords the infant the opportunity to grow and thrive.

Currently there is no known prevention.

Coarctation of the Aorta

This defect is characterized by a narrowed aortic lumen, causing a partial obstruction of the flow of blood through the aorta (Fig. 2–12). The result is increased left ventricular pressure and workload, with decreased blood pressure distal to the narrowing. Signs and symptoms can be evident shortly after birth or may not surface until adolescence. They include signs of left ventricular failure with pulmonary edema. The patient is pale and **cyanotic** with weakness, **dyspnea,** and **tachycardia.** Systemic blood pressure is elevated when measured in the arms, yet no pulse is felt in the leg vessels because pressure in them may be decreased.

Atrial Septal Defect

ASD is an abnormal opening between the right and left atria (Fig. 2–13). Although the de-

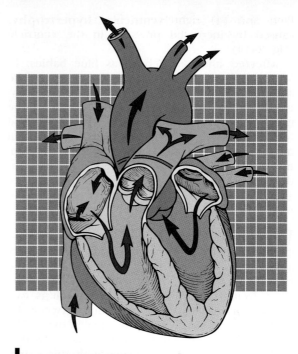

Figure 2–13

Atrial septal defect. (Used with permission of Ross Products Division, Abbott Laboratories, from *Congenital Heart Abnormalities* [Clinical Education Aid no. 7], 1992.)

fect can vary in size and location, left to right shunting of blood generally occurs in all atrial septal defects. Small defects may be undetected or cause symptoms such as fatigue, shortness of breath, and frequent respiratory tract infections. A large defect causes pronounced **cyanosis,** dyspnea, and **syncope.** A classic systolic cardiac murmur can be heard with a stethoscope. This condition often is associated with prematurity and PDA, and closure is achieved with surgical repair.

CYANOTIC DEFECTS

Central cyanosis is a sign that the atrial blood is not fully oxygenated.

Tetralogy of Fallot

The most common cyanotic cardiac defect is a combination of four congenital heart defects: (1) ventricular septal defect, an abnormal opening in the ventricular septum; (2) pulmonary **stenosis,** a tightening of the pulmonary valve or vessel; (3) dextroposition (displacement to the right) of the aorta, which overrides the ventricular septal de-

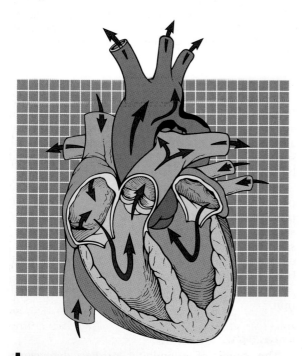

Figure 2–12

Coarctation of the aorta. (Used with permission of Ross Products Division, Abbott Laboratories, from *Congenital Heart Abnormalities* [Clinical Education Aid no. 7], 1992.)

43

fect; and (4) right ventricular **hypertrophy,** caused by increased pressure in the ventricle (Fig. 2–14).

Affected infants are born as blue babies. In severe defects, deoxygenated blood enters the aorta, causing the symptoms of **hypoxia:** tachycardia, **tachypnea,** dyspnea, and seizures. Bone marrow hypoxia causes polycythemia, increased total red blood cell mass. Physical examination may reveal delayed physical growth and development and clubbing of the fingers and toes. Cardiac murmurs can be heard. Older children assume a squatting position after exercise to relieve breathlessness caused by hypoxia.

Transposition of the Great Arteries

In this defect, the aorta and the pulmonary artery are reversed: the aorta originates from the right ventricle, and the pulmonary artery originates from the left ventricle. The result is two closed-loop circulatory systems: one between the heart and the lungs, and the other between the heart and systemic circulation (Fig. 2–15). Within a few hours of birth, neonates with this defect exhibit cyanosis and tachypnea, followed by signs of heart failure.

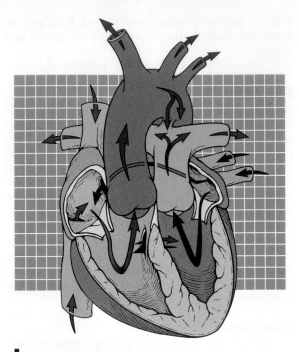

Figure 2–15

Transposition of the great arteries. (Used with permission of Ross Products Division, Abbott Laboratories, from *Congenital Heart Abnormalities* [Clinical Education Aid no. 7], 1992.)

Immediate surgical intervention is indicated. Prostaglandins are administered to the infant in an effort to keep the ductus arteriosus patent and the foramen ovale from closing. As soon as surgery is possible, the blood flow is redirected by correction of the defect.

Prognosis for these infants is poor unless a pediatric surgical unit is readily available and transportation to it is swift. Another factor in the survival of infants with this condition is the response to the drug therapy to maintain the fetal circulation from altering into the normal postbirth circulatory system.

There is no known prevention of this condition.

ETIOLOGY

The cause of congenital cardiac defects remains unknown. They may be the result of several factors, including chromosomal abnormalities and environmental conditions such as maternal infections and the mother's use of certain drugs during gestation. Several congenital disorders result from the failure of the circulatory system to

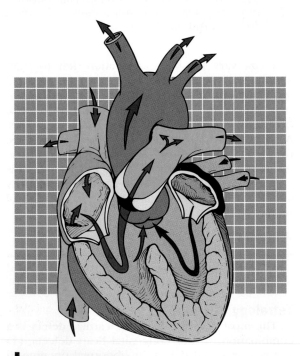

Figure 2–14

Tetralogy of Fallot. (Used with permission of Ross Products Division, Abbott Laboratories, from *Congenital Heart Abnormalities* [Clinical Education Aid no. 7], 1992.)

shift from the fetal route of blood flow at the time of birth.

DIAGNOSIS

Physical examination and patient history are essential. The physician palpates the neck vessels and auscultates for blood pressure and murmurs. Diagnostic procedures depend on the initial findings and may include radiographic chest films, blood tests, cardiac catheterization, echocardiogram, and electrocardiogram. The diagnostic investigation determines the presence and severity of any structural or functional abnormality or defect.

TREATMENT

Medical management of congenital cardiac defects is determined by the type of defect, the degree of symptoms and signs, and the presence of life-threatening complications. Advances in surgical techniques enable surgeons to close septal defects, to reconstruct or replace a valve, and to repair or join blood vessels. These procedures make it possible to save, improve, and extend the lives of persons born with congenital cardiac defects. Medications are available to strengthen and regulate the heartbeat. Supportive measures include prophylactic antibiotic administration to ward off infection. Parents and caretakers need understanding, encouragement, and teaching to cope with changes in individual and family lifestyle imposed by the disease.

Musculoskeletal Diseases

CLUBFOOT (TALIPES EQUINOVARUS)

SYMPTOMS AND SIGNS

Clubfoot is an obvious, nontraumatic deformity of the foot of the newborn in which the anterior half of the foot is adducted and inverted. The heel is drawn up, with the lateral side of the foot being convex and the medial aspect being concave (Fig. 2-16). A true clubfoot cannot be manipulated to the proper position, whereas distortions that are caused by intrauterine position usually can be.

ETIOLOGY

Some sources indicate that fetal position is the cause, and other studies implicate genetic factors because of an abnormal development of the germ plasma during the embryonic stage.

DIAGNOSIS

The deformity is obvious at birth, with a resistance of the foot to return to a neutral position during manipulation. A shortening of the Achilles tendon is involved.

TREATMENT

Treatment consists of either cast application or the use of splints. Treatment must start early in the neonatal period. Casts are reapplied at frequent intervals as the correction increases and the infant grows. Splints involve a bar affixed to shoes; the infant is placed in the shoes, which hold the feet and legs in position. Many physicians employ a combination of manipulative methods, with cast application followed by the use of splints as the child matures. The child must be observed throughout childhood for regression of the improvement. If casting and splinting are unsuccessful, surgery may be indicated to correct the condition.

CONGENITAL HIP DYSPLASIA

SYMPTOMS AND SIGNS

Congenital hip dysplasia (CHD) is an abnormal development of the hip joint that ranges from an unstable joint to dislocation of the femoral head from the acetabulum. Physical examination reveals asymmetric folds of the thigh of the newborn with a limited abduction of the affected hip. A shortening of the femur is noted when the knees and hips are flexed at right angles (see Fig. 2-16).

ETIOLOGY

The exact cause is unknown. Typical CHD occurs shortly before, during, or shortly after birth, possibly as a result of softening of the ligaments from effects of the maternal hormone relaxin. CHD may result from a breech presentation and is more common in female infants.

DIAGNOSIS

Abnormal signs, including a positive **Ortolani's sign,** may be detected at birth. Diagnosis is made during the physical examination and is confirmed by radiographic studies.

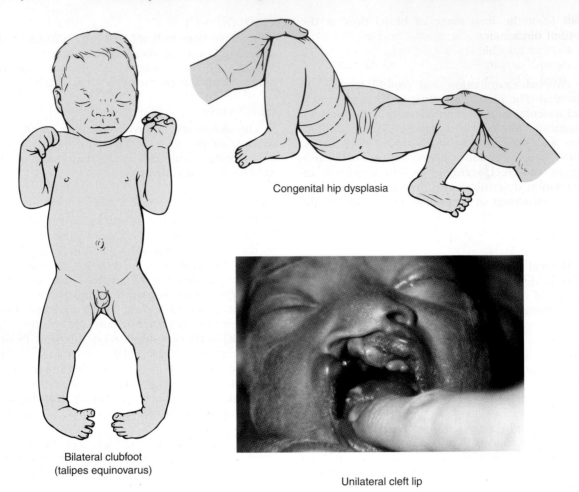

Congenital hip dysplasia

Bilateral clubfoot
(talipes equinovarus)

Unilateral cleft lip

Figure 2–16

Congenital musculoskeletal diseases. (From Behrman RE, Kliegman RM, Arvin AM: Slide set for Nelson Textbook of Pediatrics, 15/E. Philadelphia, WB Saunders, 1996.)

TREATMENT

Treatment involves the use of various devices to reduce the congenital hip dislocation. After replacement of the femoral head into its proper position in the acetabulum is achieved, the legs are held in place by a Pavlik harness, a splint, or a cast, allowing stable maintenance of the hip in a position of flexion and abduction. Early treatment offers the best results and may avoid the necessity of surgical intervention.

CLEFT LIP AND PALATE

SYMPTOMS AND SIGNS

Cleft lip (harelip) is a congenital birth defect consisting of one or more clefts in the upper lip (see Fig. 2-16). Cleft palate is a birth defect in which there is a hole in the middle of the roof of the mouth (palate). The cleft may extend completely through the hard and soft palates into the nasal area. The defects appear singularly or may be linked and vary in severity. Some infants have difficulty with nasal regurgitation and feeding because of air leaks around the cleft. A major problem is the infant's appearance.

ETIOLOGY

The cause is a failure in the embryonic development of the fetus. It is considered a multifactorial genetic disorder and occurs in approximately 1 in 10,000 births.

DIAGNOSIS

Cleft abnormalities are obvious during clinical inspection at birth.

TREATMENT

Cleft deformities usually are repaired surgically as soon as possible. Extensive deformities require a second repair. Special feeding devices can be tried. The child frequently requires speech therapy.

Genitourinary Diseases

CRYPTORCHIDISM (UNDESCENDED TESTES)

SYMPTOMS AND SIGNS

Cryptorchidism, or failure of the testicles to descend into the scrotum, is detected at birth or shortly thereafter. The condition may be unilateral or bilateral. During infancy and early childhood, there are no symptoms, just the absence of the testes. The condition is more common in premature infants.

ETIOLOGY

What causes failure of the testes to descend during the final fetal developmental stages is not clearly understood. Some experts suspect that hormones play a role.

DIAGNOSIS

Diagnosis is by visual inspection and by palpation, starting above the inguinal ring and pushing downward on the inguinal canal toward the scrotum. The examination reveals no evidence of one or both testes in the scrotal sac. When the condition is bilateral, the scrotum appears underdeveloped.

TREATMENT

Often, the testes descend spontaneously during the first year of life. If this does not happen by 4 years of age, the treatment is to place the undescended testes into the scrotum by either surgical manipulation (orchiopexy) or hormonal drug therapy. Treatment is important because untreated cryptorchidism may lead to sterility in the adult male. There is an increased risk of testicular cancer in untreated cryptorchidism.

WILMS' TUMOR

SYMPTOMS AND SIGNS

Wilms' tumor is a highly malignant tumor of the kidney affecting children younger than 5 years of age. A mass in the kidney region may be discovered accidentally by a parent or the examining physician. The patient experiences **hematuria,** pain, vomiting, and hypertension.

ETIOLOGY

Wilms' tumor is an **adenosarcoma** arising from abnormal fetal kidney tissue that is left behind during early embryonic life. The tissue begins unrestrained cancerous growth after the child is born.

DIAGNOSIS

Physical examination reveals a palpable kidney mass. **Intravenous pyelography** shows displacement and distortion of the pelvis of the kidney.

TREATMENT

Prompt recognition and treatment are imperative because the tumor is locally invasive and has the propensity to metastasize. Removal of the tumor and accessible metastatic sites is followed by radiation therapy and chemotherapy. The prognosis is uncertain but has greatly improved with modern treatment methods.

PHIMOSIS

SYMPTOMS AND SIGNS

Phimosis is stenosis, or narrowing, of the opening of the foreskin in the male infant. He may experience difficulty with urination, or the parents may have difficulty with cleaning the area under the prepuce of the glans penis, resulting in an accumulation of secretions. These symptoms may develop later in uncircumcised males.

ETIOLOGY

Many male infants are born with phimosis; the cause is unknown.

DIAGNOSIS

Diagnosis is made by visual examination and the inability to slide the prepuce back over the glans penis.

TREATMENT

Treatment is circumcision, the surgical removal of the prepuce. This procedure, which used to be routine for male newborns, is usually done in the first few days of life.

Diseases of the Digestive System

CONGENITAL PYLORIC STENOSIS

SYMPTOMS AND SIGNS

Pyloric stenosis is a gastric obstruction associated with narrowing of the pyloric sphincter at the exit of the stomach. The infant has episodes of projectile vomiting after feedings (Fig. 2–17). There is a failure to gain weight. The onset of symptoms normally occurs at 2 to 3 weeks of age. The infant appears hungry, continues to feed, and yet fails to gain weight. If left untreated, the infant becomes dehydrated and experiences electrolyte imbalances. A small olive-shaped hard mass may be palpated in the region of the pyloric sphincter, and left to right peristalsis may be noted, followed by reverse peristalsis. The emesis contains no bile.

ETIOLOGY

There is a slight hereditary tendency, but the exact cause is unknown. It occurs four times more frequently in male than in female infants.

DIAGNOSIS

Diagnosis is made from the history and the patient's physical condition. Diagnostic studies include upper gastrointestinal radiographic studies and ultrasonographic study of the pylorus.

TREATMENT

Treatment consists of surgical intervention in which the constricted pylorus is incised and sutured to relieve the obstruction.

HIRSCHSPRUNG'S DISEASE (CONGENITAL AGANGLIONIC MEGACOLON)

SYMPTOMS AND SIGNS

Hirschsprung's disease is an impairment of intestinal motility that causes obstruction of the distal colon. The symptoms and signs differ slightly depending on the age of the child experiencing an exacerbation of the condition. In the neonatal period, the newborn fails to pass **meconium** within 48 hours after birth. The infant may have bile-stained or fecal vomitus and does not want to feed. The abdomen becomes distended.

After the neonatal period, the symptoms and signs include a failure to thrive, with obstinate constipation, vomiting, and abdominal distention. When the condition worsens, the infant may become feverish and may have explosive, watery diarrhea.

The older child exhibits more chronic symptoms such as constipation, abdominal distention, ribbon-like stools that are foul smelling, easily palpable fecal masses, and visible peristalsis. The child appears malnourished and anemic.

ETIOLOGY

The defect lies in the abnormal innervation of the **intrinsic** musculature of the bowel wall. In Hirschsprung's disease, there is an absence of the parasympathetic nerve ganglion cells in a seg-

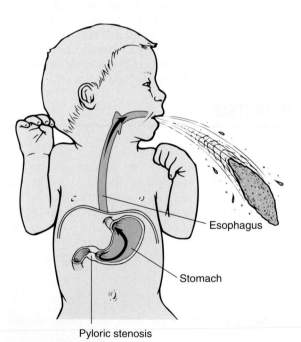

Esophagus

Stomach

Pyloric stenosis

Figure 2–17

Congenital pyloric stenosis. The abnormal narrowing of the opening of the pylorus causes episodes of projectile vomiting.

ment of the colon, usually in the rectosigmoid area. This deficiency of innervation results in lack of peristalsis in the affected portion of the colon and the succeeding backup of fecal material. The proximal portion of the colon becomes grossly distended, and intestinal obstruction results.

Statistics indicate that males are more likely than females to have a megacolon and that the risk is increased in children with Down syndrome. It is believed to be a familial congenital disease.

DIAGNOSIS

Diagnosis is based on family history, the clinical picture, radiographic studies of the bowel, and finally, biopsy that confirms the absence of the ganglionic cells.

TREATMENT

Treatment consists of relief of the obstruction by surgical intervention; the affected bowel is excised, and the normal colon is joined to the anus. A temporary colostomy is performed proximal to the aganglionic section of the colon. Electrolyte and fluid balance must be maintained. After the colon recovers function (6 months to 1 year), the colostomy is closed.

Metabolic Disorders

CYSTIC FIBROSIS

SYMPTOMS AND SIGNS

Cystic fibrosis (CF) is a chronic dysfunction of the exocrine glands (glands that secrete through ducts) affecting multiple body systems; it is the most common fatal genetic disease. Symptoms may become apparent soon after birth or may develop in childhood. The disease primarily attacks the lungs and the digestive system, with the production of copious thick and sticky mucus that accumulates and blocks glandular ducts. The clinical effects of CF can be immense, including a dry paroxysmal cough, exercise intolerance, pneumonia, bulky diarrhea, vomiting, and bowel obstruction. Pancreatic changes occur, with fat and fibrous replacement of normal tissue. Involvement of sweat glands causes increased concentrations of salt in sweat. Normal

growth and ability to thrive are diminished (Fig. 2–18).

ETIOLOGY

CF is an inherited disorder and is transmitted as an autosomal recessive trait.

DIAGNOSIS

The diagnostic workup includes a family history, a pulmonary function test, radiographic chest film, and stool studies. Sweat test reveals elevated levels of sodium and chloride and confirms the diagnosis.

TREATMENT

CF is considered a fatal disease. However, with early diagnosis and treatment, life expectancy has improved greatly during the past few decades. The treatment is directed at supportive measures that help the child to lead as normal a life as possible and prevention of pulmonary infections. These measures include the use of a high-calorie, high–sodium chloride diet; chest physiotherapy; and pancreatic enzyme supplementation to aid in digestion. Broad-spectrum antibiotics are used aggressively to treat infection, and drugs that thin the mucus are given. Oxygen therapy may be required. The family needs emotional support and teaching about the disease; referral for genetic counseling is helpful.

PHENYLKETONURIA

SYMPTOMS AND SIGNS

Phenylketonuria (PKU) is an inborn error in the metabolism of amino acids that causes brain damage and mental retardation when not corrected. In this defect, an enzyme needed to change an amino acid (phenylalanine) in the body into another substance (tyrosine) is lacking. As a result, phenylalanine accumulates in the blood and urine and is **toxic** to the brain. The onset of symptoms may not occur until the infant is 4 months old, when a characteristic musty odor of the child's perspiration and urine is noted. Other signs include rashes, irritability, hyperactivity, personality disorders, and evidence of arrested brain development.

ETIOLOGY

PKU is inherited as an autosomal recessive trait and causes defective enzymatic conversion in protein metabolism, resulting in the accumulation of phenylalanine in the blood.

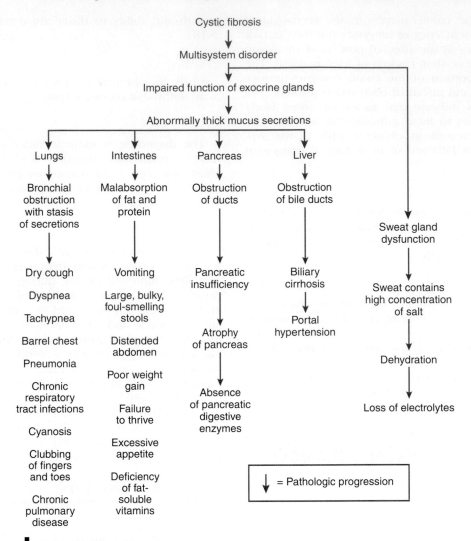

Figure 2–18

Major clinical manifestations of cystic fibrosis in a child.

DIAGNOSIS

The detection of PKU is achieved by mandatory screening of the newborn blood. A positive **Guthrie test** result indicates the presence of phenylalanine in the blood. The urine is tested for phenylalanine derivatives.

TREATMENT

Prognosis is excellent when the infant is placed on a diet free of phenylalanine early postnatally. Late dietary intervention does not reverse brain damage. Because natural proteins contain phenylalanine, the patient must remain on a protein-restricted diet. Close follow-up with testing for phenylalanine levels in the blood may allow some modifications in the difficult dietary restrictions. Emotional support is important for the child and the parent. Genetic counseling is advised.

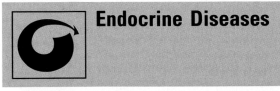

Endocrine Diseases

Klinefelter's syndrome and Turner's syndrome are examples of genetic, chromosomal diseases that are not inherited. They result from nondisjunction, or the failure of a chromosome pair to separate, during **gamete** production.

Humans normally have 46 chromosomes, 22 pairs of **autosomes** and 2 sex chromosomes. The technical notation for a human female is 46,XX and for a male, 46,XY. In a fertilized ovum, one chromosome from each pair of autosomes originates from the mother's ovum, the other from the father's sperm. Each ovum normally contains a single X chromosome. Sperm cells may contain either an X or a Y chromosome. If a sperm bearing the X chromosome fertilizes the ovum, the fetus develops into a female. A sperm carrying the Y chromosome produces a male fetus. Sometimes, through what may be described as an accident of nature, extra chromosomes or absent chromosomes in the fertilized ovum cause congenital syndromes with a variety of physical and mental developmental effects.

KLINEFELTER'S SYNDROME

SYMPTOMS AND SIGNS

Klinefelter's syndrome is a chromosomal disorder that affects an estimated 1 in 1000 liveborn males and is characterized by the presence of an extra X chromosome (typically the 47,XXY pattern). The presence of two X chromosomes in affected males causes abnormal development of the testes and decreased levels of the male hormone testosterone. Puberty begins at the usual time and results in a normal-sized penis, but the testes are small and body hair is scant. In general, the person appears normal, except for exceptionally long legs, above average height, and decreased muscle development. The most significant problem associated with Klinefelter's syndrome is infertility due to **azoospermia.** Other alterations include mild delay in language acquisition and increased risk of behavioral and learning disabilities. Some affected persons have mild to more significant intellectual impairment. The mammary glands may be enlarged in about one half of the cases. Possible complications include osteoporosis and chronic pulmonary disease.

ETIOLOGY

Klinefelter's syndrome results from the presence of at least two X chromosomes, typically the 47,XXY pattern. Other variants include

XXYY, XXXY, and XXXXY. The disease is not inherited but results from a nondisjunction during gamete formation.

DIAGNOSIS

The diagnostic workup includes a physical examination, serum and urine gonadotropin level determination, and semen analysis. A chromosomal smear analysis confirms the diagnosis.

TREATMENT

At the time of normal puberty, long-term hormone replacement with testosterone by injection or a transdermal patch is given, usually under the supervision of an endocrinologist. Testosterone is necessary for maintaining normal sexual function and normal muscle and bone mass. However, fertility cannot be restored. Many patients report an improvement in energy and emotional stability with hormone therapy. Support group meetings are available for psychological support.

TURNER'S SYNDROME

SYMPTOMS AND SIGNS

Turner's syndrome is a chromosomal disease that occurs in females with a single sex chromosome, 45,XO. It is the most common disorder of gonadal dysgenesis in females. At birth, the ovaries are immature or absent, and the female infant appears short, with swollen hands and feet; there may be webbing of the neck. As these children grow, there is absence of sexual maturation, amenorrhea, sterility, dwarfism, impaired intelligence, and cardiac defects.

ETIOLOGY

Turner's syndrome results from loss of the second X chromosome caused by nondisjunction during gamete formation.

DIAGNOSIS

Chromosomal smear studies show only one X chromosome instead of the normal 46,XX chromosomal pattern.

TREATMENT

Symptoms can be reduced by estrogen and growth hormone therapy. Emotional support for the patient and the family helps them to develop strategies for coping with low self-esteem, body image disturbance, and impaired intelligence.

Childhood Diseases

Nothing causes more anxiety than a seriously ill child. Pathologic processes in children pose special threats because children constantly are changing physically and functionally. Normally, the journey through childhood results in maturation and expansion of the body's natural immune defense mechanisms. Additionally, rapid advances in treatment and preventive medicine enable the control of many infectious diseases that formerly caused serious illness and disabling complications, even death. However, various infections and disease syndromes can interrupt the normal growth and development of any child. The following material addresses the characteristics of common diseases that affect children.

over the extremities; they can be distributed everywhere on the body and even have been found internally. A day or two before the rash appears, the patient may experience fever, malaise, and anorexia. The lesions can continue to erupt for 3 to 4 days and cause intense itching. Recovery is usually complete within 2 weeks, leaving the person with lifetime immunity. Some possible complications include secondary bacterial infec-

 ## Infectious Diseases

Although limited natural immunity is acquired by the infant from the mother, the growing child is vulnerable to many infectious diseases and the disabilities that they cause. Many of these communicable diseases can be prevented. Dramatic results have been achieved in pediatric medicine through routine prophylactic immunization with vaccines that build specific and prolonged protection. To prevent epidemics of contagious diseases, all states in the United States require that children have inoculations before entering school (Table 2–2).

CHICKENPOX (VARICELLA)

SYMPTOMS AND SIGNS

Chickenpox is a highly contagious, acute viral infection that is common in children and young adults. It is a systemic disease with superficial cutaneous lesions that begin as red **macules** that progress to **papules** and then finally become **vesicles** that form crusts. The lesions first are seen on the face or the trunk and then spread

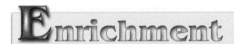

VACCINES

A vaccine is a suspension of dead or attenuated organisms given to stimulate an active immune response that affords more or less permanent resistance to pathogenic organisms and viruses. Booster doses are smaller amounts of the original vaccine given at specified intervals to maintain serum antibody levels. Vaccines are controlled for potency and stability and are tested for safety and effectiveness. Some vaccines are grown in bird eggs or in animal organs or are weakened with chemicals. The person is screened for certain allergies or previous reactions to vaccines. Local responses of soreness, redness, and swelling at the site of injection are common. Untoward responses include high fever, generalized swelling, difficult breathing, severe headache, arthralgia, and seizures; any of these occurrences should be reported immediately to the physician.

Toxoids use an altered form of a bacterial toxin to stimulate antibody production and therefore impart protection against toxins.

TABLE 2–2 ➤ Typical Immunization Schedule for Normal Children

NAME OF VACCINE	NAME OF DISEASE	NUMBER OF DOSES	AGE GIVEN
Diphtheria and tetanus toxoids and pertussis vaccine (DTP)	Diphtheria, tetanus, pertussis	5	2 mo 4 mo 6 mo 15–18 mo 4–6 yr
Oral poliomyelitis vaccine (OPV)	Poliomyelitis	4	2 mo 4 mo 15 mo 4–6 yr
Measles, mumps, and rubella virus vaccine (MMR)	Measles, mumps, rubella	2	15 mo 4–6 yr, or before starting kindergarten or 1st grade
Haemophilus b conjugate vaccine (HibCV)	Meningitis	3	2, 4, 6 mo
Diphtheria and tetanus toxoids (Td)	Diphtheria	1	14–16 yr
Varicella virus vaccine	Chickenpox (varicella)	1	1–12 yr
Hepatitis B vaccine	Hepatitis B	3	birth–2 mo 1–4 mo 6–18 mo

Special schedules are recommended for older children, adults, and people at special risk. The chronically ill, immigrants, foreign travelers, or those with lifestyle risks may need additional immunizations.
The American Academy of Pediatrics recommends routine hepatitis B vaccination of infants.
See text for additional information on varicella vaccine.

tion, viral pneumonia, conjunctival ulcers, and Reye's syndrome.

ETIOLOGY

The causative organism is the varicella-zoster virus (VZV), a member of the herpesvirus group. The virus is transmitted by direct or indirect droplet nuclei spread from the respiratory tract of the infected person or a carrier. Fluid from the cutaneous lesions is also infectious, but dried crusty lesions are not contagious. The patient is considered contagious for 1 to 2 days before the eruptions until about 6 days after the eruptions. The incubation period is 2 to 3 weeks. A varicella virus vaccine (Varivax) currently is available for protection against chickenpox. For children, a single injection of the vaccine at 1 to 12 years of age is recommended. For adolescents and adults, a second dose is administered 4 to 8 weeks after the first dose. The need for booster doses has not been defined because the duration of protection of varicella vaccine presently is unknown.

DIAGNOSIS

The diagnosis of chickenpox usually is made by the history of exposure and by the presence of characteristic cutaneous eruptions. Although laboratory testing is not usually necessary, the VZV can be visualized when a culture of vesicular fluid is examined microscopically. After the infection, antibodies are found in the serum.

TREATMENT

Palliative treatment to alleviate **pruritus** includes cool bicarbonate of soda baths followed by a cornstarch dusting or the application of calamine lotion. This helps to control scratching that can lead to secondary infection and scarring. Other comfort measures include the administration of acetaminophen for fever and pain. *Caution:* Aspirin is *not* given to children with chickenpox because of the possibility of Reye's syndrome. Isolation of the patient is required until all lesions have crusted.

The patient who is immunocompromised, or other high-risk persons, can be given the varicella-zoster immune globulin within 4 days of exposure.

DIPHTHERIA

SYMPTOMS AND SIGNS

Diphtheria is an acute communicable disease that causes necrosis of the mucous membrane in the respiratory tract. The patient, most frequently a child, has sore throat, **dysphagia,** a cough, hoarseness, and chills; fever, swollen regional lymph nodes, and foul breath can be noted. As the bacteria invade the nasopharynx, they multiply and produce a powerful **exotoxin** that travels in the blood throughout the body. Locally, the infection and inflammation cause grayish patches of thick mucous membrane to appear along the respiratory tract known as pseudomembrane, or false membrane. The membrane, which can be extensive, is composed of bacteria, inflammatory cells, dead tissue, and **fibrin;** it is surrounded by inflammation and swelling that can interfere with the airway, impairing swallowing and speech. As the toxin is absorbed, it affects other vital organ systems, with many possible complications, including otitis media, pneumonia, myocarditis, and paralysis.

Carriers, although infected, remain asymptomatic and do not contract active infection.

ETIOLOGY

The causative bacteria, *Corynebacterium diphtheriae,* is present in the nasopharynx of infected persons or carriers and is transmitted by airborne respiratory droplets. The incubation period is 2 to 5 days. The patient is contagious for 2 to 4 weeks if untreated or for 1 to 2 days after initiating antibiotic treatment. Carriers of the disease remain asymptomatic but can infect the inadequately immunized individual.

DIAGNOSIS

The presence of the characteristic membrane adhering to the throat is diagnostic. Culture of the throat and laboratory stains are positive for *C. diphtheriae,* and antibodies are present in the serum. Immunity or susceptibility can be determined by the **Schick test.**

TREATMENT

Diphtheria antitoxin is given as soon as possible. The administration of antibiotics, such as penicillin and erythromycin, is indicated to kill the organism. The patient is isolated, restricted to bed rest, and given a diet as tolerated. The patient is observed for the possible complications related to systemic involvement. Carriers are given antibiotics to eliminate the organisms from their respiratory tract.

Diphtheria, once common in North America and Europe, can be prevented by the administration of diphtheria toxoid to produce active immunity. Inoculation begins at 2 to 3 months, with booster doses given at appropriate intervals during childhood.

MUMPS (EPIDEMIC PAROTITIS)

SYMPTOMS AND SIGNS

Mumps is an acute communicable disease causing inflammation and swelling of one or both parotid glands. The patient, usually a child, has tenderness in the neck in front of and below the ears in the region of the parotid glands and pain on swallowing. Patients also may experience a headache and a low-grade fever, with loss of appetite and an earache that is aggravated by chewing. A common complication of the disease in the male adult is mumps **orchitis.** Often, the infection is a subclinical illness without noticeable symptoms.

ETIOLOGY

The causative agent of mumps is an airborne virus, which is spread by droplet nuclei from the respiratory tract. The incubation period is long, usually 14 to 21 days. The patient is contagious for 1 to 7 days before the swelling of the parotid glands and up to 9 days thereafter. Lifelong immunity develops after a clinical or subclinical infection; active immunization with the mumps vaccine also affords prolonged immunity.

DIAGNOSIS

Diagnosis is made from a history of exposure and a clinical picture that includes swelling of the parotid glands. The male patient is assessed for tenderness of the testes.

TREATMENT

Acetaminophen is given, and warm or cold compresses are applied for pain. A soft or liquid diet can help to minimize discomfort when eating. Scrotal support may be necessary in the male patient who is experiencing testicular tenderness and swelling.

Meningitis and encephalitis are possible complications of mumps. Childhood immunization is the best prevention. An unimmunized person should be referred to a physician for active immunization within 48 hours of contact to prevent or alter the severity of the disease.

PERTUSSIS (WHOOPING COUGH)

SYMPTOMS AND SIGNS

Whooping cough is a highly contagious bacterial infection of the respiratory tract. There are three stages of the disease: (1) the highly contagious catarrhal stage, when the child seems to have a common cold; (2) the paroxysmal stage, when the cough becomes violent, ending in a high-pitched inspiratory whoop, often followed by vomiting of thick mucus; and (3) a convalescent period, when the cough gradually decreases.

ETIOLOGY

The pertussis bacillus *Bordetella pertussis* reproduces in the respiratory tract, where it releases a toxin that leads to **necrosis** of the mucosa with a thick exudate. It is transmitted by droplet nuclei spread and direct or indirect contact with nasopharyngeal secretions of the contagious patient.

DIAGNOSIS

Bacterial studies of nasopharyngeal mucus are positive for the pertussis bacillus. The patient's WBC count usually is increased.

TREATMENT

Erythromycin is the antibiotic of choice for treatment. Intake of fluids is encouraged to prevent dehydration. A nutritious diet is important to prevent weight loss. Quiet and rest are required because the episodes of prolonged coughing cause exhaustion and weakness. The patient should be observed closely for respiratory distress. Bronchopneumonia, convulsions, or hemorrhages are possible complications of severe disease. If untreated, pertussis can be fatal. Pertussis is preventable by immunization with the pertussis vaccine.

MEASLES (RUBEOLA)

SYMPTOMS AND SIGNS

Measles is an acute, highly contagious viral disease occurring in children who have not been vaccinated. Early symptoms include cold-like

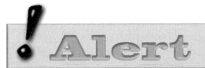

SUBACUTE SCLEROSING PANENCEPHALITIS

Parents are encouraged to have their children immunized against measles.

Subacute sclerosing panencephalitis (SSPE), an infectious condition of the CNS, is considered a rare disorder and, as such, is listed in the National Organization for Rare Disorders, Inc (NORD). SSPE, one of three forms of encephalitis occurring secondary to measles virus, evolves after the reactivation of the dormant measles virus. Symptoms of this progressive neurologic disorder emerge with an insidious onset and are identified by progressive motor and mental or intellectual deterioration, including personality changes and neurologic deterioration subsequently resulting in severe dementia. Seizures, blindness, and fever are additional symptoms. Motor involvement leads to periodic involuntary movements and eventual decerebrate rigidity. The patient usually is 5 to 20 years of age and has experienced an attack of measles in the prior 2 to 10 years. Occasionally, the onset of this inappropriate immune response may follow measles immunization.

The reactivation of the latent measles virus causes a cerebral infection. This infectious process causes atrophy of the cortical areas of the brain, demyelination of the nerves, or ventricular dilation. There is a diffuse inflammation of the brain tissue.

Diagnosis is made from symptoms and history of previous occurrence of measles or recent measles immunization. CSF shows elevated gamma globulin levels. The antibody titer is elevated to measles.

There is no effective therapy or cure for SSPE. Treatment includes supportive measures including drug therapy for seizure control. Duration of this disorder is several years, with progressive deterioration of the CNS. The patient usually is nonresponsive and unable to care for him- or herself for a period of time before death intervenes.

The mother of a young English singer who was afflicted by this rare disorder at the age of 18 years urges all parents to have their children immunized against measles, hopefully preventing the condition that left her daughter blind and unable to speak. The daughter died 14 years after the onset of SSPE.

symptoms, tracheobronchitis, conjunctivitis, and photophobia. The child has a fever, which is followed in 3 to 7 days by a red blotchy rash. The rash starts behind the ears, hairline, and forehead and then progresses down the body. Before the eruption of the rash, Koplik's spots can be detected on the oral mucosa as tiny white spots on a red background.

ETIOLOGY

The causative agent of measles is the measles virus. The infection is airborne, spread by direct contact with secretions from the nose or throat. The patient is contagious from about 4 days before the onset of the rash until about 4 days after the onset. The incubation period is 8 to 12 days after exposure.

DIAGNOSIS

Diagnosis is based on a history of exposure and the clinical picture, which includes the presence of Koplik's spots on the oral mucosa and the rash.

TREATMENT

Uncomplicated measles runs its course in 7 to 10 days. Acetaminophen is given to treat the fever. If the fever is persistently high, tepid sponge baths may be given. Protection of the eyes from bright light is a comfort measure. If secondary infection occurs, antibiotics are prescribed to treat the infection. Pneumonia, otitis media, conjunctivitis, and encephalitis are complications of measles.

Inoculation with the live measles vaccine is given during childhood to protect the individual and prevent epidemics of the disease. Measles immune globulin given 5 days after exposure to the disease affords passive immunity for high-risk unimmunized individuals. An attack of the disease usually affords immunity for life.

Enrichment

CONGENITAL RUBELLA SYNDROME

Women of childbearing age who have not been immunized against rubella or who have not had the disease can transmit rubella to their infant if they become infected during pregnancy. When the virus is transferred to the fetus during the first trimester of pregnancy, a variety of congenital deformities, known as congenital rubella syndrome, occur in approximately 25% of births. The risk is less if infection transpires later in pregnancy. Anomalies caused by congenital rubella syndrome include congenital cardiac disease, blindness, deafness, and mental retardation.

It is recommended that pregnant women be isolated from persons infected with rubella to prevent perinatal infection; pregnant women must not be given the rubella vaccine. The best protection against congenital rubella syndrome is routine immunization of all persons with live rubella vaccine during infancy or as soon as possible in adulthood (Fig. 2–19).

Rubella causes great danger to the unborn children of pregnant women who contract the disease.

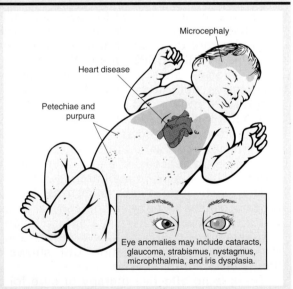

Figure 2–19

Congenital rubella syndrome. (From Damjanov I: Pathology for the Health-Related Professions. Philadelphia: WB Saunders, 1996.)

RUBELLA (GERMAN MEASLES, THREE-DAY MEASLES)

SYMPTOMS AND SIGNS

Rubella resembles measles clinically, but it has a shorter course and fewer complications. In this viral disease, the child has a rose-colored, slightly elevated rash, which appears first on the face and head and then progresses downward on the body. Additionally, there is a low-grade fever, and there can be tenderness and enlargement of the lymph nodes. Complications include a transient arthritis, myocarditis, and hemorrhagic manifestations.

Rubella causes great danger to the unborn children of pregnant women who contract the disease.

ETIOLOGY

The causative agent is the rubella virus, which is spread by direct contact with nasal or oral secretions. The patient is contagious from 1 week before eruption of the rash until 1 week after the onset of rash. The incubation period after exposure is 14 to 21 days. Although preventable with immunization, sporadic epidemic occurrences of rubella still arise.

DIAGNOSIS

Diagnosis is made from a history of exposure and the clinical picture, including the rash. Because rubella resembles other diseases, a definitive diagnosis includes throat culture for the rubella virus and serologic studies to detect antibodies.

TREATMENT

Treatment consists of supportive measures, including the administration of a mild analgesic for fever and joint pain. The patient is isolated until the rash disappears. Active immunity with rubella vaccine in a patient older than 12 months of age prevents the disease.

TETANUS

SYMPTOMS AND SIGNS

Tetanus is an acute, potentially deadly, systemic infection characterized by painful involuntary contraction of skeletal muscles. The patient is extremely febrile, is irritable, and sweats profusely. He or she has a stiff neck, a tight jaw (lockjaw), spasms of the facial muscles, and difficulty with swallowing. As the infection progresses, the muscles of the back and abdomen become rigid, with generalized convulsive muscle spasm (opisthotonos). These tonic spasms may cause death from asphyxiation.

ETIOLOGY

The bacillus *Clostridium tetani* is found in contaminated soil or animal excreta and enters the skin through a puncture wound, laceration, abrasion, burn, or other injury. Puncture wounds are excellent breeding grounds for the bacillus because they do not have a good oxygen supply and the bacillus thrives in dead tissue, producing a powerful exotoxin that attacks the nervous system. The incubation period is 3 to 21 days, with the onset commonly occurring at about 8 days. Tetanus antitoxin immunizations followed by booster doses every 10 years afford immunity.

DIAGNOSIS

The patient's history may indicate inadequate immunization. The patient is fiercely ill as described previously. Laboratory test results do not always provide conclusive data for diagnosis.

TREATMENT

The medical management is chiefly supportive, with the administration of sedatives and muscle relaxants to relieve spasms and seizures; a quiet, dark environment promotes rest. If convulsions occur, respiratory integrity must be preserved. The unimmunized patient is given human tetanus immune globulin (TIG) within 72 hours of injury for temporary immunity. A booster injection of tetanus toxoid is needed if the injured person has not had tetanus immunization within 5 years. Tetanus carries a 35% mortality rate, so prevention is important. The best course is childhood immunizations, with timely booster doses, and prompt cleaning of wounds with hydrogen peroxide.

INFLUENZA

Influenza is an acute, highly contagious viral infection of the respiratory tract. Its highest incidence is in school children, and it is more severe in young children. Influenza occurs sporadically or as an epidemic and is transmitted by droplet nuclei or direct contact with moist secretions. Children tend to have high fevers with influenza and are susceptible to pulmonary complications and Reye's syndrome. Because of the latter, acetaminophen, and *not* aspirin, is given to children and adolescents for fever and pain. A full description of influenza can be found in Chapter 9.

COMMON COLD

Young children have several colds a year, and most colds are self-limiting and run their course in 4 to 5 days. In infants, the nasal congestion can cause difficulty with eating and breathing. Supportive treatment consists of rest, increased fluid intake, and diet as tolerated. The possibility of secondary bacterial infection or extension of the infection into the lower respiratory tract or into the middle ear is potentially dangerous for the child. These complications warrant antibiotic therapy. For a complete discussion of the common cold, see Chapter 9.

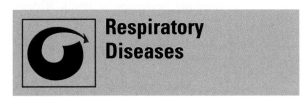

Respiratory Diseases

SUDDEN INFANT DEATH SYNDROME

SYMPTOMS AND SIGNS

Known causes and contributing factors for the sudden death of an infant are ruled out. These may include an immature respiratory control system, the susceptibility to deadly arrhythmias, congenital heart disease, or myocarditis.

Sudden infant death syndrome (SIDS), formerly called crib death, is defined officially as the sudden death of an infant under the age of 1 year for which a cause cannot be established. It is the number one cause of death among infants from 1 to 12 months of age; 1 in 500 infants dies mysteriously during the first year of life. Death occurs within seconds during sleep and without sound or struggle, and the baby does not suffer. Most SIDS infants appeared healthy before death. When found, the dead infant may have a mottled complexion and cyanotic lips and fingertips. There is often a trace of blood-tinged fluid coming from the mouth or the nose.

ETIOLOGY

Although there are many theories and much misinformation about SIDS, the exact cause is uncertain. Research studies and autopsies point to certain pathologic findings in some SIDS infants that lead to the suspicion of more than one

cause. Numerous maternal and infant risk factors are known: mother's age younger than 20 years, poor prenatal care, smoking and drug abuse during pregnancy, prematurity, recent upper respiratory tract infection in the infant, and a sibling with apnea. The incidence is higher in males and during the winter months.

DIAGNOSIS

A complete postmortem investigation, including autopsy, a review of the child's medical history, and examination of the scene of death, fail to identify the cause of death.

TREATMENT

Resuscitation attempts fail. At this time, SIDS is not predictable or preventable. The American Academy of Pediatrics has added sleeping in the prone position to the list of risk factors. To reduce that risk, the recommendation is to put babies to sleep on their sides or their backs instead of on their stomachs. A home apnea machine and cardiac monitor may be recommended during the peak age of vulnerability.

Survivors of SIDS should be offered sensitive interventions to help them to deal with the grief and possible feelings of guilt and anger. The Sudden Infant Death Syndrome Alliance is a national voluntary organization in the United States dedicated to eliminating SIDS through medical research.

Recent studies have isolated risk factors for SIDS. Although these risk factors may play a role in SIDS, parents must understand that by themselves these factors do not cause SIDS.

As previously mentioned, a supine sleeping position carries the lowest risk for SIDS. Exposure to cigarette smoke should be limited. Firm bedding materials in a safety-approved crib are prudent. Research indicates that overheating an infant with too much clothing, especially during illness, is to be avoided. Other important factors include good prenatal care and breast-feeding.

CROUP

SYMPTOMS AND SIGNS

Croup is an acute, severe inflammation and obstruction of the respiratory tract. It usually is preceded by an upper respiratory tract infection. The symptoms include hoarseness, fever, a harsh high-pitched cough, and **stridor** during inspiration caused by narrowing of the upper airways. The child may be anxious and frightened by the respiratory distress.

ETIOLOGY

Croup is usually a viral disease that involves the larynx, trachea, and bronchi. The clinical manifestations are caused by edema and spasm of the vocal cords, creating varying degrees of obstruction.

DIAGNOSIS

Croup must be distinguished from epiglottiditis. If necessary, blood or throat cultures may be done to determine certain bacterial causes. Laryngoscopy may be done.

TREATMENT

The patient is treated symptomatically, with the administration of antipyretic agents, rest, increased fluid intake, cool humidification of air, and antibiotic therapy if the cause is bacterial. In severe cases, hospitalization is necessary for endotracheal intubation and oxygen therapy until the respiratory crisis passes. In most instances, the illness subsides in 3 to 4 days.

EPIGLOTTIDITIS

SYMPTOMS AND SIGNS

Epiglottiditis is an inflammation of the epiglottis, the thin, leaf-shaped structure that covers the entrance of the larynx during swallowing. It typically strikes children between ages 3 and 7 years. The symptoms include a sore throat, croupy cough, fever, and respiratory distress from laryngeal obstruction. Visual inspection reveals a red and swollen epiglottis. Rapidly increasing dyspnea and drooling are the most significant signs of a critical respiratory emergency.

ETIOLOGY

Epiglottiditis may follow an upper respiratory tract infection. The most common cause is *Haemophilus influenzae* type B bacteria.

DIAGNOSIS

Radiographic films of the neck may reveal the enlarged epiglottis. If the obstruction is not significant, a throat examination is done to inspect the epiglottis.

TREATMENT

If the airway is obstructed, the child is hospitalized and given intensive care. The airway is established with tracheostomy or endotracheal intubation. Antibiotics, usually ampicillin, are given parenterally, and the patient is closely monitored. Prompt treatment affords a good prognosis. The American Academy of Pediatrics recommends that all children receive the *Haemophilus* B conjugate vaccine.

ACUTE TONSILLITIS

SYMPTOMS AND SIGNS

Tonsillitis, or inflammation of the tonsils, usually has a sudden onset. The patient has a mild to severe sore throat, chills, fever, headache, malaise, **anorexia,** and muscle and joint pain. The tonsils appear inflamed and swollen, with yellowish exudate projecting from crypts. Lymph glands in the submandibular area are tender and enlarged (Fig. 2–20).

ETIOLOGY

Tonsillitis is caused by many organisms, with group A beta-hemolytic streptococci the most common cause.

DIAGNOSIS

The throat is examined, and a throat culture is done to identify the causative organism. The WBC count may be elevated in response to the infection.

TREATMENT

When the throat culture is positive for streptococci, a full 10-day course of penicillin is given. This strict regimen is necessary to prevent rheumatic fever, rheumatic heart disease, and kidney complications. The child is placed on bed rest, is given a liquid diet, and is given saline throat irrigations. Tonsillectomy may be recommended for chronic tonsillitis or peritonsillar abscess.

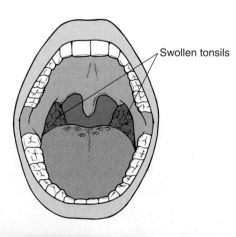
Swollen tonsils

Figure 2–20
Tonsillitis.

ADENOID HYPERPLASIA

SYMPTOMS AND SIGNS

Adenoids (and tonsils) are present at birth and play a role in the formation of immunoglobulins. After puberty, they normally atrophy. Adenoid hyperplasia is an abnormal enlargement of the lymphoid tissue located in the space above the soft palate of the mouth, causing partial breathing blockage, especially in children. Adenoid hyperplasia also can contribute to recurrent otitis media and conductive hearing loss, owing to obstruction of the eustachian tube. The child is usually a mouth breather and snores during sleep. The child's speech has a nasal quality.

ETIOLOGY

The cause of adenoid hyperplasia is unknown. Contributing factors include repeated infection, chronic allergies, and heredity.

DIAGNOSIS

The abnormal enlargement may be visualized on lateral pharyngeal radiographic films or with nasopharyngoscopic examination.

TREATMENT

Adenoidectomy is indicated for obstructive adenoids with recurrent otitis media or chronic serous otitis media with conductive hearing loss.

ASTHMA

SYMPTOMS AND SIGNS

Asthma is a chronic disease caused by increased reactivity of the tracheobronchial tree to various stimuli. It is a leading cause of chronic illness and school absenteeism in children. The child presents with an incessant productive or nonproductive cough, a pronounced expiratory wheeze, and rapid shallow respirations. The la-

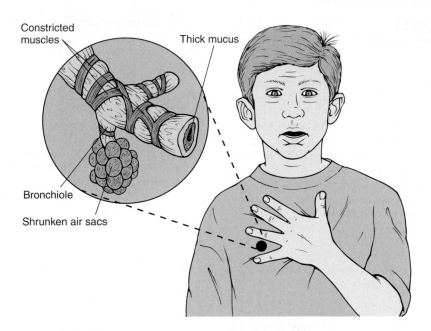

Constricted muscles

Thick mucus

Bronchiole

Shrunken air sacs

Symptoms
• Shortness of breath
• Wheezing
• Difficult breathing
• Cough
• Anxiety

Physical findings
• Rapid, shallow respirations
• Rapid pulse
• Pallor or cyanosis
• Diminished breath sounds
• Generalized retractions
• Frequent pausing to catch the breath when talking
• Hyperexpansion of the chest

Figure 2–21

An asthma attack with respiratory distress.

bored breathing results in a rapid pulse, pallor, profuse perspiration, and an inability to speak more than a few words without halting for "more air." The patient is frequently anxious, is exhausted, and reports a "tight chest." The examining physician hears diminished breath sounds with wheezes and rhonchi in the lungs. The bronchial spasms trap air and thick mucus in the lungs. An asthmatic episode (Fig. 2–21) can be mild to severe, can last minutes or days; and may become a medical emergency. The attack may or may not have been preceded by a respiratory infection.

ETIOLOGY

There is a strong hereditary factor associated with the disease. Asthma is the result of "twitchy," or hyperactive and hypersensitive, bronchial tubes. The bronchial spasms of asthma can be triggered by many extrinsic (allergic) or intrinsic (nonallergic) factors, including stress, heavy exercise, infection, and inhalation of allergens or other substances.

DIAGNOSIS

The best tool available to reveal the degree of airway obstruction is the pulmonary function test. However, it is possible for this test to be normal between attacks. Radiographic chest films may show hyperinflation and changes in the lungs associated with mucous plugging. Specialists may order intradermal skin testing to identify inhalant and food allergies. Blood tests include a CBC with differential leukocyte count, which may show an increased eosinophil count and elevated serum immunoglobulin E (IgE) levels.

TREATMENT

Many persons with chronic asthma require medical management under the care of an expert. Strict compliance with a regimen of medications to relax and widen the bronchi and to release excessive mucus is important. Some of the drugs used are cromolyn sodium, albuterol, theophylline, and aerosol corticosteroids. Results from allergy evaluation and skin testing may indicate immunotherapy by desensitization injections, commonly called allergy shots. Avoidance of infection and known allergens and other triggers is strongly advised.

Severe acute asthma attacks are treated with injections of epinephrine and inhalation therapy. When a severe attack is unresponsive to drug therapy, a condition called status asthmaticus may lead to fatal respiratory failure. The patient requires hospitalization for aggressive medical treatment and follow-up.

Gastrointestinal Disorders

INFANTILE COLIC

SYMPTOMS AND SIGNS

Colic is intermittent abdominal distress in the newborn or during early infancy. The infant intermittently draws up the legs, clenches the fists, and cries as if in pain. During the episode, the infant may pass gas by mouth and rectum. The episodes of colic are likely to occur in the late afternoon and evening. These babies usually thrive, gain weight, and appear to tolerate the formula or mother's milk.

ETIOLOGY

The etiology of colic is unknown, although several theories have been advanced. One hypothesis suggests that improper feeding techniques may be responsible, whereas another theory blames overeating or the swallowing of excessive air. Sensitivity to cow's milk may be the causative factor, even for the nursing infant. In this case, it is suggested that the nursing mother eliminate cow's milk from her diet. Another sensitivity may be to iron, necessitating the elimination of supplemental iron from either the infant's formula or the lactating mother's diet. Whatever the cause, the infant is extremely uncomfortable and cries a great deal, with sleep pattern disturbance.

DIAGNOSIS

Diagnosis is made by the symptoms and a physical examination to rule out other causes of the apparent abdominal spasms.

TREATMENT

Investigation into possible causes is the first step in treatment. Eliminating any of the possible causative factors may help to lessen the symptoms. Characteristically, the infant outgrows the condition at about 3 months of age. Occasionally, in severe cases, an anticholinergic or antispasmodic drug may be given.

HELMINTH (WORM) INFESTATION

SYMPTOMS AND SIGNS

Worm infestations in children occur as they introduce eggs into their mouths from contaminated hands. After pinworm (*Enterobius vermicularis*) eggs are swallowed, they hatch in the intestine. The female worms migrate to the perianal area at night, where they lay their eggs. This process causes mild to intense itching and irritation in the area. The itching and scratching contaminates the fingers with the eggs and allows reingestion by the host.

ETIOLOGY

E. vermicularis (pinworm) is one of many possible parasitic worms. It is the most common cause of helminth infestation in the United States, and most patients are preschool or school-aged children and the mothers of infected children. Pinworms are transmitted directly or indirectly from human to human (Fig. 2–22).

DIAGNOSIS

The diagnosis is made by detection of eggs or worms in the anal opening by transparent adhesive tape placed in the perianal area. A stool specimen examined microscopically may be positive.

TREATMENT

A complete course of anthelmintic agents is given; some physicians treat the entire family. Frequent showering and hand washing are advised. The worms and eggs also can be destroyed by the process of laundering clothing and linens.

DIARRHEA

SYMPTOMS AND SIGNS

Diarrhea is rapid passage of stool through the intestinal tract, with a noticeable change in the frequency, fluid content, appearance, and consistency. Diarrhea may be mild or severe, acute or chronic. In the infant or child, diarrhea rapidly can cause dehydration and electrolyte imbalance when fluid loss is profuse. Severe or prolonged diarrhea can produce metabolic **acidosis;** the patient may be lethargic and may hyperventilate. Depending on the cause, the symptoms could include intestinal cramping, weakness, nausea, irritability, and fever. Stool passage may become painful from excoriation of the anus or skin in the diaper area.

ETIOLOGY

Diarrhea has multiple causes: infection (viral, bacterial, or parasitic), medications, allergic reactions, emotions, anatomic abnormalities, malabsorption syndromes, mechanical or chemical irritation from diet, and toxicity. The cause may be unknown.

DIAGNOSIS

The clinician attempts to determine the degree of diarrheal disease, the underlying cause, and the fluid and electrolyte status of the patient. This requires a specific history of the onset and severity of symptoms, laboratory blood testing, stool cultures, and analysis of the stools.

TREATMENT

The treatment of diarrhea is directed at the cause, if known. Blood components are monitored for fluid and electrolyte balances. The frequency, color, consistency, and general composition of the stool is observed. Oral intake may be restricted to rest the intestinal tract and to reduce intestinal irritability. When infection is the cause, appropriate antibiotics may be given. It is dangerous to ignore prolonged diarrhea in the infant or small child. The patient may require hospitalization for IV fluid and electrolyte therapy.

VOMITING

SYMPTOMS AND SIGNS

Vomiting, or ejection through the mouth of stomach contents, is a common symptom in infants and children. When chronic or severe, it deserves special attention as a warning sign of disease or possible dehydration. Vomiting can range from a mild regurgitation to projectile expulsion. The infant has a distended abdomen, is irritable, and has a fever. Aspiration of vomitus into the lungs can result in pneumonia.

ETIOLOGY

Vomiting, which is more common in infants than in children, usually results from trivial or temporary factors. However, it has a host of possible causes: overfeeding, food allergy, gastric irritation, infection, drug poisoning, intracranial pressure, genetic defects such as pyloric stenosis, and habitual voluntary vomiting.

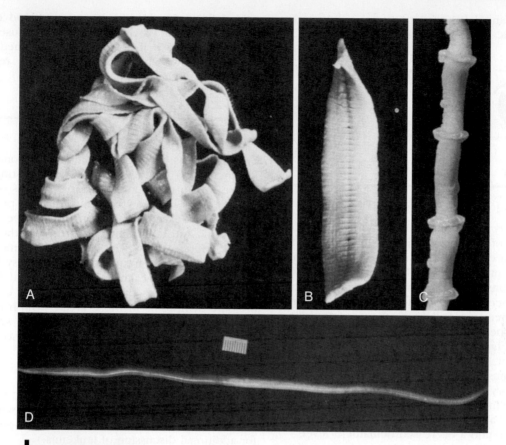

Figure 2-22

Intestinal worms. *A,* Tapeworms. Part of the tapeworm *Diphyllobothrium latum.* The total length of the worm is greater than 30 feet. The head is about 1 mm in diameter, and the immature segments (proglottides) are much smaller than are the segments shown (x 1.5). *B,* Part of the worm shown in *A.* It is made up of many segments, each of which is wider than it is long. *C,* Part of the tapeworm *Taenia saginata.* Each segment is longer than it is wide. *D, Ascaris lumbricoides.* This worm is the largest roundworm parasite of humans and superficially resembles an earthworm (from the Latin *lumbricus,* an "earthworm"). It ranges in length from 15 to 35 cm. The specimen was approximately 20 cm (8 inches) in length. Other common roundworms are considerably smaller: *Trichuris trichiura,* 3 to 5 cm; *Enterobius vermicularis,* 8 to 13 mm; and *Ancylostoma duodenale,* up to 1 cm. (The scale above the roundworm shown is 1 cm.) (From Walter JB; An Introduction to the Principles of Disease, 3rd ed. Philadelphia: WB Saunders, 1992.)

DIAGNOSIS

Vomiting in the infant or child always must be evaluated in the context of the child's total state of health. Causative factors are assessed by performing a physical examination, taking the history, and monitoring the patient's vital signs, weight, nutritional status, and fluid and electrolyte balance. Radiographic studies of the intestinal tract may be indicated.

TREATMENT

Most vomiting can be expected to abate spontaneously. Food may be withheld for a time to rest the upper GI tract and to decrease gastric irritation. When treatment is indicated, it depends on the cause and the severity and nature of the vomiting. Infant feeding problems require changes in technique or intake. Other more serious causes, such as infection, poisoning, and congenital anomalies of the GI tract, may require direct medical or surgical intervention.

Blood Disorders

ANEMIA

SYMPTOMS AND SIGNS

Anemia is an abnormal reduction of the concentration of red blood cells (RBCs) or of the hemoglobin content of circulating blood; it is not a disease, but a symptom of various diseases. The manifestations of anemia are the result of tissue hypoxia. (See Chapter 10 for additional information on anemias.) Pallor, weakness, fatigability, and listlessness are noted initially in the anemic child or infant. Palpitation, tachycardia, cardiac enlargement, jaundice, and mental sluggishness are symptoms of severe anemia.

Laboratory signs indicating anemia vary with the underlying cause or type of anemia and are reflected in abnormal hemoglobin concentrations in the blood and a decreased hematocrit level.

ETIOLOGY

Iron deficiency is the most common cause of anemia in children. Other causes include acute or chronic blood loss, decreased blood formation, nutritional deficiency disorders, hemolytic diseases, inhibition or loss of bone marrow, and sickle-cell disease.

DIAGNOSIS

Diagnosis is based on physical examination and laboratory testing for signs and symptoms of anemia. Diagnostic tests include determination of hemoglobin concentration, hematocrit levels, serum iron levels, RBC count, and mean corpuscular hemoglobin levels and bone marrow studies. The appearance of abnormal RBCs may be seen microscopically.

TREATMENT

The first priority of treatment is to determine the cause of anemia. For iron deficiency anemia, iron-rich foods and oral preparations of ferrous iron are administered. When blood loss is the cause, blood volume is restored by transfusion. Replacement therapy is indicated in deficiency states (e.g., vitamin B_{12}, folic acid, and ascorbic acid deficiency). Specific hemolytic blood disorders are treated when the anemia is caused by excessive blood cell destruction. A planned program of activity balanced with rest is recommended during treatment.

LEUKEMIA

SYMPTOMS AND SIGNS

Leukemia is the most common childhood malignancy. It is characterized by an abnormal increase in the number of immature WBCs or undifferentiated blastocytes. Leukemia, a primary malignant disease of bone marrow, can be acute or chronic and is classified according to the type and aberration of WBCs. Acute symptoms may begin with a fever, frequent infection, easy bruising, pallor, and weakness. The abnormal blood cells invade various organs of the body, causing pressure symptoms in those areas. Lymph nodes and the spleen may be enlarged. Night sweats, weight loss, and anemia result as the disease progresses.

ETIOLOGY

The cause is unknown. Predisposing factors include congenital disorders such as Down syndrome, radiation, and viruses. (See Chapter 10 for additional discussion of leukemia.)

DIAGNOSIS

Diagnostic studies and findings vary with the type of leukemia. Immature WBC forms are found in the circulating WBCs. The diagnosis is confirmed by microscopic examination of the bone marrow.

TREATMENT

The disease is treatable with systemic chemotherapy to eradicate leukemic cells and to induce remission. Bone marrow transplantation is possible. Transfusions of blood components and antibiotic therapy may be employed. Psychological support for the child and the family must be provided.

ERYTHROBLASTOSIS FETALIS (HEMOLYTIC DISEASE OF THE NEWBORN)

SYMPTOMS AND SIGNS

Erythroblastosis fetalis stems from an incompatibility of fetal and maternal blood, resulting in excessive rates of RBC destruction. It is characterized by anemia, jaundice, **kernicterus,** and enlargement of the liver and spleen. In the most severe form, called hydrops fetalis, the fetus or infant is in great jeopardy because of extreme **hemolysis.** If the infant survives, the condition is marked by heart failure, edema, pulmonary congestion, lethargy, seizures, and mental retardation.

ETIOLOGY

The cause is Rh factor incompatibility. Rh factor is the antigen found on RBCs of the Rh-positive individual. The mother, through prior pregnancy, has become sensitized to the Rh factor (Rh isoimmunization) of the fetal RBCs. When sensitized maternal blood finds its way into fetal circulation, particularly during delivery, the antibodies in the mother's blood destroy the RBCs of the fetus (Fig. 2–23).

If an Rh-negative woman has children with an Rh-positive man, some or all of the infants will be Rh positive. During pregnancy, blood from the Rh-positive fetus may move from fetal circulation into the mother's bloodstream, where it can stimulate the mother's body to form antibodies against the Rh factor. When sufficient quantities of the antibodies pass back into the infant's circulation, the antibodies are capable of clumping and destroying Rh-positive cells, causing the symptoms of erythroblastosis fetalis.

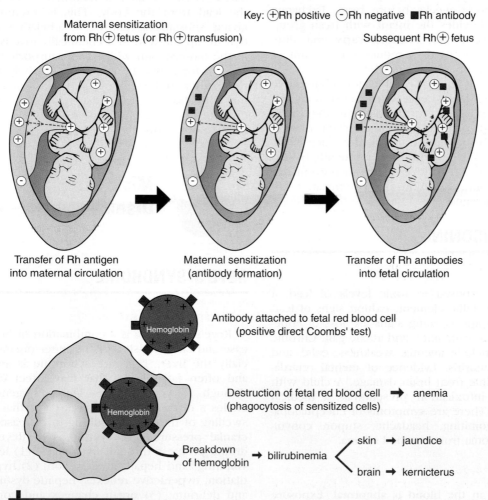

Key: (+)Rh positive (−)Rh negative ■Rh antibody

Maternal sensitization
from Rh(+) fetus (or Rh(+) transfusion)

Subsequent Rh(+) fetus

Transfer of Rh antigen
into maternal circulation

Maternal sensitization
(antibody formation)

Transfer of Rh antibodies
into fetal circulation

Antibody attached to fetal red blood cell
(positive direct Coombs' test)

Destruction of fetal red blood cell ➡ anemia
(phagocytosis of sensitized cells)

Breakdown
of hemoglobin ➡ bilirubinemia 〈 skin ➡ jaundice
                                    brain ➡ kernicterus

Figure 2–23

Etiology of erythroblastosis fetalis (hemolytic disease of the newborn). (Redrawn with permission of Ross Products Division, Abbott Laboratories, from *Congenital Heart Abnormalities* [Clinical Education Aid no. 7], 1992.)

DIAGNOSIS

Blood typing of mother and father is essential. The maternal history includes pregnancy, elective and spontaneous abortions, and blood transfusions. A direct Coombs' test of umbilical cord blood measures Rh-positive antibodies in the newborn; a bilirubin test for **bilirubinemia** and hematocrit determination also are done on the infant's blood. Amnionic fluid analysis for hemolysis may be performed.

TREATMENT

The treatment is dictated by the degree of erythroblastosis fetalis and its effect on the fetus or newborn. Intrauterine transfusions may be indicated when the fetus shows signs of distress. When necessary, the delivery of the infant is planned 2 to 4 weeks before term. Exchange transfusion provides the infant with fresh group O Rh-negative blood. **Phototherapy** and albumin infusion are used to reduce the amount of circulating bilirubin in the newborn.

Protection is now available for Rh-negative mothers who have never been sensitized, preventing the possibility of harm to an Rh-positive baby. $Rh_O(D)$ immune globulin is given as soon as possible to the woman at risk after each exposure to Rh-positive blood (most frequently by giving birth to an Rh-positive infant) to prevent maternal Rh isoimmunization and complications in subsequent pregnancies.

LEAD POISONING

SYMPTOMS AND SIGNS

Children exposed to toxic levels of lead, a poisonous metallic element, exhibit signs of lead poisoning. Some warning signs are loss of appetite, vomiting, irritability, and ataxic gait. Chronic symptoms include anemia, weakness, colic, and peripheral neuritis. Evidence of mental retardation is possible from brain damage. A child with acute lead intoxication presents as a medical emergency. There are symptoms of encephalopathy with vomiting, headache, stupor, convulsions, and coma from cerebral edema.

ETIOLOGY

Any lead in the blood is abnormal. Exposure results from breathing or swallowing substances containing lead. The condition has developed in children who eat flakes of peeling lead paint, drink water from lead pipes, or ingest lead salts in certain foods. Lead taken into the body is stored in many tissues; it is released into the blood and excreted in the urine.

DIAGNOSIS

The diagnosis is suspected from the history of lead exposure and the presence of symptoms previously listed. Blood tests reveal anemia and a blood lead level greater than 5 μg/dl. There is increased excretion of lead in the urine. Characteristic changes in the ends of growing bones are noted on radiographic films.

TREATMENT

The source of poisoning first must be eliminated. Then the goal of treatment is to remove the lead from the body. This is attempted by giving substances, known as chelating agents, that tie up the lead in a chemically inactive form in the bloodstream while it is transported to the kidneys for elimination. Antiemetics help to control nausea and vomiting, and sedation is given for convulsions. After acute therapy, penicillamine (a chelating agent for lead) is given orally for 3 to 6 months.

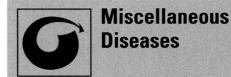

Miscellaneous Diseases

REYE'S SYNDROME

SYMPTOMS AND SIGNS

Reye's syndrome is a combination of brain disease and fatty invasion of the inner organs, especially the liver. This rare syndrome is an acute and often fatal illness that may affect children through 15 years of age. The pathogenesis includes a disruption in the urea cycle that causes swelling of the brain, resulting in increased intracranial pressure. The symptoms of Reye's syndrome progress through five stages: (1) lethargy, vomiting, and hepatic dysfunction; (2) hyperventilation, hyperactive reflexes, hepatic dysfunction, and delirium; (3) organ changes and coma; (4) deeper coma and loss of cerebral functions; and (5) seizures, loss of deep tendon reflexes, and respiratory arrest.

ETIOLOGY

The cause of Reye's syndrome is unknown. However, it typically follows infection with influenza A or B viruses or chickenpox. It has been linked to the use of aspirin during these infections.

DIAGNOSIS

The medical history and the patient's clinical features suggest the disease. Laboratory blood studies show elevated serum ammonia levels. Liver function tests show elevated enzyme levels. Other tests include liver biopsy and CSF analysis.

TREATMENT

The early recognition and treatment of Reye's syndrome has cut the mortality rate from 90% to 20%. Hospitalization is required to stabilize the patient, to control cerebral edema, to monitor blood chemistries, to manage seizures, and to provide mechanical ventilation if needed. Recovery can be complete. For prevention, the use of nonsalicylate analgesics and antipyretics, such as acetaminophen, is recommended instead of aspirin.

FETAL ALCOHOL SYNDROME

SYMPTOMS AND SIGNS

Fetal alcohol syndrome (FAS) refers to birth defects and other associated problems in infants born to alcoholic mothers who consume alcohol during the gestational period. Intrauterine exposure to sufficient levels of alcohol has been associated with fetal growth retardation; the infants are short and below average in weight. Facial characteristics include smaller eye openings with eyes spaced widely apart and a thin upper lip. FAS also is associated with mental retardation. The infant may exhibit signs of alcohol withdrawal shortly after birth.

ETIOLOGY

FAS is caused when alcohol enters the fetal blood as a result of chronic, excessive use of alcohol during gestation.

DIAGNOSIS

Typical clinical features present in the newborn, and a maternal history of chronic alcoholism determine the diagnosis (Fig. 2-24).

TREATMENT

The treatment depends on the defects in the newborn. Much of the treatment is supportive because neurologic damage cannot be reversed. Proper nutrition is vital. Because the baby may have poor sucking reflex, special adaptation may be necessary to ensure proper intake. The psychosocial needs of the infant and the mother must be addressed. Preventive measures include prenatal care and education. Because experts do not agree on a safe minimal amount of alcohol intake during pregnancy, women generally are advised not to drink during gestation.

DIAPER RASH

SYMPTOMS AND SIGNS

Diaper rash, considered a contact dermatitis, is evident in the diaper area as an irritation or rash. It can vary from mild to severe and can be self-limiting or a chronic source of discomfort to the infant and dismay to the parent or caretaker. Diaper rash takes multiple forms from a mild excoriation, or **maculopapular** rash, to blisters and ulceration.

ETIOLOGY

Infants with sensitive skin seem to have a hereditary predisposition to irritant dermatitis, or diaper rash. Diaper rash may be triggered by friction or prolonged exposure to moisture, feces, or the ammonia produced by bacterial action on urine. Poorly washed or rinsed diapers or the use of occlusive plastic pants over the diapers may contribute. Poor hygiene or overzealous cleaning could irritate the diaper area.

DIAGNOSIS

Diaper rash may need to be differentiated from seborrheic dermatitis, eczema, and secondary skin infection.

TREATMENT

In addition to frequent diaper changing and proper cleaning and drying of the diaper area, a bland protective agent such as zinc oxide or topical hydrocortisone may promote healing. Careful application of dry heat, as directed by the physician, may improve the condition. Topical antimicrobial agents are used for secondary skin infection. Cloth diapers should be rinsed of irritating residue.

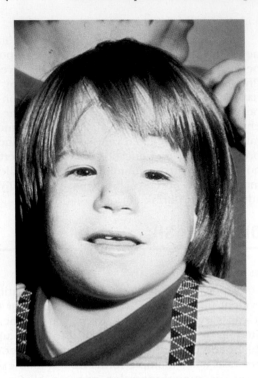

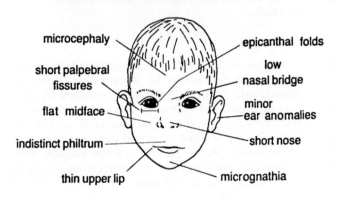

microcephaly

short palpebral fissures

flat midface

indistinct philtrum

thin upper lip

epicanthal folds

low nasal bridge

minor ear anomalies

short nose

micrognathia

Figure 2–24

Fetal alcohol syndrome (FAS). Affected children have typical features that, when accompanied by mental retardation, are diagnostic of FAS. The features on the left are those most frequently seen in patients with FAS, whereas those on the right are features that are seen with increased frequency in this population compared with the general population. (From Jones KL, Smith DW, Ulleland CN, et al: Pattern of malformation in offspring of chronic alcoholic mothers. Lancet 1:1267, 1973.)

Summary

- Some pathologic conditions in children are caused by congenital diseases that are present at birth or are detected later. The cause may not be known or may be genetic, nongenetic, or a combination of both.
- Advancements in technology are making possible the survival of more very low birth weight and early gestational infants.

- Prematurity can evolve from numerous causes, resulting in associated disorders.
- Certain congenital diseases affecting the nervous system can be the result of trauma, as in cerebral palsy, or the result of a genetic defect, as in muscular dystrophy.
- Neural tube defects include spina bifida, meningocele and myelomeningocele; they can result

in neurologic impairment or damage. Surgical repair frequently is indicated.

- Down syndrome is a common chromosomal disorder that affects many areas of the body. The condition is usually apparent at birth because of certain distinct characteristics and entails mild to severe mental retardation.
- Congenital heart diseases are defects involving the heart or the large vessels. The signs and symptoms may be evident at birth or appear during infancy or childhood. Examples are ventricular septal defect, which allows shunting of blood from the left to the right side of the heart, and tetralogy of Fallot, which is a combination of four congenital defects.
- Congenital diseases of the musculoskeletal system described in this chapter are deformities usually detected at birth and can be treated with corrective devices or surgery.
- Wilms' tumor, a highly malignant tumor of the kidney in young children, requires early intervention with surgery, radiation, and chemotherapy.
- Congenital diseases of the digestive system may involve obstructive anomalies that require surgery.
- Cystic fibrosis and phenylketonuria (PKU) are

congenital disorders that pose serious threats to life and health. All newborns are screened for PKU.

- Klinefelter's syndrome and Turner's syndrome are chromosomal disorders that affect males and females respectively; both conditions respond favorably to hormone therapy.
- Many serious childhood infections are preventable with routine prophylactic immunization.
- Sudden infant death syndrome (SIDS) is not predictable or preventable because the cause remains uncertain. The American Academy of Pediatrics recommends putting babies on their sides or backs for sleeping (instead of their stomachs) to reduce the risk of SIDS.
- Asthma requires strict medical management to control symptoms and reduce the need for hospitalization.
- Anemic blood disorders are treated with replacement therapy. Leukemia requires cancer therapy.
- Reye's syndrome, a rare but life-threatening disease, requires early recognition and treatment.
- Prenatal care and education about the use of alcohol during pregnancy can prevent fetal alcohol syndrome.

Review Challenge

REVIEW QUESTIONS

1. List the possible causes of congenital anomalies.
2. What is the purpose of amniocentesis? Describe the procedure.
3. Trace fetal circulation.
4. Describe the condition of prematurity and list its causes. List the associated disorders, identifying their causes, and discuss the treatment options.
5. Explain the differences between muscular dystrophy and cerebral palsy.
6. Describe patent ductus arteriosus and its treatment.
7. Name and describe the most common congenital cyanotic cardiac defect.
8. List the major clinical manifestations of cystic fibrosis.

9. Explain the differences between Klinefelter's syndrome and Turner's syndrome.
10. Describe the clinical condition of congenital rubella syndrome.
11. Discuss the incidence, etiology, and treatment of asthma.
12. List the symptoms and signs of anemia; describe the pathology of leukemia.
13. Explain the etiology of erythroblastosis fetalis.
14. Name some warning signs of lead poisoning.
15. Describe the infant born with fetal alcohol syndrome.
16. Discuss the importance of childhood immunizations and list the schedule for the first year of life.

REAL-LIFE CHALLENGE

Asthma

A 6-year-old male presents coughing with audible expiratory wheezes and dyspnea. The child is pale, skin is moist and cool, and he has difficulty speaking more than a few words before stopping to catch his breath. Parents state that the difficult breathing had a rapid onset approximately 1 hour earlier when he was playing with the neighbor's dog. The child has a history of previous asthma attacks, primarily after visiting his aunts' homes, where there are cats.

Assessment of the child shows T 98.6, P 120, R 40 and labored. Bilateral rales are heard on auscultation, louder on expiration but also present on inspiration. Cromolyn sodium had been prescribed prophylactically before visits to aunts' homes. Child also has an Alupent inhaler to be used PRN. The use of the inhaler brought no relief.

Questions

1. Which diagnostic procedures would be ordered to reveal the degree of airway obstruction?
2. Explain patient teaching involved with cromolyn sodium usage.
3. What changes in vital signs would be expected with the use of an Alupent inhaler?
4. Which immediate intervention may be ordered to relieve symptoms and provide comfort to the child?
5. What future testing may be ordered?
6. What is the cause of the dyspnea?
7. List allergens commonly responsible for asthma attacks.
8. Explain why asthma attacks are considered as medical emergencies and what steps should be taken on arrival of a patient in the midst of an asthma attack.

REAL-LIFE CHALLENGE

Patent Ductus Arteriosus

A premature infant weighing 1 pound, 10 ounces, and 1 week old begins exhibiting reduced oxygen saturation levels, bradycardia, and cyanosis. The infant's respirations are being maintained with mechanical ventilation. Increased oxygen concentration is required to maintain oxygen saturation levels at 90%. The chest radiograph reveals IRDS as resolving. The echocardiogram indicates a PDA.

Questions

1. Explain the two treatment options, drug therapy, or a surgical procedure used to close the PDA.
2. Explain the complication that could occur because of high-concentration levels of oxygen.
3. What is the prognosis for the cardiac status of this child once closure has been achieved?
4. Which other congenital cardiac defect may be present?
5. Trace fetal circulation and explain the role of the ductus arteriosus before birth.

RESOURCES

American Sudden Infant Death Syndrome Institute
6065 Roswell Rd, Ste 876
Atlanta, GA 30328
800-232-SIDS
800-847-SIDS in Georgia
(http://www.sids.com)

National SIDS Foundation
1314 Bedford Ave, Ste 210
Baltimore, MD 21208
800-221-SIDS

United Cerebral Palsy Association
Fax 800-872-1827

Cystic Fibrosis Foundation
6931 Arlington Rd
Bethesda, MD 20814-5200
1-800 FIGHT-CF

National Down's Syndrome Congress
16105 Chantilly Dr, Ste 250
Atlanta, GA 30324
800-232-NDSC

National Down's Syndrome Society Hotline
666 Broadway
New York, NY 10012
800-221-4602
For information, enclose SASE: 9×12″ with $1.75 postage
attached

National Easter Seal Society, Inc.
230 W Monroe, Ste 1800
Chicago, IL 60606-4802
800-221-6827
(http://www.seals.com)

American Cleft Palate Association
1829 E Franklin St, Ste 1022
Chapel Hill, NC 27514
800-24-CLEFT

American Association on Mental Retardation
444 N Capital St NW, Ste 846
Washington, DC 20001
800-424-3688

Muscular Dystrophy Association
3300 E Sunrise Dr
Tucson, AZ 85718
800-572-1717

National Reye's Syndrome
426 North Lewis
PO Box 829
Bryan, OH 43506
800-233-7393

Spina Bifida Information and Referral
Spina Bifida Association of America
4590 MacArthur Boulevard NW, Ste 250
Washington, DC 20007-4226
1-800-621-3141

Centers for Disease Control and Prevention
1600 Clifton Rd NE
Atlanta, GA 30333

Hydrocephalus Association
2040 Polk St
San Francisco, CA 94109

March of Dimes–Birth Defects Foundation
1275 Mamaroneck Ave
White Plains, NY 10605

Blind Children's Fund
2875 Northwind Dr, Ste 211
East Lansing, MI 48823-5040
517-333-1725
Fax 517-333-1730

National Organization for Parents of Blind Children
1800 Johnson St
Baltimore, MD 21230
410-659-9314
Fax 410-685-5653

Shriners Hospitals for Children
PO Box 31356
Tampa, FL 33631-3356
1-800-237-5055 USA
1-800-361-7256 Canada
(http://www.shrinershq.org)

American Academy of Allergies, Asthma, and Immunology
611 E Wells St
Milwaukee, WI 53202
800-822-ASMA
(http://www.aaaai.org)

Asthma and Allergy Foundation of America
1125 15th St NW
Washington, DC 20005
800-7-ASTHMA
(http://www.aafa.com)

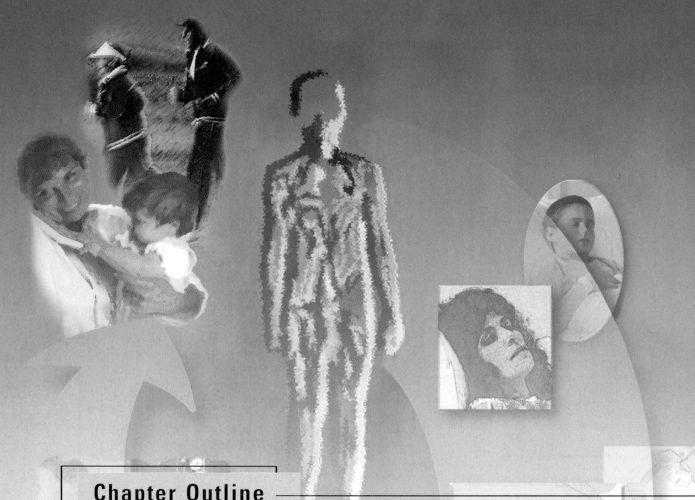

Chapter Outline

Immunologic Diseases and Conditions

Key Terms

anticholinesterase   (**an**–tee–koh–lyn–**ES**–ter–ase)

autoimmune
candidiasis   (**aw**–toh–im–**YOON**)
(**kan**–dih–**DIE**–ah–sis)

collagen	(**KOLL**–ah–jen)
hematopoietic	(**hem**–ah–toh–poy–**ET**–ik)
hypogammaglobulin-emia	(**hye**–poh–**gam**–a–**glob**–you–lyn–**EE**–me–ah)
immunocompetence	(**im**–you–no–**KOM**–peh–tens)
immunodeficiency	(**im**–you–no–deh–**FISH**–en–see)
immunoelectrophore-sis	(im–**you**–no–ee–**lek**–troh–foh–**REE**–sis)
immunogen	(**IM**–you–no–jen)
immunoglobulin	(**im**–you–no–**GLAHB**–you–lyn)
immunosuppressive	(**im**–you–no–sup–**PRESS**–iv)
keratoconjunctivitis	(**ker**–ah–toh–kon–**junk**–tih–**VIE**–tis)

lymph	(limf)
lymphadenopathy	(lim–**fad**–eh–**NOP**–ah–thee)
lymphocyte	(**LIM**–foh–sight)
macrophage	(**MACK**–roh–fayj)
megakaryocyte	(mega–**KAIR**–ee–oh–syte)
phagocytes	(**FAG**–oh–sights)
phagocytosis	(**fag**–oh–sigh–**TOH**–sis)
reticuloendothelial	(re–**tik**–you–loh–en–doh–**THEE**–lee–ohl)
retrovirus	(**ret**–roh–**VIE**–rus)
tetany	(**TET**–ah–nee)
thrombocytopenia	(**throm**–boh–**sigh**–toh–**PEE**–nee–ah)
xerostomia	(**zeh**–roh–**STOH**–mee–ah)

74

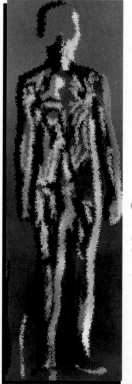

Orderly Function of the Immune System

The immune system, a major defense mechanism, is responsible for a complex response to the invasion of the body by foreign substances. This immune response assists the body in maintaining its functional integrity. The ability to generate an immune response is controlled by one's genetics. The immune system includes bone marrow, lymphoid tissues (**lymph** nodes, tonsils, adenoids, spleen, Peyer's patches, appendix, and thymus gland), their products (**lymphocytes** and antibodies), and **macrophages** (**phagocytes** found in the blood, liver, brain, lymph nodes, spleen, and other organs) (Fig. 3-1). The three major functions of the immune system are

- Protecting the body against foreign organisms or substances (**antigens**) through normal body structure and function, such as the action of healthy cells, mucous membranes, and tears.
- Maintaining **homeostasis** by the elimination of damaged cells from the circulation in a process called **phagocytosis.**
- Recognizing and guarding against the development, growth, and distribution of abnormal cells within the body in a response known as the inflammatory response.

When the immune system reacts appropriately to an antigen and homeostasis is maintained, it is called **immunocompetence.** If the immune system's response is inappropriate, either too weak

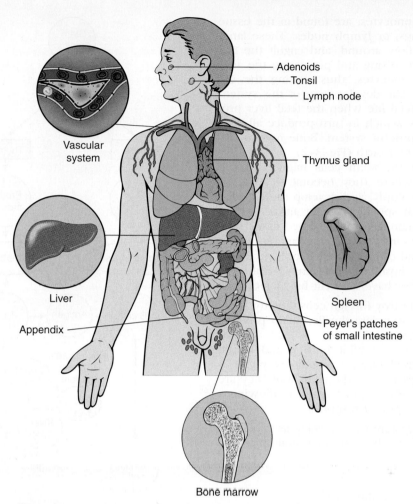

Adenoids
Tonsil
Lymph node

Vascular system

Thymus gland

Liver

Spleen

Appendix

Peyer's patches of small intestine

Bone marrow

Figure 3–1

Immune system.

or too strong, disruption of homeostasis results, causing a malfunction in the system, or immunoincompetence. Disruption of homeostasis can cause many diseases. Inappropriate responses or malfunctioning of the immune system are classified as

- Hyperactive responses (e.g., allergies), in which the immune response is excessive;
- **Immunodeficiency** disorders (e.g., acquired immunodeficiency syndrome), in which the immune response is inadequate;
- **Autoimmune** disorders (e.g., SLE), in which the immune response is misdirected; or
- Attacks on beneficial foreign tissue (e.g., reaction to blood transfusions or transplanted organ rejection).

The immune response normally is activated whenever foreign substances or antigens enter the body. The body recognizes the antigen or **immunogen,** usually a protein, as foreign, or non-self, and produces **antibodies** in response to the specific antigen. If local barriers fail to contain or destroy the foreign invader or are inadequate and if the inflammatory process is unable to halt the assault against the body, an immune response evolves to recognize the antigen and originates a humoral or a cell-mediated response.

The mononuclear phagocytic system or what used to be termed the **reticuloendothelial** system initiates the immune response, working to defend against infection and disposing of the products of cell destruction. Macrophages, which develop from monocytes, are found in the tissue of the liver, lungs, or lymph nodes. These large cells intercept, flow around, and engulf the foreign invader, processing and presenting the antigen to the lymphocytes, thus starting the immune response. The development of this system begins early in fetal life when the fetal liver produces stem cells, which in turn produce all cells of the **hematopoietic** system. Bone marrow assumes this role after birth (Fig. 3–2).

A portion of the stem cells migrate to the thymus gland, where they become T cells (T lymphocytes), multiply, and develop the capacity to combine with specific foreign antigens from viruses, fungi, tumors, or transplanted tissue (Fig. 3–3). This results in a sensitization and an immunity that is termed cell mediated. T cells go out to meet the foreign invaders. There are several types of T cells, and they have different functions:

- Killer T cells destroy foreign cells directly.
- Helper T cells stimulate the B cells to produce more antibodies.
- Suppressor T cells inhibit both B and T cell activities and moderate the immune response.
- Memory T cells remain dormant until they are reactivated by the original antigen, allowing a rapid and more potent response.

The remaining stem cells develop as B cells (B lymphocytes) to produce humoral immunity that

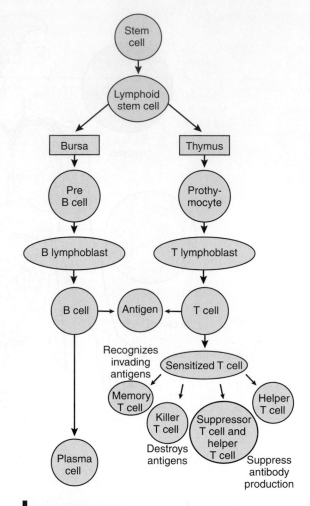

Figure 3–3

T cell and B cell formation.

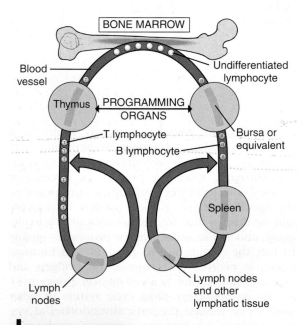

Figure 3–2

Bone marrow formation of lymphocytes.

protects the body against bacterial and viral infections and reinfections (see Fig. 3–3). As plasma cells, the B cells are responsible for producing antibodies that attach to invading foreign antigens, thus marking the antigens accessible for destruction by other cells of the immune system. Some of the B cells become memory B cells, having the ability to produce small amounts of antibodies for a period of years.

B cells are coated with **immunoglobulins,** providing them with the ability to recognize foreign protein, stimulating antigen–antibody reaction. The five classes of immunoglobulins or antibodies are IgM, IgG, IgA, IgD, and IgE (Table 3–1). These immunoglobulins are usually all present during an antigenic response, although in varying

TABLE 3-1 ➤ Classes of Antibodies

CLASS	PERCENT OF TOTAL	LOCATION	FUNCTION
IgG	75–85	Blood plasma	Major antibody in primary and secondary immune responses; inactivates antigen; neutralizes toxins; crosses placenta to provide immunity for newborn; responsible for Rh reactions
IgA	5–15	Saliva, mucus, tears, breast milk	Protects mucous membranes on body surfaces; provides immunity for newborn
IgM	5–10	Attached to B cells; released into plasma during immune response	Causes antigens to clump together; responsible for transfusion reactions in the ABO blood typing system
IgD	0.2	Attached to B cells	Receptor sites for antigens on B cells; binding with antigen results in B cell activation
IgE	0.5	Produced by plasma cells in mucous membranes and tonsils	Binds to mast cells and basophils, causing release of histamine; responsible for allergic reactions

From Applegate EJ: The Anatomy and Physiology Learning System: Textbook. Philadelphia: WB Saunders, 1996, p 300. Used with permission.

amounts, depending on the stimulant and the health of the patient. Defense mechanisms of the antigen–antibody complex include

- Inactivation of the pathogen or its toxin
- Stimulation of phagocytosis
- Activation of the complement system (complement fixation)

Complement fixation includes the activation of several normally inactive proteins found in plasma or body fluids. The antigen–antibody reaction initiates a series or cascade of reactions that activate the complement system, fixing the complement and consequently permitting the complement system to destroy the pathogens by the process of phagocytosis or lysis of the pathogen's cell membrane. This activation occurs during an immune reaction with IgG or IgM.

Immunity is classified as either natural or acquired. Natural immunity is a genetic feature and is specific to race, sex, and the individual's ability to respond. This natural immunity results partly from the presence of natural antibodies in the blood's plasma that have the ability to combine with the invading antigen. Acquired immunity means that the body has developed an ability to defend itself against foreign antigens.

Acquired immunity can be active or passive. *Active* immunity results when a person has had previous exposure to a disease, which was possibly asymptomatic and therefore unrecognized, or receives *immunizations* against a disease to stimulate the production of a specific antibody. Active immunity affords acquired permanent protection. *Passive* immunity bypasses the body's immune response to afford the benefit of immediate immune substances created outside the body for temporary immunity (e.g., colostrum and breast milk). Passive immunity is gained from receiving immune substances created outside the body, such as immune globulin (Fig. 3–4).

Immunodeficiency Diseases

An absent or inadequate response of the immune system results in immunodeficiency diseases and increased susceptibility to other diseases. Although the deficiency may be in either the humoral or the cell-mediated realm, the consequences are similar: the individual does not have the capability to dispose of foreign and harmful substances. Some of the flaws are genetic and are present at birth, whereas other defects do not manifest themselves until later in life. Acquired immunoincompetence may result from a bacterial or viral insult to the body, malnutrition, exposure to radiation or certain drugs, and the inability of the body to respond to immunodeficiency disease. The severity of the immunodeficiency disease depends on the area of the immune response that is affected and can range from annoying chronic infections to severe life-threatening or fatal conditions. **Opportunistic infections** can emerge as a result of deficiencies of the immune system.

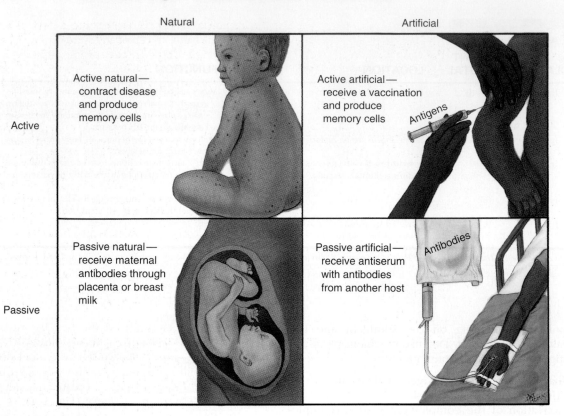

Natural   Artificial

Active

Active natural—
contract disease
and produce
memory cells

Active artificial—
receive a vaccination
and produce
memory cells

Antigens

Passive

Passive natural—
receive maternal
antibodies through
placenta or breast
milk

Passive artificial—
receive antiserum
with antibodies
from another host

Antibodies

Figure 3–4

Acquired immunity. (From Applegate EJ: The Anatomy and Physiology Learning System: Textbook. Philadelphia: WB Saunders, 1996, p 300. Used with permission.)

ACQUIRED IMMUNODEFICIENCY SYNDROME

SYMPTOMS AND SIGNS

Acquired immunodeficiency syndrome (AIDS) is a progressive impairment of the immune system caused by HIV. This gradual destruction of the immune system affects many organ systems with ultimate fatal consequence for the person infected. This deadly disease eradicates resistance to infection and disease by infecting helper T lymphocytes (T cells) and replicating itself therein, destroying the lymphocyte, and then invading other lymphocytes.

Initially it is not possible to tell by looking at someone whether they are infected with HIV. They may remain healthy for years in the latent period and may unknowingly transmit the virus to other people. Within 1 to 2 weeks after exposure, the patient may experience a sore throat with fever and body aches. **Lymphadenopathy**, weight loss, fatigue, diarrhea, and night sweats are common as the clinical course unfolds. The body's resistance is lowered, and this leads to frequent infections, pneumonia, fever, malignancies, and a number of opportunistic infections. See Enrichment for Malignancies and Common Opportunistic Infections and Conditions in AIDS. Frequently, in the later stages, encephalopathy and malignancy lead to dementia and death (Fig. 3-5).

ETIOLOGY

AIDS is caused by HIV (type I or type II), a **retrovirus** that contains **RNA;** it cannot survive apart from human cells. It is spread most readily by direct contact with the blood or semen of an infected person. HIV attacks helper T lympho-

Enrichment

MALIGNANCIES AND COMMON OPPORTUNISTIC INFECTIONS AND CONDITIONS IN AIDS

- **Kaposi's sarcoma** is an aggressive malignancy of the blood vessels that appears as purple or blue patches on the skin, in the mouth, or anywhere on the body.
- **Lymphomas** are cancerous lesions of lymphoid tissues.
- *Pneumocystis carinii* pneumonia (PCP) is a lung infection that can progress to be life threatening. It is the most common lung disease in persons with AIDS.
- **Tuberculosis** is a tumorous infection of the lungs or other organs.
- **Herpes simplex** consists of painful blister-like lesions of the mouth, genitalia, or anus, caused by the herpesvirus.
- **Herpes zoster** (shingles) is characterized by clusters of red blister-like skin lesions that follow an inflamed nerve path.
- *Candida albicans* causes a fungal infection of the mucous membrane of the mouth, genitalia, or skin.
- **Toxoplasmosis** is an infection caused by a protozoan intracellular parasite. There can be a rash and lymphadenopathy, and the central nervous system, heart, or lungs can become involved.
- **Neurologic complications** include inflammation of nerves, neuropathy, neoplasms, and AIDS dementia complex.
- **Diarrhea** is a symptom of a host of bacterial and viral infections of the gastrointestinal tract, liver, or gallbladder.

cytes, the body's safeguard against tumors, viruses, and parasites. The destruction of T cells and the proliferation of HIV leave the body defenseless against infection and malignancy. The virus also directly damages the nervous system. AIDS first was recognized in the United States in 1981. Since then, it has become a top killer of young men and a worldwide threat to humankind. The time from infection with HIV to death is approximately 10 years. To date, neither a cure nor an effective vaccine has been found for this disease.

Sexual contact is the primary means of transmission. Although AIDS initially was associated with homosexual activity, more recent statistics show an increase in the number of women infected through heterosexual transmission. AIDS also can be transmitted through blood and blood products. Infants of infected mothers can contract the disease in utero, through the placenta, during the birth process and postpartum, and from breast milk. Sharing of needles by intravenous drug users also leads to infection. The risk of transmission of HIV to and from health-care workers and patients is minimized by strict adherence to the universal precautions for infection control.

DIAGNOSIS

The laboratory screening test to detect the presence of HIV antibodies in the blood is the **enzyme-linked immunosorbent assay (ELISA).** If the findings are positive, the test is repeated, and the result then is confirmed by using a **Western blot test.** A positive P24 antigen test indicates circulating HIV antigen. The lymphocyte count is monitored for the evaluation of immunocompetence; for example, as the disease progresses, the T cell count decreases. Other tests can detect impairment of the immune system and monitor the total health status of the HIV-infected person. Transmission of HIV is possible during all stages of infection, even early, before it can be detected by laboratory tests.

TREATMENT

Currently, no cure exists for AIDS. The goal of medical management is to maintain the best possible immune status with immunizations and anti-infective therapy. The antiviral drug zidovudine (AZT) has had some favorable results in certain patients. This drug and other antiretroviral drugs used to suppress HIV actions in the body are associated with a number of toxicities and serious side effects. Drugs used in combinations with protease inhibitors, sometimes referred to as "drug cocktails," have successfully extended life for some persons with AIDS. Surgery for the removal of **neoplasms** may be suggested to prolong life and to provide some comfort. Individu-

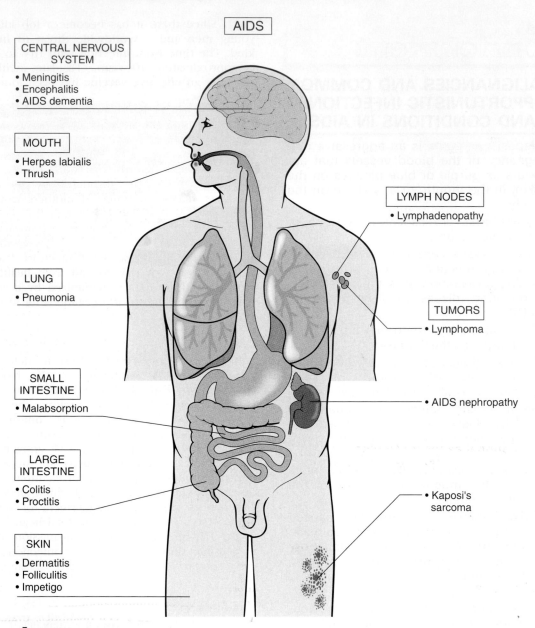

AIDS

CENTRAL NERVOUS
SYSTEM
• Meningitis
• Encephalitis
• AIDS dementia

MOUTH
• Herpes labialis
• Thrush

LYMPH NODES
• Lymphadenopathy

LUNG
• Pneumonia

TUMORS
• Lymphoma

SMALL
INTESTINE
• Malabsorption

• AIDS nephropathy

LARGE
INTESTINE
• Colitis
• Proctitis

• Kaposi's
  sarcoma

SKIN
• Dermatitis
• Folliculitis
• Impetigo

Figure 3–5

Pathologic changes associated with acquired immunodeficiency syndrome (AIDS). (From Damjanov I: Pathology for the Health-Related Professions. Philadelphia: WB Saunders, 1996, p 71. Used with permission.)

alized supportive treatment plans vary with the body systems affected and the needs of each patient. Addressing the psychological needs of the patient with AIDS is essential.

HIV is not transmitted by casual contact such as touching, handshaking, and hugging. Health-care practitioners who are involved in various forms of patient care with exposure to body fluids and blood should follow the principles of infection control and universal precautions. See Alert for Infection Control and Universal Precautions. All body fluids and blood should be han-

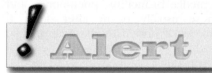

INFECTION CONTROL AND UNIVERSAL PRECAUTIONS

Guidelines: Treat blood and body fluids as if infected and remember to use the following precautions:

1. Practice frequent and thorough hand washing.
2. Report any accidental needle sticks.
3. Wear personal protective equipment, including mask, gown, gloves, and goggles.
4. Use caution with laboratory specimens.
5. Dispose of contaminated sharps in designated biohazard containers. *Caution:* Do not recap or break needles.
6. Use proper linen disposal containers.
7. Use clean mouthpieces and resuscitation bags.
8. Obtain hepatitis B vaccination for occupational exposure to blood.
9. Use proper decontamination techniques.
10. Blood spills should be absorbed with paper towels, then the area cleaned with soap and water, followed by disinfecting the area with a 1:10 solution of household bleach.

dled with extreme care, as if the patient were known to be infected with HIV.

Because HIV is transmitted directly from human to human, prevention measures relate directly to avoiding risk factors for sexually transmitted diseases and infection control by using universal precautions.

Although AIDS is considered a fatal disease, the number of Americans dying of AIDS has dropped and it is no longer 1 of the top 10 killers, although the number of new infections has decreased only slightly. Better access to care and more aggressive use of newer drugs are

thought to be reasons that people with AIDS are living longer.

COMMON VARIABLE IMMUNODEFICIENCY (ACQUIRED HYPOGAMMAGLOBULINEMIA)

SYMPTOMS AND SIGNS

The person with common variable immunodeficiency (CVID), a condition in which there is an absence of antibody production and or function, has a history of chronic infections. The **sinopulmonary** symptoms include sinus tenderness, cough, fever, runny nose, abnormal sputum, and **dyspnea.** Gastrointestinal symptoms include diarrhea, abdominal pain, and weight loss. **Lymphadenopathy, splenomegaly,** and **hepatomegaly** frequently are observed. Recurrent **otitis media** is experienced. When CVID is associated with **autoimmune** disorders, rashes, bleeding, bruising, fatigue, arthralgia (painful joints), muscle weakness, and pain may be noted. As the disease progresses and T cell involvement occurs, susceptibility to opportunistic and viral infections and malignancies escalates.

ETIOLOGY

Although the exact cause of acquired hypogammaglobulinemia is not known, circulating B cells are present, but dysfunctional, thereby curtailing the synthesis and release of immunoglobulins.

DIAGNOSIS

A history of repeated and chronic infections along with the clinical picture leads to further investigation of immunoglobulin levels, B cell titers, and B cell and T cell quantities. Evaluations of sinopulmonary status include cultures, radiographic studies, and pulmonary function tests. Abnormal findings in any of these studies necessitate a **biopsy** of lymph tissue. Decreased plasma cell presence is indicative of the disease.

TREATMENT

Treatment is aimed at preventing infections and implementing early treatment with appropriate antibiotic administration when infections occur. Proper nutrition and adequate rest are encouraged. Immune globulin replacement on a regular basis is helpful, and fever is treated with acetaminophen. Sinus and ear infections may be treated surgically to ensure proper drainage. Care must be taken *never to immunize these persons with live virus vaccines.*

SELECTIVE IMMUNOGLOBULIN A DEFICIENCY

SYMPTOMS AND SIGNS

The patient with selective IgA deficiency, the most common form of immunoglobulin deficiency, experiences chronic sinopulmonary infections with subsequent respiratory allergy. Celiac disease, ulcerative colitis, regional enteritis, and other autoimmune diseases often are associated with this condition. Children with selective IgA deficiency undergo recurrent otitis media and respiratory tract disease. IgA may begin to be produced spontaneously, and this usually is followed by the subsiding of ear and respiratory tract problems.

ETIOLOGY

Autosomal dominant or recessive inheritance appears to play a role in the etiology of this condition, in which B cells are apparently not secreting IgA.

DIAGNOSIS

Immunologic studies indicate below-normal levels of circulating IgA along with an absence of IgA in saliva and nasal, bronchial, and intestinal secretions. Circulating B cells have a normal appearance.

TREATMENT

There is no known cure for this condition, although some patients may spontaneously begin to produce IgA. Treatment is geared to symptoms of gastrointestinal and respiratory tract conditions. Immune globulin must never be administered to these patients because sensitization can lead to anaphylaxis if blood products are administered later.

X-LINKED AGAMMAGLOBULINEMIA

SYMPTOMS AND SIGNS

The infant with X-linked agammaglobulinemia, a condition of severe B cell deficiency, has recurrent severe gram-positive infections, including

bacterial otitis media, bronchitis, pneumonia, and meningitis. These usually occur after 4 to 6 months of age, when the natural transplacental immunity from the mother is depleted. Additional symptoms may include conjunctivitis (**purulent**), dental caries, and rheumatoid arthritis–type symptoms. Lymphadenopathy and splenomegaly are noticeably absent.

ETIOLOGY

This congenital X-linked disorder affects only males. All five immunoglobulin classes are thought to be absent, along with the absence of circulating B cells and the presence of normal numbers of circulating T cells. Parents of these children are encouraged to seek genetic counseling regarding future pregnancies.

DIAGNOSIS

The clinical picture, along with a thorough history of age at onset and family history of relatives who died of severe infections, leads to the suggestion of X-linked agammaglobulinemia. Immunoelectrophoresis indicates decreased levels of serum IgM, IgA, and IgG; however, this method of diagnosis is not valid before the infant is 6 to 8 months of age.

TREATMENT

Because this condition cannot be cured, treatment is directed at improving the child's immune defenses, controlling infections, and relieving rheumatoid arthritis–like symptoms. Immune globulin injections, occasional infusions of fresh frozen plasma, and appropriate antibiotics are administered. These children must never be immunized with live virus vaccines, nor should corticosteroids or immunosuppressive drugs be administered.

SEVERE COMBINED IMMUNODEFICIENCY DISEASE

SYMPTOMS AND SIGNS

Severe combined immunodeficiency disease (SCID), an X-linked recessive condition, manifests in an unusual susceptibility to infection. SCID is characterized by the complete absence of normal cell-mediated (T cell) and antibody-mediated (B cell) immunity. This occurs by the age of 3 to 6 months, when the natural maternal placental immunity begins to be depleted. In addition, the infant fails to thrive and experiences chronic otitis media, diarrhea, recurrent pulmonary infections, thrush, and sepsis. The infant usually has a low-grade fever until the natural maternal acquired immunity is depleted, and then severe infections erupt.

ETIOLOGY

The exact cause of the genetic defect is not known; however, it is thought that there may have been a failure of the stem cell to differentiate into B cells and T cells.

DIAGNOSIS

The difficulty of not being able to detect defective antibody-mediated immunity in a child before the age of 6 months to 1 year complicates the diagnosis. Many of these children die of overwhelming infection before the age of 1 year. Abnormally low or absent B cell and T cell immunity, along with absence of lymphocytes, plasma cells, and lymphoid follicles in lymph node biopsy, indicates this condition.

TREATMENT

Preventing exposure to infection and assisting the immune response through bone marrow transplantation are the goals of treatment. Compatible bone marrow donors are usually siblings. Children with SCID are placed in completely sterile environments to prevent infection.

DIGEORGE SYNDROME (THYMIC HYPOPLASIA OR APLASIA)

SYMPTOMS AND SIGNS

DiGeorge syndrome, a congenital condition of immunodeficiency, is identified in young children by a set of structural anomalies. These anomalies include abnormally wide-set, downward slanting eyes; low-set ears with notched pinnas; a small mouth; and cardiovascular defects, possibly tetralogy of Fallot. There is an absence or underdevelopment of the thymus and parathyroid glands. The infant exhibits signs of **hypocalcemia** and **tetany.**

ETIOLOGY

This congenital disorder also is known as thymic hypoplasia or aplasia. It is thought to originate during the 12th week of gestation as an abnormal development of the third and fourth pharyngeal pouches. This causes the thymus gland to be underdeveloped or absent. If the thymus gland is underdeveloped, it is abnormally located.

DIAGNOSIS

Diagnosis is made by the clinical picture; the radiographic confirmation of absence, hypoplasia, or abnormal placement of the thymus gland; and the absence of or decreased number of functional T cells. B cell function is normal. **Hypoparathyroidism** is diagnosed by low serum calcium levels, elevated serum phosphorus levels, and lack of parathyroid hormone.

TREATMENT

Aggressive treatment of the hypocalcemia with intravenous infusion to replace calcium is essential to restore the electrolyte balance and to reduce the risk of seizures. Vitamin D and parathyroid hormone replacement therapy are also necessary. Repair of cardiac anomalies may be attempted. Occasionally, a human fetal thymus may be transplanted. Parents are taught to control exposure of the infant to prevent infections. Generally, the child dies of infection before the second year of life.

83

CHRONIC MUCOCUTANEOUS CANDIDIASIS

SYMPTOMS AND SIGNS

Chronic mucocutaneous candidiasis (CMC) is a chronic syndrome of persistent and recurrent candidal (fungal) infections of the skin, nails, and mucous membranes. Symptoms usually develop during the first 2 or 3 years of life or, if onset is later, in young adulthood. Large circular lesions appear on the skin, mucous membranes, nails, or vagina. Sores in the mouth make eating difficult. Recurrent thrush or diaper rash is often the first symptom of the disease in infants. Older children exhibit lesions, often beginning on the scalp and also involving the nails. Patients in late stages of the disease experience recurring respiratory tract infections.

Glands can become involved (endocrinopathies), and the particular symptoms of hypofunction, such as hypocalcemia, hypoparathyroidism, and pernicious anemia, are related to the specific glands or organs affected. Some patients experience severe viral infections before the onset of the endocrinopathies.

Syndromes of chronic mucocutaneous candidiasis are chronic oral candidiasis (disease affecting the mucosa of the lips, tongue, and buccal cavity), chronic mucocutaneous candidiasis with endocrinopathy (hypoadrenalism, hypothyroidism, hypoparathyroidism, and ovarian failure in females), chronic localized candidiasis (cutaneous lesions with hyperkeratosis), chronic diffuse candidiasis (widespread infection of the skin, nails, and mucous membranes), and candidiasis with thyoma (candidiasis accompanied by hypogammaglobulinemia, neutropenia, aplastic anemia, or myasthenia gravis).

ETIOLOGY

There appears to be an inherited defect in the T cell–mediated immune system that permits autoantibodies to develop against target organs. This is associated with the endocrinopathies. Siblings and cousins often are affected; however, parents and offspring do not appear to have the tendency for the disease to develop.

DIAGNOSIS

Blood studies indicate normal T cell circulation and normal antibody response to all organisms except *Candida.* Other immunodeficiency diseases need to be ruled out, and all endocrine functions should be evaluated. Any other abnormalities are evaluated according to the organs involved.

TREATMENT

Treatment is directed at eliminating the infections along with correcting the immunologic defects. Treatment is systemic, and the drug of choice is amphotericin B. Topical treatment with antifungal agents appears to improve skin and nail lesions. Symptoms arising from other organs and glands are addressed according to the organ or gland involved. Treatment of the immunologic defect includes thymus transplantation, thymic extract injections, lymphocyte infusions, and administration of transfer factor.

WISKOTT-ALDRICH SYNDROME

SYMPTOMS AND SIGNS

The child with Wiskott-Aldrich syndrome, an immunodeficiency disorder characterized by inadequate B and T cell function, experiences eczema and **thrombocytopenia** with severe bleeding. These youngsters also display an increased susceptibility to bacterial, viral, and fungal infections. Infants experience bleeding with **petechiae** and **purpura.** By the age of 1 year, the bleeding subsides and eczema develops. These children are predisposed to the development of leukemia and lymphoma.

ETIOLOGY

This rare immunodeficiency disorder is inherited as an X-linked trait affecting only males. The thymus gland is normal at birth but decreases in size as the child becomes older, resulting in decreased B and T cell functions. This compromises the child's immunity and increases the risk of infection.

Additionally, there are metabolic defects in platelet synthesis, causing platelets to be short lived, and incompetent phagocytes.

DIAGNOSIS

Diagnosis is made by the decreased activity of B and T cells along with the clinical picture and history of lowered resistance to infections. Platelet count is decreased, and bleeding time is prolonged.

TREATMENT

Treatment consists of appropriate antibiotic therapy for infections. Administration of transfer factor derived from activated lymphocytes helps to increase resistance to infections and resolves the eczema. Transfusions of platelets, immune globulin injections, and steroid administration are additional means of treatment.

Autoimmune Diseases

Autoimmune diseases occur when autoantibodies develop and begin to destroy the body's own cells. Tolerance to self-antigens is believed to commence during fetal life. As the body ages or experiences various disease processes, the immune system misidentifies body cells and develops antibodies against its own cells and tissues, resulting in self-destruction. Present theories consider **autoimmunity** acquired, not congenital; however, certain genetic markers identify patients at increased risk for many autoimmune diseases. Currently, the specific gene products involved are mostly indeterminate.

Autoimmune diseases can occur in many body systems because lymphocytes and antibodies are sensitized to develop against self. The production of the autoantibodies may occur by several mechanisms to initiate changes, including disease, injury, metabolic change, and a mutation of immunologically competent cells. Additionally, vi-

TABLE 3–2 ➤ Autoimmune Diseases

BODY SYSTEM OR TISSUE	DISEASE
Hematopoietic system	Autoimmune hemolytic anemia
	Pernicious anemia
	Idiopathic thrombocytopenic purpura
	Idiopathic neutropenia
Kidney	Goodpasture's syndrome
	Immune complex glomerulonephritis
Rheumatoid and collagen	Systemic lupus erythematosus
	Progressive scleroderma (systemic sclerosis)
	Sjögren's syndrome
	Rheumatoid arthritis
	Juvenile rheumatoid arthritis
Endocrine system*	Graves' disease
	Hashimoto's disease (chronic thyroiditis)
	Insulin-dependent diabetes
Neurologic system	Multiple sclerosis
	Myasthenia gravis
Vascular system	Small vessel vasculitis
	Systemic necrotizing vasculitis

See Chapter 4.

ral infection, trauma, and certain drugs or chemicals may alter specific body proteins, thwarting recognition and terminating in their rejection as foreign.

Systems or body tissue particularly affected by autoimmunity and some of the resulting disease entities are listed in Table 3-2.

HEMATOPOIETIC DISORDERS

Autoimmune Hemolytic Anemia

SYMPTOMS AND SIGNS

Autoimmune hemolytic anemia, an autoimmune condition in which red blood cells (RBCs) are destroyed by antibodies, causes the patient to experience fatigue, weakness, chills, fever, dyspnea, and itching. The skin is pale and **jaundiced** and bruises easily. Additionally, the patient may be hypotensive.

ETIOLOGY

Because of failure of the immune response, B cell–produced antibodies are not able to identify RBCs as self, resulting in an attack on and destruction of the red corpuscles.

DIAGNOSIS

A direct Coombs' test indicates antibody-coated RBCs that agglutinate when antiglobulin is added to the medium. Some RBCs are spherical; serum bilirubin levels are elevated; and RBC count, platelet count, hemoglobin concentration, and **hematocrit** all usually are decreased. In mild or sporadic disease, these previously mentioned results may not be evident when the patient is tested.

TREATMENT

Immunosuppressive drugs and/or corticosteroids may be administered. Transfusions of plasma, washed RBCs, and platelets may be attempted. Splenectomy is a last resort if the RBC destruction cannot be arrested.

Pernicious Anemia

SYMPTOMS AND SIGNS

The patient with pernicious anemia, a **megaloblastic** anemia caused by decreased gastric production of hydrochloric acid and the resulting shortage of intrinsic factor, has a sore tongue, weakness, and tingling and numbness in the extremities. The lips, tongue, and gums appear pale, whereas the sclera and skin appear slightly jaundiced (Fig. 3-6). Because of the decreased hydrochloric acid production and atrophy of the gastric mucosa, the patient experiences disturbances in digestion such as **anorexia,** nausea, vomiting, diarrhea, constipation, flatulence, and weight loss. Vitamin B_{12} deficiency causes demyelination of the peripheral nerves and eventually the spinal cord. This is the cause of the neuritis, peripheral weakness, numbness, and **paresthesia.** Ataxia (muscular incoordination), lightheadedness, altered vision, **tinnitus,** and optic muscle **atrophy** are additional symptoms as the anemia progresses. Central nervous system changes may cause headaches, irritability, and depression. Reduced hemoglobin levels are responsible for decreased oxygen-carrying capacity, leading to fatigue, weakness, and lightheadedness. The patient may experience palpitations, dyspnea, **tachycardia,** premature ventricular contractions, and even congestive heart failure.

ETIOLOGY

Because of the frequent presence of anti–intrinsic factor antibodies, pernicious anemia is be-

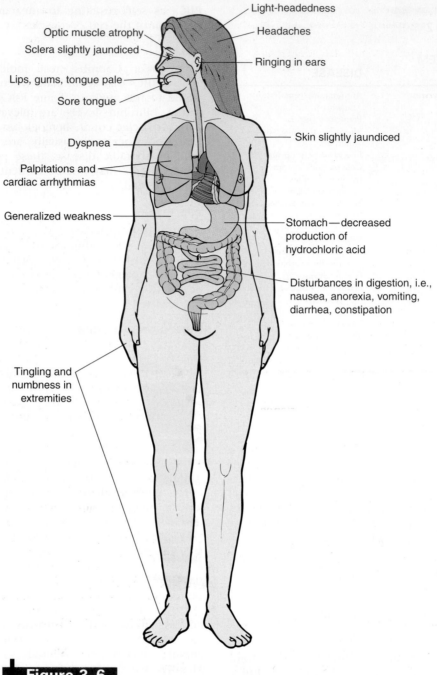

Light-headedness

Headaches

Optic muscle atrophy

Sclera slightly jaundiced

Ringing in ears

Lips, gums, tongue pale

Sore tongue

Dyspnea

Skin slightly jaundiced

Palpitations and cardiac arrhythmias

Generalized weakness

Stomach—decreased production of hydrochloric acid

Disturbances in digestion, i.e., nausea, anorexia, vomiting, diarrhea, constipation

Tingling and numbness in extremities

Figure 3–6

Symptoms and signs of pernicious anemia.

lieved to be associated with an autoimmune response. The intrinsic factor must be present in the gastric mucosa for vitamin B_{12} absorption to occur. Vitamin B_{12} is necessary for RBC formation, and a deficiency causes RBCs to be deformed and reduced in number.

DIAGNOSIS

Diagnosis is confirmed by the clinical picture and laboratory tests. Blood tests reveal decreased hemoglobin (Hb) level, decreased RBC count, increased mean cell volume (MCV), and decreased **white blood cell (WBC) count** and platelet count. Similar to the case for the RBCs, the platelets are large and malformed. Bone marrow studies indicate abnormal RBC production and other changes typical of vitamin B_{12} deficiency. Reduced amounts or absence of gastric acid is found on gastric analysis. Vitamin B_{12} is also necessary for proper **myelin** formation; a myelin deficiency can cause damage to the nerves.

TREATMENT

Injections of vitamin B_{12} are the primary treatment of this type of anemia, and they must be continued for life. Blood replacement may be indicated in severe cases. There is no known cure for pernicious anemia.

Idiopathic Thrombocytopenic Purpura

SYMPTOMS AND SIGNS

The patient with idiopathic thrombocytopenia purpura, a deficiency in platelets and a primary immune disorder, exhibits symptoms of inability of the blood to clot. These symptoms include spontaneous hemorrhages in the skin, mucous membranes, or internal organs. Petechiae, small spider-like hemorrhages under the surface of the skin, and ecchymoses, larger hemorrhagic areas, are apparent. The patient may experience **epistaxis** (nosebleeds), gastrointestinal bleeding, **hematuria,** and easy bruising.

ETIOLOGY

Thrombocytopenic purpura often is considered **idiopathic** (unknown cause), although antibodies that reduce the life of platelets have been found in most cases. Some cases may follow a viral infection, especially rubella or mumps. Additionally, the spleen may be destroying the damaged platelets.

DIAGNOSIS

The clinical symptoms, along with prolonged bleeding time and reduced platelet count, suggest the diagnosis. The size and shape of the platelets may be abnormal. Bone marrow studies indicate an increase in **megakaryocytes** (precursors of platelets). Circulating platelet time is reduced to hours instead of the normal days.

TREATMENT

Corticosteroid administration increases capillary integrity for a short time. Anemia needs to be corrected with blood transfusion, and vitamin K administration improves clotting mechanism. Therapeutic plasma exchange occasionally is at-

tempted. Splenectomy is a last resort; however, this treatment is effective, with platelet numbers increasing after the procedure.

Idiopathic Neutropenia

SYMPTOMS AND SIGNS

The patient with idiopathic neutropenia, a decreased number of circulating neutrophils, experiences malaise, fatigue, weakness, fever, stomatitis, and various infections, even to the point of **septicemia.**

ETIOLOGY

This condition is characterized by a diminished number to almost complete absence of neutrophils in the blood. It may be associated with infection, acute rheumatoid arthritis, acute leukemia, chronic splenomegaly, or vitamin B_{12} deficiency.

DIAGNOSIS

Diagnosis is confirmed by the significantly reduced numbers of neutrophils displayed in a WBC count. Bone marrow aspiration demonstrates an increased ratio of immature to mature neutrophils along with defective development of the neutrophils, which have an abnormal appearance.

TREATMENT

The cause of this condition must be established and, if possible, eliminated. Appropriate antibiotics are administered to treat bacterial infections. Transfusions of WBC concentrates may be indicated. Care must be taken to avoid exposure to any type of infection.

RENAL DISORDERS

Goodpasture's Syndrome

SYMPTOMS AND SIGNS

The patient with Goodpasture's syndrome, an autoimmune kidney disease, experiences **hemoptysis,** hematuria, dyspnea, and **proteinuria.**

ETIOLOGY

The cause of this rare disease is obscure. Antibodies cause complement-mediated tissue damage in the glomerular and alveolar basement membranes, resulting in glomerulonephritis and pulmonary hemorrhage. Progression of the disease frequently leads to renal failure.

DIAGNOSIS

A host of diagnostic studies and findings help to make a differential diagnosis to rule out the many other diseases that manifest similar signs. Urinalysis indicates the presence of protein and blood in the urine.

TREATMENT

Corticosteroid and immunosuppressive drugs are administered to patients with mild forms of the disease. Hemodialysis and kidney transplants are last resorts for severely compromised patients.

COLLAGEN DISEASES

The main component of connective tissue, the essential part of all structures in the body, is a fibrous, insoluble protein called collagen. Collagen constitutes 30% of the total body protein. With collagen diseases, inflammation results from damage of the collagen in certain areas of connective tissue.

Collagen diseases are known as autoimmune disorders. In autoimmune disorders, the immune system works abnormally against itself. In this case, the immune system attacks and destroys the collagen, resulting in damage to some of the body's connective tissue. The reason for the malfunction of the immune system is unknown. Somehow the immune system wrongly identifies the body's own tissues as foreign.

There are no cures for collagen diseases, and treatment is frequently only **palliative.** Death usually results from damage to the heart, lungs, or kidneys.

Collagen diseases are numerous, but systemic lupus erythematosus and scleroderma are two well-known examples.

Systemic Lupus Erythematosus

SYMPTOMS AND SIGNS

SLE, also called disseminated lupus erythematosus, can inflame and damage connective tissue anywhere in the body. SLE most commonly produces inflammation of the skin, joints, nervous system, kidneys, lungs, and other organs. A characteristic butterfly rash, or erythema, may be present on the face, spreading from one cheek, across the nose, to the other cheek (Fig. 3–7). Similar rashes may appear on other exposed areas of the body. Exposure to the sun aggravates the rash. SLE may begin acutely with fever, joint pain, and malaise, or may develop slowly over a period of years, with intermittent fever, malaise, joint deformities, and weight loss. This disease occurs most frequently in young women in their 30s or 40s.

ETIOLOGY

The cause of SLE is unknown; however, it is thought to be an autoimmune disorder. Genetic, environmental, and hormonal factors may predispose a person to this disease. Events that can precipitate SLE include stress, immunization reactions, pregnancy, and overexposure to ultraviolet light.

DIAGNOSIS

The diagnosis of SLE can be made if four or more of these symptoms are present either at the same time or sequentially: a butterfly rash on the face, a **discoid** skin lesion, **Raynaud's phenomenon,** alopecia, photosensitivity, nasopharyngeal ulceration, arthritis without deformity, chronic pleuritis or pericarditis, a false-positive serologic test result for syphilis, more than 35 g of protein in the urine in a 24-hour period, the presence of cellular casts in the urine, hemolytic anemia, thrombocytopenia, the presence of abnormal antibodies in the bloodstream, and the characteristic leukocytes (WBCs) called LE cells, which are not found in the circulation but are created in the laboratory as part of the testing. Diagnostic tests include a complete blood count (CBC) with differential leukocyte count, platelet count,

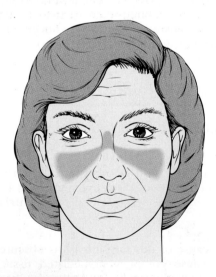

Figure 3–7

Typical butterfly rash of systemic lupus erythematosus.

erythrocyte sedimentation rate (ESR), antinuclear antibody determination, and anti-DNA test. The anti-DNA test is the most specific test for SLE, but it is reliably positive only with active disease.

TREATMENT

In mild cases, anti-inflammatory drugs, including aspirin, may be all that is needed for the fever and joint pain. For severe cases, antimalarial therapy and corticosteroids are indicated. Immunosuppressive medications are useful when life-threatening or severe crippling disease is present. Immunosuppressive agents are also helpful when the patient fails to respond to conventional therapy or when intolerable side effects develop. *IBProfen, Naprosin*

The prognosis for SLE is guarded. It improves slightly with early detection and treatment, but remains poor for persons with renal, cardiovascular, or neurologic complications or a serious bacterial infection. The death rate is high with SLE, with death usually occurring within 5 years from the onset of the disease. There are no preventive measures for SLE.

Scleroderma (Systemic Sclerosis)

SYMPTOMS AND SIGNS

Scleroderma is a chronic, progressive, systemic disease of the skin. It is characterized by sclerosis (hardening) and shrinking of the skin and certain internal organs, including the gastrointestinal tract, heart, lungs, and kidneys. The skin becomes taut, firm, and edematous and is attached to the subcutaneous tissue. The skin feels tough and leathery, it may itch, and pigmented patches may occur. Raynaud's phenomenon (see Raynaud's disease in Chapter 10) is usually the first symptom of scleroderma. This is followed by swelling, stiffness, and pain of the joints.

ETIOLOGY *(cause)*

The cause of scleroderma is unknown, but it appears to be an autoimmune disease. It occurs 4 times as frequently in women as men. It is found especially in women between 30 and 50 years old.

DIAGNOSIS

Physical examination, patient history, urinalysis (UA), and radiographic studies of the chest and gastrointestinal tract are all necessary for the diagnosis. A skin biopsy also may be performed.

TREATMENT

There is no specific treatment for scleroderma. A large number of drugs have been tried, including corticosteroids, vasodilators, and immunosuppressive agents, but they are just palliative. Physical therapy helps to maintain muscle strength but does not change the course of joint disease.

The prognosis for individuals with scleroderma is poor. Death usually results from cardiac, pulmonary, or renal failure. It is not known how to prevent the disease.

Sjögren's Syndrome

SYMPTOMS AND SIGNS

Sjögren's syndrome occurs in postmenopausal women. Its symptoms include rheumatoid arthritis, **xerostomia,** and **keratoconjunctivitis sicca.** This dryness of the nasal, oral, and laryngeal pharynx causes difficulty with talking, chewing, and swallowing. The patient may experience sores on or in the mouth and nose.

ETIOLOGY

Sjögren's syndrome is thought to be a form of collagen disease. It usually follows the onset of rheumatoid arthritis.

DIAGNOSIS

The enlargement of the salivary glands leads to further investigation, including a lower lip biopsy, which indicates an infiltration of lymphocytes. The blood studies demonstrate anemia, decreased WBC count, and elevated ESR. Additional studies show autoantibodies and high **rheumatoid factor** titers.

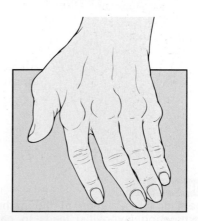

Figure 3–8

Joints affected by rheumatoid arthritis.

TREATMENT

Treatment is symptomatic, especially for the dryness in the oral cavity and eyes. Increasing fluid intake, chewing sugarless gum, and using oral sprays help to relieve oral dryness. Artificial tears are used in the eyes, and the wearing of sunglasses is recommended.

Rheumatoid Arthritis

SYMPTOMS AND SIGNS

Rheumatoid arthritis (RA) is a chronic, inflammatory, systemic disease affecting the joints (Fig. 3–8). It is one of the most severe forms of arthritis, affecting 5 to 8 million Americans, women 3 times more frequently than men. RA may begin at any age, but it most commonly strikes individuals in their 30s and 40s, with the frequency of the disease increasing with advancing age.

The disease leads to inflammation and edema of the synovial membranes surrounding a joint. Eventually, this inflammation spreads to other parts of the affected joint and, if untreated, has the capacity to destroy cartilage, deform joints, and in severe cases, destroy adjacent bone. Only one or two joints may be affected, or the disease rapidly can become widespread. If the neck is involved, the interlocking mechanism of the top two vertebrae may become affected so badly that it causes damage to the spinal cord. There is a risk that paralysis or death could result from this damage. In many cases, RA is not limited to the joints. It also can cause generalized inflammation in the cardiac muscle, in blood vessels, and within the layers of the skin.

RA may begin without any obvious symptoms in the joints. The person may have unexplained weight loss, fatigue, a persistent low-grade fever, and general malaise. This may accompany or precede joint stiffness, which is noticed especially on wakening and during periods of inactivity. Edema, pain, tenderness, erythema, and warmth in one or more joints occurring in a symmetric pattern gradually emerge as the principal symptoms. Joints generally affected are those of the fingers, wrists, knees, ankles, and toes. RA occurs less often in the spine or the hips, which are

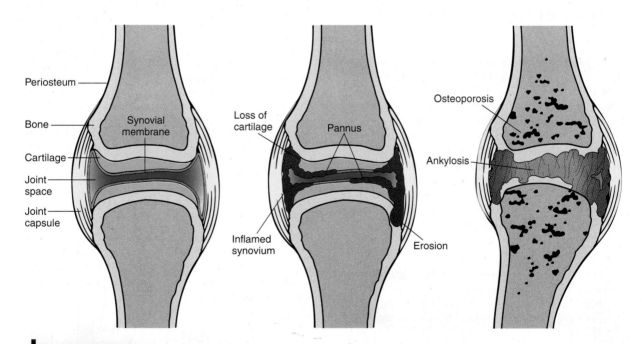

Periosteum
Bone
Cartilage
Joint space
Joint capsule
Synovial membrane
Loss of cartilage
Pannus
Inflamed synovium
Erosion
Osteoporosis
Ankylosis

Figure 3–9

Schematic presentation of the pathologic changes in rheumatoid arthritis. The inflammation (synovitis) leads to pannus formation, obliteration of the articular space, and, finally, to ankylosis. The periarticular bone shows diffuse atrophy in the form of osteoporosis. (From Damjanov I: Pathology for the Health-Related Professions. Philadelphia: WB Saunders, 1996, p 470. Used with permission.)

more susceptible to osteoarthritis (see Osteoarthritis in Chapter 7).

In some patients, the joint symptoms appear suddenly without any previous symptoms. In other cases, joint symptoms are accompanied by bursitis or anemia. Some persons may have only one mild attack, whereas others may have several episodes that may or may not leave them increasingly disabled.

ETIOLOGY

The exact cause of RA is unknown, although it is thought to be an autoimmune disorder. Heredity may predispose some persons to the disease; in other patients, a viral infection can trigger the disease process (Fig. 3–9).

DIAGNOSIS

Diagnosis is based on a review of the symptoms, family history, radiographic studies, and blood tests that show elevated levels of rheumatoid factor. Other useful laboratory tests include a CBC, synovial fluid analysis, serum protein electrophoresis, ESR, and antinuclear antibody titer. Occasionally, the only way to make a positive diagnosis of RA is to observe the disease progression for several weeks or months.

TREATMENT

The primary objectives of treatment are the reduction of inflammation and pain, the preservation of joint function, and the prevention of joint deformity. These require a combination of medication, rest, special exercises, and joint protection. Anti-inflammatory medications, including high doses of aspirin, are among the first choice to ease pain and stiffness, to reduce edema, and to control inflammation. Nonsteroidal anti-inflammatory drugs (NSAIDs) are prescribed as an alternative to aspirin. Corticosteroids often are given to control acute flare-ups. Even more potent drugs, such as gold compounds, penicillamine, and immunosuppressive agents, may slow the disease process or produce a remission in patients with severe RA.

Special splints and other devices to make dressing, bathing, cooking, eating, and performing other daily activities easier often are recommended to prevent, or at least reduce, deformities. Surgery is not often required, but it may be used to correct a deformity, relieve severe pain, and improve range of motion in persons with severe disease. For patients who no longer have adequately functioning joints, replacement with artificial joints may be recommended.

Juvenile Rheumatoid Arthritis

SYMPTOMS AND SIGNS

Juvenile rheumatoid arthritis (JRA), also known as Still's disease, is a form of RA that affects children. It usually involves the large joints and begins most commonly between the ages of 2 and 5 years. The attacks each last for several weeks and tend to lessen in severity, usually disappearing by puberty.

The child may have the following symptoms: a temperature fluctuating from normal in the morning to about 103°F in the evening; poor appetite, with resulting weight loss; a blotchy, red rash over the limbs and trunk of the body; anemia; and swollen, stiff, and painful joints, most commonly involving the neck, elbows, knees, and ankles. Other symptoms include red, painful eyes; swollen cervical or axillary lymph glands; and acute pericarditis. Skeletal development may be impaired if the **epiphyseal,** or growth, plates of the long bones are damaged owing to the inflammation around the joints.

Sites of JRA development vary considerably from child to child, and girls are affected 4 times as often as boys. The inflammation develops gradually but can be abrupt. In a few cases, the inflammation in the joints leads to partial or crippling deformity as a result of the recurring attacks. Complete remission occurs in approximately 75% of affected children.

effects large joints

ETIOLOGY

The specific cause of JRA is unknown, but it generally is believed that the pathologic changes in the joints are related to an autoimmune disorder. Heredity may play a role in some children.

DIAGNOSIS

Diagnosis is based on history and physical examination, which may show a lack of or delayed physical growth appropriate for the age of the child, and the results of blood tests for the rheumatoid factor.

TREATMENT

Treatment of children with JRA is essentially the same as that of an adult with RA (see Rheumatoid Arthritis). Medication dosages are based on the child's weight. Parents should encourage the child's independence. Participation in school and social activities that do not increase joint pain or cause undue fatigue are also important

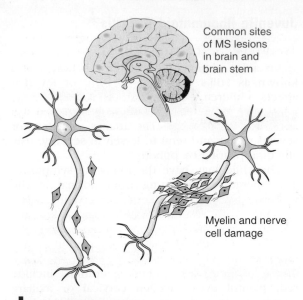

Common sites of MS lesions in brain and brain stem

Myelin and nerve cell damage

Figure 3–10

Myelin degeneration in multiple sclerosis (MS).

for the child. A well-balanced diet with plenty of protein is essential. Physical therapy exercises are crucial to minimizing the pain and reducing the crippling effects of arthritis. Braces or splints may be needed for growth disturbances.

NEUROLOGIC DISORDERS

Multiple Sclerosis

SYMPTOMS AND SIGNS

Multiple sclerosis (MS) is an inflammatory disease of the central nervous system. It attacks the myelin sheath, a fatty substance covering most of the nerves in the brain and spinal cord, causing scarring (sclerosis) (Fig. 3–10). The scarring prevents the transmission of stimuli to the brain and spinal cord and causes the following sensory and motor abnormalities:

- Weakness or numbness in one or more limbs
- Optic neuritis
- Loss of vision in one eye or **diplopia**
- Unsteady gait
- Vertigo
- Difficulty with urinating, leading to increased urinary tract infections
- Facial numbness or pain
- Speech problems

- **Dysphagia**
- Hearing loss
- Impotence in men
- Emotional disturbances, including depression, irritability, and short-temperedness

The symptoms once were thought to develop gradually, but this is not always true. In approximately 40% of cases, the onset may occur within a few hours. MS is rare in children; in about two thirds of cases, it develops between the ages of 20 and 40 years; and it occurs rarely in people older than 60 years. MS occurs only slightly more often in women than in men.

MS can be one of two types: the exacerbating-remitting type, in which episodes of neurologic dysfunction are followed by recovery, and the chronic progressive type, in which there is a steady progression of neurologic dysfunction. The duration of MS is variable, with some patients dying within a few months after onset of the disease. The average duration is 30 years or longer. Recurrent urinary tract infections pose a danger of eventual renal failure.

ETIOLOGY

The cause of MS is unknown. It is thought that the immune system is involved somehow, and there also may be an inherited trait that increases one's susceptibility to the disease. A common theory holds that an unknown virus triggers the immune system to turn against the body and attack the myelin, which eventually results in MS.

DIAGNOSIS

MS is difficult to diagnose because the symptoms are so variable and sporadic. A physical examination done in the early stages may have completely normal findings. Often, the diagnosis is discovered by eliminating other possible causes of the symptoms. This process may involve a variety of tests, including computed tomography (CT), radiographic studies of the skull and spine, magnetic resonance imaging (MRI), and brain scans. Brain lesions can be detected in most cases. Certain tests, such as **ophthalmoscopy,** cerebrospinal fluid analysis, and **lumbar puncture** (LP), also can aid in the diagnosis.

TREATMENT

There is no cure for MS, but the administration of drugs such as corticotropin and prednisone, which suppress inflammation, and cyclophosphamide, which slows the immune system's response, may decrease the severity of attacks and benefit patients. If started early in the disease, the use of an experimental drug called co-polymer 1 (COP 1) (a polymer of various amino acids) has had a favorable effect on the exacer-bating-remitting form of MS. Otherwise, the disease is treated symptomatically. This may include the patient's taking muscle relaxants; taking vita-min supplements to prevent a vitamin B deficiency, which might contribute to nerve damage; undergoing physical therapy to help to preserve as much muscle function as possible; wearing braces; and using a cane, walker, or wheelchair. Adequate rest and a well-balanced diet are also important.

Myasthenia Gravis

SYMPTOMS AND SIGNS

Myasthenia gravis is a chronic, progressive neuromuscular disease that mainly affects women between the ages of 20 and 40 years. The disease is characterized by extreme muscular weakness (without atrophy) and progressive fatigue. The onset, although usually gradual, may be sudden, with symptoms of muscular weakness generally appearing first and most noticeably in the face. Drooping eyelids, diplopia, and difficulty with talking and swallowing may be the first signs that something is wrong. The degree of weakness varies considerably from hour to hour, day to day, and year to year. Muscle weakness typically occurs late in the day or after strenuous exercise. Short periods of rest characteristically restore muscle function. Muscle weakness is progressive in myasthenia gravis, and eventually paralysis occurs. A myasthenic crisis (sudden inability to swallow and respiratory distress) may be so severe that mechanical ventilation becomes necessary. Prolonged exposure to sunlight, cold, infections, and emotional stress exacerbate the symptoms.

ETIOLOGY

The disease is thought to be caused by an autoimmune mechanism in which there is a faulty transmission of nerve impulses to and from the central nervous system, especially at the neuromuscular junction. In about one fifth of cases, the cause of myasthenia gravis appears to be related to the development of a thymus gland tumor.

DIAGNOSIS

The diagnosis can be made after obtaining blood tests to detect the presence of antibodies characteristically present with myasthenia gravis, radiographic chest studies, and **electromyography.** Improvement of muscle strength after rest or after an injection of **anticholinesterase** drugs also helps to confirm the diagnosis.

TREATMENT

The treatment of myasthenia gravis is **symptomatic** and supportive. Restricted activity, complete bed rest for severe cases, and a soft or liquid diet may be necessary. Anticholinesterase drugs are effective for the fatigue and muscle weakness, but they become less effective as the condition worsens. Pyridostigmine bromide (Mestinon) is the drug of choice for treatment. If a thymus gland tumor (thymoma) is present, a thymectomy is needed. Corticosteroids are effective in patients who have not been aided by the thymectomy. A useful adjunct to alternate-day therapy with corticosteroids is immunosuppression.

Unexplained, spontaneous remissions can occur; however, the disease is usually a lifelong condition characterized by remissions and exacerbations. Prolonged remissions may occur, but the course of the disease is variable.

VASCULITIS

Vasculitis, an immune complex (antigen–antibody)–mediated response, is an inflammation of blood vessels; it may be accompanied by progressive **necrosis** of the vessels. The vessel becomes necrotic when it is obstructed by a thrombus, and an **infarct** is the outcome of the inflammatory response. Biopsies of involved vessel walls have shown the presence of immunoglobulins. Any blood vessel can be involved, and vasculitis is classified into two types, small vessel vasculitis and systemic necrotizing vasculitis.

Small Vessel Vasculitis

SYMPTOMS AND SIGNS

Inflammation of the small vessels (arterioles, venules, and capillaries) causes petechiae (non-blanching), purpura, erythema, ulcerations, and edema; these are found most frequently on the skin of the lower extremities. Pain and a burning sensation accompany these lesions. Additionally, depending on the type of small vessel syndrome that the patient experiences, symptoms include ocular lesions, genital or oral ulcerations, abdominal pain, arthralgia, and weakness.

ETIOLOGY

Although the exact cause is unknown, vasculitis frequently accompanies other immune disorders. Exposure to certain chemicals, foreign proteins, drugs, foods, and infections have been suggested as etiologic.

DIAGNOSIS

Diagnosis is confirmed by immunofluorescent studies of biopsied tissue and confirmation of the presence of the immunoglobulins and complement as well as of the pattern of vascular involvement and cell types present.

TREATMENT

Treatment consists of recognizing and avoiding exposure to the causative agent or managing the underlying disease. Corticosteroid therapy may afford relief, analgesics are given, and rest is encouraged.

Systemic Necrotizing Vasculitis

SYMPTOMS AND SIGNS

Systemic necrotizing vasculitis occurs in numerous cutaneous and systemic conditions and causes involvement of both small and medium-sized arteries. Symptoms differ depending on the body system involved and include headaches, fever, weakness, fatigue, **malaise,** anorexia, and weight loss. Patients also may experience muscle and joint pain, **angina,** dyspnea, hypertension, and visual disturbances. Impaired tissue **perfu-**

sion causes **ischemic** pain in the system or tissues involved.

ETIOLOGY

It is not clear how the inflammation and necrosis of blood vessels develop. Each syndrome has specific clinical features with several probable mechanisms involved. Autoimmune responses constitute the causes and are mediated by antibodies, T cells, or IgA.

DIAGNOSIS

A complete history and a thorough physical examination are important. Comprehensive blood studies, including CBC, ESR, RA factor determination, and serum tests for immunoglobulins are done. The CBC indicates anemia and usually elevated WBC and platelet counts. The ESR is elevated during the acute stage. Biopsy specimens of involved vessels display the invasion of leukocytes. When the pulmonary system is involved, radiographic chest films show pulmonary infiltrates. Hematuria and proteinuria are present with renal involvement. Aneurysms and myocardial ischemia are indicators of cardiac involvement.

TREATMENT

Treatment addresses the underlying causative factors and the systemic involvement. Corticosteroids and analgesics afford relief. Hypertension is treated with antihypertensive drugs, usually **angiotensin-converting enzyme (ACE)** inhibitors. Ocular problems should be monitored, and patients should be taught good skin care. Patients who smoke are encouraged to stop.

Summary

The immune system is composed of a variety of specific and nonspecific defense mechanisms to counteract the threat of pathogens and other harmful agents. This system consists of lymphoid tissue and its products, as well as barriers and mechanisms that destroy and eliminate foreign particles. Healthy immune responses, such as inflammation, maintain the body's homeostasis; inappropriate, absent, or insufficient respon-

ses leave the body vulnerable to disease and disorder.

Malfunctions of the immune system include hyperactive responses, immunodeficiency disorders, and rejection responses.

An absent component of the immune system or inadequate response of the immune system induces immunodeficiency diseases, resulting in increased susceptibility to other diseases. Some of these flaws are genetic and are present at birth, whereas others manifest themselves later in life. The result is impaired resistance, recurrent infections, and increased incidence of cancer, as seen in AIDS or CVID. Other forms of immunodeficiency occur with an insufficient secretion of immunoglobulins (selective IgA deficiency), B cell deficiency (X-linked agammaglobulinemia), or a combined absence of T cell and B cell immunity (SCID). Congenital absence or underdevelopment of the thymus and parathyroid glands leaves a child with structural abnormalities and seriously compromised immunity (DiGeorge syndrome).

Often the etiology of immunodeficiency diseases is uncertain or unknown. Diagnostic tests reveal immunoglobulin levels or the titer of specific antibodies. Treatment may include anti-inflammatory and antibiotic therapies. In certain cases, replacement therapy with gamma globulin is indicated. Bone marrow transplants may be tried.

Autoimmune diseases occur when autoantibodies develop and begin to destroy the body's own cells. These diseases can occur in many body systems, resulting in anemias (autoimmune hemolytic anemia and pernicious anemia), kidney disorders, endocrine system diseases, and neurologic and vascular diseases as well. SLE and RA are thought to be autoimmune disorders; they are systemic, inflammatory, progressive syndromes. MS and myasthenia gravis, each a neurologic disorder, are presumed to be of autoimmune origin. Both these incurable disorders have remissions and exacerbations of neurologic symptoms.

Review Challenge

REVIEW QUESTIONS

1. Name the functional components of the immune system.
2. Describe the three major functions of the immune system.
3. List examples of inappropriate responses of the immune system.
4. Explain the difference between natural and acquired immunity and give examples of each.
5. Trace the formation of T cells and B cells from stem cells.
6. Explain how T cells and B cells specifically protect the body against disease.
7. List the five immunoglobulins.
8. Explain complement fixation and its importance in the immune system.
9. Describe the invasion of human immunodeficiency virus (HIV) into the T helper cells.
10. Explain the ways that HIV is transmitted.
11. List the guidelines for universal precautions and infection control.
12. Describe the primary absent or inadequate response of the immune system in the following diseases:
    Common variable immunodeficiency
    Selective immunoglobulin A deficiency
    Severe combined immunodeficiency disease
13. Explain the destructive mechanisms in autoimmune diseases.
14. Describe the symptoms and signs of pernicious anemia. Name the primary treatment.
15. Describe the systemic features of SLE. Recall the diagnostic criteria.
16. Detail the pathology of rheumatoid arthritis (RA).
17. Specify the primary objectives of the treatment for RA.
18. Compare the pathology of multiple sclerosis to that of myasthenia gravis.

REAL-LIFE CHALLENGE

Pernicious Anemia

A 46-year-old female patient reports fatigue, loss of appetite with occasional nausea and vomiting, a sore tongue, and weight loss. She also mentions weakness and numbness and loss of feeling in her hands, lower arms, feet, and lower legs. Recently, she has experienced light-headedness, visual complaints, ringing in the ears, shortness of breath, rapid pulse, and palpitations. Additionally she mentions experiencing headaches, irritability, and depression. Examination shows pale-appearing lips, tongue, and gums. Her skin and sclera appear jaundiced.

Hematology tests reveal decreased hemoglobin, RBC, WBC, and platelets and increased MCV. The RBCs and platelets appear large and malformed. Studies of bone marrow are indicative of abnormal RBC production. Gastric acid presence is either reduced or absent.

Questions

1. What is meant by megaloblastic anemia?
2. What is the importance of the intrinsic factor?
3. Why would the patient experience gastrointestinal-type symptoms?
4. What is the cause of the neurologic symptoms?
5. Why would the patient experience light-headedness, fatigue, and weakness?
6. How long must the patient continue treatment once the symptoms abate?
7. Why is the patient unable to take the vitamin B_{12} orally?
8. At the present time, what is the cure for pernicious anemia?

REAL-LIFE CHALLENGE

Rheumatoid Arthritis

A 33-year-old woman reports recent onset of pain in the joints of her fingers and hands. She recently has experienced weight loss, fatigue, and a persistent low-grade fever. On examination, the joints of the hands and fingers display tenderness, redness, warmth, and swelling. Blood tests indicate an elevated level of the rheumatoid factor. Further observation over a period of a few months shows a continuation of the symptoms with involvement of additional joints. The patient is diagnosed with rheumatoid arthritis.

Questions

1. Compare the incidence of rheumatoid arthritis in males and females.
2. Compare the symptoms and signs of rheumatoid arthritis and osteoarthritis. (See Chapter 7 for osteoarthritis.)
3. If rheumatoid arthritis is left untreated, describe the projected course.
4. What is the cause of rheumatoid arthritis?
5. Which diagnostic tests usually are ordered when rheumatoid arthritis is suspected?
6. With the primary treatment being to decrease inflammation and pain, preserve joint function, and prevent deformities, what is the usual prescribed treatment?
7. Explain the side effects the patient may experience from NSAID therapy.

RESOURCES

Lupus Foundation of America
800-558-0121
301-670-9292 in Maryland

American Lupus Society
23751 Madison St
Torrance, CA 90503
213-373-1335

National Lupus Erythematosus Foundation (NLEF)
5430 Van Nys Blvd, Ste 206
Van Nys, CA 91401
213-885-8787

National Patient Organization for Primary Immunodeficiencies (IPOPI)
(http://www.ipopi.org/)

Sjögren's Syndrome Foundation, Inc.
382 Main St
Port Washington, NY 11050
1-800-475-6473

Arthritis Foundation
3400 Peachtree Rd NE
Atlanta, GA 30329
404-320-3333
1-800-283-7800

Myasthenia Gravis Foundation
222 S. Riverside, Ste 1540
Chicago, IL 60606
1-800-541-5454

National AIDS Hotline, 24 hours a day
PO Box 13827
RTP, NC 27709
1-800-342-AIDS
(http://www.hivmail@cdc.gov)

Family AIDS Network
678 Front St NW
Grand Rapids, MI 49504

National Multiple Sclerosis Society
733 Third Ave
New York, NY 10077
(http://www.info@nmss.org)

International MS Support Foundation
PO Box 90154
Tucson, AZ 85752-0154

National Prevention Information Network
PO Box 6003
Rockville, MD 20849-6003
1-800-458-5231
(http://info@cdcnpin.org)

Primary Immunodeficiency Association
(http://www.pia.org.uk)

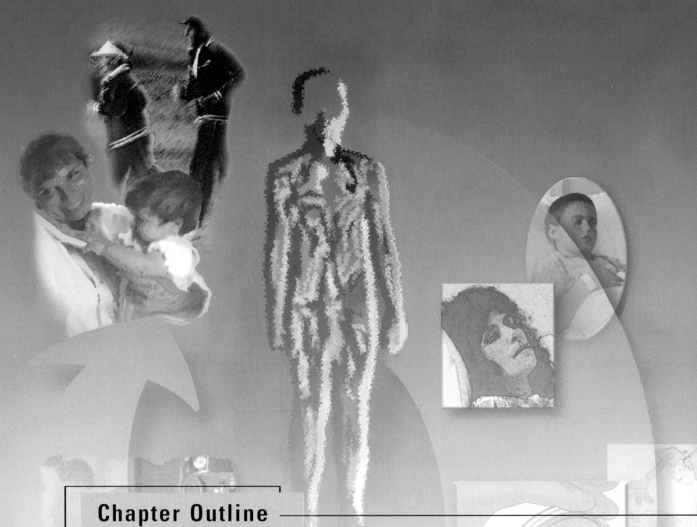

Chapter Outline

Diseases and Conditions of the Endocrine System

Learning Objectives

After studying Chapter 4, you should be able to:

1. List the major glands of the endocrine system.
2. Describe the importance of hormones and explain some of the critical body functions that they control.
3. Explain the importance of normal pituitary function.
4. Compare gigantism to acromegaly.
5. Describe the condition of dwarfism and its etiology.
6. Explain the cause of diabetes insipidus.
7. Explain the treatment of a simple goiter.
8. List the signs and symptoms of Graves' disease.
9. Distinguish between cretinism and myxedema.
10. Explain the pathogenesis involved in diabetes mellitus.
11. Classify the three types of diabetes mellitus.
12. Distinguish between diabetic coma and insulin shock.
13. Explain the medical management of all three types of diabetes mellitus.
14. Explain why hypoglycemia can be a serious medical condition.
15. Compare the signs and symptoms of thyroid hypofunction to thyroid hyperfunction.

Key Terms

acidosis	(**ass**–ih–**DOE**–sis)	hypothalamus	(**hye**–poh–**THAL**–ah–mus)
corticotropin	(**kor**–tih–ko–**TRO**–pin)		
epiphyseal	(**eh**–pih–**FEEZ**–e–al)	panhypopituitarism	(pan–**high**–poh–pih–**TOO**–ih–tair–ism)
gonadotropin	(**go**–nad–oh–**TRO**–pin)		
hyperglycemia	(**hye**–per–gli–**SEE**–me–ah)	polydipsia	(**pahl**–ee–**DIP**–see–ah)
		polyphagia	(**pahl**–ee–**FAY**–jee–ah)
hyperkalemia	(**hye**–per–ka–**LEE**–me–ah)	polyuria	(**pahl**–ee–**U**–ree–ah)
		pruritus	(pruh–**RI**–tus)
hypocalcemia	(**hye**–poh–kal–**SEE**–me–ah)	radioimmunoassay	(**ray**–dee–oh–**IM**–u–no–**ass**–a)

somatotropin	(**soh**–mat–oh–**TROH**–pin)	thyroxine	(thye–**ROKS**–in)
thyrotoxicosis	(**thye**–roh–tox–ih–**KOH**–sis)	triiodothyronine	(**try**–eye–oh–doh–**THYE**–row–neen)
thyrotropin	(thye–**ROT**–roe–pin)	vasopressin	(**vaz**–oh–**PRES**–in)

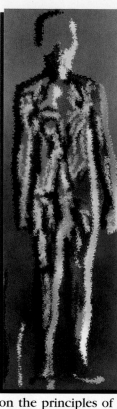

Orderly Function of the Endocrine System

Body activities, **home-ostasis,** and response to stress are controlled by two distinct interacting systems: the nervous system and the endocrine system. The systems interact as one system initiates, terminates, or extends the activity of the other. The nervous system (discussed in Chapter 13) provides an immediate but short-lived response, operating on the principles of electricity, with impulse conduction. The endocrine system has a slightly slower onset, with a more prolonged duration of action, which uses highly specific and powerful hormones to mediate its response chemically. Hormones are chemical messengers classified as either amino acids (protein) or steroids.

The endocrine system is composed of many glands scattered throughout the body; these glands secrete unique and potent chemicals called hormones directly into the blood stream (Fig. 4–1). The action of most hormones is directed to target glands or tissues at a distant receptor site, thereby regulating critical body functions such as urinary output, cellular metabolic rate, and growth and development. Hormonal secretions typically are regulated by negative feedback; information regarding the hormone level or its effect is fed back to the gland, which then responds accordingly.

Certain endocrine glands are stimulated to secrete hormones in response to other hormones. Hormones that stimulate secretion of other hormones are called *tropic* hormones. For example, the gonadotropins stimulate ovarian hormones. In diagnostic analysis, when excessive hormones

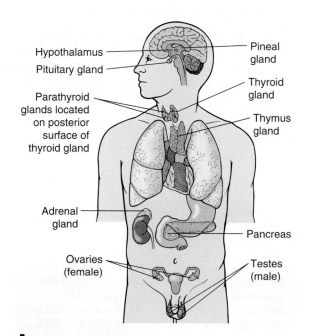

Figure 4–1

Major glands of the normal endocrine system.

result from an ectopic source (such as a malignant tumor), the tropic hormones are low. Other secreting cells that perform endocrine function may be scattered in the tissue, as in the digestive tract, where local hormones regulate its motility and secretions.

Endocrine diseases are the result of abnormally decreased or increased secretion of hormones. Manifestations of disease vary with the degree of increase or decrease of hormonal secretion and the age of the patient. This alteration in normal hormone quantities may be the result of hyperplasia, **hypertrophy,** or **atrophy** of an endocrine gland. Alterations in gland size affecting the hormone production and secretion are frequently the consequences of an insult to the gland, such as infection, radiation, trauma, surgical intervention, and inflammation. Dysfunction of an endocrine gland is associated with many physical and mental manifestations. Some common symptoms include:

- Growth abnormalities
- Emotional disturbances or psychiatric problems
- Skin, hair, and nail changes
- Edema
- Hypertension or hypotension
- **Arrhythmia**
- Changes in urinary output
- Muscle weakness and atrophy
- Menstrual irregularity or amenorrhea
- Changes in libido or impotence
- Sharp changes in energy level

To appreciate the influence of endocrine gland function on health and disease, a review of the main glands and their primary hormones is recommended (Table 4-1). The pituitary gland, called the master gland of the endocrine system, has a cascading effect on the glands it stimulates. Many activities of the pituitary gland are controlled by the hypothalamus, a part of the brain that also has endocrine functions. Pituitary dysfunction can affect some or all of the target glands of pituitary hormones, thereby indirectly influencing body structure and function.

The diagnosis of endocrine disorders depends on a correct match of the patient's symptoms with a specific hormone dysfunction and with laboratory confirmation of overproduction or underproduction of a particular hormone or hormones. Hormone levels commonly are detected by blood tests, **radioimmunoassay** (RIA), and 24-hour urine tests. Scans, ultrasound, and magnetic resonance imaging (MRI) are helpful in determining the type and location of a lesion. Bi-

opsy is used to determine whether a lesion is malignant.

Once an endocrine problem is identified, the treatment is specific to replace the hormone deficit or reduce a lesion by surgical removal or radiation therapy. Other medical therapies have emerged that inhibit the synthesis of hormones. However, therapeutic drugs may have substantial side effects.

Pituitary Gland Diseases

HYPERPITUITARISM

Hyperpituitarism, a chronic and progressive disease, is a condition caused by increased production and secretion of pituitary hormones, particularly human growth hormone (hGH). The excessive hGH results in one of two distinct conditions, gigantism or acromegaly, depending on the time of life when the dysfunction begins.

Gigantism

SYMPTOMS AND SIGNS

When the hypersecretion of hGH occurs before puberty, gigantism, a proportional overgrowth of all body tissue, occurs. The child experiences abnormal and accelerated growth, especially of the long bones, because **epiphyseal** closure has not begun. The very young child may have an arched palate and slanting eyes. Frequently, sexual and mental development are retarded.

ETIOLOGY

An anterior pituitary **adenoma** is frequently the cause of oversecretion of hGH that results in gigantism. Although a genetic link has not been determined, gigantism occasionally affects multiple members of a family.

DIAGNOSIS

The clinical picture of the abnormal growth of the prepubescent child leads the physician to perform diagnostic investigations. Levels of hGH are elevated on RIA. Various forms of imaging of the skull, such as radiography, computed tomography (CT), and arteriography, indicate the pres-

TABLE 4-1 ➤ Major Endocrine Gland Secretions and Functions

ENDOCRINE GLAND	HORMONE	TARGET ACTION
Anterior pituitary	Growth hormone (GH)	Promotes bone and tissue growth
	Thyrotropin (thyroid-stimulating hormone [TSH])	Stimulates thyroid gland and production of thyroxine
	Corticotropin (adrenocorticotropic hormone [ACTH])	Stimulates adrenal cortex to produce glucocorticoids
	Gonadotropins	
	Follicle-stimulating hormone (FSH)	Initiates growth of eggs in ovaries; stimulates spermatogenesis in testes
	Luteinizing hormone (LH)	Causes ovulation; stimulates ovary to produce estrogen and progesterone; stimulates testosterone production
	Prolactin	Stimulates breast development and formation of milk during pregnancy and post partum
	Melanocyte-stimulating hormone (MSH)	Regulates skin pigmentation
Posterior pituitary	Vasopressin (antidiuretic hormone [ADH])	Stimulates water resorption by renal tubules; has antidiuretic effect
	Oxytocin	Stimulates uterine contractions, stimulates ejection of milk in mammary glands; causes ejection of secretions in male prostate gland
Thyroid	Thyroxine (T_4) and triiodothyronine (T_3)—thyroid hormone (TH)	Regulates rate of cellular metabolism (catabolic phase)
	Calcitonin	Promotes retention of calcium and phosphorus in bone; opposes effect of parathyroid hormone
Parathyroid	Parathyroid hormone (parathormone, PTH)	Regulates metabolism of calcium; elevates serum calcium levels by drawing calcium from bones
Adrenal cortex	Mineralocorticoids (MC), primarily aldosterone	Promote retention of sodium by kidneys; regulate electrolyte and fluid homeostasis
	Glucocorticoids (GC): cortisol, corticosterone, cortisone	Regulate metabolism of carbohydrates, proteins, and fats in cells
	Gonadocorticoids: androgens, estrogens, progestins	Govern secondary sex characteristics and masculinization
Adrenal medulla	Catecholamines: epinephrine and norepinephrine	Produce quick-acting "fight or flight" response during stress; increase blood pressure, heart rate, and blood glucose level; dilate bronchioles
Pancreas	Insulin	Regulates metabolism of glucose in body cells; maintains proper blood glucose level
	Glucagon	Increases concentration of glucose in blood by causing conversion of glycogen to glucose
Ovaries	Estrogens	Cause development of female secondary sex characteristics
	Progesterone	Prepares and maintains endometrium for implantation and pregnancy
Testes	Testosterone	Stimulates and promotes growth of male secondary sex characteristics and is essential for erections
Thymus	Thymosin	Promotes development of immune cells (gland atrophies during adulthood)
Pineal gland	Melatonin	Regulates daily patterns of sleep and wakefulness
		Inhibits hormones that affect ovaries; other functions unknown

ence of a pituitary lesion. Bone radiographic films show thickening of the cranium and long bones.

TREATMENT

The object of treatment is to decrease the amount of hGH that is secreted. This is accomplished by either radiation of the pituitary gland or surgical intervention to reduce its size. Yearly follow-up examinations are recommended.

Acromegaly

SYMPTOMS AND SIGNS

When the hypersecretion of hGH occurs after puberty and epiphyseal closure, acromegaly (an overgrowth of the bones of the face, hands, and feet) occurs, along with an excessive overgrowth of soft tissue (Fig. 4-2). The patient notices that it is necessary to wear larger gloves or shoes or

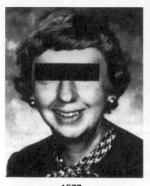
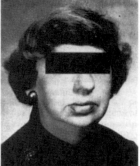
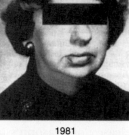

1977

1981

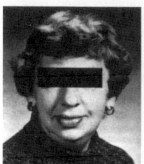
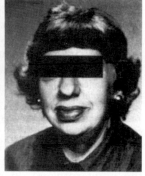

1983

1988

Figure 4–2

Clinical features of acromegaly. (From Bennett JC, Plum F: Cecil Textbook of Medicine, 20th ed, vol 2, Philadelphia: WB Saunders, 1996, p 1212. Used with permission.)

both. An increase in the size of the jaw causes larger spaces between the teeth.

ETIOLOGY

As with gigantism, a pituitary tumor or adenoma often is the cause of acromegaly.

DIAGNOSIS

The clinical picture of abnormal thickening of the bones of the face, hands, and feet leads the physician to perform diagnostic tests. Levels of hGH are elevated on RIA. Various forms of imaging of the skull, such as radiography, CT, and arteriography, indicate the presence of a pituitary lesion along with a thickening of the bones.

TREATMENT

The object of treatment is to decrease the amount of hGH that is secreted. Correction of the disorder prevents further disfigurement and

reduces mortality that results from excess growth hormone production. This is accomplished by either radiation of the pituitary gland or surgical intervention to reduce its size.

HYPOPITUITARISM

SYMPTOMS AND SIGNS

Hypopituitarism is a condition caused by deficiency or absence of any of the pituitary hormones, especially those produced by the anterior pituitary lobe. Because the anterior pituitary secretes several major hormones, the syndrome can be complex, marked by metabolic dysfunction, sexual immaturity, or growth retardation. Physical findings vary with the specific hormone deficiency. Deficiency of pituitary hormones that stimulate other endocrine glands can result in the atrophy of those glands. When thyrotropin (thyroid-stimulating hormone [TSH]) secretion is diminished, the functioning of the thyroid gland is affected and the patient experiences symptoms of hypothyroidism. Salt balance and metabolism of nutrients are affected when the secretion of corticotropin (adrenocorticotropic hormone [ACTH]) dwindles. Gonadotropin deficiency causes sexual functions, including sexual development, menstruation, and libido, to become diminished.

Hypopituitarism produces growth retardation in children. Headache and blindness are signs of infringement on the optic nerve resulting from tumor growth.

ETIOLOGY

The cause of hypopituitarism may be a pituitary tumor or a tumor of the hypothalamus. In some instances, hypopituitarism results from damage to the pituitary gland caused by radiation or surgical removal or from **ischemia** of the gland owing to **infarct,** tumor, or basilar skull fracture. If the ischemia is severe and not reversed, permanent destruction of glandular tissue ensues. Destruction of the entire anterior lobe is termed **panhypopituitarism,** and none of the important anterior pituitary hormones are secreted. The condition is most common in women, and sometimes the cause is unknown.

DIAGNOSIS

When the patient presents with the clinical symptoms of hyposecretion of any of the anterior pituitary hormones, a complete medical evaluation is necessary to pinpoint the diagnosis. A

103

history of head trauma, previous radiation, or a surgical procedure to the gland or nearby tissue is significant in the diagnosis. Plasma levels of all or some of the pituitary hormones are low. Radiographic films of the skull, cranial CT, and MRI scans are used to identify tumors. The clinical investigation must rule out disease of the target glands themselves.

TREATMENT

The age of the patient, the severity and type of deficiency, and the underlying cause of hypopituitarism determine the course of treatment. When neoplasia is the cause, removal of the tumor eases the symptoms. Replacement therapy with hormonal supplements, including thyroxine, cortisone, somatrem or somatropin (hGH), and sex hormones, is usually effective. Continued monitoring of hormone levels is required during hormone replacement therapy.

DWARFISM

SYMPTOMS AND SIGNS

Dwarfism is the abnormal underdevelopment of the body, or hypopituitarism, occurring in children. Hyposecretion of the pituitary gland hormones, especially hGH, results in growth retardation. As a result, the child is extremely short, with a body that is small in proportion. The prepubescent child does not develop secondary sex characteristics. The condition may be linked to other defects and a varying degree of mental retardation.

ETIOLOGY

Dwarfism can be congenital or the result of a cranial hemorrhage after the birth process. Occasionally, there is no identifiable cause. A deficiency of the growth hormone–releasing hormone (GH-RH) produced by the hypothalamus is termed secondary hypopituitarism and results from head trauma, tumor, or infection.

DIAGNOSIS

Physical examination shows that the child fails to grow at a normal rate and is short in stature. The child's general health appears to be good. However, secondary tooth eruption is delayed, and fat deposits may be noted in the lower trunk area. Persistently low serum hGH levels are found. A CT scan may confirm the presence of a cranial tumor.

TREATMENT

Somatotropin (hGH) is administered until the child reaches a height of 5 feet. These children also may need replacement of thyroid and adrenal hormones. As they approach puberty, sex hormones are administered, if necessary.

DIABETES INSIPIDUS

SYMPTOMS AND SIGNS

Diabetes insipidus is a deficiency in the release of vasopressin (antidiuretic hormone [ADH]) by the posterior pituitary gland, resulting in the excretion of copious amounts of colorless and dilute urine. The patient experiences excessive thirst, fatigue, and symptoms of dehydration, including dry mucous membranes, hypotension, dizziness, constipation, and poor skin turgor.

ETIOLOGY

In diabetes insipidus, the posterior pituitary gland releases reduced amounts of vasopressin. The condition may be hereditary, or it may be the result of an insult to the hypothalamus or to the pituitary gland. In many cases, the cause is unknown. When there is a deficiency of vasopressin, the distal tubules of the nephron do not reabsorb water from the filtrate back into the blood stream; consequently, the volume of urine is excessive.

DIAGNOSIS

The presence of polyuria and polydipsia leads the clinician to investigate the composition of the urine by laboratory tests. Urinalysis that reveals an almost colorless urine that has a low specific gravity (<1.005) suggests diabetes insipidus as a diagnosis. To confirm the diagnosis of diabetes insipidus, the person is given a water restriction test during which the kidneys exhibit the inability to concentrate urine when the person is deprived of fluid intake for several hours. After the patient has lost 3% of his or her body weight or hypotension becomes severe, vasopressin is administered. Urine volume and specific gravity amounts are compared. Decreased urine output and increased specific gravity after vasopressin administration indicate diabetes insipidus.

TREATMENT

Treatment consists of the administration of vasopressin injections or nasal spray therapy with lypressin (Diapid) or desmopressin acetate

(DDAVP). The presence of any underlying cause should be determined and treated. When the excessive diuresis is the outcome of trauma to the pituitary gland, the symptoms begin to subside as the insult resolves and inflammation is reduced.

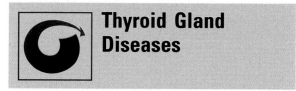

Thyroid Gland Diseases

Thyroid diseases present as functional disturbances that cause individuals to suffer from excessive or diminished secretions of thyroid hormones thyroxine (T_4) and triiodothyronine (T_3). Table 4-2 illustrates a comparison of thyroid diseases and their signs and symptoms.

SIMPLE GOITER

SYMPTOMS AND SIGNS

Simple goiter, a hyperplasia of the thyroid gland, may be **asymptomatic** in the early stages. The patient, who is usually female, may be unaware of the condition until the anterior aspect of the neck enlarges with a conspicuous swollen mass, called a goiter (Fig. 4-3). As the hyperplasia increases, pressure is exerted on the trachea, producing **dyspnea,** and on the esophagus, pro-

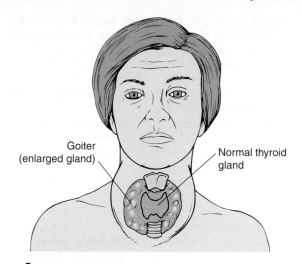

ducing difficulty in swallowing. A large goiter can cause dizziness or **syncope.**

ETIOLOGY

Simple, or nontoxic, goiter results from inadequate amounts of iodine in the diet. Iodine is necessary for the synthesis of both triiodothyronine (T_3) and thyroxine (T_4), together known as thyroid hormone, which are produced by the

Figure 4–3

Thyroid enlargement typical of goiter.

TABLE 4–2 ➤ Comparison of Hypothyroid and Hyperthyroid Disorders

	HYPOFUNCTION OF THYROID	HYPERFUNCTION OF THYROID
Names or Types	Congenital, untreated can become cretinism or thyroid dwarfism	Hyperthyroidism
	Thyroiditis–Myxedema	Thyrotoxicosis
	Hashimoto's disease	Graves' disease–autoimmune with or without exophthalmos
	Iodine deficiency–simple goiter	Toxic nodular hyperplasia
	Idiopathic hypothyroidism	Toxic adenoma, thyroid tumors
Symptoms and Signs	Decreased activity, sleepy, lethargic	Restlessness, irritability, easily fatigued, nervousness
	Decreased mental alertness	
	Tires easily	Tremors
	Skin and hair dry, decreased sweating	Skin moist, increased sweating
	Cold intolerance	Heat intolerance
	Bradycardia	Tachycardia and palpitations
	Constipation	Diarrhea
	Weight gain	Weight loss, increased appetite
	Edema, bloated face, puffy eyelids	Polydipsia
	Poor circulation, extremity edema	Loss or thinning of hair
	TSH levels increased	TSH levels decreased
	T_3, T_4 levels decreased	T_3, T_4 levels increased
	I^{131} uptake decreased	I^{131} uptake increased

I^{131}, radioactive iodine; T_3, triiodothyronine; T_4, thyroxine; TSH, thyroid-stimulating hormone.

thyroid gland. The inadequate blood level of thyroid hormone causes the anterior pituitary gland to secrete increased amounts of thyrotropin. Thyrotropin keeps attempting to stimulate the thyroid gland to produce thyroid hormone. This continued stimulation in turn causes the thyroid gland to increase in size.

Geographic regions in which the soil had low levels of iodine and where seafood was not readily available had high rates of simple goiter. The advent of rapid refrigerated transportation of seafood and fresh vegetables from areas in which soil and water iodine levels are high has decreased the **endemic** aspects of this condition. Sporadic occurrence of a simple goiter can result from ingestion of large amounts of **goitrogenic** foods such as turnips and cabbage or drugs such as lithium.

DIAGNOSIS

Diagnosis is made by examination of the neck, noting the enlargement of the thyroid gland (goiter). Blood studies indicate elevated thyrotropin levels and decreased levels of T_3 and T_4.

TREATMENT

Treatment in the early stages is simple: the administration of one drop per week of saturated solution of potassium iodide. Prevention calls for the addition of iodine to the diet, including the use of iodized salt. Sporadic goiter requires avoidance of goitrogenic drugs or food. When a large goiter is unresponsive to treatment, a subtotal **thyroidectomy** may be required.

HASHIMOTO'S DISEASE

SYMPTOMS AND SIGNS

Hashimoto's disease (chronic thyroiditis) is a chronic disease of the immune system that attacks the thyroid gland; it occurs in women 8 times as often as men and is the leading cause of nonsimple goiter and hypothyroidism. The outstanding clinical feature is the goiter, which causes a feeling of pressure in the neck and difficulty with swallowing. Symptoms of hypothyroidism, such as sensitivity to cold, weight gain, and mental apathy, appear as the disease progresses.

ETIOLOGY

The cause of Hashimoto's disease is unknown; a genetic factor is suspected. Autoimmune factors play a prominent role because antibodies appear to destroy thyroid tissue instead of stimulating it. The gland enlarges as a result of an inflammatory process, with massive infiltration by lymphocytes and plasma cells, resulting in replacement of gland tissue with fibrous tissue.

DIAGNOSIS

Thyroid function is measured by a radioactive iodine uptake (RAIU) test. Autoantibodies against thyroid tissue are present in the blood. In Hashimoto's disease, characteristic changes can be seen in the thyroid gland with needle biopsy and examination of the gland tissue.

TREATMENT

The treatment is lifelong replacement of thyroid hormone. This also prevents further growth of the goiter.

HYPERTHYROIDISM

Graves' Disease

SYMPTOMS AND SIGNS

Graves' disease, a condition of primary hyperthyroidism, occurs when the entire thyroid gland hypertrophies, resulting in a goiter. Overproduction of thyroid hormone causes increased metabolism and multisystem changes. The patient has rapid heartbeat and palpitations, nervousness, excitability, and insomnia. Despite excessive appetite and food ingestion, the patient loses weight. Profuse perspiration and warm moist skin cause the person to be intolerant of hot weather. Other symptoms include excessive thirst, nausea and vomiting, muscular weakness, and dermopathy. As the condition advances, the eyes develop exophthalmos, an outward protrusion, which gives the patient a staring expression (Fig. 4-4). A sudden exacerbation of symptoms may signal **thyrotoxicosis,** or thyroid storm, which can be life threatening.

ETIOLOGY

The cause of Graves' disease is uncertain; however, it is believed to be an autoimmune response. The hyperactivity of the thyroid gland is stimulated by antibodies to thyroid antigens. There is a familial predisposition that strongly suggests genetic causation.

DIAGNOSIS

The clinical picture and a thorough history are the first steps in the diagnosis. Serum T_3 and T_4 levels are increased, and a thyroid scan indicates increased uptake of radioiodine. Blood tests may reveal elevated levels of certain antithyroid immunoglobulins.

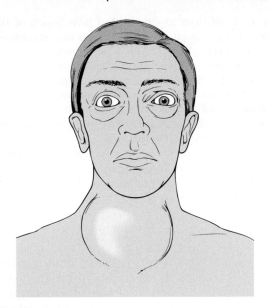

Figure 4–4

Exophthalmos and goiter in Graves' disease.

TREATMENT

Treatment begins with the administration of antithyroid drugs such as propylthiouracil and methimazole (Tapazole) to block thyroid hormone synthesis. Beta-blockers such as propranolol hydrochloride (Inderal) and atenolol (Tenormin) are given to treat **tachycardia** and hypertension. In nonresponsive or severe cases, radioactive iodine therapy or surgery is used to reduce the activity of the thyroid gland. Patients require ongoing medical supervision to monitor thyroid hormone levels. Some patients need help to cope with the anxiety and physical discomforts associated with Graves' disease.

HYPOTHYROIDISM

Cretinism

SYMPTOMS AND SIGNS

Cretinism is a congenital hypothyroid condition in which the thyroid gland is lacking or thyroid hormone is not synthesized by the thyroid gland; this causes mental and growth retardation in the infant or young child. The child develops as a dwarf, stocky in stature with a protruding abdomen. Other physical characteristics include the following: a short forehead, a broad nose, small wide-set eyes with puffy eyelids, a wide-open mouth with a thick, protruding tongue, an expressionless face, and dry skin. The sex organs fail to develop. Growth and physical and mental capabilities are retarded. A lack of muscle tone contributes to an inability to stand or walk.

ETIOLOGY

An error in fetal development may cause the thyroid gland not to develop or to be nonfunctional. There may be a congenital absence of one of the enzymes necessary for T_3 and T_4 synthesis. Antithyroid drugs taken during pregnancy may be an etiologic factor.

DIAGNOSIS

A blood test that indicates a lack of or abnormally low amounts of T_4 in the presence of an elevated level of thyrotropin is indicative of cretinism. Thyroid scan shows decreased levels of iodine uptake and confirms the absence of thyroid tissue. If cretinism is not detected during the neonatal period, the infant will be slow to smile and eventually will be developmentally retarded.

TREATMENT

The prognosis is good when cretinism is discovered early in life and replacement of thyroxine is begun. Even skeletal abnormalities are reversible with treatment. This replacement therapy needs to continue throughout the life of the patient.

Myxedema

SYMPTOMS AND SIGNS

Myxedema, severe hypothyroidism with reduced levels of T_4, has its onset in adult life. As levels of T_4 decrease, metabolism is slowed and there is the insidious onset of systemic conditions. The patient, who is usually female, experiences **menorrhagia.** The skin becomes dry and scaly, with little or no perspiration. The face becomes bloated, the tongue thick, and the eyelids puffy (Fig. 4–5). Muscular weakness, excessive tiredness, and fatigue are common symptoms. Weight gain, loss of hair, constipation, and intolerance to cold are experienced. Speech becomes slow and slurred, with mental apathy, and there are diminished physical capabilities. In severe cases, myxedema coma, a rare but life-threatening emergency, can occur; this is best treated with intensive care.

ETIOLOGY

The thyroid gland's ability to synthesize T_4 is impaired. This can be the result of reduced

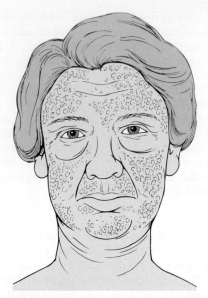

Figure 4–5

Typical facial appearance of a myxedematous woman.

amounts of thyrotropin, radiation destruction of the thyroid gland, surgical removal of the gland without T_4 replacement therapy, tumor, or failure of the thyroid gland to function. The disorder also may be secondary to failure of the pituitary to produce thyrotropin.

DIAGNOSIS

The retardation of physical and mental capabilities leads the physician to perform diagnostic tests. Blood studies indicate abnormally low levels of T_4 or thyrotropin, or both. Radioactive iodine uptake tests may indicate no response to thyrotropin.

TREATMENT

Levothyroxine sodium (T_4), a therapeutic agent, is administered. Response to hormone replacement therapy is usually good, and the symptoms improve. The patient should be informed that replacement therapy likely will be required for the rest of his or her life.

CANCER OF THE THYROID GLAND

SYMPTOMS AND SIGNS

Palpation of a hard painless lump or nodule on the thyroid gland is often the first indication of thyroid cancer. The **pathogenesis** varies with

the form of thyroid cancer and how much of the gland is destroyed by tumor. Signs and symptoms of hypothyroidism result when enough thyroid tissue is destroyed; mental apathy and sensitivity to cold develop. Some tumors trigger secretion of excessive thyroid hormones, which cause symptoms of hyperthyroidism, such as nervousness, irritability, tachycardia, weight loss, and heat intolerance. **Dysphagia** and **stridor** may indicate pressure on neck structures by a space-occupying lesion. Some thyroid cancer **metastasizes** quickly to distant sites and causes severe hormonal alteration.

ETIOLOGY

As with many forms of cancer, the etiology is unknown. It has been associated with radiation therapy to the neck. Metastasis to the thyroid of breast, lung, or kidney cancer or of malignant melanoma is possible. Some forms of thyroid cancer are thought to be inherited.

DIAGNOSIS

Suspicion of thyroid gland cancer arises with the presence of the palpable lump or nodule. The diagnosis is confirmed with needle aspiration biopsy. Thyroid profile blood tests and RAIU studies may indicate abnormal levels. Ultrasonography shows a lesion that has an irregular display. Thyroid cancer is staged and classified by size, site of origin, extent of lymph node involvement, and metastasis.

TREATMENT

Surgical removal of the thyroid gland usually is indicated for all types of thyroid cancer. Radiation or radioactive iodine therapy may be attempted along with chemotherapy if metastasis is widespread. Lifetime T_4 replacement therapy is required.

Parathyroid Gland Diseases

HYPERPARATHYROIDISM

SYMPTOMS AND SIGNS

Hyperparathyroidism is a condition caused by overactivity of one or more of the four parathyroid glands and results in the overproduction of parathyroid hormone (parathormone [PTH]). Hyperparathyroidism increases the breakdown of bone (demineralization) with the subsequent release of excessive calcium into the blood (hypercalcemia) and extracellular fluid. Hypercalcemia is responsible for the symptoms of hyperparathyroidism. Hypercalcemia decreases the irritability of nerve and muscle tissue, and this causes the patient to experience muscle weakness and atrophy, gastrointestinal pain, and nausea and vomiting. High serum calcium levels increase the irritability of the cardiac muscle, causing arrhythmias. Increased deposit of calcium in soft tissue causes low back pain and **renal calculi.** Bone tenderness, arthritis-type pain, and easy fracturing of the bones is the result of demineralization of the bone.

ETIOLOGY

The cause of primary hyperparathyroidism is increased activity of the parathyroid gland, usually as a result of a parathyroid tumor (adenoma) or an **idiopathic** hyperplasia of the gland. Secondary hyperparathyroidism may be caused by an increased secretion of PTH induced by a low level of serum calcium due to renal disease or other disorders.

DIAGNOSIS

A high concentration of serum PTH is noted on RIA. Blood calcium, chloride, and alkaline phosphatase levels are elevated, and serum phosphorus levels are decreased. The calcium level in urine is increased. Diffuse demineralization of bones along with bone cysts is evident on radiographic films; cortical bone absorption also is noted along with erosion of the middle phalanx.

TREATMENT

The treatment plan for hyperparathyroidism varies with the cause. If the hypersecretion of PTH is caused by an adenoma, the tumor is removed. If hypertrophy is the origin of the hypersecretion, part or all of a gland is removed. Limitation of dietary intake of calcium is helpful, as is **diuresis** by forcing fluid intake and administering loop diuretics (furosemide [Lasix] or ethacrynic acid [Edecrin]), with resulting excretion of calcium and sodium. When the condition is secondary, the underlying cause must be treated and the blood serum calcium levels lowered. Drugs that increase the excretion of calcium by the kidneys or inhibit the reabsorption of calcium from bone may be used.

HYPOPARATHYROIDISM

SYMPTOMS AND SIGNS

Hypoparathyroidism is an insufficient secretion of PTH by the parathyroid glands. PTH promotes calcium retention by the bones. When this hormone level is insufficient, circulating levels of calcium are reduced, resulting in hypocalcemia, with excessive deposit of calcium into bone tissue. A consequence of the hypocalcemia is a hyperexcitable nervous system, resulting in an overstimulation of the skeletal muscles. Initial symptoms include numbness and tingling of fingertips, toes, ears, or nose, followed by muscular spasms or twitching of the hands and feet; **tetany,** or severe sustained muscular contractions, may develop. Emotional changes, confusion, and irritability may be experienced. Sustained hypocalcemia leads to laryngospasm, arrhythmias, respiratory paralysis, and death.

ETIOLOGY

The cause may rest in the parathyroid gland itself or stem from raised blood calcium levels, which, by negative feedback, cause decreased PTH output. Acquired hypoparathyroidism can be the result of injury to one or more of the parathyroid glands, ischemia from an infarct, accidental radiation, **neoplasia,** or various disease processes. Accidental surgical removal of the parathyroid gland during thyroidectomy can induce hypocalcemia. The condition may originate from an **autoimmune** genetic disorder or from a congenital absence of the glands.

DIAGNOSIS

The clinical picture of neuromuscular hyperexcitability, along with a history of possible insult to the parathyroid glands, leads the physician to further investigation. The presence of **Trousseau's phenomenon** is a sure indication of hypocalcemia. Blood studies indicate decreased serum calcium levels and increased serum phosphate levels. Increased bone density is evident on radiographic films. An **electrocardiogram** discloses increased QT and ST intervals. PTH levels are decreased on RIA.

TREATMENT

Replacement therapy of calcium along with vitamin D reduces hypocalcemia. This replacement therapy is usually lifelong unless the condition is reversible. In the case of a life-threatening deficiency (tetany), intravenous calcium gluconate is administered. The patient is encouraged to follow a high-calcium, low-phosphorus diet.

Adrenal Gland Diseases

CUSHING'S SYNDROME

SYMPTOMS AND SIGNS

Cushing's syndrome is caused by hypersecretion of the adrenal cortex, which results in excessive circulating cortisol levels. The patient with Cushing's syndrome experiences fatigue, muscular weakness, and changes in body appearance. Fat deposits form in the scapular area (buffalo humps) and in the trunk, causing a protruding abdomen. Salt and water retention results not only in hypertension and edema, but also in the characteristic moon face noted in the patient with Cushing's syndrome. The patient may show clinical evidence of **hyperlipidemia,** osteoporosis, and atherosclerosis. Psychiatric problems are common. The skin becomes thin, has a tendency to bruise easily, and develops red or purple striae (stretch marks). Other symptoms includes excessive hair growth, amenorrhea, and impotence. The person also may have diabetes mellitus.

ETIOLOGY

Excessive circulating cortisol levels can be caused by hyperplasia of the adrenal gland, excessive secretion of **corticotropin** from the pituitary gland, a tumor of the adrenal cortex, or production of corticotropin in another organ (because of extrapituitary tumors). Prolonged administration or large doses of corticosteroids used to treat other diseases can induce Cushing's syndrome.

DIAGNOSIS

The typical picture of the moon face, buffalo hump, and gross obesity of the trunk, particularly the abdomen, leads the physician to further investigation. Continuous elevation of serum cortisol levels is found in Cushing's syndrome. Elevated free cortisol levels are present in 24-hour urine collections.

TREATMENT

Treatment of Cushing's syndrome depends on the cause of the oversecretion of cortisol. When

a tumor is the cause, surgical removal or radiation of the tumor is indicated (Fig. 4-6). Drug therapy to suppress ACTH secretions can be employed separately or as an adjunct to radiation.

ADDISON'S DISEASE

SYMPTOMS AND SIGNS

Addison's disease, adrenal insufficiency or hypoadrenalism, is manifested as symptoms of fatigue, weakness, weight loss, and gastrointestinal disturbances. A typical bronze color of the skin is exhibited. The patient can experience cardiovascular difficulties, including irregular pulse, decreased cardiac output, and orthostatic (postural) hypotension. Decreased levels of aldosterone cause an inability to retain salt and water. When dehydration, hyperkalemia, and electrolyte imbalance occur, the condition is life threatening.

ETIOLOGY

The onset of Addison's disease is usually gradual, with progressive destruction of the adrenal gland and diminishment of its many important hormones. The destruction can be the result of an autoimmune process, tuberculosis, hemorrhage, fungal infections, **neoplasms,** or surgical removal. Familial tendencies exist. It also can be secondary to hypopituitarism, in which there is a decreased output of corticotropin.

DIAGNOSIS

Blood and urine cortisol levels are low, as are serum sodium and fasting glucose levels. Serum potassium, blood urea nitrogen, lymphocyte, and eosinophil levels and **hematocrit** are elevated. Adrenal calcification is identified by radiographic film, as is a smaller-than-normal heart.

TREATMENT

Treatment includes replacement of the natural hormones with glucocorticoid and mineralocorticoid drugs, increased fluid intake, control of salt and potassium intake, and a diet high in carbohydrate and protein. Hormone replacement therapy with close medical supervision must continue for life. The patient must be educated regarding symptoms of overdosage and underdosage and the role of stress and infection in Addison's disease. Insufficiency or a sudden decrease in adrenocortical hormone levels, such as from a sudden withdrawal of glucocorticoid therapy, can result in a life-threatening emergency, called an *addisonian crisis.*

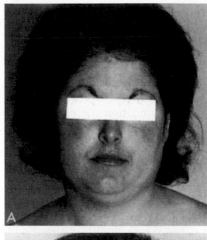
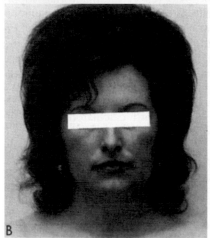
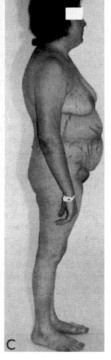

Figure 4–6

The appearance of a patient with Cushing's syndrome: *A*, before, and *B*, 1 year after removal of an adrenal adenoma; *C*, profile before treatment. (From Wyngaarden J, Smith L, Bennett J: Cecil Textbook of Medicine, 19th ed. Philadelphia: WB Saunders, 1992, p. 1285 Used with permission.)

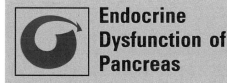

Endocrine Dysfunction of Pancreas

DIABETES MELLITUS

SYMPTOMS AND SIGNS

Diabetes mellitus is a chronic disorder of carbohydrate, fat, and protein metabolism caused by inadequate production of insulin by the pancreas or faulty utilization of insulin by the cells. Insulin lowers levels of glucose in the blood by transporting glucose into the cells for use as energy and storage as glycogen. Decreased insulin results in **hyperglycemia.** Cells therefore are deprived of fuel, and they begin to metabolize fats and proteins; this process allows wastes called ketone bodies to accumulate in the blood (ketosis). Hyperglycemia and ketosis then are at the root of the principal symptoms: polyuria, polyphagia, polydipsia, weight loss, and fatigue. The patient may have **pruritus,** especially in the genital area, and a fruity odor to the breath may be noted. Diagnostic tests of the blood and urine point to the common signs of diabetes mellitus.

There are two primary forms of diabetes mellitus:

1. Type I. Juvenile onset is insulin dependent with an early onset, usually before 30 years of age, with little or no insulin being secreted by the patient, and can be difficult to control. Also referred to as insulin-dependent diabetes mellitus (IDDM).

2. Type II. Adult onset, is non-insulin dependent having a gradual onset in adults older than

40 years of age. Non-insulin dependent diabetes (NIDDM) is the more common form where some pancreatic function permits control of symptoms by dietary management.

There are many systemic complications of untreated or poorly managed diabetes. Even with good compliance with treatment, diabetics are prone to retinopathy, which leads to blindness. Other complications include neuropathy, atherosclerosis, infection, myocardial infarction, and cerebrovascular accidents.

ETIOLOGY

In most instances, the cause of diabetes mellitus, although an ancient disease, is unknown. Both forms seem to be linked genetically. In type I, IDDM, an autoimmune process may be triggered by infection early in life, which produces antibodies that destroy the beta cells of the pancreas. Type II, NIDDM, tends to occur in older, overweight adults. Destruction of the pancreas by tumor, trauma to the pituitary gland, or other endocrine disorders can induce diabetes mellitus. Suppression of insulin production also may be drug induced. Some genetic disorders render the body's insulin receptors insensitive to insulin.

DIAGNOSIS

The diagnosis of diabetes mellitus is straightforward. The patient is assessed carefully for the cardinal symptoms. A positive fasting blood glucose test result and the presence of glucose and acetone in the urine confirm the diagnosis. Other tests include blood insulin level determination and an ophthalmic examination for diabetic retinopathy.

TREATMENT

The goal of treatment is to normalize blood glucose levels and thus prevent complications. Management of diabetes is multifactorial, incorporating a well-balanced diet that is closely related to insulin administration, if needed, exercise, blood and urine testing, and hygienic measures. Patient compliance and education are vital to the control of symptoms and complications.

Type I diabetics may require insulin injections that correlate closely with calculated caloric intake on a regular schedule and consistent, moderate exercise. Type II diabetics (NIDDM) usually do not require insulin injections to control blood glucose levels; their therapeutic regimen includes restricted caloric intake and exercise, although some require oral medications.

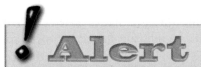

HYPOGLYCEMIC AGENTS: INFORMATION AND WARNINGS

Glucophage. Glucophage should not be taken by patients with a history of kidney disease, congestive heart failure, history of liver disease, and alcoholism. Patients should be instructed to stop taking Glucophage before any imaging procedures with injectable contrast agents. Also, the surgeon is to be notified of Glucophage use before any surgery so that he or she may decide whether to discontinue the medication until after the surgical procedure.

A rare but serious side effect of Glucophage is lactic acidosis. Therefore, patients for whom Glucophage is prescribed must be cautioned about symptoms and signs of lactic acidosis and must be provided with warning for an awareness of certain side effects.

The symptoms and signs of lactic acidosis are weakness, fatigue, unusual muscle pain, dyspnea, unusual stomach discomfort, dizziness or lightheadedness, and bradycardia or cardiac arrhythmias. *Stop* the Glucophage immediately and contact the physician.

Various forms of oral drug therapy currently are used to treat type II diabetes (NIDDM). The sulfonylureas (oral hypoglycemic drugs) such as glipizide (Glucotrol) and glyburide (DiaBeta or Micronase) stimulate the pancreas to produce insulin. These medications are usually taken once a day, and blood glucose levels need to be monitored on a regular schedule. Because sulfonylureas stimulate increased insulin production by the pancreas, the increased levels of insulin have a tendency to lower blood glucose levels, often resulting in symptoms and complications of hypoglycemia.

Metformin hydrochloride (Glucophage) approaches NIDDM with a trilateral concept. It prevents the liver from producing hepatic glucose, decreases intestinal absorption of glucose, and increases available insulin utilization. Under normal circumstances, metformin hydrochloride does not elevate blood insulin levels and therefore does not produce hypoglycemia.

Acarbose (Precose), an alpha-glucosidase inhibitor, works in the gastrointestinal tract to delay the digestion of carbohydrates and lengthens the time it takes for carbohydrates to convert to glucose, mainly affecting blood sugar levels after eating. An annoying side effect is the formation of intestinal gas and resulting flatus.

Diabetic control is monitored daily mainly by blood glucose determination using a blood glucose level device and by testing of urine glucose and acetone levels. These monitoring techniques are taught to patients so that they can use them at home. With experience, the patient can interpret the results and make simple modifications in insulin dosage and caloric intake to maintain precise blood glucose control. All diabetic persons are encouraged to reach and maintain appropriate body weight. Also, patients must be made aware that the balance between insulin and glucose requirements is upset easily by trauma and infection. Regular medical supervision is encouraged, especially for insulin-dependent persons. The patient and family members must be educated to recognize the symptoms of diabetic coma (high blood glucose levels) and insulin shock (too much insulin) and to implement immediate action to correct these serious complications (Table 4–3).

TABLE 4–3 ➤ **Warning Signs and Interventions for Diabetic Coma and Insulin Reaction**	
DIABETIC COMA	**INSULIN REACTION**
Causes	
Undiagnosed diabetes	Too much insulin
Skipped insulin dose	Delayed meal
Too much food	Insufficient food
Infection or stress	Excessive exercise
Symptoms and Signs	
Slow onset	Rapid onset
Thirst	Hunger
Increased urination	Trembling and paleness
Nausea and vomiting	Feeling faint
Abdominal pain	Cold sweat
Drowsiness	Headache
Lethargy	Anxiety
Flushed appearance	Rapid heartbeat
Dry skin	Irritability
Fruity breath odor	Impaired vision
Dehydration	Hypoglycemia
Heavy respirations	Confusion
Dilated, fixed pupils	Seizures
Hyperglycemia	Loss of consciousness
Ketoacidosis	
Loss of consciousness	
Coma	
Intervention	
Give insulin, fluids, and salt	If awake, give simple sugar, candy, orange juice, or soda
If severe, give intravenous fluids, insulin, and sodium bicarbonate	If unconscious, give intravenous dextrose or glucagon

GESTATIONAL DIABETES

SYMPTOMS AND SIGNS

Gestational diabetes mellitus (GDM), or type III diabetes, is the damaged ability to process carbohydrate, which has its onset during pregnancy. The pregnant patient may be asymptomatic or she may exhibit the usual signs of diabetes mellitus: polyuria, polydipsia, and polyphagia. Routine urine screening, done during each prenatal visit, indicates the presence of glucose. The condition usually disappears after delivery. Thirty to forty percent of women who have had GDM develop type II diabetes within 5 to 10 years later.

ETIOLOGY

There are signs that destruction of insulin by the placenta plays a role in causing GDM. Increased maternal insulin production results in increased placental production of human placental lactogen (hPL). This is followed by the diminished effectiveness of maternal insulin. The fetus takes its glucose from the mother, stressing the balance of glucose production and glucose utilization. Elevated levels of estrogen and progesterone block the action of insulin.

DIAGNOSIS

The first indication of GDM is when the routine prenatal urine glucose test demonstrates the presence of glucose in the urine. A fasting blood glucose determination indicates elevated levels of glucose. Other serum tests are glucose tolerance tests, 2-hour **postprandial** (oral glucose tolerance) tests, and glycohemoglobin tests. Elevations above normal levels yield a positive diagnosis.

TREATMENT

The medical management of GDM is similar to the treatment of any diabetes; the diet is controlled, and intake of simple sugars is limited. Consistent moderate exercise, such as walking, is encouraged. Oral hypoglycemic agents may be prescribed, or insulin may be indicated. The patient is instructed to monitor blood glucose levels with finger sticks and glucometer testing. If delivery of the infant and placenta does not terminate the condition, a therapeutic diabetic regimen needs to continue.

HYPOGLYCEMIA

SYMPTOMS AND SIGNS

Hypoglycemia, a deficiency of glucose (sugar) in the blood, can be a serious condition. It occurs when excessive insulin enters the blood stream or when the glucose release rate falls behind tissue demands. This condition may exist despite adequate food intake. The symptoms include sweating, nervousness, weakness, hunger, dizziness, trembling, headache, and palpitations. Because glucose is the primary fuel of the brain, the consequences of hypoglycemia can be severe. Extremely low blood glucose levels can cause central nervous system manifestations, including confusion, visual disturbances, behavior that may be mistaken for drunkenness, stupor, coma, and seizures. Hypoglycemic syndromes are classified as drug induced (the most common) or non–drug induced.

ETIOLOGY

The major cause of drug-induced hypoglycemia is insulin overdosage in a diabetic subject; failure to eat a meal or too much exercise also can trigger hypoglycemia in the insulin-dependent diabetic. A person with a significantly elevated blood alcohol level can experience alcoholic hypoglycemia. **Sulfonylureas** can induce hypoglycemia. Non–drug-induced hypoglycemia can result from fasting, delayed or excessive secretion of insulin by the pancreas, adenoma or carcinoma of the pancreas, gastrointestinal disorders, or various hereditary or endocrine disorders.

DIAGNOSIS

The diagnosis requires evidence that the symptoms correlate with a low blood glucose level and are remedied by raising the blood glucose level. The glucometer, or a blood reagent strip, can be used as a quick screening test for abnormally low blood glucose levels in patients with symptoms of hypoglycemia. The blood glucose level is further evaluated by a glucose tolerance test. An abnormally low plasma glucose level usually is defined as less than 40 mg/dl in men or less than 45 mg/dl in women after a period of fasting. The diagnosis is uncomplicated when the initial assessment suggests a probable cause, such as a history of insulin use, excessive ingestion of alcohol, and the use of sulfonylureas in treatment.

TREATMENT

In acute hypoglycemia, the priority is to restore a normal blood glucose level with intravenous infusion of glucose. The hormone glucagon also may be given to counteract the effects of insulin. As the patient's condition is stabilized, a complex carbohydrate and protein snack is given to keep the blood glucose level within normal limits. Identification of the underlying cause of hypoglycemia dictates the long-term management of the disorder. An insulin-dependent diabetic always should be prepared to ward off an attack of hypoglycemia by carrying glucose tablets to take at the first sign of hypoglycemia. Hypoglycemia associated with tumors may require surgery. Dietary modifications are made to correct hereditary fructose intolerance or gastrointestinal conditions that provoke symptoms.

Precocious Puberty

PRECOCIOUS PUBERTY IN BOYS

SYMPTOMS AND SIGNS

Precocious, or earlier than expected, sexual maturity in the male is manifested by early development of secondary sex characteristics, gonadal development, and spermatogenesis. The patient's history may include altered growth pattern or emotional disturbances. Pubic hair and the beard begin to grow, the gonads and the penis increase in size, and sebaceous gland activity is increased. The onset of male puberty usually occurs between 13 and 15 years; the onset is considered precocious before 10 years of age.

ETIOLOGY

Idiopathic precocity may be transmitted genetically. Normally, the hypothalamus initiates puberty by stimulating the pituitary gland. Because the pituitary gland secretes vital gonadotropic hormones that stimulate the testes to produce sex hormones, many problems involving sexual development can be traced to pituitary dysfunction. Intracranial pituitary or hypothalamic neoplasia can cause excessive or premature secretion of gonadotropin. Testicular tumors and other endocrine disorders can induce precocious development.

DIAGNOSIS

Obvious physical and emotional signs of precocity are noted. Diagnostic tests include blood tests for elevated hormone levels, brain scans and electroencephalographic (EEG) studies, skull and bone radiographic studies, chromosomal **karyotype** studies, and testing of a 24-hour urine specimen for steroid excretion levels.

TREATMENT

The therapy depends on the cause of precocious puberty. When the boy's condition is idiopathic, no specific treatment may be needed. Taking hormones known as progestogens may suppress sexual maturity until the appropriate time for the onset of puberty. When the cause is testicular tumor or brain tumor, the treatment is more invasive and the prognosis is guarded. Other endocrine disorders may require lifelong hormone therapy. Genetic counseling and psychological care are important.

PRECOCIOUS PUBERTY IN GIRLS

SYMPTOMS AND SIGNS

Precocious, or earlier than expected, sexual maturity in the female is marked by increased growth rate, breast enlargement, and the appearance of pubic hair and underarm hair before 8 years of age; the onset of menstruation (menarche) may occur before 10 years of age. Ovarian function makes pregnancy a possibility. Emotional problems may occur.

ETIOLOGY

In most cases, precocious puberty in girls is idiopathic, without associated abnormalities. Uncommon causes include intracranial tumors, encephalopathy, **meningitis,** and endocrine disorders. The ingestion of oral contraceptives, other estrogen-containing drugs, or meat with a high estrogen content is a rare cause. Infrequently, hormone-secreting ovarian or adrenal neoplasms are causative.

DIAGNOSIS

Blood serum levels of follicle-stimulating hormone (FSH), luteinizing hormone (LH), and sex steroids are in the normal adult range. Urinalysis for hormone levels and excretion of 17-ketosteroids shows elevated levels. RIA for both FSH and LH demonstrates elevated concentrations of the hormones in blood plasma. Other diagnostic studies to determine the cause include ultrasonography, electroencephalography, CT, and MRI.

TREATMENT

As in male precocity, the treatment of precocious female puberty depends on the cause. Tumors, if treatable, may require surgery or radiation. Hormone therapy may be used to suppress the secretion of gonadotropins and to prevent menstruation in true precocious female puberty. The girl and her family may benefit from mental health counseling to develop coping skills for emotional problems. Parents need to understand that there is a contradiction between physical maturity and psychological immaturity and that precocious puberty does not necessarily trigger sexual behavior.

Summary

The primary function of the endocrine system is to produce hormones that are carried in the bloodstream throughout the body to affect certain cells. Endocrine diseases are the result of abnormally increased or decreased secretions of hormones. Causes and effects of these changes vary with the age of the patient and the severity of dysfunction. Major endocrine pathology frequently relates to hyperfunction of a gland, hypofunction of a gland, or a tumor.

- Diseases that affect the widespread influence of the pituitary gland produce many clinical and mental manifestations. Hyperpituitarism resulting from oversecretion of human growth hormone (hGH) produces gigantism before puberty and acromegaly after puberty.
- Deficiency of pituitary hormones can cause a complex set of conditions because the anterior pituitary gland secretes several major hormones.
- A comparison of hypofunction and hyperfunction of the thyroid gland reveals many opposite signs and symptoms.

- Hyperthyroidism may have several causes, including Graves' disease or cancer of the thyroid gland.
- Cretinism is a congenital hypothyroid condition that causes mental and growth retardation in the infant or child; myxedema has its onset of hypothyroidism in adult life.
- Hyperfunction or hypofunction of the parathyroid glands causes disturbances in the balance of calcium in the body.
- Disease conditions of the adrenal cortex induce metabolic disturbances that manifest as an excess (e.g., Cushing's syndrome) or a deficiency (e.g., Addison's disease) of adrenal steroids.
- There are three forms of diabetes mellitus: type I, or insulin-dependent (IDDM), type II, or non–insulin-dependent (NIDDM), and type III, or gestational diabetes mellitus (GDM).
- Hyperglycemia and ketosis are the cardinal signs of diabetes mellitus and are responsible for many of the symptoms.
- Insulin overdosage can precipitate the onset of acute hypoglycemia.

Review Challenge

REVIEW QUESTIONS

1. Name the major glands of the endocrine system.
2. What are some ways in which the endocrine system influences health and disease?
3. Describe two conditions that are the result of increased production and secretion of pituitary human growth hormone (hGH).
4. What pathologic changes may be experienced from hypopituitarism? Why is the age of the individual significant?
5. What causes diabetes insipidus?
6. What causes the thyroid gland to enlarge in the individual with a simple goiter?
7. Which hypothyroid condition (or chronic thyroiditis) is thought to be caused by autoimmune factors?
8. Describe the signs and symptoms of Graves' disease.
9. Explain the relationship of hypoparathyroidism to hypocalcemia.
10. What disease may be induced by prolonged administration or large doses of corticosteroids?
11. What are the possible causes of Addison's disease?
12. Compare the cause and treatment of type I, type II, and type III diabetes mellitus.
13. Distinguish between diabetic coma and insulin shock.
14. How are hypoglycemic syndromes classified?
15. What are the possible causes of precocious puberty in boys and girls?

REAL-LIFE CHALLENGE

Hypothyroidism

A 40-year-old woman reports being tired, loss of hair, and weight gain. She has not had a menstrual period for 3 months. Her skin appears dry and scaly. On questioning, the patient reports episodes of constipation and tells of being unable to tolerate cold. Her speech is somewhat slow and slightly slurred. Blood test for thyroid functioning indicates low thyrotropin levels. Thyroid scan shows no uptake of thyrotropin. The diagnosis of this patient is hypothyroidism.

Questions

1. Hypothyroidism with maturity onset also often is termed *myxedema*. What is hypothyroidism with onset in infancy or early childhood called?
2. What causes the insidious onset of the various complaints and conditions of the patient with hypothyroidism?
3. What can be the cause of the reduced production of T_4 by the thyroid gland?
4. Hormone replacement is the usual drug therapy of choice. Research Synthroid (levothyroxine sodium) and explain its side effects.
5. For patient teaching, how long will the patient have to take the medication?

REAL-LIFE CHALLENGE

Diabetes Mellitus

A 50-year-old man became lethargic and drowsy with flushed dry skin after eating a large meal. His family became concerned when he was difficult to rouse, and he had a fruity odor to his breath. He was transported to an emergency facility, where he gave a history of extreme thirst, hunger, and frequent urination. He recently had an upper respiratory infection that had been slow to clear. Adult maturity onset diabetes mellitus is suspected.

Questions

1. Which blood test would be ordered?
2. What are normal blood glucose levels?
3. What are some of the possible causes of adult onset NIDDM?
4. In addition to the symptoms previously described, what else might be observed?
5. What determines the course of the treatment prescribed?
6. Why is glucose level monitoring important?
7. What patient teaching should be considered?
8. Why is diet important?
9. Explain how insulin works.
10. What is the therapeutic action of the sulfonylureas?
11. How does Glucophage (metformin hydrochloride) lower blood glucose levels?

RESOURCES

National Diabetes Information Clearinghouse (NDIC)
PO Box NDIC
Bethesda, MD 20892
301-468-2162
(http://www.niddk.nih.gov)

American Diabetes Association
800-ADA-DISC
703-549-1500 in Virginia and
Washington, DC, metro area
(http://www.diabetes.org)

Juvenile Diabetes Foundation International Hotline
120 Wall St, 19th Floor
New York, NY 10005
800-223-1138
212-785-9595 in New York

Children with Diabetes
(http://www.chilrenwithdiabetes.com)

American Thyroid Association
Mayo Clinic
200 First St NW
Rochester, MN 55905
(http://www.thyroid.org)
(http://www.thyroid.com)

Endocrine Society
9650 Rockville Pike
Bethesda, MD 20814
(http://www.endo-society.org)

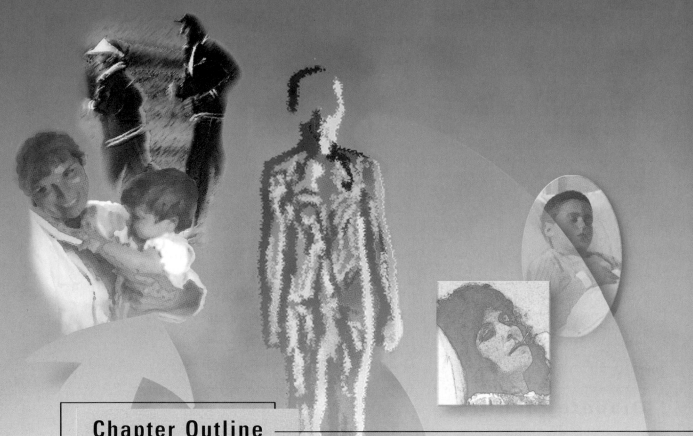

Chapter Outline

Diseases and Disorders of the Eye and Ear

Learning Objectives

After studying Chapter 5, you should be able to:

1. Describe the process of vision and hearing.
2. Recall and define the four main refractive errors of vision.
3. Compare the pathology and etiology of nystagmus to that of strabismus.
4. Explain the importance of early treatment of glaucoma.
5. Name the possible causes of conjunctivitis.
6. List the causes of cataracts.
7. Explain the susceptibility of diabetics to diabetic retinopathy.
8. Characterize the visual disturbance caused by macular degeneration.
9. Explain why early diagnosis and treatment is important for retinal detachment.
10. Compare conductive hearing loss to sensorineural hearing loss.
11. List the symptoms of otitis externa.
12. Describe the treatment of otitis media.
13. Explain the signs and symptoms of Meniere's disease.
14. Consider the importance of prevention of sensorineural deafness.

Key Terms

amblyopia	(**am**–blee–**OH**–pee–ah)	otoscopy	(oh–**TOSS**–ko–pee)
blepharitis	(**blef**–ar–**RIE**–tis)	retinopathy	(**ret**–ih–**NOP**–ah–thee)
cryotherapy	(kry–o–**THER**–ah–pee)	seborrhea	(seb–oh–**RHEE**–ah)
diplopia	(dih–**PLO**–pee–ah)	sensorineural	(**sen**–so–ree–**NEU**–rol)
iridotomy	(ir–ih–**DOT**–oh–me)		
labyrinth	(**LAB**–ih–rinth)	tinnitus	(tih–**NIE**–tus)
macula	(**MACK**–you–la)	tonometry	(tohn–**AHM**–eh–tree)
meibomian	(my–**BO**–mee–an)	tympanoplasty	(**tim**–pan–oh–**PLAS**–tee)
myringotomy	(mir–in–**GOT**–oh–me)		
orthoptic	(or–**THOP**–tic)	vertigo	(**VER**–tih–go)

Disorders of the Eye

Functioning Organs of Vision

Major organs of special sense include the eye and the ear. The functional process of vision takes place in the presence of light in the following manner: (1) an image is formed on the retina (refraction); (2) the rods and cones are stimulated, and (3) nerve impulses are conducted to the brain. The portion of the brain that deals with sight is much larger than the portions that deal with the other senses. Before the pathophysiology of ocular disease is discussed, the complex structure of the eye is reviewed (Fig. 5–1).

The eyeball, similar in shape to a sphere, has a wall of primary structures in three concentric layers—the sclera, the choroid, and the retina—and is connected to the brain by way of the optic nerve.

The sclera, the outermost layer, consists of tough fibrous connective tissue that is visible as the white of the eye. Attached to the sclera are the extrinsic muscles that move the eye. The cornea, the colorless transparent structure on the front of the eye, is continuous with the sclera on the anterior aspect of the globe. This transparent structure, the window of the eye, helps to focus the light rays as they enter the eye.

Next to the sclera is the middle layer of tissue called the choroid. The choroid has dark pigment cells whose function it is to absorb excess light rays that interfere with vision. Anteriorly, this layer is continuous with the ciliary body and the iris. These vascular structures supply the tissues of the eye with oxygen and nutrients. Anteriorly, the choroid joins the ciliary body, which contains ciliary muscles used to focus the lens of the eye. The ciliary processes in the ciliary body secrete aqueous humor, the fluid found in the anterior portion of the eye. The ciliary body is connected by suspensory ligaments to the biconvex, transparent lens of the eye. Contraction of the ciliary muscles causes the suspensory ligaments to relax. The lens then bulges, allowing for focusing necessary for close vision.

Also attached to the ciliary body is the iris, or colored portion of the eye, which helps to regu-

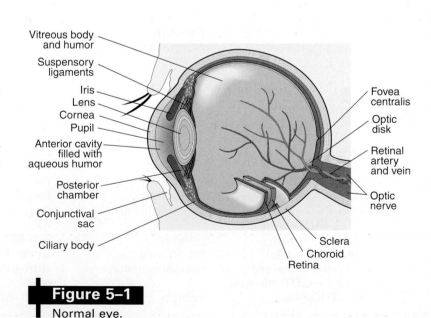

Figure 5–1

Normal eye.

late the amount of light entering the eye. In brightness, the iris contracts, causing the opening in the center of the iris, the pupil, to become smaller. In limited light, the iris relaxes and the pupil enlarges, permitting more light to enter the eye.

The innermost layer, covering the posterior three quarters of the eye, is called the retina. The retina is a light-sensitive layer made up of sensor-receptive cells called rods and cones. The rods function best in dim light, enabling night vision, whereas the cones function in bright light and also detect color and fine detail. Within the rods and cones, the image initiates a chemical reaction, sending a message through the nerve fiber layer of the retina to the optic nerve. The optic nerve penetrates the fibrous layers at the optic disk and continues to the brain. The optic disk contains no receptor cells and often is called the blind spot of the eye. The optic nerve transmits the image to the portion of the brain that is used for vision. The brain interprets the impulses from each eye and produces a single three-dimensional image. The **macula** lutea, a yellow spot, lies lateral to the optic disk. In the center of the macula lutea is the fovea centralis, the area that produces the sharpest image.

Covering the anterior visible portion of the sclera is a thin transparent membrane called the conjunctiva. It begins at the edge of the cornea and extends over the exposed sclera and turns anteriorly to line the inside portion of the lids. This creates both a superior cul-de-sac and an inferior cul-de-sac where the conjunctiva reflects from the sclerae to the lids. The space between the iris, the colored portion of the eye, and the anterior clear cornea is called the anterior chamber. The space immediately behind the iris and anterior to the lens is called the posterior chamber. The fluid occupying the anterior and posterior chambers is a watery substance called the aqueous humor. This is produced by the ciliary body and exits the anterior chamber through a drainage system located at the junction of the

base of the iris and the cornea. Appropriate pressure within the eye is maintained by the aqueous humor, which eventually enters the general circulation of the body. The large cavity behind the lens is the vitreous body; it contains a jelly-like fluid called the vitreous humor. It helps to maintain the globular shape of the eyeball while aiding the refraction of images.

The internal lens of the eye is elastic and therefore can focus images both near and distant. The focusing is carried out by contraction and relaxation of the muscles of the ciliary body. This permits the lens to assume either a more spherical or a flatter shape, depending on the focus required. The lens is attached to the ciliary body by small strands of tissue called zonules. These are attached 360° around the lens. When the ciliary body relaxes, the zonules are pulled, causing a flattening of the lens, which is used for focusing a distant image.

Light rays are the key to sight. The light rays enter the eye and pass through the cornea, aqueous humor, lens, and vitreous humor. These rays can travel either in a straight line or they can be bent. The process of bending lights rays is known as refraction. A concave surface causes the light rays to scatter or diverge whereas a convex surface does the opposite, bringing the light rays closer together and causing them to converge. The cornea, aqueous humor, lens, and vitreous humor all have the capability of bending or refracting the light rays so that they can focus on the retina. The image that forms on the retina is backward and upside down. The image is turned around in the brain, and the visual concept is interpreted in the correct manner. Another step in the process of vision includes accommodation. Adjustments must be made in the eye for the focusing or sharpness of vision according to the distance of the object being viewed. The process of accommodation involves changing the shape of the lens, making it either flat or bulging. The ciliary muscle and the sus-

TABLE 5-1 ➤ The Extrinsic Muscles of the Eye

MUSCLE	FUNCTION	CRANIAL INNERVATION
Inferior rectus	Causes the eye to look down	Oculomotor nerve (III)
Lateral rectus	Rotates eye laterally	Abducens nerve (VI)
Medial rectus	Rotates eye medially	Oculomotor nerve (III)
Superior rectus	Causes eye to look up	Oculomotor nerve (III)
Inferior oblique	Causes eye to roll, to look up and to the side	Oculomotor nerve (III)
Superior oblique	Causes eye to roll, to look down and to the side	Trochlear nerve (IV)

pensory ligaments contract and relax in opposition to accomplish this task.

There are six extrinsic muscles involved in controlling the movements of the eye by pulling on the eyeballs, making the two move together to center in on one visual field (Table 5–1). Normally, the eyes work together; an assessment of the functioning of these muscles often is included in a neurologic assessment.

Common symptoms of eye diseases and conditions that should be called to the attention of the physician include:

- Redness of the eye
- Pain or burning in or around the eye
- Visual disturbances.

Refractive Errors

There are four main refractive errors that result when the eye is unable to focus light effectively on the retina.

HYPEROPIA (FARSIGHTEDNESS)

Hyperopia (farsightedness) occurs when light that enters the eye focuses behind the retina, which requires an extra amount of focusing of the internal lens or the use of a corrective lens to place the object on the retina to obtain a sharp image. Near vision is strained whereas distance vision is usually clear. Hyperopia occurs when the eyeball is abnormally short (Fig. 5–2).

MYOPIA (NEARSIGHTEDNESS)

Myopia (nearsightedness) results when light rays entering the eye focus in front of the retina, causing the vision to be blurred. Near objects can be seen clearly; however, distant objects are blurry, and the image cannot be sharpened by the internal lens of the eye. Myopia occurs when the eyeball is abnormally long (Fig. 5–3).

ASTIGMATISM

Astigmatism is an irregular focusing of the light rays entering the eye. It usually is caused by a cornea that is not spherical. The front of the cornea may be more egg shaped than spherical, causing light rays to be unevenly or diffusely fo-

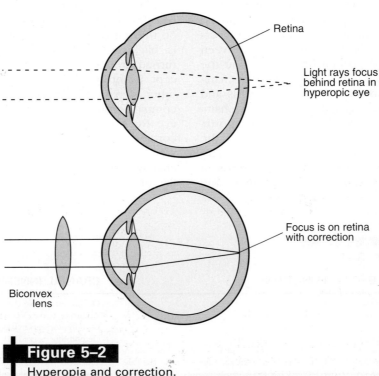

Figure 5–2

Hyperopia and correction.

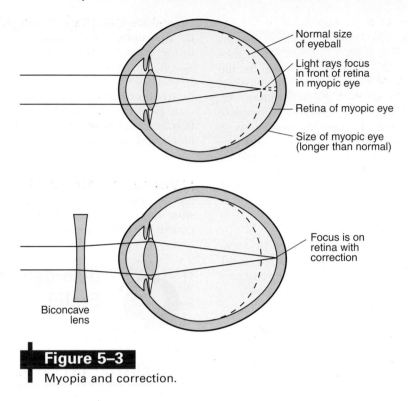

- Normal size of eyeball
- Light rays focus in front of retina in myopic eye
- Retina of myopic eye
- Size of myopic eye (longer than normal)
- Focus is on retina with correction
- Biconcave lens

Figure 5–3
Myopia and correction.

123

cused across the retina. This causes some images to appear clearly defined, whereas others appear blurred.

PRESBYOPIA

Presbyopia is the inability to focus quickly and refocus with the internal lens because of loss of its elasticity, which generally is caused by aging. This usually occurs in the mid-40s.

SYMPTOMS AND SIGNS

The primary symptom of a refractive error is blurred vision. This can lead to squinting, frequent rubbing of the eyes, and headaches. These symptoms are in addition to the previously mentioned refractive errors.

ETIOLOGY

Some refractive errors seem to be familial, which suggests a genetic link.

DIAGNOSIS

Tests for visual acuity, **ophthalmoscopic** examination, and evaluation with various lenses are used in the diagnosis of refractive errors.

TREATMENT

The correction of refractive errors involves the use of artificial lenses in the form of eyeglasses or contact lenses. A surgical procedure can be done to correct myopia and astigmatism; it is called a radial keratotomy. It involves making small, shallow incisions in the outer portion of the cornea, causing it to flatten in desired areas. This is an invasive procedure and has been successful; however, there is the potential for significant complications.

 Nystagmus

SYMPTOMS AND SIGNS

Any repetitive or involuntary movement of one or both eyes is called nystagmus. Eye movements that are horizontal, vertical, or circular, or a combination of these, are symptoms of nystagmus. Blurred vision also can be a symptom.

ETIOLOGY

Brain tumors and cerebrovascular lesions cause nystagmus. Acquired nystagmus results when a disease process produces lesions in the brain or inner ear. Alcohol use and abuse of certain drugs also may cause this condition. Acquired nystagmus always necessitates a complete neurologic evaluation. Congenital nystagmus is the most common type and often accompanies poor vision arising from congenital abnormalities. Nystagmus is not necessarily associated with brain lesions and may consist of abnormal development of the retina.

DIAGNOSIS

Nystagmus usually can be diagnosed by viewing the eyes externally and observing any involuntary movement. Other, more specific, complex tests are also available for definitive diagnosis.

TREATMENT

Nystagmus is managed by treating the underlying cause of the condition. Congenital nystagmus often remains present for the life of the individual and cannot be treated successfully.

Strabismus

SYMPTOMS AND SIGNS

A failure of the eyes to look in the same direction at the same time, which occurs because of weakness in the muscles controlling the position of one eye, is called strabismus. In esotropia (convergent strabismus, or cross-eye), one eye turns inward; in exotropia (divergent strabismus, or wall-eye), one eye turns outward. With either form, the main symptom is **diplopia** if strabismus is acquired in an adult. In congenital strabismus, diplopia is usually not present.

ETIOLOGY

Esotropia usually develops in infancy or early childhood and may be associated with **amblyopia.** Amblyopia is reversible until the retina is fully developed at about 7 years of age. In almost all cases, esotropia that develops in adults is caused by a condition or disease elsewhere in the body. Either the nerves between the brain and the eye muscles or the muscles themselves are affected. These diseases and conditions in-

clude diabetes mellitus, temporal arteritis, muscular dystrophy, high blood pressure, and trauma to the brain.

DIAGNOSIS

To discover the underlying cause, the physician performs a complete ophthalmic examination and orders various radiographic studies and blood and urine tests.

TREATMENT

Strabismus should be treated early. Corrective glasses, **orthoptic training,** or surgery to restore the eye muscle balance may be used in the course of the treatment.

Disorders of the Eyelid

HORDEOLUM (STYE)

SYMPTOMS AND SIGNS

Styes are inflammatory infections of the hair follicles of the eyelids (Fig. 5-4). They occur most often at the outside edge of the lid. Pain, swelling, redness, and the formation of pus at the site are the main symptoms of a stye. Patients may report a feeling of having "something in the eye."

ETIOLOGY

Styes usually result from a staphylococcal infection. They often are associated with and sec-

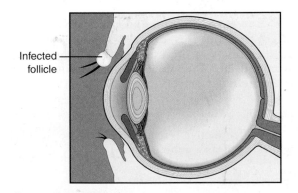

Figure 5–4
Hordeolum (stye).

ondary to blepharitis (see Blepharitis). Recurrence is common.

DIAGNOSIS

Visual examination is usually sufficient for the diagnosis. To confirm that the infection is caused by staphylococci, a culture may be taken.

TREATMENT

To hasten the relief from pain, hot compresses may be applied to the eye as soon as the inflammation appears. If recurrence becomes a problem, topical or systemic antibiotics may be needed.

CHALAZION

SYMPTOMS AND SIGNS

A chalazion, also called a meibomian cyst, is a painless, slow-growing mass or swelling on the margin or body of the eyelid. It can vary in size from barely visible to the size of a pea. Chalazions can become infected, producing redness, swelling, and pain.

ETIOLOGY

Chalazions are caused by a blockage of fluid from one of the meibomian glands, which lubricate the eyelid margin.

DIAGNOSIS

Visual examination and patient history are all that is necessary for the diagnosis.

TREATMENT

Small chalazions usually disappear spontaneously over a month or two. Larger pea-sized chalazions do not spontaneously disappear and need to be removed surgically. This is a minor procedure that often can be done in the ophthalmologist's office or in an outpatient setting.

KERATITIS

SYMPTOMS AND SIGNS

Inflammation with superficial ulceration of the cornea is known as keratitis. Symptoms are decreased visual acuity, irritation, tearing, **photophobia,** and mild redness of the conjunctiva. Pain or numbness of the cornea soon follows and is an important sign.

ETIOLOGY

Keratitis frequently is caused by an infection resulting from the herpes simplex virus. This is

especially likely when it is preceded by an upper respiratory infection (URI) with facial cold sores (see Herpes Simplex [Cold Sores] in Chapter 8). Certain bacteria and fungi also can be responsible for keratitis. Other forms of keratitis can be caused by corneal trauma or exposure of the cornea to dry air or intense light, as occurs during welding.

DIAGNOSIS

Examination of the cornea using a slit lamp confirms the diagnosis. Medical history may indicate a recent URI, and visual acuity may be decreased.

TREATMENT

Ophthalmic ointments and eyedrops may be prescribed, and the administration of a broad-spectrum antibiotic prevents any secondary infections. An eye patch may be necessary for comfort because of the photophobia.

BLEPHARITIS

SYMPTOMS AND SIGNS

Blepharitis is inflammation of the margins of the eyelids involving hair follicles and glands. It can be either ulcerative or nonulcerative. Blepharitis causes an unattractive, persistent redness and crusting on and around the eyelids. Symptoms may include itching, a burning sensation, or a feeling of a foreign body present in the eye. In severe cases, **ulcers** can develop on the eyelid margins, eyelashes can fall out, and the scales can flake from the eyelids and get into the eye, causing conjunctivitis (see Conjunctivitis).

ETIOLOGY

The ulcerative form is usually the result of a staphylococcal infection. Nonulcerative blepharitis can be caused by allergies or exposure to smoke, dust, or chemicals. This condition also can be secondary to **seborrhea** of the eyelid's sebaceous glands, and there is often a history of repeated hordeolum (see Hordeolum [Stye]) and chalazions (see Chalazion).

DIAGNOSIS

Visual examination of the eyelids and a culture of the material found around the eyelids may be necessary to determine the presence of staphylococci.

125

TREATMENT

If the condition does not improve within 2 weeks of cleaning the eyes twice a day with warm salt water, a physician should be consulted. Antibiotic or sulfonamide ophthalmic ointments may be needed.

ENTROPION

SYMPTOMS AND SIGNS

In this condition, the eyelid margins, more often the lower lid, turn inward, causing the lashes to rub the conjunctiva (Fig. 5–5). The patient has a foreign body sensation, tearing, itching, and redness. Continuous rubbing may cause conjunctivitis (see Conjunctivitis) or corneal ulcers (see Corneal Abrasion or Ulcer). Entropion damages the cornea and causes vision problems if not corrected.

ETIOLOGY

This condition most often affects older people. With aging, the fibrous tissue on the lower eyelids becomes loose, resulting in excessive contraction of the eyelid muscle. This excessive contraction causes the eyelids to turn inward, allowing the lashes to irritate the conjunctiva.

DIAGNOSIS

Visual examination reveals the inversion of the eyelid. The lashes are visible on the conjunctiva, along with the redness resulting from the irritation.

TREATMENT

If the condition does not clear up on its own, a physician should be seen. A minor surgical procedure on the eyelid corrects the problem.

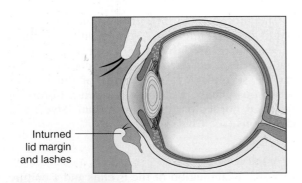

Inturned lid margin and lashes

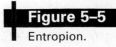
Figure 5–5
Entropion.

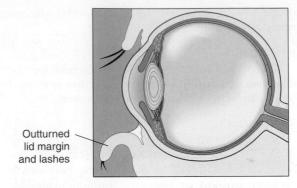

Outturned lid margin and lashes

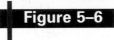
Figure 5–6

ECTROPION

SYMPTOMS AND SIGNS

With ectropion, in which the lower eyelid everts from the eyeball, the exposed surface of the eyeball and the lining of the eyelid become dry and irritated (Fig. 5–6). Tears are prevented from entering the tear duct and run down the cheeks. The patient reports dryness in the eye and tearing.

ETIOLOGY

This condition usually occurs in the elderly because the muscle in the lower eyelid becomes weak. Ectropion also can be caused by a scar on the eyelid or cheek that contracts, pulling down on the eyelid. If it is not treated, ectropion can cause the development of corneal ulcers and permanent damage to the cornea.

DIAGNOSIS

Visual examination indicates the problem, and a history of symptoms confirms the diagnosis.

TREATMENT

The condition rarely disappears on its own; therefore, a physician should be consulted. A minor surgical procedure corrects the condition.

BLEPHAROPTOSIS

SYMPTOMS AND SIGNS

Blepharoptosis, also called ptosis, is a permanent drooping of the upper eyelid so that it partially or completely covers the eye (Fig. 5–7). It usually affects one eye, but both can be involved. The condition can vary in severity

126

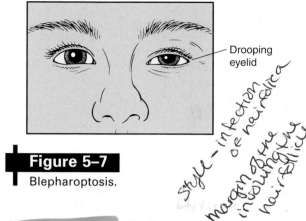

Drooping eyelid

Figure 5–7
Blepharoptosis.

style — infection of hair follicle
margin of the involving the hair follicle

throughout the day. Blepharoptosis occurs at any age, is often familial, and, if severe, blocks the vision of the affected eye.

ETIOLOGY

This condition is caused by a weakness of the muscle that raises the eyelid. It also can occur when the muscle of the eyelid or the nerve that controls the muscle is damaged by secondary trauma. Several diseases, such as diabetes mellitus, muscular dystrophy, myasthenia gravis, and brain tumor can cause ptosis.

DIAGNOSIS

If vision is affected, or if a previously normal upper eyelid begins to droop, a physician should be consulted. In addition to an ophthalmic examination, blood tests may be ordered to rule out underlying disease.

TREATMENT

Surgery

An operation can be performed to strengthen the muscle of the eyelid, or a support to keep the eyelid raised can be incorporated into glasses. Successful treatment of any underlying disease should correct the blepharoptosis.

CONJUNCTIVITIS

SYMPTOMS AND SIGNS

pinkeye and highly contagious

Inflammation of the conjunctiva, the mucous membrane that covers the anterior portion of the eyeball and lines the eyelids is called conjunctivitis. Conjunctivitis can be either unilateral or bilateral and is common. Symptoms include redness, swelling, and itching of the sclera and conjunctiva. The eyes may tear excessively and be extra sensitive to light. In cases of infectious conjunctivitis, pus is discharged from the eye, and this condition (pinkeye) is highly contagious.

ETIOLOGY

Conjunctivitis can be caused by infection, either viral or bacterial, and also by irritation from allergies, chemicals, or ultraviolet light. Infections often are transmitted when contaminated fingers, washcloths, or towels touch the eyes. Except in rare instances, conjunctivitis is usually not a serious condition, although recurrences are common.

DIAGNOSIS

Trachimus

Ophthalmic examination reveals inflammation of the conjunctiva. To identify bacterial or viral organisms, samples of the discharge are taken for culture and sensitivity tests.

TREATMENT

The treatment varies depending on the causative agents. The eyes should be kept free from discharge. This can be accomplished with warm compresses applied to the eyes 3 or 4 times a day for about 10 to 15 minutes at a time. For bacterial infections, antibiotics are needed. They can be in the form of ophthalmic preparations or systemic medications. Usually, 1 to 2 weeks of treatment clears up this type of infection. Viral infections usually are self-limiting.

10–14 days w/o treatment

Disorders of the Globe of the Eye

CORNEAL ABRASION OR ULCER

SYMPTOMS AND SIGNS

The transparent outer covering of the eye is called the cornea. Because of its position, it is susceptible to injury and infection. Symptoms of abrasion and ulcer include pain, redness, and tearing. The patient may describe a sensation of having something constantly in the eye. The patient may report vision impairment as well. There may be a history of a foreign body or ocular trauma.

ETIOLOGY

Abrasions may be caused by the trapping of foreign bodies between the cornea and the eyelid, by direct trauma to the cornea, such as from a fingernail, or by the use of contact lenses that are scratched or poorly cleaned. Poorly fitting

127

contact lenses also can cause corneal abrasions. If abrasions are not treated promptly, an ulcer can develop. Ulcers can, in turn, become infected. A corneal ulcer is always a serious problem, and the patient should be referred to an ophthalmologist immediately.

DIAGNOSIS

The diagnosis is confirmed by the presence of characteristic symptoms as well as by a visual examination of the patient. Corneal abrasions and ulcerations stain with fluorescein, which makes them readily detectable.

TREATMENT

If a foreign body is present, it needs to be removed promptly to prevent ulceration and infection. An ophthalmic antibiotic ointment often is prescribed to prevent a secondary infection. Application of an eye dressing may be needed to promote healing if an abrasion is present. The dressing reduces the amount of movement of the cornea against the eyelid. Abrasions can be prevented by wearing protective eyewear while working in hazardous situations or when engaging in sports that might contribute to ocular injuries.

SCLERITIS

SYMPTOMS AND SIGNS

Inflammation of the sclera, the white outermost covering of the eyeball, is called scleritis. It can affect either one or both eyes, with dull pain and intense redness in one or more areas of the sclera. Inflammation can occur in the posterior portion of the eye, which may cause some loss of vision. If scleritis is left untreated, there is a chance of perforation of the globe and loss of the eye.

ETIOLOGY

The inflammation often is associated with rheumatoid arthritis (see Rheumatoid Arthritis in Chapter 3) and certain digestive disorders, such as Crohn's disease (see Crohn's Disease [Regional Enteritis] in Chapter 8).

DIAGNOSIS

An ophthalmologist should be seen as soon as possible if symptoms develop, because of the possibility of perforation. A thorough ophthalmic examination is needed, and blood tests may be necessary to uncover any underlying causes.

TREATMENT

Mild cases of scleritis usually respond well to topical drops. For severe cases, **immunosuppressive** drugs may be prescribed. Perforation of the sclera necessitates a surgical repair, called a scleroplasty.

CATARACT

SYMPTOMS AND SIGNS

A **cataract** is a cloudy or opaque area in a normally clear lens of the eye. Cataracts usually develop slowly and progressively reduce visual acuity. The primary symptom is the deterioration of vision in the affected eye. Blurring of vision and photosensitivity are also common. In advanced cases, the cataract may become readily visible, giving the pupil a white, opaque appearance and blocking light, impairing vision.

ETIOLOGY

The most common cause of cataracts is deterioration of the lens caused by the aging process. They also may be congenital or may result from ocular trauma, lightning injury, drug toxicity (prolonged high-dose corticosteroid administration), or systemic disease such as diabetes mellitus, or as a complication of other ocular diseases. Cataracts often have a familial occurrence; however, they are a common condition in the general population.

DIAGNOSIS

Examination by an ophthalmologist should be considered if vision becomes distorted or seems to be deteriorating. A simple penlight or slit-lamp examination confirms the presence of a cataract.

TREATMENT

The treatment depends on the amount of visual impairment and the age, health, and occupation of the patient. Surgery is advised when the cataracts begin to interfere with the lifestyle of the patient. The two most common methods of removing a cataract are intracapsular and extracapsular extraction and phacoemulsification. Contrary to general belief, at present, cataracts are not removed routinely with the laser. In extracapsular surgery, the nucleus, or center, of the cataract is removed in one piece. This necessitates a larger incision and more sutures. With phacoemulsification, an ultrasonic probe vibrates to break up the cataract, which subsequently is aspirated through the small incision. With this method, only one or two, or possibly no, sutures are required for wound closure.

In both extracapsular cataract extraction and phacoemulsification, the posterior capsule of the lens is left in place. This membrane helps to support an artificial lens, which is placed into the eye after removal of the cataract. Frequently, the posterior membrane becomes cloudy 1 to 3 years after surgery, which again reduces the visual acuity. If this occurs, a laser can be used to make an opening in the center of the cloudy membrane, thus immediately restoring good vision. This outpatient procedure entails no anesthesia and no significant postoperative care.

After cataract surgery, the patient needs a change in eyeglass prescription. Cataract surgery currently is quite successful; however, as with all surgery, there is a chance of significant complications.

GLAUCOMA

One of the most common and severe ocular diseases is glaucoma. Glaucoma is a major cause of blindness. It is more common in patients older than 60 years of age; however, it can occur at any age. Glaucoma, an increased intraocular pressure (IOP), results in atrophy of the optic nerve and blindness. Risk factors include age older than 60 years, nearsightedness, blood relatives of persons with glaucoma, and African Americans.

There are two types of glaucoma: chronic open-angle, or simple, glaucoma and acute angle-closure glaucoma (Fig. 5–8).

Chronic Open-Angle Glaucoma

SYMPTOMS AND SIGNS

Chronic open-angle glaucoma, a silent disease, is the most common form of glaucoma and is the most treatable cause of blindness. Patients can have open-angle glaucoma for a significant period of time before symptoms appear. By the time that symptoms appear, there usually has been considerable damage. The best way to detect glaucoma is by having periodic routine ophthalmic examinations, which include intraocular pressure readings as well as optic nerve evaluations. If the intraocular pressure is somewhat elevated or the optic nerve appears to be becoming atrophic, glaucoma needs to be considered. If chronic open-angle glaucoma goes untreated, the patient gradually loses peripheral (side) vision. The central vision may remain clear for a considerable period of time. However, if the condition progresses, the central vision is also lost, causing complete blindness.

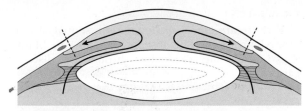

A Open-angle glaucoma

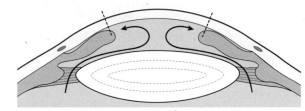

B Closed-angle glaucoma

Figure 5–8

Glaucoma. *A*, In open-angle glaucoma, the obstruction occurs in the trabecular meshwork. *B*, In closed-angle glaucoma, the trabecular meshwork is covered by the root of the iris or adhesions between the iris and the cornea. (From Damjanov I: Pathology for the Health-Related Professions. Philadelphia: WB Saunders, 1996, p 528. Used with permission.)

ETIOLOGY

The ciliary body in the eye continually produces fluid called the aqueous humor. This fluid circulates freely between the posterior and anterior chambers of the eye and passes through the trabecular meshwork and drains into the general circulation. In chronic open-angle (simple) glaucoma, there is a malfunction of the drainage system, which subsequently causes the IOP to be elevated. The channels that drain the fluid do not do so properly. With the elevated IOP, optic nerve damage can be sustained. In chronic open-angle glaucoma, the opening of the drainage system is adequate; however, the drains themselves are not. In chronic glaucoma, the circulation of aqueous humor gradually is blocked over a number of years. Eventually, this creates an internal pressure that affects the blood supply to the retina and the optic nerve.

Chronic open-angle glaucoma can occur secondary to trauma, even years later. Overuse of topical steroids also can cause the condition.

DIAGNOSIS

The diagnosis is determined by ophthalmic examination with **tonometry,** patient history, and symptoms.

TREATMENT

Early treatment of glaucoma is essential; if not treated promptly, the disease can lead to blindness because any vision lost through the disease cannot be regained. This condition usually is treated with medication (miotics) to help open the drainage system or decrease the production of aqueous humor (carbonic anhydrase inhibitors, beta blockers, and alpha-adrenergic agents). Laser treatment also can be beneficial in opening the drainage system; occasionally, even surgery is necessary to bypass the chronically defective draining system. Fortunately, most of the time chronic open-angle glaucoma can be controlled with eyedrops.

Acute Angle-Closure Glaucoma

SYMPTOMS AND SIGNS

Acute angle-closure glaucoma usually is associated with blurred vision, severe pain, headaches, and redness of the eye. The patient becomes photophobic and sees "halos" around light. With the full attack of acute glaucoma, the symptoms persist and become worse. Often, severe pain develops, associated with nausea and vomiting. The cornea of the eye becomes hazy because of the elevated pressure. The elevation of pressure in acute angle-closure glaucoma is usually significantly higher than that associated with chronic open-angle (simple) glaucoma. If acute angle-closure glaucoma is left untreated, the patient rapidly loses his or her vision and becomes completely blind within a few days.

ETIOLOGY

In acute angle-closure glaucoma, the mouth or opening of the drainage system is narrow and can close completely, causing a marked increase in the IOP during a short time.

DIAGNOSIS

The diagnosis is made by the history as well as a marked increase in the IOP. With a special lens called a goniolens, the ophthalmologist can view directly the opening of the drainage system to determine whether it is open or closed. The eye is usually red, and the cornea can be hazy.

TREATMENT

Treatment of acute angle-closure glaucoma is primarily by laser iridotomy, which creates a small opening between the anterior and the posterior chambers, allowing the filtering angle to open. Often, the IOP is lowered with medication before the laser treatment. However, the definitive treatment of angle-closure glaucoma is virtually always a laser iridotomy.

MACULAR DEGENERATION

SYMPTOMS AND SIGNS

The area in the retina near the optic nerve that defines fine details, in the center of the field of vision, is known as the macula lutea. An early symptom of macular degeneration may be a mild distortion of central vision. The condition is usually painless, develops slowly, and does not affect the peripheral vision. In most cases, both eyes are affected, either at the same time or one after the other. As the condition worsens, reading and activities that require sharp vision become impossible. Eventually, the central vision disappears altogether.

ETIOLOGY

This condition usually is age related. When age related, it usually is caused by degenerative changes in the pigment epithelium of the retina. There may be associated atherosclerotic changes in the vessels as well. Hemorrhage may occur in some cases. As a result, the macula does not receive sufficient blood, causing it to degenerate and central vision to become blurred.

DIAGNOSIS

The diagnosis of macular degeneration is made after a thorough examination by an ophthalmologist, using ophthalmoscopy and **fluorescein angiography,** coupled with the patient history.

TREATMENT

There is no known medical cure; however, the age-related form of this disease may be helped with a procedure called **laser photocoagulation.** Some researchers believe that increasing the amount of zinc in the diet also may be beneficial; however, this has not been definitively proved. Visual aids, such as strong magnifying lenses in glasses, also may be beneficial.

DIABETIC RETINOPATHY*

SYMPTOMS AND SIGNS

Diabetes can have an abnormal effect on the retina, called diabetic retinopathy. This consists of microaneurysms, hemorrhages, dilation of retinal veins, and the formation of abnormal new vessels (neovascularization). This condition usually occurs in both eyes, affecting the sharpness and clarity of vision. Diabetic retinopathy is a major cause of blindness.

ETIOLOGY

Diabetic retinopathy usually occurs about 8 to 10 years after the onset of diabetes mellitus. It occurs most often in diabetics who do not control their blood glucose levels, but all diabetics are susceptible. Diabetes causes some of the tiny blood vessels in the retina to become constricted and die. The remaining vessels may leak blood into the retina and cause a permanent reduction in the sharpness of vision. Sometimes, fragile new blood vessels (neovascularization) can grow

on the retina and, in turn, leak blood into the vitreous humor. This may markedly reduce vision. In either case, the blood usually is reabsorbed by the retina; however, scar tissue forms on the retina and may cause partial or permanent loss of vision (Fig. 5–9).

DIAGNOSIS

Complete ophthalmoscopic examination detects the retinal effects of diabetes. As with other ocular disorders, a thorough ophthalmic examination should be done regularly, especially when diabetes is a factor.

TREATMENT

Treatment with laser photocoagulation and **vitrectomy** is usually effective in controlling retinopathy. The condition has a tendency to recur, but with repeated treatments, vision may be maintained.

RETINAL DETACHMENT

SYMPTOMS AND SIGNS

A retinal detachment is an elevation of the retina from the choroid (Fig. 5–10). This may be partial or complete and usually is associated with a retinal tear, or a hole in the retina. Early symptoms of detachment consist of many new floaters as well as light flashes. This persists and worsens and is followed by a dark shadow extending from the periphery inward. This may begin in the lower or upper field of vision or one of the side fields of vision. This completely opaque shadow nearly always indicates the presence of a retinal detachment. If the detachment extends to the central retina, the central vision also is

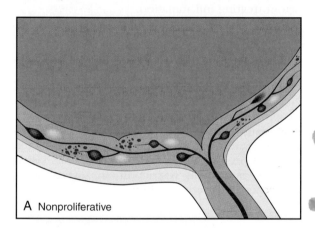

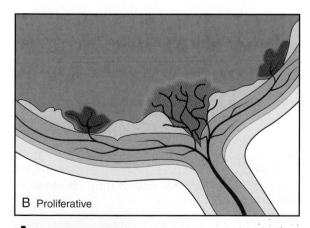

Figure 5–9

Diabetic retinopathy. *A,* Nonproliferative retinopathy shows edema, microaneurysm, and exudates. *B,* Proliferative retinopathy shows new blood vessel formation. (From Damjanov I: Pathology for the Health-Related Professions. Philadelphia: WB Saunders, 1996, p 527. Used with permission.)

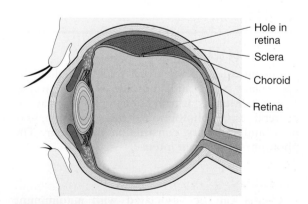

Figure 5–10

Retinal detachment.

blocked. The detachment often happens suddenly and without pain.

ETIOLOGY

People who are extremely nearsighted are more susceptible to retinal detachments than the general population. Ocular trauma also can predispose a person to retinal detachments. A retinal detachment usually begins with a tear in the retina. Fluid then leaks under the retina and separates the choroid. After the retina is separated from the choroid, this portion of retina no longer permits vision. As the retina continues to elevate, more and more vision is lost.

DIAGNOSIS

An ophthalmoscopic examination readily reveals the retinal detachment.

TREATMENT

Early treatment and sedation are advised until intervention can take place. Treatment of a retinal detachment virtually always consists of surgery. This should be done without delay to prevent additional portions of the retina from detaching. When the detached retina is repositioned, it regains most of its function. If the detachment has extended to the macula, the central retina, there is often some permanent reduction in central acuity. Photocoagulation or **cryotherapy** can be used to treat retinal tears if there is no associated detachment. Photocoagulation is a relatively simple procedure, which can be used to seal retinal tears before the development of retinal detachment. Early diagnosis is important in such cases.

UVEITIS

SYMPTOMS AND SIGNS

Inflammation of the uveal tract, including the iris, ciliary body, and choroid, is called uveitis. The condition is usually unilateral but may be bilateral. Pain, photophobia, blurred vision, redness, and pupillary constriction can occur. The photophobia is often intense.

ETIOLOGY

Uveitis can be associated with autoimmune disorders. Infections such as syphilis, tuberculosis, toxoplasmosis, and histoplasmosis also may

be causative. Frequently, an exact cause for uveitis cannot be determined.

DIAGNOSIS

A complete examination with the slit lamp is necessary for the diagnosis. To detect some forms of disease, skin tests for tuberculosis, **toxoplasmosis,** and **histoplasmosis** may be needed. Certain blood tests also may aid in the diagnosis.

TREATMENT

Treatment is specific for the particular type of uveitis. Any underlying cause should be treated. Cycloplegic agents and steroids are often beneficial in treating inflammation.

EXOPHTHALMOS

SYMPTOMS AND SIGNS

Protrusion of one or both eyeballs is known as exophthalmos. The condition exposes an abnormally large amount of the anterior eye. Patients report dryness and a gritty feeling in the affected eye or eyes. They also may note double vision and eye movement restriction. In severe cases, vision becomes seriously blurred.

ETIOLOGY

Exophthalmos is caused by edema of the soft tissue that lines the bony orbit of the eye. This condition may be caused by an overproduction of thyroid hormone (see Hyperthyroidism in Chapter 4). Sudden unilateral onset is usually a sign of hemorrhage or inflammation. Slower onset of edema indicates the presence of a tumor.

DIAGNOSIS

A complete ophthalmic examination, along with blood tests, radiographic studies, computed tomography (CT), and echography, is done to find the underlying cause.

TREATMENT

The diagnosis determines the therapy. If the condition is caused by hyperthyroidism, the disorder needs to be corrected. Severe cases may require surgical decompression of the orbit, and systemic steroids are beneficial in controlling edema.

Disorders of the Ear

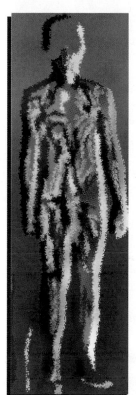

Functioning Organs of Hearing

The ear is the organ of balance as well as the organ of hearing. There are three sections to the ear: the outer, the middle, and the inner ear (Fig. 5-11).

The outer section is made up of the external ear, also called the pinna or auricle, and the external auditory canal. The latter's function is to collect sound waves or vibrations from the air, channel them to the **tympanic membrane** (eardrum), and make it vibrate.

The middle section contains the tympanic membrane and three ossicles (tiny bones) called the malleus (hammer), the incus (anvil), and the stapes (stirrup). Also in the middle ear is a canal, called the eustachian tube, that leads to a cavity (the pharynx) at the back of the nose. At the innermost region of the middle ear is the oval window, the opening to the inner ear. The middle ear's function is to receive the sound waves from the vibrating eardrum and pass them along the three bones to the oval window.

The inner ear contains two membrane-lined chambers, each filled with fluid, called the cochlea and the labyrinth. The cochlea contains tiny hairs that change the sound waves in the fluid into nerve impulses, which then are transmitted to the brain via the auditory nerve. The labyrinth is responsible for maintaining balance. It consists of three connected tubes bent into half circles, called the semicircular canals. Their function is to detect movement of the head and relay this information to the brain.

Common symptoms of ear diseases and conditions that should receive attention from healthcare professionals include

- Hearing loss
- Ear pain or pressure
- **Tinnitus** (ringing or buzzing noise)
- Vertigo (dizziness)
- Nausea and vomiting

Hearing loss or deafness is divided into two basic types: conductive loss and sensorineural loss. Conductive deafness is caused by an impairment of the eardrum or bones in the middle ear, which conduct sound waves to the cochlea in the inner ear. Sensorineural, or nerve, deafness results from impairment of the cochlea or the auditory nerve (see Enrichment on Cochlear Implants).

Central deafness results when the central nervous system (CNS) cannot interpret impulses because of a cerebrovascular accident (CVA) or brain tumor. See Alert on ototoxicity for chemical causes of temporary or permanent hearing loss.

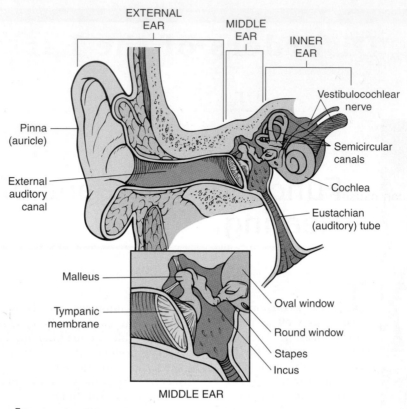

EXTERNAL EAR

MIDDLE EAR

INNER EAR

Vestibulocochlear nerve

Pinna (auricle)

Semicircular canals

External auditory canal

Cochlea

Eustachian (auditory) tube

Malleus

Tympanic membrane

Oval window

Round window

Stapes

Incus

MIDDLE EAR

Figure 5–11
Normal ear.

Enrichment

COCHLEAR IMPLANTS

Individuals experiencing severe sensorineural hearing loss that is not helped by hearing aids may have partial hearing restored by cochlear implants. Cochlear implants are electronic devices using minute electrical currents to stimulate the auditory nerve and help the currents travel to the auditory cortex to be perceived as sound.

Cochlear implant systems are complex and include an electrode array, a receiver, a speech processor, a transmitting coil, and a microphone. The electrode array is placed surgically in the cochlea, and the receiver is implanted and fixed to the skull behind the mastoid bone. The surgical incision is allowed to heal for 4 to 6 weeks, after which the external components are fit and the patient is connected to the microphone, transmitting coil, and speech processor. Fitting includes calibration of the transmitting coil and programming of the speech processor. Auditory and speech training are provided to the implant recipient.

Cochlear implants do not restore normal hearing; however, they do assist a deaf person to have increased functioning in a hearing world. Candidates are selected carefully for the implants and should have a severe to profound bilateral sensorineural hearing loss and be older than 2 years of age. Many still employ lip reading and American Sign Language (ASL) as adjunct therapies in order to communicate.

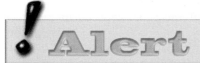

OTOTOXICITY

Ototoxicity occurs when a drug or chemical causes damage to the eighth cranial (acoustic) nerve or to the inner ear, resulting in temporary or permanent hearing loss or disturbances in balance. Symptoms and signs of ototoxicity usually have an insidious onset and include tinnitus, a feeling of fullness or pressure in the ears, hearing loss, vertigo, and occasionally nausea.

Drugs that can cause ototoxicity include salicylates (aspirin and aspirin-containing products), nonsteroidal anti-inflammatory drugs (NSAIDs), certain antibiotics (aminoglycosides, erythromycin, vancomycin), loop diuretics (furosemide [Lasix], bumetanide [Bumex], ethacrynic acid [Edecrin]), chemotherapeutic agents (cisplatin, vincristine, vinblastine), and quinines (quinidine and quinine). The physician should be notified of any of the aforementioned symptoms when the individual is taking or receiving any of the previously mentioned medications.

Discontinuing aspirin, aspirin-containing products, and NSAIDs often reverses the ototoxic effects of these drugs. Any of the other drugs should not be discontinued unless so ordered by the physician. Quinine ototoxicity, like aspirin-induced ototoxicity, usually can be reversed when the medication is stopped. Large dosages of antibiotics that may be ototoxic usually are administered in life-threatening situations.

Chemotherapeutic agents are monitored for any ototoxic side effects. In normal dosages, the loop diuretics usually have very few ototoxic side effects; it is when they are given in massive doses for treatment of acute kidney failure or acute hypertension that ototoxicity may occur.

Environmental chemicals include, but are not limited to, butyl nitrite, carbon disulfide, hexane, styrene, toluene, trichloroethylene, and xylene.

There is no way to reverse the damage once it has become permanent. Hearing loss may be helped by hearing aids or cochlear implants, and the loss of balance may require physical therapy.

Disorders of Conduction

IMPACTED CERUMEN

SYMPTOMS AND SIGNS

The normal, soft, yellowish brown, wax-like secretion produced by the glands of the external ear canal is called cerumen, or ear wax. If this secretion accumulates excessively, there may be a gradual loss of hearing, a feeling of the ear's being plugged, tinnitus, or sometimes an earache (otalgia). Impacted cerumen is a frequent cause of conductive hearing loss.

ETIOLOGY

ear wax

Abnormal accumulation of cerumen can be caused by dryness and scaling of the skin or by excessive hair in the ear canal. Some people have abnormally narrow ear canals, which may predispose them to this condition.

DIAGNOSIS

The physician or specialist does an otologic examination, and the patient history of symptoms confirms the diagnosis.

TREATMENT

If impacted cerumen is found, it must be removed. If the cerumen adheres to the wall of the ear canal, it may have to be softened with oily drops or hydrogen peroxide and irrigated with water to be removed (Fig. 5–12). Any hearing loss caused by the impaction is alleviated after

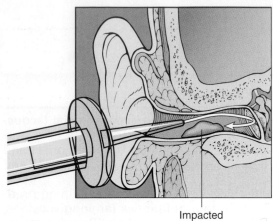

Impacted
cerumen

Figure 5–12

Irrigation of the ear for impacted cerumen. Irrigation of the ear also is used to remove foreign bodies.

136

removal of cerumen. This condition can recur, so periodic examinations may be necessary.

OTITIS EXTERNA (SWIMMER'S EAR)

SYMPTOMS AND SIGNS

Inflammation of the external ear canal is called otitis externa, or swimmer's ear. Severe pain; a red, swollen ear canal; hearing loss; fever, and **pruritus** are common symptoms. Any drainage from the ear may be either watery or **purulent.**

ETIOLOGY

Accumulation of cerumen in the ear canal, when mixed with water (as during swimming), acts as a culture medium for bacteria or fungi. Otitis externa also may be caused by dermatologic conditions such as seborrhea and psoriasis. Trauma to the ear canal, from attempts to clean or scratch inside the ear with a foreign object or frequent use of earphones and earplugs can predispose a person to the development of otitis externa.

DIAGNOSIS

Otoscope

An otologic examination and a history of symptoms confirms the diagnosis. If a bacterial infection is suspected, a culture of the material found in the canal may be needed to determine how to properly treat the infection.

TREATMENT

The ear canal must be kept clean and free from water. Antibiotic or steroid eardrops and systemic antibiotics may be prescribed, depending on the severity. Otitis externa tends to recur and can become chronic.

OTITIS MEDIA

SYMPTOMS AND SIGNS

Otitis media is inflammation of the normally air-filled middle ear with the accumulation of fluid behind the tympanic membrane (eardrum), occurring either unilaterally or bilaterally. It is the most frequent reason for visits to physicians by children and also can be experienced by adults.

Otitis media is classified as either serous or suppurative, according to the composition of the accumulating fluid. In serous otitis media, the fluid is relatively clear and sterile. With suppurative otitis, the fluid is purulent. Symptoms vary according to the type. With serous otitis media, the only symptoms may be a feeling of fullness or pressure and some degree of impaired hearing. Suppurative otitis media, however, is painful. General symptoms of infection, fever, chills, nausea, and vomiting usually accompany this type. Children often rub or pull at the affected ear and lean the head sideways toward the affected side. Dizziness can be a symptom in either type. Muffled hearing may be present, or there may be a significant loss of hearing.

ETIOLOGY

Serous otitis media may be either acute or chronic. With acute serous otitis media, the cause is usually a virus from a URI that has spread through the eustachian tube into the middle ear. It can occur spontaneously or may result from an allergic reaction. Chronic otitis media can develop from an acute attack, hypertrophy of the adenoids, or chronic sinus infections. Suppurative otitis media is caused by bacteria, which also can enter the middle ear through the eustachian tube from the nose or throat or from a ruptured tympanic membrane. This condition often follows a bout of influenza or mumps. Variations in the normal structure of the eustachian tube can predispose a person to this disease.

DIAGNOSIS

Otoscopy reveals the presents of a fluid-filled middle ear. The normally pearl-gray eardrum is inflamed and may be bulging. Fluid bubbles may be visible through the membrane. If a culture of the fluid taken from the ear shows bacteria and there is an elevated **white blood cell (WBC) count,** suppurative otitis media is present. Audiometry may reveal mild to severe hearing loss. Measurement of the pressure in the middle ear by a tympanogram provides the physician with an idea of how well the eustachian tube is functioning.

TREATMENT

Analgesics and decongestants may be ordered to provide pain relief and to promote drainage in both types of otitis media. Antibiotics are ordered for cases of suppurative otitis media. In severe cases, or patients who fail to respond to medical treatment, surgical evacuation of the fluid (myringotomy) is necessary to prevent permanent hearing loss and the possible development of mastoiditis (see Mastoiditis) or a cholesteatoma (see Cholesteatoma). To keep the middle ear air filled and to prevent fluid from accumulating, tympanostomy tubes may need to be inserted after the myringotomy (Fig. 5–13).

OTOSCLEROSIS

SYMPTOMS AND SIGNS

With this condition, an abnormal growth of spongy bone forms around the oval window, causing **ankylosis** of the stapes, the third ossicle (small bone) in the middle ear. Ankylosis produces conductive deafness because the ossicles cannot conduct the sound vibrations as they enter the ear. Symptoms of otosclerosis are a gradual hearing loss of low or soft sounds, which may be unilateral at first, but usually affects both ears at some point, and tinnitus. Patients usually report not being able to hear as well on the telephone with the affected ear. Relatives may notice that patients turn their heads to hear better. Otosclerosis is a young person's disease, with onset usually after puberty and before 35 years of age.

ETIOLOGY

Otosclerosis is **idiopathic,** but there is evidence of familial tendency, suggesting genetic factors. The condition seems to be more preva-

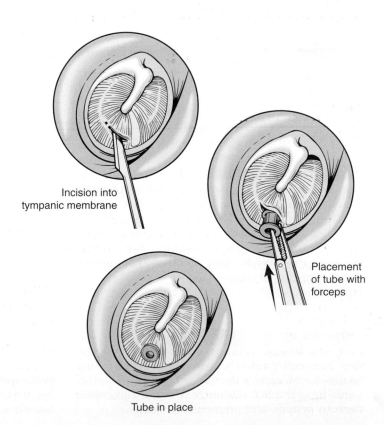

Incision into
tympanic membrane

Placement
of tube with
forceps

Tube in place

Figure 5–13

Myringotomy and insertion of a tympanoplasty tube as a treatment for otitis media.

lent in women and can be aggravated by pregnancy.

DIAGNOSIS

A diagnosis of otosclerosis is made by the physician using an **audiogram,** the patient history, and otoscopy. The audiogram shows a moderate to severe hearing loss, especially in the low range.

TREATMENT

The only treatment that cures otosclerosis is a surgical procedure called a stapedectomy. A stapedectomy is the removal of the diseased stapes and placement of a prosthesis in its place. The prosthesis may be made of metal or a ceramic or plastic material because of the advent of magnetic resonance imaging (MRI) and the inability to perform an accurate test with metal in place. If the condition is bilateral, only one ear is operated on at a time to evaluate the success of the procedure. Generally, there is improvement in hearing soon after the surgery. If surgery is not an option for the patient, a hearing aid can be tried.

Meniere's Disease

SYMPTOMS AND SIGNS

Meniere's disease is a chronic disease of the inner ear, affecting the labyrinth, and is marked by a recurring syndrome of vertigo, tinnitus, progressive hearing loss, and a sensation of fullness or pressure in the affected ear. Nausea, vomiting, sweating, and loss of balance can follow an acute attack of vertigo. These attacks can last from a few hours to several days and may become increasingly serious with each recurrence. Meniere's disease usually affects one ear, but eventually both ears may become involved. The disease usually appears in individuals between 40 and 50 years of age.

ETIOLOGY

The cause of this disease is unknown; however, the disease process seems to destroy the tiny hair cells inside the cochlea. Predisposing factors for Meniere's disease are middle ear infections, head trauma, dysfunction in the autonomic nervous system, and premenstrual edema.

DIAGNOSIS

When the four main symptoms are present, the diagnosis is easy. If symptoms are less obvious or pronounced, additional testing with audiometry, radiographic studies, and ENG (electronystagmography) may be necessary.

TREATMENT

For acute attacks of Meniere's disease, the physician usually prescribes medication to control the nausea and vomiting. Long-term treatment could include following a salt-free diet, restricting fluid intake, and using diuretics, antihistamines, and mild sedatives. If the disease does not respond to dietary restrictions and medications, surgical intervention may be needed. Surgical destruction of the affected labyrinth, using ultrasound, relieves the symptoms but also causes permanent hearing loss unless the cochlea is preserved.

Labyrinthitis

SYMPTOMS AND SIGNS

The labyrinth is a group of three fluid-filled chambers (the semicircular canals) in the inner ear that control balance (Fig. 5–14). Inflammation or infection of these chambers is called labyrinthitis. The onset of infection is often acute and is associated with fever, with temperatures of 100 to 101°F. The main symptom of this disease is extreme vertigo. Balance is affected, and there may be nausea and vomiting in some cases.

ETIOLOGY

Labyrinthitis is usually the result of a virus but can be caused by a bacterial infection that has spread from the middle ear.

DIAGNOSIS

The diagnosis of labyrinthitis is based on the results of several tests, including audiometry and blood, neurologic, caloric, and, possibly, imaging studies.

TREATMENT

Bed rest for several days may be necessary. Prescriptions for a tranquilizer, an antiemetic agent, and an antibiotic may be necessary if a bacterial infection is present. When properly

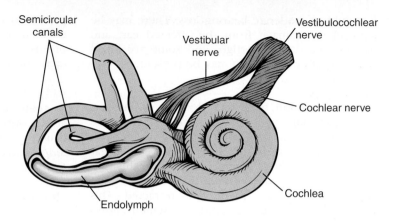

Figure 5–14

Labyrinth or inner ear. Labyrinthitis is caused by a disturbance in the fluid in the semicircular canals.

treated, labyrinthitis is not a dangerous condition; however, it can be debilitating, and the labyrinth is a delicate and easily damaged organ. In most cases, labyrinthitis completely clears up within 1 to 3 weeks.

Ruptured Tympanic Membrane (Ruptured Eardrum)

SYMPTOMS AND SIGNS

Symptoms of a ruptured tympanic membrane (eardrum) are usually slight pain and partial loss of hearing and may include a slight discharge or bleeding from the ear. These symptoms may last only a few hours. The major risk is that an infection may develop in the middle ear.

ETIOLOGY

The four most common causes of a ruptured eardrum are placement of sharp objects into the ear canal, an explosion (including lightning injuries), a severe middle ear infection, and a blow to the ear. A ruptured eardrum also can occur as a result of a fractured skull. The eardrum occasionally ruptures spontaneously.

DIAGNOSIS

A visual examination of the ear with an otoscope confirms the diagnosis of a ruptured eardrum (Fig. 5–15). Audiometry also may be used.

TREATMENT

An antibiotic may be prescribed to prevent infection, and a patch may be applied to the eardrum to aid healing and to improve hearing. This procedure is similar to a tympanoplasty (tympanoplasty involves actual grafting of tissue for eardrum repair). The eardrum heals naturally in about 1 to 2 weeks. After the eardrum has healed, hearing loss is minimal.

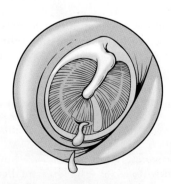

Figure 5–15

Ruptured tympanic membrane with purulent discharge.

Cholesteatoma

SYMPTOMS AND SIGNS

A cholesteatoma is a pocket of skin cells, normally shed by the eardrum, that collect into a cyst-like mass or ball and become infected. As the infected material accumulates, the bone lining the middle ear cavity erodes, and the ossicles become damaged. The most common symptom is a mild to moderate hearing loss. There may be a purulent drainage from the affected ear, and earache, headache, vertigo, and some weakness of the facial muscles also may be present.

ETIOLOGY

This condition begins to develop in infancy. The eustachian tube from the middle ear to the pharynx either fails to open properly or becomes blocked with material from recurring middle ear infections (see Otitis Media). As a result, this normally air-filled chamber develops a weak vacuum, causing the eardrum to become retracted. This forms the pocket in the eardrum, which allows the cholesteatoma to develop.

DIAGNOSIS

Patient history, otoscopy, and audiometry enable the physician to make the diagnosis. Radiographic studies also may be useful, and a culture of the purulent drainage may be necessary to determine the most effective antibiotic for treatment.

TREATMENT

If the cholesteatoma is discovered early, before eroding begins, it can be removed fairly simply by a thorough cleaning of the middle ear cavity. Inflation of the eustachian tube may produce some improvement, and treatment with steroids and antibiotics helps to prevent recurrence. If the cholesteatoma is discovered in an advanced stage, its removal becomes much more complicated. Damage to the middle ear structures may be extensive, necessitating surgical reconstruction of these structures. Badly damaged hearing may be improved with the use of a hearing aid. Untreated, a cholesteatoma erodes the roof of the middle ear cavity, producing the possibility for the development of an epidural **abscess** or **meningitis.**

Mastoiditis

SYMPTOMS AND SIGNS

Mastoiditis, whether acute or chronic, is inflammation of the mastoid bone, or mastoid process. The mastoid is a round process of the temporal bone that can be felt immediately behind each ear and is porous or honeycombed in appearance. Pain and occasionally edema are present over and around the mastoid. Fever and chills may be present. There is likely to be a profuse discharge from the external canal because of the middle ear involvement.

ETIOLOGY

Acute mastoiditis is the result of neglected acute otitis media. *Streptococcus* is the usual causative organism, but certain pneumococci and *Staphylococcus aureus* also may be involved. Chronic mastoiditis, necessitating radical or modified radical mastoidectomy, is associated with cholesteatoma.

DIAGNOSIS

The diagnosis is made from patient history, otoscopy, audiometry, radiographic studies of the mastoid, and the results of blood and culture studies.

TREATMENT

The treatment is based on the results of the sensitivity studies. Antibiotic or sulfonamide therapy is prescribed. Mastoiditis not responding to this treatment necessitates a surgical procedure, called simple mastoidectomy, to prevent further complications and to preserve hearing. A radical mastoidectomy may be needed for chronic mastoiditis.

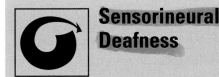

Sensorineural Deafness

SYMPTOMS AND SIGNS

In sensorineural deafness, also often referred to as occupational hearing loss, sound waves reach the inner ear but are not perceived because the nerve impulses are not transmitted to the brain. Symptoms include tinnitus and partial to severe hearing loss.

ETIOLOGY

The cause of sensorineural hearing loss is nerve failure or damage to the cochlea or the auditory nerve. This can result from the aging process; however, loud music, machinery noise, or sometimes the side effects of medications can cause damage at any age (Fig. 5-16*A* and *B*). Sensorineural hearing loss that is caused by damage to the cochlea is *irreversible.* Prevention is essential.

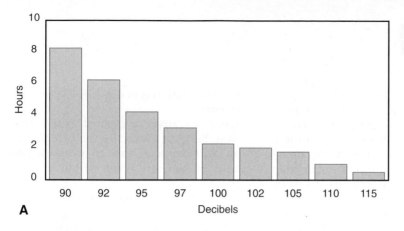

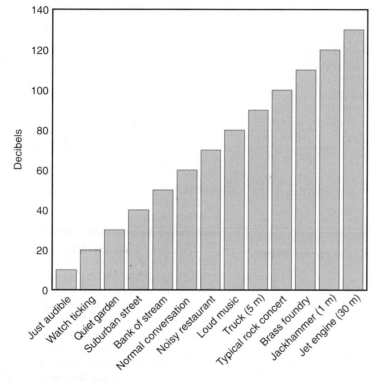

Figure 5–16

A, Maximum occupational noise exposure (in hours per day) allowed by U.S. Occupational Safety and Health Administration (OSHA) regulations. *B,* Examples of decibel levels in everyday situations.

DIAGNOSIS

The patient history and audiometry are usually all that is needed for the diagnosis. Physicians are concerned that sensorineural hearing loss, tinnitus, and vertigo may be symptoms of a space-occupying mass such as a tumor or an aneurysm; therefore, these symptoms are investigated further to rule out such masses.

TREATMENT

Regardless of the amount of damage to the cochlea, steps *must* be taken to prevent further damage. Reducing noise levels, such as by turning down the volume on loud music and wearing ear protectors at rock concerts or at work areas with high noise levels, can prevent further or future damage to the ears.

Summary

Hearing and sight are vital and complex senses of immense practical and psychological importance to all aspects of living. If there is pathology of either, the patient suffers a variety of annoying to disabling symptoms. Acute alterations in vision (as in detached retina) or hearing (as in otitis media) alert individuals to seek prompt medical investigation. Certain diseases of the eye (e.g., glaucoma) or ear (e.g., Meniere's disease) can present with a more insidious and chronic syndrome; these may result in eventual *irreversible* damage to sight or hearing.

- Refractive errors (hyperopia, myopia, astigmatism, and presbyopia) cause blurred vision that is corrected with artificial lenses or a surgical procedure called radial keratotomy.
- Repetitive, involuntary movement of one or both eyes, called nystagmus, requires complete neurologic evaluation. Although the cause may be congenital or drug related, it also can signal a brain lesion.
- Strabismus, a muscle weakness of the eye, can be congenital or acquired in adulthood from systemic disease such as diabetes mellitus or trauma to the brain.
- Infectious diseases of the eyelids include hordeolum, blepharitis, keratitis, and conjunctivitis. Chalazion (meibomian cyst) can become infected.
- Entropion and ectropion of the eyelids, more common in older individuals, can be corrected with a minor surgical procedure if necessary. Blepharoptosis, a permanent drooping of the eyelid, can be a primary weakness of the muscle that raises the eyelid or a weakness secondary to another disease.
- Corneal abrasion or ulcer can be the result of a foreign body trapped in the eye or the result of trauma.
- Cataract causes a gradual deterioration of vision. Surgical correction with replacement with an artificial lens and an eyeglass prescription may be advised when vision is seriously impaired.
- Untreated glaucoma can cause blindness because of increased intraocular pressure that damages the retina and the optic nerve.
- To prevent permanent damage and loss of vision, early diagnosis and treatment of retinal detachment is important.
- Because the ear is the organ of balance as well as the organ of hearing, common symptoms of ear disease include hearing loss and pain, as well as vertigo, nausea, and vomiting.
- The external ear can become infected (otitis externa) and/or blocked (as in impacted cerumen), causing earache, tinnitus, and conductive hearing loss.
- Otitis media, a condition of the inner ear, is suppurative or serous and acute or chronic, and is treated according to the cause. Myringotomy with insertion of a tympanostomy tube may be required in the treatment plan.
- Meniere's disease affects the labyrinth and is marked by a chronic recurring syndrome of vertigo, tinnitus, and progressive hearing loss.
- Placement of sharp objects into the external ear canal or an explosion, infection, or trauma can result in a ruptured eardrum.
- Untreated cholesteatoma can damage middle ear structures, causing hearing loss, vertigo, and weakness of facial muscles.
- Sensorineural hearing loss is caused by damage to the cochlea and is irreversible.

Review Challenge

REVIEW QUESTIONS

1. How does the process of normal vision take place?
2. What are the four main errors of refraction?
3. What is the difference between nystagmus and strabismus?
4. Name a common etiologic factor in hordeolum and blepharitis?
5. What are the presenting symptoms and signs of conjunctivitis? Is the condition contagious?
6. Name some possible causes of corneal abrasions.
7. How do cataracts interfere with vision?
8. Differentiate between the two types of glaucoma.
9. How is diabetic retinopathy detected and treated?
10. Explain the pathology involved in retinal detachment. How is this condition treated?
11. What are the possible causes of exophthalmos?
12. What is the primary symptom of refractive errors?
13. Describe the three separate parts of the ear.
14. How does impacted cerumen cause deafness?
15. Precisely define otitis media. How is it classified? How is it diagnosed?
16. What is myringotomy?
17. What symptoms may an individual with Meniere's disease experience?
18. Name the major symptom of labyrinthitis.
19. List common causes of a ruptured eardrum.
20. What causes occupational deafness?

REAL-LIFE CHALLENGE

Acute Angle-Closure Glaucoma

A 61-year-old man presents with sudden onset of blurred vision, head and eye pain, and nausea and vomiting. On questioning, he admits to seeing "halos" around lights and being extra sensitive to light. The physician examination confirms blurred vision and photosensitivity. Intraocular pressure (IOP) measures greater than 20 mm Hg on the tonometer.

The patient is diagnosed with acute angle-closure glaucoma and referred to an ophthalmologist for immediate treatment.

Questions

1. Compare the symptoms of chronic open-angle glaucoma and acute angle-closure glaucoma.
2. Compare the reason for buildup of IOP in chronic open-angle glaucoma and acute angle-closure glaucoma.
3. What history would indicate this patient to be at risk for glaucoma?
4. Which type of treatment would you expect the ophthalmologist to institute?
5. If this were chronic open-angle glaucoma, which types of medications would you expect to be prescribed?
6. How would these medications help to treat the disorder?
7. What is the danger of untreated glaucoma?

REAL-LIFE CHALLENGE

Otitis Media

A 1½-year-old male child has been brought to the physician's office by his parents, who state that he has been fussy and crying for the last 10 hours. The mother says that she is having difficulty getting him to eat and she has noticed he sits with his head held to the right side. He has a history of a cold for the past few days, with a runny nose and watering eyes.

Examination reveals a temperature of 103°F, pulse of 116, and respirations of 32. The otoscopic examination was used to evaluate the condition of the tympanic membranes. The physician examined the left ear first, a method employed to see what the asymptomatic ear

looked like. It revealed a normal translucent pearl-gray tympanic membrane. Examination of the right or symptomatic ear disclosed a red bulging eardrum. The mucous membrane of the nasal passages appeared inflamed, as did the back of the throat.

An antibiotic (amoxicillin trihydrate [Amoxil] 125 mg qid × 10 days) was prescribed. The parents were instructed to give acetaminophen or ibuprofen (Motrin) for a temperature greater than 101°F and to call if the fever and pain persisted beyond 24 hours. The child was scheduled for a follow-up visit in 1 week.

Questions

1. Why is it important to note that the child sits with his head held to the side?
2. The elevated temperature has what effect on the other vital signs?
3. Why did the physician examine the left eardrum first?
4. What patient teaching would you offer the parents concerning the medication for the elevated temperature?

5. What patient teaching would you offer the parents regarding the antibiotics?
6. Why is treatment and follow-up important?
7. Which surgical procedure may be indicated?
8. What long-term effects may the child experience if the otitis does not respond to treatment?

RESOURCES

National Institute on Deafness and Other Communication Disorders Clearinghouse
1 Communications Ave
Bethesda, MD 20892-3456
1-800-241-1044
TTY 1-800-241-1055
NIDCD@aerie.com
(http://www.nih.gov/nidcd/)

National Information Center on Deafness
Gallaudet University
800 Florida Ave NE
Washington, DC 20002-3625
202-651-5051

National Library Service for the Blind and Physically Handicapped
Library of Congress
1291 Taylor St NW
Washington, DC 20542
800-424-8567

Hearing Helpline
Better Hearing Institute
1-800-327-9355
703-642-0580 in Virginia

Dial-a-Hearing Screening Test
Hearing
PO Box 1880
Media, PA 19063
1-800-222-EARS

National Association for Hearing and Speech Action Line
800-638-8255
301-897-0039 in Hawaii, Alaska, and Maryland—call collect

National Hearing Aid Helpline
20361 Middlebelt Rd
Livonia, MI 48152
800-521-5247

Facial Plastic Surgery Information Service
American Academy of Facial, Plastic and Reconstructive Surgery
310 S Henry St
Alexandria, VA 22314
1-800-332-332-3223

American Foundation for the Blind (AFB)
800-232-5463
212-620-2147 in New York City

National Eye Care Project Helpline
American Academy of Ophthalmology
PO Box 429098
San Francisco, CA 94142-9098
800-222-EYES

National Center for Sight
National Society to Prevent Blindness
500 E Remington Rd, Ste 200
Schaumburg, IL 60173
800-221-3004

Alexander Graham Bell Association for the Deaf
3417 Volta Place NW
Washington, DC 20007

American Academy of Ophthalmology
655 Beach St
San Francisco, CA 94109
PO Box 7724
San Francisco, CA 94120
415-561-8500
fax 415-561-8575
(http://www.eyenet.org/)

Foundation for Glaucoma Research
490 Post St
San Francisco, CA 94102

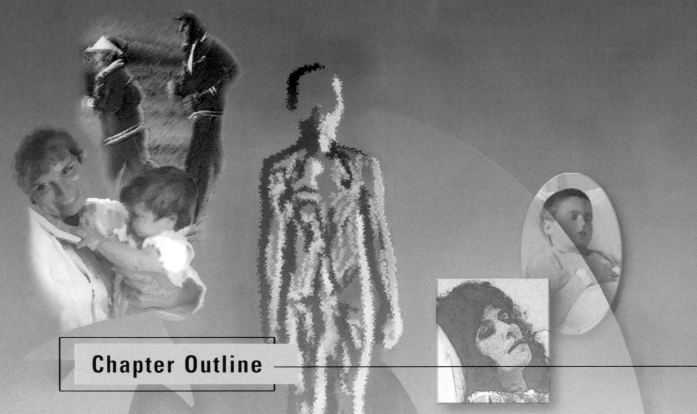

Chapter Outline

Diseases and Conditions of the Integumentary System

Learning Objectives

After studying Chapter 6, you should be able to:

1. Explain the functions of the skin.
2. Recognize common skin lesions.
3. Describe how seborrheic dermatitis affects the skin.
4. Discuss the possible causes of contact dermatitis, atopic dermatitis, and psoriasis.
5. Describe the treatment of acne vulgaris.
6. Explain the pathologic course of herpes zoster.
7. Name the etiology of impetigo.
8. Explain why the treatment of cellulitis is important.
9. Site examples of how fungal infections of the skin are classified.
10. List preventive measures for decubitus ulcers.
11. Name the two most common parasitic insects to infest man. Describe how infestation can occur.
12. Name two common premalignant tumors.
13. Differentiate between the three types of skin cancer.
14. Recite the guidelines to avoid excessive sun exposure.
15. Describe some conditions that are caused by the abnormal development or distribution of melanocytes.
16. Name some possible causes of alopecia.
17. State the cause of warts.
18. List some of the likely causes of deformed or discolored nails.

Key Terms

bulla	(**BUL**–la)	electrodesiccation	(ee–leck–tro–**des**–ih–**KA**–shun)
cellulitis	(sell–you–**LIE**–tis)		
comedo	(**KOM**–ee–doe)	erythema	(**eh**–rih–**THEE**–ma)
débride	(dah–**BREED**)	exudate	(**EKS**–you–date)
dermatome	(**DER**–mah–tome)	exudative	(**EKS**–you–**day**–tive)

fissure	(**FIS**–ur)	plaques	(plaks)
keratolytic	(ker–ah–toe–**LIT**–ik)	sebaceous	(seh–**BAY**–shus)
keratosis	(ker–ah–**TOE**–sis)	vesicle	(**VES**–ih–kl)
nevus	(**NEE**–vus)	vesicular	(veh–**SIK**–you–lar)
papule	(**PAP**–youl)	wheal	(**WHEEL**)

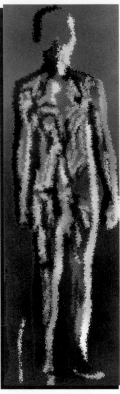

Orderly Functioning of the Integumentary System

The system comprising the skin and its accessory organs (hair, nails, and glands) is called the integumentary system. The skin, one of the largest organs, protects the body from trauma, infections, and **toxic** chemicals, and when exposed to sunlight, the skin **synthesizes** vitamin D. Within the skin are millions of tiny nerve endings called receptors. These receptors sense touch, pressure, pain, and temperature. In addition to its roles in protection, sensation, and synthesis of vitamin D, the skin assists in the regulation of body temperature and in excretion.

The skin has three main structural layers (Fig. 6–1). The epidermis (outer layer) is a thin, cellular, multilayered membrane that is responsible for the production of **keratin** and **melanin.** The dermis, or corium (middle layer), is a dense fibrous, connective tissue layer that gives skin its strength and elasticity. Within the dermis are blood and lymph vessels, nerve fibers, hair follicles, and sweat and sebaceous glands. Third is the subcutaneous layer, a thick, fat-containing section that provides insulation for the body against heat loss.

Skin diseases frequently are manifested by cutaneous lesions, or alterations of the skin surface. The diagnosis of a cutaneous disease often is based on the appearance of a specific type of lesion or group of lesions (Fig. 6–2).

Common presenting symptoms that need attention from health-care professionals include:

• Cutaneous lesions or eruptions
• Pruritus (itching)
• Pain
• Edema (swelling)
• Erythema (redness)
• Inflammation

Many skin conditions are known to be aggravated by stress. Cosmetically, the skin is important to appearance. Much time and money is expended in pursuit of "beauty" and disguising aging of the skin. Patients with skin conditions may experience anxiety about their appearance. The treatment of many skin diseases is tedious, requiring strict compliance. Patient education and psychological support lessen the patient's anxiety and encourage good adherence to the treatment plan.

Dermatitis

There are many types or forms of inflammation of the skin, or dermatitis. They all are manifested by pruritus, erythema, and the appearance of various cutaneous lesions. The more common

Describe S+S & causes

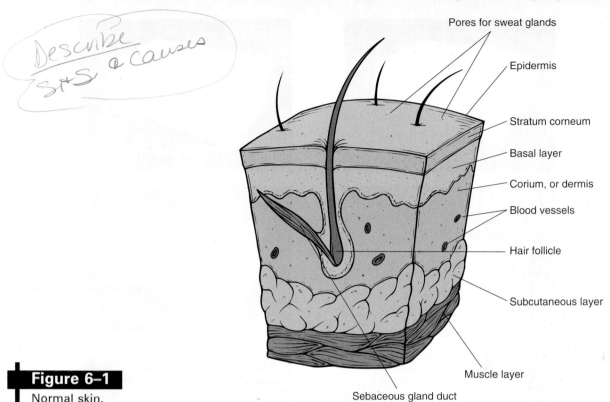

Pores for sweat glands
Epidermis
Stratum corneum
Basal layer
Corium, or dermis
Blood vessels
Hair follicle
Subcutaneous layer
Muscle layer
Sebaceous gland duct

Figure 6–1
Normal skin.

forms are seborrheic dermatitis, contact dermatitis, and atopic dermatitis (eczema). All forms of dermatitis can be acute, subacute, or chronic.

SEBORRHEIC DERMATITIS

SYMPTOMS AND SIGNS

Seborrheic dermatitis, one of the most common skin disorders, is an inflammatory condition of the sebaceous, or oil, glands. This condition is marked by an increase in the amount of and a change in the quality of the **sebum** produced by the sebaceous glands. The inflammation occurs in areas with the greatest number of sebaceous glands. These include the scalp, eyebrows, eyelids, sides of the nose, the area behind the ears, and middle of the chest. Affected skin is reddened and covered by yellowish, greasy-appearing scales (Fig. 6–3). Itching may occur and, if present, is usually mild.

Seborrheic dermatitis can occur at any age but is most common during infancy, when it is called cradle cap. Cradle cap usually clears without treatment by 8 to 12 months of age. There is an increased occurrence of seborrheic dermatitis in adults with disorders of the central nervous system, such as Parkinson's disease. Patients who

are recovering from stressful medical conditions, such as a myocardial infarction (heart attack); patients who have been confined to hospitals or nursing homes for long periods of time; and those who have immune system disorders such as acquired immunodeficiency syndrome (AIDS) appear to be more prone to this disorder. More intense forms of seborrheic dermatitis can be seen in patients with psoriasis (see Psoriasis). Mild forms are mainly cosmetic problems that can be easily treated or may disappear spontaneously.

ETIOLOGY

This condition is **idiopathic;** however, heredity may predispose an individual to the condition, and emotional stress may be a precipitating factor. Evidence suggests that this skin disorder may be perpetuated or intensified by a yeast-like organism normally found on the skin in small numbers. It still is not known whether diet or food allergies play a role in the development of seborrheic dermatitis in infants.

DIAGNOSIS

In most patients, blood, urine, or allergy tests are not necessary. In the rare case of chronic

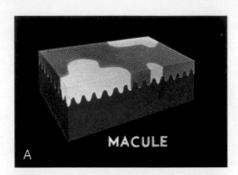

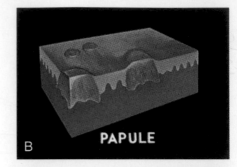

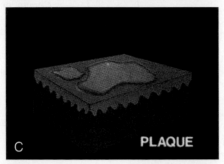

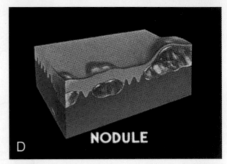

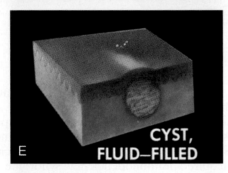

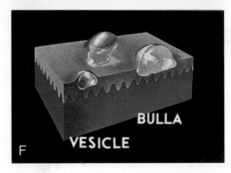

Figure 6–2

Skin lesions. *A,* Macule. A flat, colored lesion that may be white (hypopigmented), brown (hyperpigmented), or red (erythematous and purpuric). *B,* Papule. A small elevated lesion less than 0.5 cm in diameter. *C,* Plaque. A plateau-like elevated lesion greater than 0.5 cm in diameter. *D,* Nodule. A marble-like lesion greater than 0.5 cm in depth and diameter. *E,* Cyst. A nodule filled with either liquid or semi-solid material. *F,* Vesicle and bulla. Blisters containing clear fluid. Vesicles are less than 0.5 cm in diameter and bullae are greater than 0.5 in diameter.

seborrheic dermatitis that does not respond to treatment, a skin **biopsy** or more extensive testing may be performed to rule out the possibility of another disease.

TREATMENT

One of the more effective methods of treatment is the use of a low-strength cortisone or hydrocortisone cream, applied topically to the affected area. *Caution:* Prolonged use of these medications should be avoided because of the possible side effects of using steroids. If the scalp is involved, the frequent use of nonprescription shampoos containing tar, zinc pyrithione, selenium sulfide, sulfur, and salicylic acid also is recommended. Patients not responding to these treatments should consult a dermatologist who can prescribe stronger medications. Whether treated or not, this condition tends to recur.

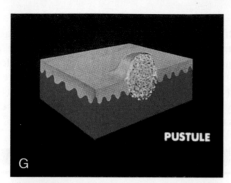

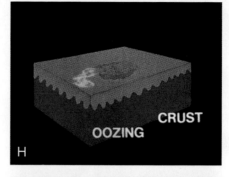

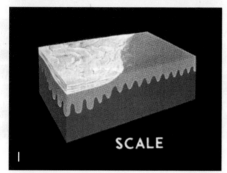

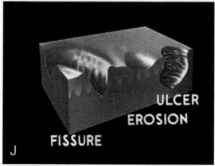

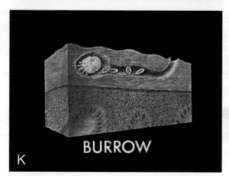

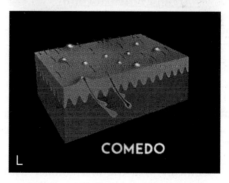

Figure 6–2 *Continued*

G, Pustule. A vesicle containing purulent or cloudy fluid. *H,* Crust. Liquid debris dried on the skin's surface, resulting from ruptured vesicles, pustules, or bullae. *I,* Scale. A thickened outer layer of skin that is dry and whitish colored. *J,* Fissure, erosion, and ulcer. A fissure is a thin tear. An erosion is a wide but shallow fissure. An ulcer involves the epidermis and dermis. *K,* Burrow. A tunnel or streak caused by a burrowing organism. *L,* Comedo. A lesion of acne. (From Lookingbill D, Marks J: Principles of Dermatology, 2nd ed. Philadelphia: WB Saunders, 1993, pp 34–36. Used with permission.)

CONTACT DERMATITIS

SYMPTOMS AND SIGNS

Contact dermatitis is an acute inflammation of the skin. It is caused either by the action of irritants on the skin's surface or by contact with a substance that causes an allergic reaction.

Symptoms include erythema, edema, and small **vesicles** that ooze, itch, burn, or sting (Fig. 6-4).

ETIOLOGY

Many substances can induce contact dermatitis, including plants such as poison ivy, oak, or sumac. Other irritants are dyes used in soaps and facial and toilet tissue, certain metals (e.g.,

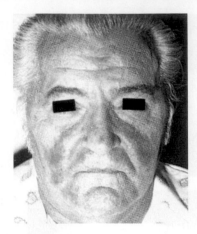

Figure 6–3

Seborrheic dermatitis. (From Lookingbill D, Marks J: Principles of Dermatology, 2nd ed. Philadelphia: WB Saunders, 1993, p 130. Used with permission.)

152

nickel) used to make jewelry, latex, drugs, detergents, cleaning compounds, cosmetics, and acids. If an irritant remains in constant contact with the skin, the dermatitis spreads.

Contact dermatitis develops in three ways.

First, it can develop by means of irritation, either chemical or mechanical, such as by latex gloves and wool fibers. If the irritant is strong, a single exposure may cause a severe inflammatory reaction.

Second, contact dermatitis may develop by sensitization. This means that the first contact with a substance causes no immediate inflammation. However, once the skin becomes sensitized, future contact or exposure results in inflammation.

Third, another interesting but uncommon mechanism for the development of this form of dermatitis is photoallergy. Some chemicals found in perfumes, soaps, suntan lotions containing *para*-aminobenzoic acid, or medications (e.g., tetracycline) can sensitize the skin to the sunlight. The next time the individual uses the products and is exposed to sunlight, a rash develops.

DIAGNOSIS

Diagnosis of a contact dermatitis is based on the appearance of the affected area; a medical history, including prior outbreaks and their locations; and identification of the specific irritant or allergen with a **patch test.**

TREATMENT

If a patient has come in contact with a known irritant, a thorough cleaning of the skin surface should be the first step. This should be followed by the topical application of a steroid cream. An oral steroid such as methylprednisolone (Medrol) may be prescribed for 6 days, with a decreasing dosage.

ATOPIC DERMATITIS (ECZEMA)

SYMPTOMS AND SIGNS

Atopic dermatitis (eczema) is an inflammation of the skin that tends to occur in persons with a family history of allergic conditions. A rash, with vesicular and exudative eruptions in children and dry, leathery vesicles in adults, develops (Fig. 6–5). The rash occurs in a characteristic pattern on the face, neck, elbows, knees, and upper trunk of the body and is accompanied by pruritus.

ETIOLOGY

Eczema is an idiopathic disease. The tendency for this condition to develop is inherited, and it is assumed that there is an allergic connection. Eczema in some infants is believed to be traceable to a sensitivity to milk, orange juice, or some other foods.

A flare-up of eczema can be triggered by stress, anxiety, or conflict. Stress actually can make the condition worse. Climate, especially sudden or extreme changes in temperature, can

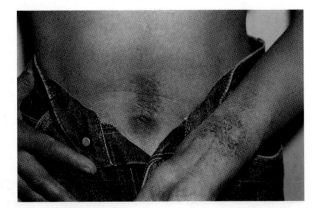

Figure 6–4

Contact dermatitis. (From Lookingbill, D, Marks J: Principles of Dermatology, 2nd ed. Philadelphia: WB Saunders, 1993. Used with permission.)

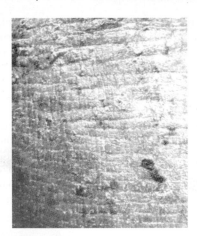

Figure 6–5

Atopic dermatitis (eczema). (From Lookingbill D, Marks J: Principles of Dermatology, 2nd ed. Philadelphia: WB Saunders, 1993, p 127. Used with permission.)

affect or aggravate the condition. High humidity also may aggravate eczema.

Eczema in infants usually subsides by the age of 2 years. The rash may resolve during adolescence or persist into adulthood. Generally, eczema tends to improve with time.

DIAGNOSIS

A medical history, including family history, along with examination of the skin, confirms the diagnosis. On occasion, skin testing for specific allergies may be indicated to identify underlying causes.

TREATMENT

The main objective in treating atopic dermatitis is decreasing the frequency and severity of eruptions and relieving the pruritus. Unfortunately, no medications can eliminate eczema. Topical ointments and creams containing a cortisone derivative are the primary treatment of eczema. Local and systemic medications, such as antihistamines, tranquilizers, and other sedatives, may be prescribed to prevent or control the pruritus.

Secondary bacterial or viral infections can result from scratching the rash or lesions. A secondary bacterial infection is the most common complication. The physician likely prescribes an antibiotic to control the infection. A more serious complication of eczema can be caused by infection with certain viruses, specifically herpes simplex virus.

  # Urticaria

SYMPTOMS AND SIGNS

Urticaria, or hives, is associated with severe itching followed by the appearance of redness and an area of swelling (**wheal**) in a localized area of skin. Hives of various sizes can erupt as a few lesions anywhere on the skin or frequently are scattered over the body or the mucous membrane. In gastrointestinal involvement, the patient complains of abdominal colic. When hives develop in the pharyngeal mucosa, the airway can become obstructed, causing asphyxiation. When the swelling involves deeper tissues, the condition is called *angioedema*, a more serious condition. Urticaria is common, frequently acute, and self-limiting, lasting a few hours. In other instances, hives continue over months or years, becoming a chronic condition.

ETIOLOGY

Urticaria affects the dermis, resulting from an acute hypersensitivity and the release of histamine. This causes local inflammation and vasodilatation of capillaries with marked edema. Allergic reactions to foods (such as shell fish, strawberries, or peanuts), drugs (such as penicillin), or insect stings (frequently from a bee) are some more common causes. Infection can precipitate an attack of hives, as can some inhalants, sunlight, or temperature extremes. Sometimes the cause is not identified.

DIAGNOSIS

Visual inspection of the urticaria is diagnostic. A prior episode, in conjunction with a particular exposure to a known allergen, is significant in the patient's history. If the medical history is void of clues to the cause, sensitivity testing and blood tests for antibodies may help distinguish the causative agent.

TREATMENT

If known, the antigenic factor is removed and then avoided if possible. Antihistamines bring quick relief of symptoms. An injection of epinephrine is used in more severe cases. In persistent cases, a course of prednisone is therapeutic.

153

Psoriasis

SYMPTOMS AND SIGNS

Psoriasis is a chronic skin condition marked by thick, flaky, red patches of various sizes, covered with characteristic white, silvery scales (Fig. 6-6). These scales develop into dry **plaques** (see Fig. 6-2 *C*), sometimes progressing to **pustules** (see Fig. 6-2 *G*). They usually do not cause discomfort but might be slightly itchy or sore. Affected skin typically appears dry, cracked, and encrusted. The most common areas for psoriasis to develop are the scalp; the outer sides of the arms and legs, especially the elbows and knees; and the trunk of the body. Also, the palms of the hands and soles of the feet may be affected. In some individuals, psoriasis spreads to the nail beds, causing the nails to thicken and crumble. Psoriasis can occur at any age but is more common between 10 and 30 years of age. It is noninfectious and does not affect general health.

ETIOLOGY

The cause of psoriasis is unknown, but it seems to be genetically determined. Psoriasis may be an **autoimmune** disorder and is more common among the white race. Precipitating fac-

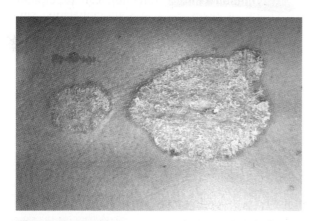

Figure 6–6

Psoriasis. (From Lookingbill D, Marks J: Principles of Dermatology, 2nd ed. Philadelphia: WB Saunders, 1993, p 138. Used with permission.)

tors for the development of psoriasis include hormonal changes such as those occurring with pregnancy, climate changes, emotional stress, or a period of generally poor health.

DIAGNOSIS

The white, silvery scales of psoriasis are recognizable, making the condition easy to diagnose. A careful patient history, observation of the skin, or a skin biopsy may be helpful when the scales are not evident, as with patients who bathe and scrub frequently. Scratching the lesions reveals the telltale scales.

TREATMENT

There is no cure for psoriasis; however, it is controllable. Remissions and **exacerbations** occur frequently. Treatment options include exposure to ultraviolet light to help to retard cell reproduction, the use of steroid creams (methoxsalen) in combination with ultraviolet light, the application of coal tar preparations, the administration of low-dosage antihistamines, and oatmeal baths. Severe cases of psoriasis may require chemotherapy or the use of etretinate, which is related to vitamin A. *Caution:* Pregnant women and nursing mothers should never take etretinate.

10-30 more mens then females

Rosacea

SYMPTOMS AND SIGNS

Rosacea, a disorder of the facial skin, causes redness, primarily in the areas where individuals blush or flush. The onset is insidious and often is mistaken for a complexion change, a sunburn, or even acne. The redness becomes more noticeable and does not go away. This may be followed by the skin exhibiting a dryness and pimples that may become inflamed or pus filled. Additionally, small blood vessels of the cheeks and face enlarge and show through the skin as red lines remaining even after the redness decreases (Fig. 6-7). Occasionally, mostly in the male with rosacea, small knobby bumps appear on the nose, causing it to look swollen.

154

cise, extreme heat or cold, stress, spicy foods, hot drinks, and alcohol. Sun exposure, hot weather, cold weather, and wind all have been identified as trip wires, as have abrupt changes of the seasons and weather extremes. The physician may prescribe medications to control the redness. Sometimes antibiotics are prescribed. Mild cleansers should be used, and moisturizers that do not contain alcohol or drying agents should be applied routinely. Sunscreens are helpful. Consistent treatment is necessary to avoid flare-ups.

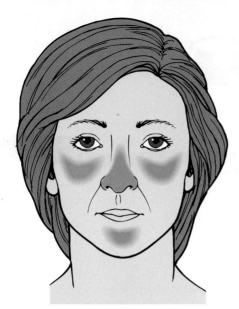

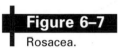
Figure 6–7
Rosacea.

ETIOLOGY

The etiology of rosacea, a chronic and often cyclic condition, is unknown. A possible correlation with the frequency of the individual's blushing or facial flushing has been suggested. Also, those with lighter complexions appear to have a greater incidence of the disorder, and rosacea possibly may be inherited. Rosacea is not considered to be infectious or contagious and is not spread by skin contact.

DIAGNOSIS

Diagnosis is made from the history of facial blushing and flushing. Although rosacea often has many of the same symptoms as acne, the individual experiencing episodes of rosacea does not have the blackheads or whiteheads (comedones) typical of acne. A dermatologist should be consulted for a definite diagnosis.

TREATMENT

There is no cure for rosacea, although symptoms can be controlled by medical treatment and modification of lifestyles. It is helpful for the patient to identify situations that cause him or her to blush or experience facial flushing and attempt to avoid these triggers or trip wires. These events may be different for various rosacea sufferers, so it is wise to avoid sunlight, hard exer-

 Acne Vulgaris

SYMPTOMS AND SIGNS

Acne vulgaris is an inflammatory disease of the sebaceous glands and hair follicles. It is marked by the appearance of **papules,** pustules, and **comedones** (see Fig. 6–2 *B, G,* and *L*). Sometimes, deeper boil-like lesions called nodules can occur. Scars may develop if the chronic irritation and inflammation continue for a long period. Acne is found most commonly on the face but also can occur on the neck, shoulders, chest, and back. Acne can appear at any age but is more common in adolescents. In girls, it is usually at its worst between the ages of 14 and 17 years. In boys, it reaches its peak in the late teens.

ETIOLOGY

The cause of acne vulgaris is unknown. Research on the cause, however, links it to hormonal changes taking place in adolescence that affect the activity of the sebaceous glands. Hereditary tendencies also are known to be predisposing factors. Precipitating factors may include food allergies, endocrine disorders, psychological factors, fatigue, and the use of steroid drugs.

Sebum, an oily substance produced by the sebaceous glands, reaches the skin surface through the hair follicle. The oil seems to stimulate the follicle walls, causing a more rapid shedding of skin cells. This causes the cells and sebum to stick together and to form a plug, which promotes the growth of bacteria in the follicles. This is the process by which pimples and bumps form.

DIAGNOSIS

Examination of the characteristic lesions and patient history confirm the diagnosis.

TREATMENT

Therapy may include the use of topical or systemic antibiotics, or both. Topically applied **keratolytic** agents may prove appropriate for many cases of acne. Ultraviolet light treatments and the topical application of medications chemically related to vitamin A reduce the skin's natural oils and promote drying and peeling of the acne lesions (e.g., tretinoin [Retin-A]).

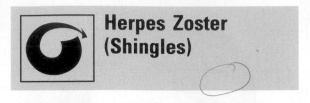

Herpes Zoster (Shingles)

SYMPTOMS AND SIGNS

Herpes zoster, or shingles, is an acute inflammatory dermatomal eruption of extremely painful vesicles. Shingles occurs in a band-like unilateral pattern along the course of the peripheral nerves

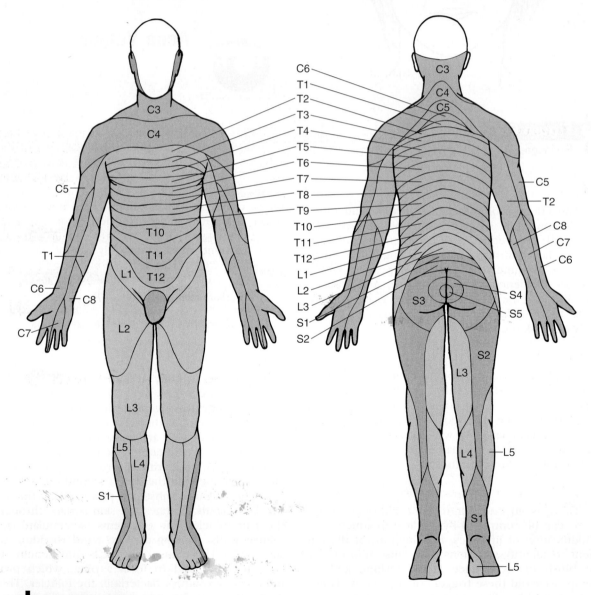

Figure 6–8
Dermatomes.

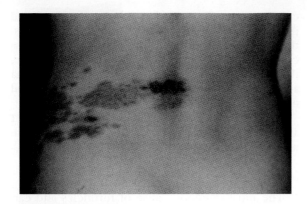

Figure 6–9

Herpes zoster (shingles). (From Callen J, Greer K, Hood A, et al: Color Atlas of Dermatology. Philadelphia: WB Saunders, 1993, p 273. Used with permission.)

or **dermatomes** that are affected and does not cross the midline of the body (Fig. 6–8). Pain beginning about 2 or 3 days before the appearance of the lesions sometimes is accompanied by a fever. The eruptions begin as a rash that rapidly develops into vesicles (Fig. 6–9). The skin that overlies the affected dermatome or dermatomes becomes reddened and blistered. These vesicles often are grouped on a reddened area of the skin. After several days, the vesicles appear pustular, develop a crust, and then a scab.

The incubation period is from 7 to 21 days. The duration of the disease, from onset to recovery, is usually 10 days to 5 weeks. If all the vesicles appear within 24 hours, the total duration is usually shorter. Although the commonly affected site is the skin overlying thoracic dermatomes, any area of the body may be affected. Occasionally, shingles may occur on the face, neck, and scalp. When nerves supplying the eye are involved, the disease may cause serious damage to the structure of the eye.

ETIOLOGY

The cause is the herpes varicella-zoster virus (VZV), the same virus that causes chickenpox. For unknown reasons, after lying dormant in the dorsal root ganglia, it becomes reactivated in later years. Stress appears to be a precipitating factor.

DIAGNOSIS

Shingles is diagnosed by its characteristic pattern and painful vesicles. The confirmation can be made by culturing the virus from vesicle scrapings. A blood sample containing the varicella-zoster antibodies also aids in the diagnosis. Although shingles can affect any age group, those older than 55 years of age are more frequently affected.

TREATMENT

Treatment of shingles is directed toward making the patient comfortable. Analgesics, mild tranquilizers or sedatives, antipruritics, steroids (e.g., methylprednisolone, prednisone, and betamethasone [Celestone Soluspan]) and a drying agent to be applied directly to the vesicles may be prescribed. Acyclovir (Zovirax) used orally, parenterally, or topically also is prescribed and is quite effective. Other antiviral agents that may be prescribed include famciclovir (Famvir), valacyclovir (Valtrex), or foscarnet sodium (Foscavir). Antibiotic therapy may be necessary to prevent a secondary infection. If the eye is affected, early treatment with idoxuridine is necessary. The latter therapy should be supervised by an ophthalmologist.

A common complication for some patients is postherpetic neuralgia. This chronic pain may persist for as long as a month after the skin lesions have healed.

When the pain is intolerable, lidocaine injections and nerve block injections may be attempted. If these steps do not provide relief, permanent nerve blocks with alcohol or nerve resection may be used as a last resort. Shingles also may reoccur at later dates.

Impetigo

SYMPTOMS AND SIGNS

Impetigo is a common, contagious, superficial skin infection. It manifests with early vesicular or pustular lesions that rupture and form thick yellow crusts (Fig. 6–10). The lesions commonly develop on the legs and are found less frequently on the face, trunk, and arms. They usually are accompanied by pruritus. Adjacent lesions may develop as a result of autoinoculation from scratching, but systemic symptoms are uncommon. Ulcerations with erythema and scarring also may occur from scratching or abrading the skin.

157

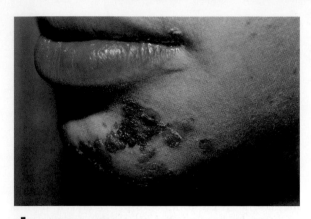

Figure 6–10

Impetigo. (From Lookingbill D, Marks J: Principles of Dermatology, 2nd ed. Philadelphia: WB Saunders, 1993, p 198. Used with permission.)

158

ETIOLOGY

Impetigo is caused by either *Streptococcus* or *Staphylococcus aureus*. The infection is thought to originate from insect bites, scabies infestation, poor hygiene, anemia, and malnutrition. Cases of impetigo are prevalent in temperate climates and occur more frequently in warm weather.

DIAGNOSIS

The diagnosis is made on the appearance of the characteristic lesions. To differentiate impetigo from other skin diseases, a **Tzanck test** and a **Gram stain** may be useful.

TREATMENT

Systemic use of antibiotics, Bactroban ointment, and proper cleaning of lesions 2 or 3 times a day are effective treatments for impetigo. Avoidance of infected individuals is essential.

Furuncles and Carbuncles

SYMPTOMS AND SIGNS

A furuncle, or boil, is an **abscess** that involves the entire hair follicle and adjacent subcutaneous tissue. A carbuncle is either an unusually large furuncle or multiple furuncles that develop in adjoining follicles, connected by many drainage canals. The affected area is red, swollen, and painful (Fig. 6-11). Eventually, over several days, the abscess either bursts through the skin or, less commonly, discharges internally. In either case, the pain is relieved and the boil heals. Erythema and edema may persist at the site for several more days or weeks.

Boils are extremely common. They can affect almost everyone at some time. Carbuncles are much more rare. Both tend to recur.

ETIOLOGY

The most common cause of furuncles and carbuncles is bacterial infection with *Staphylococcus.* Both are localized infections and usually heal uneventfully. Predisposing factors include diabetes mellitus, nephritis, and other underlying diseases (e.g., digestive or gastrointestinal conditions). In some cases, furuncles and carbuncles are the result of poor resistance to infection or poor hygiene.

DIAGNOSIS

A diagnosis is made by observing the characteristic lesion. An abscess may be cultured to isolate the causative organism. If recurring boils are a problem, the physician may order blood

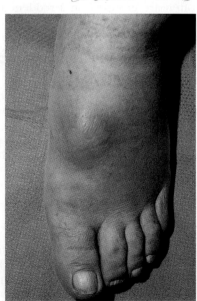

Figure 6–11

Furuncle. (From Lookingbill D, Marks J: Principles of Dermatology, 2nd ed. Philadelphia: WB Saunders, 1993, p 234. Used with permission.)

and urine analyses to rule out any underlying disease.

TREATMENT

Applying hot compresses every few hours helps to relieve the discomfort and to hasten the draining. Surgical incision and drainage (I & D) may be necessary. Antibiotic treatment also may be needed for several weeks.

Erysipelas (Cellulitis)

SYMPTOMS AND SIGNS

Cellulitis is an acute, diffuse, bacterial infection of the skin and subcutaneous tissue. It occurs most commonly in the lower extremities; however, any part of the body can be infected. Clinically, erythema and pitting edema develop, and the skin becomes tender and hot to the touch (Fig. 6–12). The infection develops and spreads gradually over a couple of days. Red lines or streaks may occur proximal to the infec-

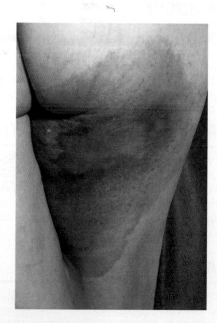

Figure 6–12

Erysipelas (cellulitis). (From Lookingbill D, Marks J: Principles of Dermatology, 2nd ed. Philadelphia: WB Saunders, 1993, p 232. Used with permission.)

tion and run along lymph vessels to nearby lymph glands. If the lymph glands become edematous, systemic symptoms of fever and malaise may be present.

ETIOLOGY

The cause of cellulitis is either *Streptococcus* or *Staphylococcus* that enters the skin's surface via a small cut or lesion. The bacteria produce enzymes that break down the skin cells. As a result of the release of enzymes, the infection spreads locally. These enzymes prevent body responses that normally would reduce local spread of infection by closing off the site.

DIAGNOSIS

Examination of the affected part of the body, checking for pitting edema and other symptoms, and a blood culture aid the physician in making the diagnosis.

TREATMENT

The affected limb should be immobilized and elevated. Cool magnesium sulfate solution compresses may be used for discomfort. Warm compresses should be applied to increase circulation to the affected part. Systemic antibiotics, with penicillin being the drug of choice, are prescribed for the infection. Aspirin or acetaminophen alone or in combination with codeine is given for pain. Hospitalization is indicated when cellulitis is severe.

Dermatophytoses

SYMPTOMS AND SIGNS

Dermatophytosis (tinea) is a chronic superficial fungal infection of the skin. Dermatophyte infections are classified by the body region they inhabit. All dermatophytosis lesions are characterized by an active border and are marked by scaling with central clearing. Dermatophytosis occurring on the scalp is called tinea capitis; the body, tinea corporis; the nails, tinea unguium; the feet, tinea pedis; and the groin region, tinea cruris.

TINEA CAPITIS

Tinea capitis is characterized by round, gray, scaly lesions on the scalp (Fig. 6–13). It is conta-

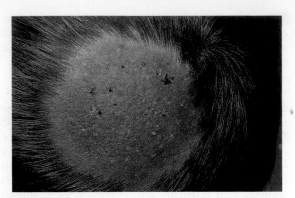

Figure 6–13

Tinea capitis. (From Callen J, Greer K, Hood A, et al: Color Atlas of Dermatology. Philadelphia: WB Saunders, 1993, p 106. Used with permission.)

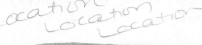

gious and often epidemic among children. The infected child may have a slight pruritus of the scalp or may be **asymptomatic.**

TINEA CORPORIS (RINGWORM)

Tinea corporis is characterized by lesions that are round, ringed, and scaled with vesicles (Fig. 6–14). This infection can occur in anyone who has skin contact with infected domestic animals, especially cats. It is more common in rural settings and in hot and humid climates.

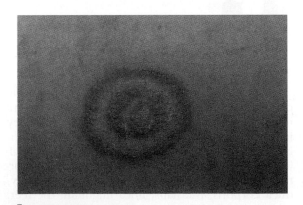

Figure 6–14

Tinea corporis (ringworm). (From Callen J, Greer K, Hood A, et al: Color Atlas of Dermatology. Philadelphia: WB Saunders, 1993, p 106. Used with permission.)

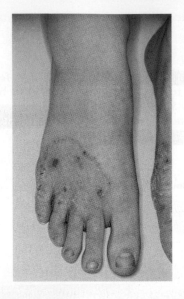

Figure 6–15

Tinea pedis (athlete's foot). (From Callen J, Greer K, Hood A, et al: Color Atlas of Dermatology. Philadelphia: WB Saunders, 1993. Used with permission.)

TINEA UNGUIUM

Tinea unguium frequently begins at the tip of toenails, affecting one or more nails at a time. It also can affect fingernails, but this is less common. The affected nail or nails appear hypertrophic or thickened, brittle, and lusterless.

TINEA PEDIS (ATHLETE'S FOOT)

Tinea pedis is characterized by intense, burning, stinging pruritus between the toes and on the soles of the feet (Fig. 6–15). The skin can become inflamed, dry, and peeling and fissures (see Fig. 6-2 J) may develop. This condition is rare in children.

TINEA CRURIS (JOCK ITCH)

Tinea cruris is characterized by raised, red, pruritic vesicular patches, with well-defined borders, located in the groin area (Fig. 6–16). It can be associated with athlete's foot and occurs more commonly in adult men. Flare-ups are frequent in summer months and are aggravated by physical activity, perspiration, and tight-fitting clothes.

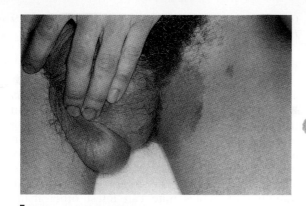

Figure 6–16

Tinea cruris (jock itch). (From Callen J, Greer K, Hood A, et al: Color Atlas of Dermatology. Philadelphia: WB Saunders, 1993, p 33. Used with permission.)

ETIOLOGY

Dermatophytosis is caused by several species of fungi that can invade the skin or nails, especially if the integrity of the skin is compromised. The infection is transmitted by direct contact with the fungus or its spores.

DIAGNOSIS

The diagnosis is made by the appearance and location of the lesions. To isolate the causative fungus, a culture of the lesions is necessary.

TREATMENT

Antifungal medications are prescribed either for topical application (ointment) or for oral use, depending on the severity of the infection. The affected skin needs to be kept as clean and dry as possible; clothing should be loose fitting and clean; exercise should be limited to prevent excessive perspiration. Because all forms of dermatophytosis tend to be persistent and chronic, meticulous management is necessary to correct this condition.

Decubitus Ulcers

SYMPTOMS AND SIGNS

A decubitus ulcer, commonly called a pressure ulcer or bed sore, is a localized area of dead skin that can affect the epidermis, dermis, and subcutaneous layers (Fig. 6–17). An early sign of an ulcer is shiny, reddened skin appearing over a bony prominence in individuals with prolonged immobilization. Other signs that eventually occur include blisters, erosions, necrosis, and ulceration. If the ulcer becomes infected, a foul-smelling, purulent discharge is present. Pain may or may not accompany the decubitus ulcer.

ETIOLOGY

Decubitus ulcers are caused by impairment or lack of blood supply to the affected area of skin. This is the result of constant pressure against the surface of the skin, as seen in people who are debilitated, paralyzed, or unconscious.

DIAGNOSIS

Visual examination of the ulcer is sufficient for a diagnosis. If infection is suspected, culture and sensitivity testing may be needed to isolate the causative organism.

TREATMENT

If not treated vigorously, the ulcer progresses from a simple erosion of the skin to complete involvement of all layers of skin. Eventually, the ulcer extends to the underlying muscle and bone tissue.

Topical agents that have proved effective in the treatment of decubitus ulcers include absorbable gelatin sponges, granulated sugar, karaya gum patches, antiseptic irrigations, **débriding** agents, and antibiotics (when infection is present).

161

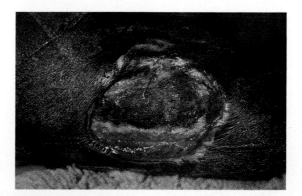

Figure 6–17

Decubitus ulcer. (From Callen J, Greer K, Hood A, et al: Color Atlas of Dermatology. Philadelphia: WB Saunders, 1993, p 226. Used with permission.)

Preventive measures include frequent inspection of the skin for signs of breakdown, alleviation of pressure points over bony prominences, good skin care, early ambulation when possible, position changes every 2 hours, passive range-of-motion exercises, and the use of special pads and mattresses.

Scabies and Pediculosis

SYMPTOMS AND SIGNS

Itch mites (scabies) and lice (pediculosis) are the two most common parasitic insects to infest humans. Human scabies infestations are caused by the human itch mite, *Sarcoptes scabiei* (Fig. 6–18 *A*). There are three species of human lice: the head louse, *Pediculus humanus capitis* (Fig. 6–19 *A*); the body louse, *P. humanus corporis*; and the pubic, or crab, louse, *Phthirus pubis* (Fig. 6–20 *A*). Both scabies and pediculosis are *highly* contagious. They produce intense pruritus and a sensation of something crawling on the skin. With scabies, the most common symptom is a rash (Fig. 6–18 *B*). It can occur anywhere on the body but usually is found on hands, breasts, armpits, waistline, and the genital area. Lice also can produce a rash or wheals, but the most common sign or symptom is the presence of nits

(eggs) on hair shafts, skin, or clothing (Figs. 6–19 *B* and 6–20 *B*).

ETIOLOGY

Itch mites and lice can infest anyone at any age. Both are spread easily from one person to another by close physical contact. Transmission occurs most commonly between children playing together, family members, and sexual partners. In addition to physical contact, transmission may occur indirectly from infected clothing, bed sheets, towels, and hair combs or brushes. Although the scabies mite can infest other mammals, it is not transmitted from pets to humans. Pubic lice, however, have been known to infest dogs and then have been retransmitted to humans. Both scabies and pediculosis are common in overcrowded areas that have inadequate facilities and where poor personal hygiene is practiced.

DIAGNOSIS

Visual examination can identify lice and nits on the hair, body, and clothing. Other skin disorders such as atopic dermatitis (see Atopic Dermatitis), contact dermatitis (see Contact Dermatitis), and psoriasis (see Psoriasis) need to be ruled out when scabies is suspected. A similar rash occurring about the same time in several family members should suggest scabies.

TREATMENT

The goals of treatment of scabies and pediculosis are to remove the mites, lice, and nits; to

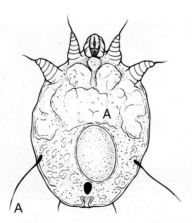

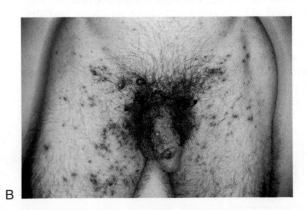

Figure 6–18

A, Itch (scabies) mite. *B*, Scabies rash. (*B* from Callen J, Greer K, Hood A, et al: Color Atlas of Dermatology. Philadelphia: WB Saunders, 1993, p 193. Used with permission.)

162

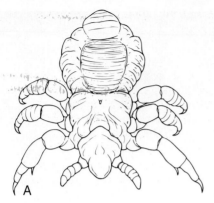

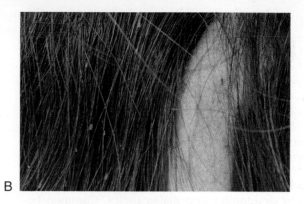

Figure 6–19

A, Pediculus humanus capitis (head louse). *B,* Lice in hair. (*B* from Callen J, Greer K, Hood A, et al: Color Atlas of Dermatology. Philadelphia: WB Saunders, 1993, p 373. Used with permission.)

eliminate the pruritus; to provide emotional support to the patient, family, and contacts; and to treat the environment to prevent reinfestation.

A special shampoo must be used to kill head lice and must be repeated in 7 to 10 days to ensure that all the nits are dead. This must be followed by meticulous combing with a special fine-toothed comb to dislodge the nits. Body lice are removed with soap and water or the same shampoo used for head lice. Pubic lice may be treated with shampoo, creams, or lotions.

Scabies treatment includes the use of special shampoos, creams, sulfur preparations, and topical steroids. Because of intense pruritus and the scratching associated with scabies and lice infestations, a secondary infection may occur, necessitating treatment with oral antibiotics.

With both scabies and pediculosis, family members and others who have had direct contact with the infected person must be treated as well. All clothing and bedding belonging to the infected person must be washed in hot water or dry-cleaned. Any furniture that the person has been using also should be cleaned either with a surface cleaner or by vacuuming.

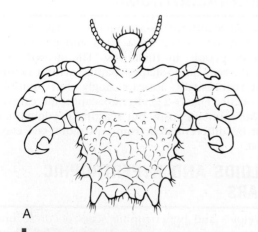

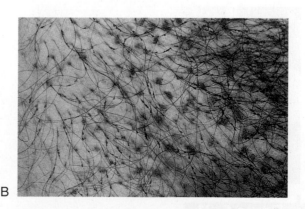

Figure 6–20

A, Phthirus pubis (pubic, or crab, louse). *B,* Pubic lice rash. (*B* from Callen J, Greer K, Hood A, et al: Color Atlas of Dermatology. Philadelphia: WB Saunders, 1993, p 332. Used with permission.)

Benign and Premalignant Tumors

SYMPTOMS AND SIGNS

Noncancerous growths or tumors of the skin fall into two categories: benign and premalignant. Benign tumors are usually a cosmetic problem only. Premalignant tumors need to be identified and treated as early as possible to prevent them from developing into malignancies. Common benign tumors include seborrheic keratoses, dermatofibromas, keratoacanthomas, keloids and hypertrophic scars, epidermal (sebaceous) cysts, and acrochordons (skin tags). Actinic keratoses and nevi (moles) are the most common premalignant tumors.

SEBORRHEIC KERATOSIS

Seborrheic keratoses are benign growths originating in the epidermis, clinically appearing as tan-brown, greasy papules or plaques (see Fig. 6-2 *B* and *C*) and having the appearance of being pasted on (Fig. 6-21). They are, for the most part, asymptomatic but may cause pruritus, especially in elderly persons. The cause of seborrheic keratoses is unknown, and although they have no potential for developing into malignancy, they should be differentiated from other potentially malignant tumors. The sudden appearance of or a sudden increase in the number or size of these growths on uninflamed skin could indicate the

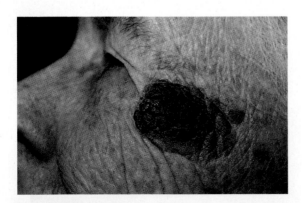

Figure 6–21

Seborrheic keratosis. (From Callen J, Greer K, Hood A, et al: Color Atlas of Dermatology. Philadelphia: WB Saunders, 1993, p 146. Used with permission.)

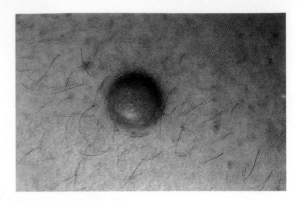

Figure 6–22

Dermatofibroma. (From Callen J, Greer K, Hood A, et al: Color Atlas of Dermatology. Philadelphia: WB Saunders, 1993, p 65. Used with permission.)

presence of an internal malignancy, most commonly of the stomach.

DERMATOFIBROMA

Dermatofibromas are benign and asymptomatic and can be found on any part of the body, particularly on the front of the lower leg. They are more prevalent in women and are thought to be caused by fibrous reactions to viral infections. These growths also can be caused by a reaction to insect bites and trauma. Dermatofibromas are scaly, hard growths that are slightly raised and pinkish brown (Fig. 6-22).

KERATOACANTHOMA

Keratoacanthoma is a benign epithelial growth that may be caused by a virus and generally is seen in people in their 60s. The growth is a smooth, red, dome-shaped papule with a central crust that usually appears singly, but multiples can occur (Fig. 6-23). Keratoacanthoma can disappear spontaneously, but scarring is common. It must be differentiated from squamous cell carcinoma.

KELOIDS AND HYPERTROPHIC SCARS

Keloids and hypertrophic scars occur secondary to trauma or surgery. At first, a keloid appears normal, but after several months, it becomes noticeably larger and thicker (Fig. 6-24). Keloids are harmless, although they can cause pruritus and sometimes deformities. They are

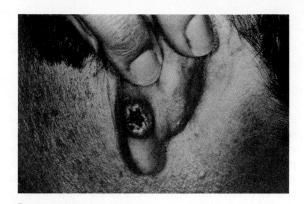

Figure 6–23

Keratoacanthoma. (From Callen J, Greer K, Hood A, et al: Color Atlas of Dermatology. Philadelphia: WB Saunders, 1993, p 226. Used with permission.)

more common in black-skinned people. Keloids extend beyond the wound site and do not regress spontaneously. Hypertrophic scars, however, do not extend, but stay confined to the site and generally regress over time.

EPIDERMAL (SEBACEOUS) CYST

Sebaceous cysts develop when a sebaceous gland slowly fills with a thick fluid. This process can take many years but is usually painless and harmless. Some cysts, usually small ones, have a blackhead in the pore connecting the cyst to the skin's surface. Larger cysts most often are closed on the surface. The cysts are palpable and moveable and range in size from millimeters to several centimeters (Fig. 6–25). Sebaceous cysts commonly are found on the scalp, on the face, at the base of the ears, and on the chest. They also can develop in any area of the body that contains sebaceous glands. If bacteria enter the pore, the cyst becomes infected and enlarges, and inflammation and tenderness occur. The cyst eventually may burst, releasing a foul-smelling pus. Inflammation recedes, but the cyst remains and can become reinfected at another time.

ACROCHORDON (SKIN TAG)

Acrochordons are common benign skin growths or tags. They are found mainly in the axilla, on the neck, and on inguinal areas of the body. They can be brown or skin colored, and are attached to the body by a short stalk (Fig. 6–26).

ACTINIC KERATOSIS

Actinic keratoses are common premalignant lesions and are seen on sun-exposed areas of the body. They are caused by long-term exposure to

165

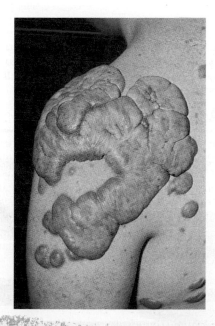

Figure 6–24

Keloid. (From Callen J, Greer K, Hood A, et al: Color Atlas of Dermatology. Philadelphia: WB Saunders, 1993, p 143. Used with permission.)

Figure 6–25

Epidermal (sebaceous) cyst. (From Lookingbill D, Marks J: Principles of Dermatology, 2nd ed. Philadelphia: WB Saunders, 1993, p 101. Used with permission.)

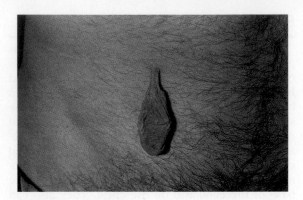

Figure 6–26

Acrochordon (skin tag). (From Callen J, Greer K, Hood A, et al: Color Atlas of Dermatology. Philadelphia: WB Saunders, 1993, p 130. Used with permission.)

sunlight, and their numbers increase with age. Light-skinned people have a higher risk. Actinic keratosis initially appears as an area of rough, vascular skin, which later forms a yellow, adherent crust (Fig. 6–27).

ETIOLOGY

The causes vary with the particular lesion.

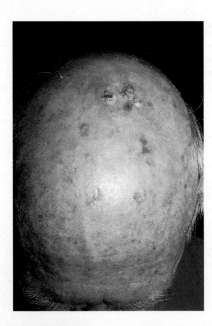

Figure 6–27

Actinic keratoses. (From Callen J, Greer K, Hood A, et al: Color Atlas of Dermatology. Philadelphia: WB Saunders, 1993, p 311. Used with permission.)

DIAGNOSIS

The diagnosis is made by visual examination; to confirm the findings, a biopsy of the tissue may be necessary.

TREATMENT

Seborrheic keratoses are treated with cryosurgery and curettage. Keratoacanthoma is treated with fluorouracil (5-fluorouracil [5-FU]) or corticosteroid injections, adrenocorticosteroids applied topically, and oral isotretinoin and etretinate administration for multiple lesions. Keloids and hypertrophic scars are treated with corticosteroids injected into the lesion once every 4 weeks or surgery with scar compression. Epidermal, or sebaceous, cysts are excised surgically and treated with antibiotics if infected. Acrochordons (skin tags) also are treated by excisional surgery. Actinic keratosis is treated with topical agents — tretinoin (Retin-A) alone or in combination with fluorouracil — and by curettage and desiccation.

Skin Carcinomas

SYMPTOMS AND SIGNS

There are three types of skin cancer: basal cell carcinoma, squamous cell carcinoma, and malignant melanoma. Of the three, basal cell carcinoma is the most common type.

BASAL CELL CARCINOMA

Basal cell carcinoma affects more than 400,000 Americans each year, with one of every four newly discovered cancers being basal cell carcinoma. Basal cell lesions can appear anywhere on the body. The most common sites are the sun-exposed areas: face, ears, back, chest, arms, and back of the hands (Fig. 6–28). There are five warning signs that could indicate the presence of basal cell cancer:

- A persistent, nonhealing, open lesion that bleeds, oozes, or crusts, remaining open for 3 weeks or longer
- A reddish, irritated area, usually on the shoulders, extremities, or chest, that may or may not be painful or cause pruritus
- A smooth growth with an indented center and elevated, rolled edge or border
- A shiny bump or nodule that is pearly or trans-

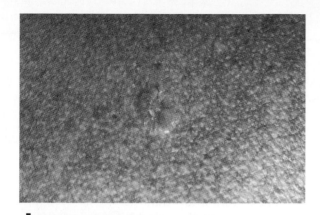

Figure 6–28

Basal cell carcinoma. (From Lookingbill D, Marks J: Principles of Dermatology, 2nd ed. Philadelphia: WB Saunders, 1993, p 81. Used with permission.)

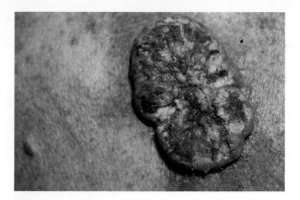

Figure 6–29

Squamous cell carcinoma. (From Callen J, Greer K, Hood A, et al. Color Atlas of Dermatology. Philadelphia: WB Saunders, 1993, p 142. Used with permission.)

lucent and white, pink, red, tan, brown, or black
- A scar-like area, often with poorly defined edges, that is white, yellow, or waxy in appearance

This form of skin cancer can develop in anyone, especially those with a history of chronic sun exposure. People at highest risk have fair skin, light-colored hair, and blue, green, or gray eyes. Basal cell carcinoma often resembles noncancerous conditions such as eczema (see Atopic Dermatitis [Eczema]) and psoriasis (see Psoriasis). This form of cancer arises from the basal (deepest) layer of the epidermis, is locally invasive, but rarely **metastasizes.** A small proportion of these cancers recur, either in the same place or nearby, usually within 2 years.

SQUAMOUS CELL CARCINOMA

Squamous cell carcinomas also develop in the epidermis. They appear as firm, fleshy, red, hard-surfaced nodules with visible scales (Fig. 6–29). Like basal cell carcinoma, squamous cell carcinoma often ulcerates and forms a crust. The lower lip, the ears, and the hands are common sites for this cancer. This is a more serious form of skin cancer because of its tendency to metastasize if allowed to reach an advanced stage.

MALIGNANT MELANOMA

Malignant melanoma is the most serious of the three types of skin cancer, but it is not as common. This type rarely occurs before adolescence.

Unlike basal cell and squamous cell carcinomas, malignant melanoma metastasizes throughout the body. The most common symptom is change, either in a new or existing pigmented area of the skin or in a mole that may have been present since birth or childhood (Fig. 6–30). Changes that may indicate the presence of malignant melanoma are

- Change in size, especially sudden or continuous enlargement
- Change in color, especially multiple shades of tan, brown, and black; mixing of red, white, and blue; or spreading of color from the border into adjacent skin
- Change in shape, especially the development of

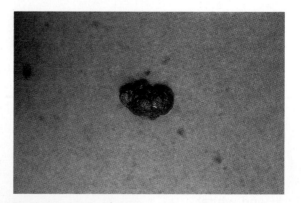

Figure 6–30

Malignant melanoma. (From Callen J, Greer K, Hood A, et al: Color Atlas of Dermatology. Philadelphia: WB Saunders, 1993, p 94. Used with permission.)

an irregular, notched border of an area with a previously regular border
• Change in the elevation of a previously flat pigmented area
• Change in the surface: scaliness, erosion, oozing, crusting, or bleeding
• Change in the surrounding skin: redness, swelling, or the development of colored areas adjacent to but not part of the pigmented area
• Change in sensation: tenderness, pain, or pruritus
• Change in consistency: softening or hardening

ETIOLOGY

Ninety-five percent of all skin carcinomas result from chronic overexposure to the sun. Geographic location is also a factor. The closer one is to the equator, the higher the frequency is, especially among fair-skinned people.

With malignant melanoma, in addition to overexposure to the sun, changes in the underlying skin cells that produce melanin can cause this life-threatening tumor to develop. Specific factors make certain individuals more prone to malignant melanoma:

• A family history of malignant melanoma
• A previous case of malignant melanoma
• The presence of large brown moles at birth
• Unusually large moles (larger than ¼ inch) that are irregular in shape and have multiple colors
• A history of painful or blistering sunburns, especially at a young age
• Indoor occupations with outdoor recreational activities

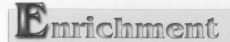

ABCDs OF MALIGNANT MELANOMA

⊃ A = Asymmetry (lack of equality in the diameter)
⊃ B = Border (notched, scalloped, or indistinct)
⊃ C = Color (uneven, variegated—ranging from tan, brown or black to red and white)
⊃ D = Diameter (usually larger than 6 mm)

* Adapted from the ABCDs of Moles and Melanoma. New York, The Skin Cancer Foundation, Copyright 1985.

Enrichment

Guidelines for Protecting the Skin Against Excessive Sun Exposure

⊃ Avoid sunlight between 10 AM and 3 PM, when ultraviolet rays are the strongest.
⊃ Plan outdoor activities for early morning or late afternoon.
⊃ Wear protective clothing, especially a hat.
⊃ Use a sunscreen with a sun protection factor (SPF) of at least 15, applied 15 to 30 minutes before exposure.

DIAGNOSIS

If any of the warning signs are observed or an unusual growth is noticed, a physician should be seen immediately. The diagnosis of each of the three types of carcinoma is confirmed by a punch, incisional, or total excisional biopsy of the suspicious lesion.

TREATMENT

The goal of treatment is to eliminate the cancerous lesions. Several effective methods to accomplish this are based on the type, size, invasiveness, and location of the tumor and the patient's age and general health. Methods of treatment include excisional surgery, electrodesiccation, cryosurgery, Mohs surgery (microscopically controlled surgery), and laser surgery. Radiation therapy is also effective, especially for elderly patients or people in poor health. Because all forms of surgical excision involve removal of skin tissue, scarring is inevitable. Cosmetically acceptable results are achieved if the tumors are small. Reconstructive surgery in the form of skin grafts or flap rotations may be required after excision of larger tumors.

Treatment of squamous cell carcinoma also may involve local application of chemotherapeutic agents. Most patients are cured completely with early treatment. Regular checkups, after treatment has been completed, are advised for the following 5 years.

Additional treatment of malignant melanoma includes chemotherapy, wide-margin excision, and possible removal of nearby lymph glands, because the tumors can metastasize through

168

them. Malignant melanomas that are less than 1/32-inch thick when removed can be cured in almost all cases. Long-term follow-up has confirmed this fact. Progressively thicker tumors have a much poorer prognosis.

Increased awareness of skin cancer and education about the dangers of sun exposure greatly enhance the prevention and early detection of skin carcinomas and the saving of lives.

See Chapter 15 for discussion of sunburn.

Abnormal Skin Pigmentation

SYMPTOMS AND SIGNS

The skin normally contains special cells called melanocytes that produce melanin, a black pigment that gives color to the skin. Several conditions cause the melanocytes to develop abnormally or to be distributed abnormally. Sometimes, melanocytes are fewer in number or less active than normal. This results in a pale area of skin that does not tan when exposed to sunlight. When melanocytes are more numerous or more active than normal, a darker area of skin that tans easily results. These abnormal conditions include albinism, vitiligo, melasma (chloasma), nevi (moles), seborrheic warts, pityriasis, and abnormal suntan.

ALBINISM

Albinism is a rare inherited condition in which the melanocytes are unable to produce melanin. The patient is pale skinned, with white hair and pink or pale blue eyes (Fig. 6–31). These people must avoid the sun to protect their eyes and skin from burning.

VITILIGO

With vitiligo, possibly an immune condition, pale irregular patches of skin appear, often evenly located on one side of the body or another (Fig. 6–32). The patches may enlarge, shrink, or stay the same size.

MELASMA (CHLOASMA)

Melasma occurs in some women during hormonal changes, as during pregnancy or with oral contraceptive administration. Patches of darker

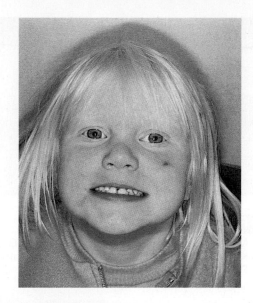

Figure 6–31

Albinism. (From Callen J, Greer K, Hood A, et al: Color Atlas of Dermatology. Philadelphia: WB Saunders, 1993, p 370. Used with permission.)

skin develop on the face, especially over the cheeks (Fig. 6–33). This condition disappears after childbirth or when the oral contraceptive use is discontinued.

HEMANGIOMAS

Hemangiomas are benign lesions of proliferating blood vessels in the dermis that produce a

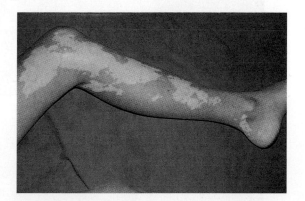

Figure 6–32

Vitiligo. (From Callen J, Greer K, Hood A, et al: Color Atlas of Dermatology. Philadelphia: WB Saunders, 1993, p 4. Used with permission.)

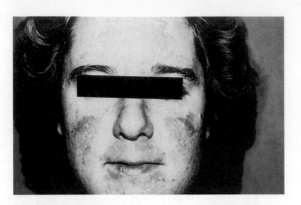

Figure 6–33

Melasma (chloasma). (From Callen J, Greer K, Hood A, et al: Color Atlas of Dermatology. Philadelphia: WB Saunders, 1993, p 310. Used with permission.)

red, blue, or purple color. Examples of hemangiomas are the nevus flammeus (port-wine stain), which is dark red to purple and usually is located on the face (Fig. 6-34 *A*); the strawberry hemangioma, which is bright red and has a protruding, rough surface (Fig. 6-34 *B*); and the cherry hemangioma, which is red to purple and is a smooth, dome-shaped, small papule 2 to 5 mm in diameter (Fig. 6-34*C*).

NEVI (MOLES)

Moles are small dark areas of skin composed of dense collections of melanocytes; some may contain hair. Occasionally, a mole may become malignant (see Malignant Melanoma).

SEBORRHEIC WARTS

Seborrheic warts are not true warts but are round or oval patches of dark-pigmented skin 1 to 3 cm across. They often develop after middle age and have a crusty, greasy-looking surface.

PITYRIASIS

Pityriasis is a fungal infection that causes patches of flaky, light or dark skin to develop on the trunk of the body. This is an uncommon condition.

ABNORMAL SUNTAN

Some drugs and certain diseases such as Addison's disease can produce a suntan without exposure to sunlight.

ETIOLOGY

The causes vary according to the abnormality.

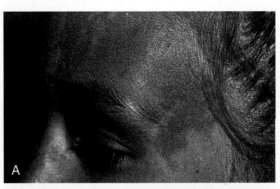

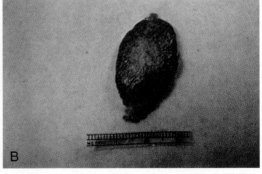

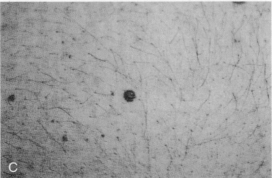

Figure 6–34

A, Port-wine stain. *B,* Strawberry hemangioma. *C,* Cherry hemangioma. (*A* from Callen J, Greer K, Hood A, et al: Color Atlas of Dermatology. Philadelphia: WB Saunders, 1993. *B* and *C* from Lookingbill D, Marks J: Principles of Dermatology, 2nd ed. Philadelphia: WB Saunders, 1993, pp 102–103. Used with permission.)

DIAGNOSIS

Most of these conditions are harmless, and visual examination by a physician confirms the diagnosis. Moles may cause concern, especially if there has been a change in size or shape. The physician may recommend a biopsy to rule out a malignancy.

TREATMENT

If the condition produces skin color variations, nonprescription depigmenting creams are available to lighten the affected skin. Vitiligo may be improved by ultraviolet lamp treatments combined with drug therapy. Pityriasis can be cured by the application of antifungal ointments. Moles can be removed surgically, and other skin blemishes can be covered with special cosmetics.

Alopecia (Baldness)

SYMPTOMS AND SIGNS

Alopecia is the loss or absence of hair, especially on the scalp. It can be either temporary or permanent. It can appear gradually, as with aging, or suddenly, occurring all at once or in patchy areas, as with alopecia areata (Fig. 6-35 A).

ETIOLOGY

In most cases, baldness is a result of the aging process or heredity. It can, however, be a consequence of certain systemic illnesses, such as thyroid diseases and iron deficiency anemia. Certain forms of dermatitis (see Dermatitis) also can cause alopecia. Chemotherapy and radiation therapy used to treat cancer and the use of some other types of medications may lead to thinning and loss of hair. The hair often grows back after treatment has been completed. More frequently, however, hair loss is not attributed to any specific disease process.

In men, alopecia tends to be part of the aging process and have a familial occurrence on the mother's side. The typical pattern is for the front hairline to recede and for the hair on the top of the head to thin. In some men, these areas eventually meet, leaving hair on only the sides of the head. This pattern of hair loss is called androgenetic alopecia (male pattern baldness) (Fig. 6-35 B). For most women, there is a gradual but slight loss of hair throughout life. Some women experience thinning of their hair about 3 months postpartum. This is a fairly common occurrence and corrects itself within a few months.

Finally, a more severe but rare form of alope-

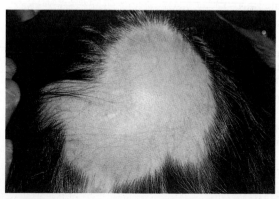

A

Figure 6-35

A, Alopecia areata. B, Androgenetic alopecia (male pattern baldness). (A from Callen J, Greer K, Hood A, et al: Color Atlas of Dermatology. Philadelphia: WB Saunders, 1993, p 364. Used with permission.)

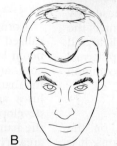 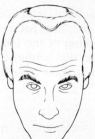 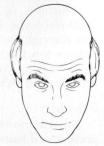

B

cia causes permanent hair loss over the entire body, including the eyebrows and eyelashes.

DIAGNOSIS

Visual examination may be all that is necessary for the diagnosis; however, the cause should be investigated as well. Blood and thyroid studies are necessary to rule out thyroid disease and anemia.

TREATMENT

Treatment of alopecia varies according to the cause. Effective treatment of any underlying disease usually restores hair growth to normal. To treat male pattern baldness, minoxidil (Rogaine) preparations used topically in cream and spray forms have been showing promise. Additional drug therapy currently includes finasteride (Propecia). Other options include wearing a toupee or wig or having a hair transplant. Transplantation is effective for certain types of hair loss, especially male pattern baldness, but transplantation and the use of minoxidil are expensive and can have side effects.

172

Folliculitis

SYMPTOMS AND SIGNS

Folliculitis is an inflammatory reaction of the hair follicles that produces erythemic, pustular lesions (Fig. 6–36). The pustules are individual and do not join. They commonly are found on the thighs and buttocks but also can occur in the beard area and on the scalp. Some patients may report mild discomfort, mainly pruritus, associated with the pustules, but folliculitis is usually asymptomatic.

This is a relatively common condition that affects primarily young adults. It can be chronic or recurrent.

ETIOLOGY

Folliculitis is a bacterial infection caused by *Staphylococcus aureus.* The bacteria enter the skin through the opening of the hair follicle and cause a low-grade infection within the epidermal layer. Shaving with a straight razor is a common precipitating factor.

DIAGNOSIS

The diagnosis of folliculitis is made on the presence of hairs within the pustular lesions. It is

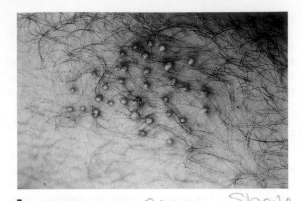

Figure 6–36 magic shave

Folliculitis. (From Callen J, Greer K, Hood A, et al: Color Atlas of Dermatology. Philadelphia: WB Saunders, 1993, p 177. Used with permission.)

confirmed when a culture of the purulent material shows the presence of *S. aureus.*

TREATMENT

For most mild cases of folliculitis, a topical antiseptic cleanser, such as povidone-iodine (Betadine), used daily or every other day for several weeks, manages the problem. More extensive involvement necessitates a systemic antibiotic, such as erythromycin, taken 4 times a day for 10 days, in addition to the topical cleansers.

Occasionally, folliculitis can result in the development of a furuncle and necessitate incision and drainage (see Furuncles and Carbuncles).

Corns and Calluses

SYMPTOMS AND SIGNS

Corns and calluses are extremely common, localized hyperplastic areas of the stratum corneum layer of the epidermis. Corns have a glassy core, are small (less than 1/5 inch), are more painful than calluses, and develop on the toes. Calluses are larger (up to 1 inch) and commonly develop on the ball of the foot and the palms of the hands. Tenderness and pain over the affected area are the common symptoms.

ETIOLOGY

Both conditions may be due to pressure or friction from ill-fitting shoes, orthopedic deformities, or faulty weight–bearing. People who play stringed instruments and manual laborers are prone to calluses because of repeated trauma. Also, people with impaired circulation in their feet because of peripheral neuropathy (sometimes caused by diabetes mellitus) are more inclined to the development of corns and calluses.

DIAGNOSIS

It is unusual for corns and calluses to become painful to the extent that a physician needs to be consulted. If a physician is consulted, a physical examination of the affected area and brief history are sufficient for diagnosis.

TREATMENT

Relieving pressure and friction points as soon as possible is the goal of treatment. Many self-help measures are available, such as pads and sponge rings, chemical agents to soften and loosen corns, and pumice stone to rub off dead skin caused from calluses. If these treatments are ineffective, a physician can trim the corn or callus surgically or with strong chemicals. *Warning:* Patients with diabetes mellitus should not use self-help measures but should seek the help of a podiatrist.

Verrucae (Warts)

SYMPTOMS AND SIGNS

Verrucae are elevated growths of the epidermis that result from hyperplasia (Fig. 6–37). There are several types of warts, but the most common type is a plantar wart. This wart is a small, hard, white or pink lump with a cauliflower-like surface. Inside the wart are small, clotted blood vessels that resemble black splinters.

A verruca can develop anywhere on the body but is most likely to be on the hands or the soles of the feet. For the most part, the wart is painless; however, a wart on the sole of a foot (plantar wart) can make a person feel as though he has a stone in his shoe. Pruritus also can accompany a wart. Verrucae are common among teenagers and children; however, there are no serious health risks associated with these warts.

ETIOLOGY

Warts are caused by viruses and are spread by touch or contact with the skin shed from a wart. Each of the five viruses known to cause warts tends to infect different parts of the body.

DIAGNOSIS

Diagnosis is made by visual examination. There are two cases of warts in which a physician should be consulted. One is if penile or vulval warts develop, and the other is a wart that develops after the age of 45 years. What looks like a wart could be a serious skin condition such as skin cancer.

TREATMENT

Most warts disappear naturally over time. There are, however, many self-help remedies in the form of paints, creams, or plasters. These medications contain chemicals that destroy the abnormal skin cells, but they also damage the surrounding healthy cells. Care must be taken to minimize soreness. Warts located on the face or genitals should not be treated with these chemicals. For persistent warts, a physician can remove them by surgical excision, cryosurgery, or electrodesiccation. Treatment is often painful and tedious.

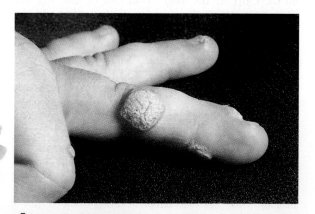

Figure 6–37

Verruca (common wart). (From Lookingbill D, Marks J: Principles of Dermatology, 2nd ed. Philadelphia: WB Saunders, 1993, p 67. Used with permission.)

Deformed or Discolored Nails

SYMPTOMS AND SIGNS

Any unusual thickening, color variations, and change in the shape of either the fingernails or the toenails can be symptoms of an underlying disease or disorder.

ETIOLOGY

Injury to the nail bed caused by continuous pressure from ill-fitting shoes or poor circulation caused by arteriosclerosis can lead to thickening of the whole nail. Many disorders can produce nail deformities. Psoriasis, lichen planus, and chronic paronychia can cause the end of the nail to separate from the underlying skin. Bacteria can enter this space and make the nail turn a blackish green. Iron deficiency anemia can cause spooning of the nails. Congenital heart disorders and lung cancer can cause clubbing, or knobby ends of the fingers or toes, and then cause the nails to grow around these ends.

Nail discoloration is caused by many illnesses. With anemia, the nail bed appears pale. A person with chronic hepatic disease has white nail beds. Small, black, splinter-like areas appear under the nails with infections of the cardiac valves, systemic lupus erythematosus, and dermatomyositis.

Injury to a nail and vitamin or mineral deficiencies may cause one or more white patches to develop in the nail. The nail of the big toe sometimes can curve under at the sides and dig into the skin, causing pain as it grows. This is known as an ingrown toenail.

DIAGNOSIS

Examination of the affected nail or nails and a medical history may be all that is needed for a diagnosis. A blood chemistry profile detects any underlying condition or illness.

TREATMENT

Deformities and discolorations caused by underlying illnesses resolve when the illness is corrected. Nails damaged from injury usually grow out or back in again in approximately 9 months. There are several self-help measures for an ingrown toenail, including wearing loose-fitting shoes, keeping the area clean and dry to prevent infection, and cutting the nail straight across the top. If these measures are not helpful, a physician should be seen. The physician can remove the ingrowing edge of the nail and the toe's nail fold and apply a chemical to the edge to relieve the discomfort and prevent the edge from regrowing under.

Paronychia

SYMPTOMS AND SIGNS

A paronychia is an infection of the skin around a nail. With an acute paronychia, the cuticle or nail fold becomes edematous, red, and painful. If the cuticle lifts away from the base of the nail, purulent material may be expressed from beneath. When the nail fold is affected, a blister of pus called a whitlow develops beside the nail (Fig. 6–38). Chronic infections produce similar symptoms, and often several nails are affected. With the cuticle lifted, the nail roots no longer are protected and become damaged. This produces deformed or discolored nails.

ETIOLOGY

The infection may be caused by bacteria or fungi. Bacteria usually cause acute infections, whereas fungi are usually responsible for chronic infections. The chronic infections develop slowly and are less painful, but are also more persistent. Paronychia occurs particularly in people who have their hands in water for long periods.

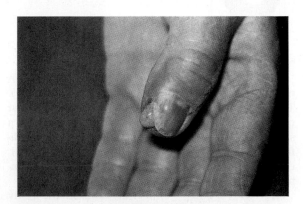

Figure 6–38

Paronychia. (From Callen J, Greer K, Hood A, et al: Color Atlas of Dermatology. Philadelphia: WB Saunders, 1993, p 354. Used with permission.)

DIAGNOSIS

A physician can diagnose a paronychia on examination of the affected areas and with a history of the symptoms. A culture of the exudate is necessary to determine a bacterial or fungal origin.

TREATMENT

Antibiotics correct a bacterial infection, and if the infection is chronic, an antifungal cream or paint is prescribed. It may take several months of treatment for the swelling to subside and the raised cuticle to return to normal.

Summary

The integumentary system is versatile and resilient in protecting the body from insults from the external environment. In addition, the skin synthesizes vitamin D, provides receptors for sensation, and assists in regulation of body temperature and excretion.

Abnormal conditions of the skin vary from flat lesions such as macules to large ulcerations, from benign to malignant, from cosmetically insignificant to severely disfiguring. More important diseases of the skin are caused by infection, autoimmune factors, trauma, and benign or malignant tumors.

- Inflammation of the skin, or dermatitis, causes itching, redness, and various lesions. It may be idiopathic or caused by an irritant (contact dermatitis) or an allergy (atopic dermatitis) and may be aggravated by stress.
- Psoriasis, characterized by white silvery scales, is a noninfectious chronic skin condition that tends to run in families.
- Rosacea, a chronic condition affecting the facial skin causing redness and pimple-like eruptions on areas where the individual normally blushes. Medical treatment and modification of lifestyles help to control symptoms.
- Acne, marked by papules, pustules and comedones, is most common in teenagers. It is controlled with antibiotics, keratolytic agents, and other topical medications.
- The extremely painful vesicles of herpes zoster, caused by the varicella zoster virus, occur along dermatomes.
- Impetigo, an infectious skin disease, causes lesions that rupture and form thick crusts.
- Furuncles (boils) and carbuncles are caused by

staphylococcus infection. The lesions usually remain localized. Antibiotic therapy or incision and drainage may be required.
- Cellulitis is an acute diffuse bacterial infection of the skin and underlying tissue that may require aggressive measures to control, if severe.
- Dermatophytosis (fungal infection of the skin) is classified by the body region infected and includes tinea corporis (ringworm), tinea pedis (athlete's foot), tinea cruris (jock itch), and tinea unguium (affects toenails).
- Constant pressure against the surface of the skin interferes with circulation and results in decubitus ulcers.
- Human scabies (itch mites) and lice are spread easily. They are the source of intense itching and a crawling sensation.
- Skin tumors, classified as benign or malignant, are distinguished by visual examination and biopsy.
- Most skin carcinomas (basal cell, squamous cell, and the most serious, malignant melanoma) result from chronic overexposure to the sun. Early warning signs must be recognized so that the cancerous lesions can be eliminated before they metastasize.
- Abnormal skin pigmentation causes areas of skin to be pale (as in vitiligo) or darker (as in melasma).
- Alopecia has possible causes other than the aging process and can be temporary or permanent.
- Folliculitis and paronychia are bacterial infections; warts are caused by viruses; corns and calluses result from repeated trauma or impaired circulation.

Review Challenge

REVIEW QUESTIONS

1. What are the functions of the integumentary system?
2. What is the difference between a macule and a cyst? A plaque and a fissure? A comedo and a pustule?
3. How is cradle cap related to seborrheic dermatitis?
4. What factors might induce the inflammation in the occurrence of contact dermatitis?
5. How is the skin likely to appear in a person diagnosed with atopic dermatitis?
6. Where are the lesions of psoriasis most likely to appear on the body?
7. What treatment might the physician prescribe for acne vulgaris?
8. What is the clinical course of herpes zoster?
9. Is impetigo contagious?
10. Are there any conditions considered predisposing to furuncles and carbuncles? If so, what are they?
11. Is cellulitis always a local infection?
12. How is dermatophytoses classified?
13. What are the early signs of a decubitus ulcer?
14. What is the comprehensive treatment plan for a human scabies infestation, or for lice?
15. What are two of the most common premalignant skin tumors?
16. What is the most serious type of skin cancer? What are the characteristics of such a lesion?
17. Besides the aging process, what are other possible causes of alopecia?
18. What are the ABCDs of malignant melanoma?

REAL-LIFE CHALLENGE

Shingles

A 57-year-old woman presents with severe pain in the left occipital region, in the left side of her neck, and in the left scapular region. The onset was approximately 36 hours ago. She describes the pain as intermittent, sharp, shooting, and severe. She has been taking ibuprofen for the pain, with little relief. She noticed small blisters forming along the painful areas in the last few hours. She is afebrile and appears quite uncomfortable.

On examination, small blister-like eruptions are noted along the left side of the neck, left anterior shoulder, and clavicular area. There also are some present at the base of the skull just in the hairline. These eruptions do not cross midline on either the front or back of the body.

The patient is diagnosed with shingles, along the C-2, C-3, C-4 peripheral nerve or dermatome area. On questioning, the patient confirms having chickenpox in childhood at approximately 8 years of age.

Medications prescribed include famciclovir (Famvir) 500 mg tid for 7 days. Acyclovir (Zovirax) cream also was prescribed for topical application to the affected areas and hydrocodone bitartrate with acetaminophen (Vicodin) for pain.

Questions

1. What is the significance of the previous occurrence of chickenpox?
2. What is the causative agent of chickenpox? Of shingles?
3. Why is the fact that the eruptions do not cross midline important?
4. Identify other medications that may be prescribed for shingles?
5. What might the patient expect as an outcome of this condition?
6. What is meant by postherpetic neuralgia?

REAL-LIFE CHALLENGE

Malignant Melanoma

A 35-year-old fair-skinned woman has noticed the enlargement of a mole on her right lower arm. The mole has been present as long as she can remember. In the past month, it appears to have doubled in size and has become darker.

The patient admits to having been exposed to direct sunlight for the past several years. She lives in southern Texas and spends several hours a day in the sun while doing garden work. She has not been consistent in the regular application of sunscreen to her lower arms and hands.

Visual examination shows a slightly elevated 7-mm irregularly shaped, dark multicolored lesion on the dorsal aspect of the right lower arm, approximately 3 inches above the wrist. Closer examination shows the lesion to be asymmetrical, with a notched border.

Family history reveals the patient's mother to have had three lesions removed from her arms and face that were diagnosed as malignant melanoma. Additionally, two maternal aunts have had malignant melanomas. One aunt recently died from metastatic cancer. The patient remembers having incurred several sunburns with blistering as a child.

Surgical excision of the lesion is performed, and the biopsy affirms the diagnosis of malignant melanoma. The patient is referred to an oncologist for possible chemotherapy.

Questions

1. What characteristics does the patient have that make her a possible candidate for malignant melanoma?
2. What symptoms distinguish malignant melanoma from basal cell or squamous cell carcinomas?
3. What is the prognosis for a patient with malignant melanoma such as this patient?
4. What patient teaching would you do in the office to patients concerning extensive exposure to sunlight?
5. What is the importance of a good family history?
6. Why was the patient referred to an oncologist?
7. Would this patient be a candidate for further surgical procedures? If so, which procedures and why?
8. List the warning signs of malignant melanoma.

RESOURCES

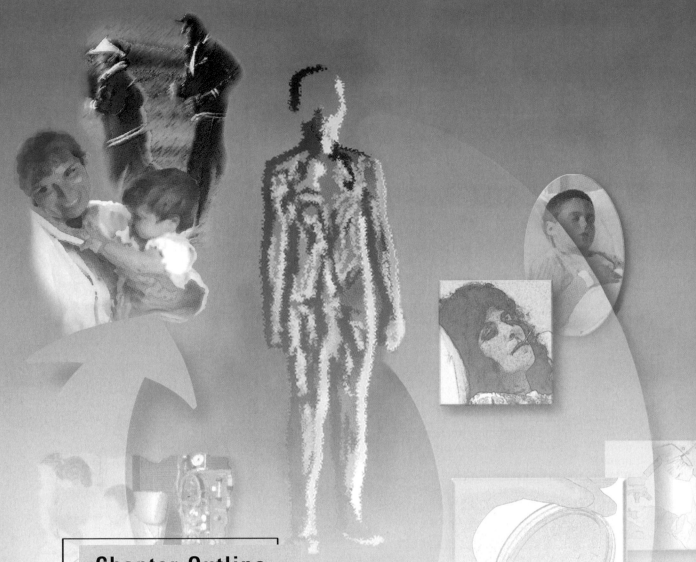

Chapter Outline

Diseases and Conditions of the Musculoskeletal System

Learning Objectives

After studying Chapter 7, you should be able to:

1. List the functions of the normal skeletal system.
2. Distinguish between the pathologic features of lordosis, kyphosis, and scoliosis.
3. Relate the signs and symptoms of the most common form of arthritis.
4. Explain the importance of early recognition and treatment of Lyme disease.
5. Compare the pathology and etiology of osteomyelitis with polymyositis.
6. Discuss the specifics of a physical examination when fibromyalgia is suspected.
7. Explain why joint disability results from gout.
8. Describe the disability that results from advanced osteoporosis.
9. Explain why osteomalacia is termed a metabolic bone disease.
10. Distinguish between hallux valgus and hallux rigidus.
11. Differentiate between a strain and a sprain.
12. Relate the importance of proper treatment of dislocations.
13. Relate the cause of shin splints.
14. List some contributing factors to the development of plantar faciitis.
15. Explain how torn meniscus is treated.
16. Characterize the signs and symptoms of rotator cuff tears.

Key Terms

avulsion	(ah–**VUL**–shun)	hematopoiesis	(**heem**–ah–toe–poy–**EE**–sis)
bursae	(**BURR**–see)		
calcitonin	(**kal**–sih–**TOE**–nin)	meniscus	(meh–**NIS**–kuss)
chemonucleolysis	(**key**–mo–new–klee–**OL**–ih–sis)	metatarsophalangeal	(**met**–ah–**tar**–so–fah–**LAN**–jee–al)
crepitation	(krep–ih–**TAY**–shun)	ossification	(**oss**–ih–fih–**KAY**–shun)
fascia	(**FASH**–ee–ah)		

| osteogenesis | (**oss**–tee–oh–**JEN**–eh–sis) | synovial | (sin–**OH**–vee–al) |
| paresthesia | (**pair**–es–**THEE**–zee–ah) | tenorrhaphy | (teh–**NOR**–ah–fee) |

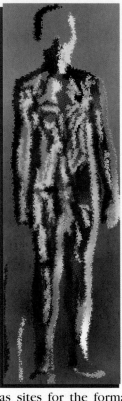

The Musculoskeletal System

Muscles, bones, and joints, along with ligaments, tendons, and cartilage, provide the body with a supportive, protective framework that allows flexibility of movement and protects the internal organs. These musculoskeletal tissues also give shape to the body; act partially as a storage and supply area for minerals, mostly calcium and phosphorus; and serve as sites for the formation of blood cells (**hematopoiesis**).

When the tissues are unable to perform their usual functions because of trauma or rheumatic, inflammatory, or degenerative conditions, a person's physical support, protection, mobility, and ability to function in normal activities are affected. Trauma is a major cause of musculoskeletal disorders, with automobile accidents and injuries (strains, sprains, dislocations, and fractures) being the leading cause of disabilities and death.

All muscles are composed of a basic cellular unit called the muscle fiber, which is made of protein. Muscles are collections or masses of tissue that cover bones, provide bulk to the body, help to hold body parts together, and help to move the various body parts (Fig. 7-1).

All movement, including the movement of the body itself and of the organs, is performed by muscle tissue. Movement of the body is accomplished through the contraction and relaxation of the skeletal muscles, aided by interaction with the nerves, the skin, connective tissues, and minerals.

There are three types of muscles: striated (skeletal), nonstriated (smooth), and cardiac (Fig. 7-2). They are classified as either voluntary or involuntary. Voluntary muscles, such as those in the limbs, are under conscious control and contract, or move at will. Involuntary muscles, such as those found in the heart and the digestive tract, function without conscious control or awareness. Muscles are attached at each end to a bone, a tendon, a ligament, or fascia. The point of muscle attachment to a stationary bone is called the origin of the muscle, and the point of attachment to a bone that moves is called the insertion of the muscle (Fig. 7-3).

The skeletal system is composed of 206 bones that provide an important support system for the many parts of the body and enable a person to stand erect (Fig 7-4).

Some bones encase and protect certain organs (e.g., the skull protects the brain, and the rib cage and the backbone protect the heart and lungs). In coordination with muscles and joints, bones assist body movement. Hematopoiesis also occurs in the bone marrow. Bones are not lifeless structures, but instead are living cells embedded in a hard framework of minerals (calcium and phosphorus). These cells are continuously forming new bone; bone formation is counterbalanced by bone reabsorption. Normally, the balance of these processes prevents bones from becoming excessively thick, as with Paget's disease, or thin, as with osteoporosis.

Bones are complete organs; they are composed mainly of connective tissue with a rich

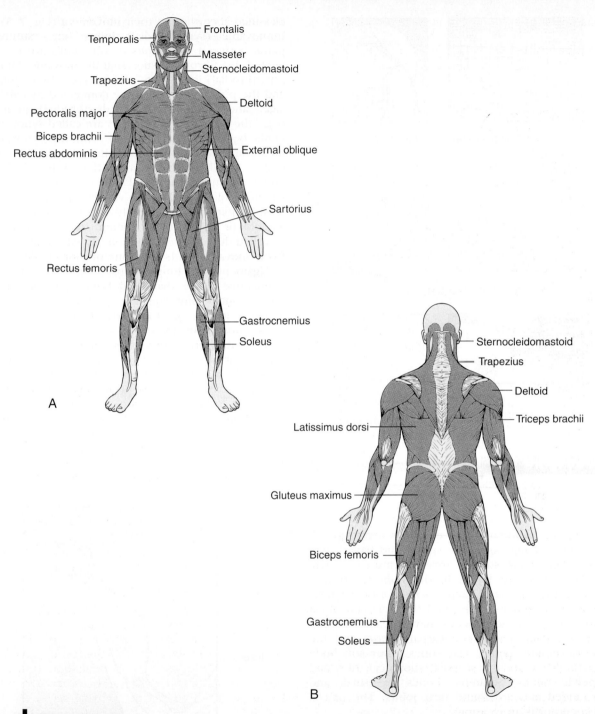

Temporalis

Frontalis

Masseter

Sternocleidomastoid

Trapezius

Deltoid

Pectoralis major

Biceps brachii

Rectus abdominis

External oblique

Sartorius

Rectus femoris

Gastrocnemius

Soleus

A

Sternocleidomastoid

Trapezius

Deltoid

Triceps brachii

Latissimus dorsi

Gluteus maximus

Biceps femoris

Gastrocnemius

Soleus

B

Figure 7–1

Normal muscular system. *A,* Anterior view. *B,* Posterior view.

supply of blood vessels and nerves. They develop through a process called osteogenesis, and the complete skeleton is formed by the end of the third month of gestation. The fetal skeleton is composed of cartilage tissue, which is replaced gradually by bone cells in a process called ossification. Ossification depends on an adequate supply of calcium and phosphorus to the bone tissue.

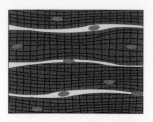
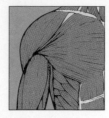

STRIATED (SKELETAL) MUSCLE

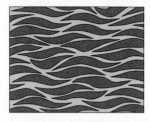
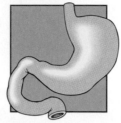

NONSTRIATED (SMOOTH) MUSCLE

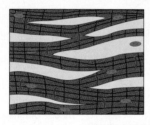
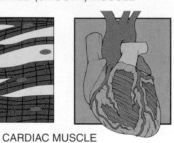

CARDIAC MUSCLE

Figure 7–2

Types of muscles.

classified according to their movement (Fig. 7-5). Immovable (synarthrodial) joints (e.g., suture joints between the bones of the skull) are connected by fibrous tissue; slightly movable (amphiarthrodial) joints (e.g., the intervertebral joints and the pubic symphysis) are connected by cartilage; and freely movable (diarthrodial) joints (e.g., the knee and the elbow) are called synovial joints because they are lined with the synovial membrane. Within synovial joints also are found bones, cartilage that covers the ends of the bones, ligaments that hold bones together, synovial fluid, blood and lymph vessels, and nerves.

Most joints are the freely movable type. The amount or degree of movement that a joint has is called its range of motion (ROM). Only the freely movable joints have one or more ROM.

Ligaments are tough, dense, fibrous bands of connective tissue that hold bones together, either around a joint capsule (e.g., the hip joint) or across a joint (e.g., the knee [Fig. 7-6]). They allow movement in some directions while restricting it in other directions. Injury to ligaments can occur in several ways; they can be overstretched, called strains; have partial tears, called sprains; or be torn loose from their attachment to a bone, called an avulsion.

Tendons are strong, tough strands, or cords, of dense connective tissue. They serve as the attachment for muscles to bones and other parts

Several different types of bones make up the skeleton. Long bones are strong and have broad ends and large surface areas for muscle attachment. They are found in the humerus (upper arm), the ulna and radius (lower arm, or forearm), the femur (thigh), and the tibia and fibula (lower leg). Short bones have small, irregular shapes and include the carpal (wrist) and the tarsal (ankle) bones. Flat bones cover soft body parts. They are the scapula (shoulder), ribs, and pelvic bones. Sesamoid bones are small and rounded and are found near joints. The patella (kneecap) is an example.

Joints are hinge-like structures or articulations where bones are joined or where two surfaces of bones come together. Assisted by the ligaments, joints hold bones firmly together yet allow movement between them. Joints are classified by the type of material found between the bones: fibrous, cartilaginous, and **synovial.** Joints also are

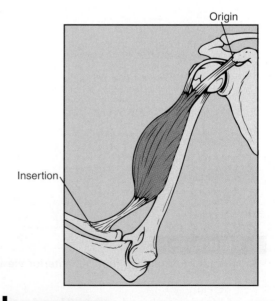

Origin

Insertion

Figure 7–3

Insertion and origin of a muscle.

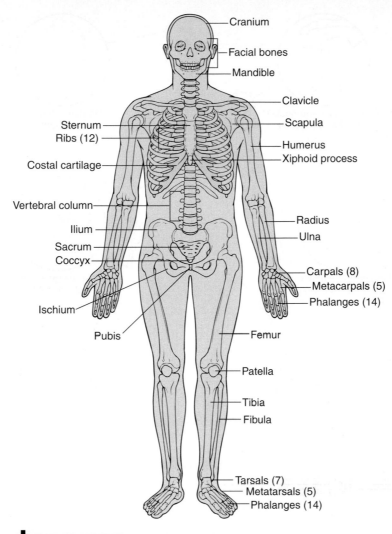

Cranium
Facial bones
Mandible
Clavicle
Scapula
Sternum
Ribs (12)
Humerus
Xiphoid process
Costal cartilage
Vertebral column
Radius
Ilium
Ulna
Sacrum
Coccyx
Carpals (8)
Metacarpals (5)
Phalanges (14)
Ischium
Pubis
Femur
Patella
Tibia
Fibula
Tarsals (7)
Metatarsals (5)
Phalanges (14)

Figure 7–4
Normal skeletal system, anterior view.

(see Fig. 7-6). Tendons are nonelastic and are capable of withstanding great forces from contracting muscles without sustaining damage to themselves.

Cartilage is a semismooth, dense, supporting connective tissue that is found at the ends of bones. It forms a cap over the ends of bones and provides support and protection for their weight-bearing activities. Cartilage absorbs weight and shock to prevent injury to joints, bones, and itself. To remain healthy, cartilage at the joints must have joint movement and weight-bearing activities. Without these activities, degenerative joint disease can result.

Also necessary to the functioning of the musculoskeletal system are the bursae. These are closed sacs or cavities of synovial fluid lined with a synovial membrane. Bursae serve as areas of cushioning between tissues, including tendons, bones, ligaments, and other tissues where friction occurs. Some bursae locations are the shoulder (see Fig. 7-15), elbow, and knee.

Another substance found throughout the musculoskeletal system is a fibrous protein called collagen. Collagen is the major supporting element, or glue, in the connective tissues. In adults, collagen makes up one third to one half of the total body protein (see Chapter 3).

184

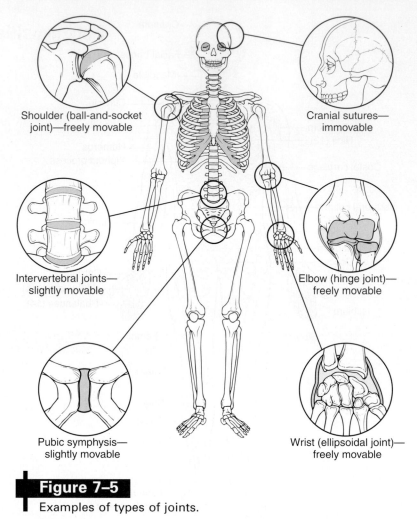

Shoulder (ball-and-socket joint)—freely movable

Cranial sutures—immovable

Intervertebral joints—slightly movable

Elbow (hinge joint)—freely movable

Pubic symphysis—slightly movable

Wrist (ellipsoidal joint)—freely movable

Figure 7–5

Examples of types of joints.

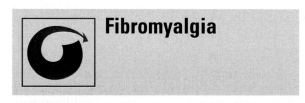

Fibromyalgia

SYMPTOMS AND SIGNS

Fibromyalgia, a painful debilitating syndrome, causes chronic pain in muscles and soft tissues surrounding joints. The patient reports diffuse aching or burning in the muscles, stiffness, fatigue, disturbed sleep patterns, and depression. Other nonspecific symptoms include headaches, jaw pain, and a sensitivity to odors, bright lights, and loud noises. Some patients experience irritable bowel syndrome or "spastic colon," including nausea, diarrhea, constipation, or abdominal pain with gas and distention. Urinary symptoms, when present, include urinary urgency or frequency brought on by bladder spasms and irritability. Frequently, patients experiencing fibromyalgia wake up feeling tired, even if they have slept all night. Others sleep lightly and wake up during the night.

ETIOLOGY

The etiology of fibromyalgia is unknown; however, it has been suggested that stress, trauma to the central nervous system, chemical or hormonal imbalances, infections, or psychological factors could be the source. The vulnerability of muscle tissue is increased because of decreased circulation, possibly resulting in the onset or exacerbation of symptoms. The condition may be aggravated by poor posture, inappropriate exercise, and smoking.

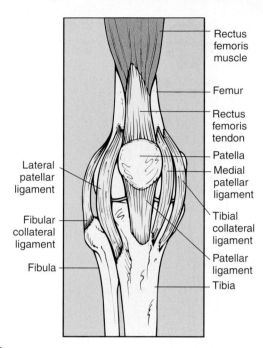

Lateral patellar ligament

Fibular collateral ligament

Fibula

Rectus femoris muscle

Femur

Rectus femoris tendon

Patella

Medial patellar ligament

Tibial collateral ligament

Patellar ligament

Tibia

Figure 7–6
Ligaments and tendons of the knee joint.

DIAGNOSIS

There are no laboratory or imaging studies that diagnose fibromyalgia. In addition to a thorough patient history, physicians rely on physical examination to reveal widespread tenderness and pain or aching in at least 11 of 18 specific tender points (Fig. 7-7). Usually found on both sides of the body in all four quadrants, the widespread pain should exist for a minimum of 3 months before being diagnosed as fibromyalgia. Regions of the neck, shoulders, chest, hips, knees, and elbows are where the 18 sites of tender points cluster. Additionally, the occurrence of sleep disorders helps to confirm the diagnosis.

TREATMENT

Although there is no known cure for fibromyalgia, treatment can help alleviate symptoms. Attempts are made to reduce pain and improve the quality of sleep. Medications to improve sleep patterns may be prescribed, as are nonsteroidal anti-inflammatory drugs (NSAIDs). Relaxation techniques, massage therapy, acupressure, and exercise also have been found to be beneficial. Regular exercise, including walking, biking, swimming, or water aerobics, is effective in reducing pain. Stress reduction, muscle relaxants, and antidepressant drugs also are included in therapy.

Polymyositis

SYMPTOMS AND SIGNS

Polymyositis is an inflammation of the muscles. The most commonly affected muscles are those of the shoulder and the pelvis. Polymyositis is a painful, progressive disease in which the muscles gradually weaken and atrophy. This disease may be accompanied by skin inflammation, which is called dermatomyositis. In such cases, a rash may appear and spread over the face, shoulders, arms, and bony prominences (e.g., knuckles, elbows, and knees). Nearly two thirds of patients with this disease are women. The person with this disease generally feels ill.

ETIOLOGY

The cause of polymyositis is unknown; however, it is thought to be an autoimmune disorder.

DIAGNOSIS

A medical history, physical examination, blood analysis, electromyography, and muscle biopsy confirm the diagnosis.

TREATMENT

Treatment of polymyositis is directed at minimizing the symptoms. High doses of steroids usually are prescribed to suppress the inflammation. Immunosuppressive agents also are used to treat some patients. Exercise therapy is taught to minimize weakness and to prevent atrophy of the muscles. In many instances, the disease disappears gradually over a few years.

Spinal Disorders

LORDOSIS

SYMPTOMS AND SIGNS

The normal anterior curve of the lumbar spine can become exaggerated by other conditions. Lordosis, also called swayback, occurs as the person compensates for additional abdominal girth

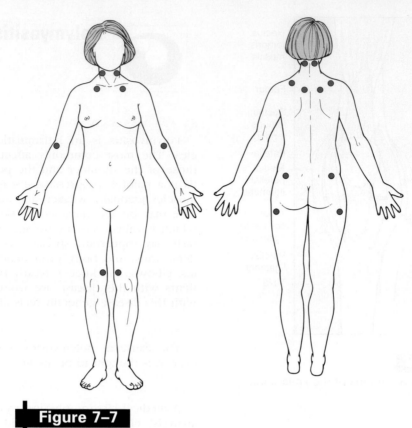

Figure 7–7

Eighteen tender points used to diagnose fibromyalgia.

caused by pregnancy, obesity, or large abdominal tumors. The patient may experience frequent back pain because of strains on the muscles and ligaments. As compared with posture with a normal spine (Fig. 7-8), lordosis results in a protruding abdomen and buttocks and an arched lower back (Fig. 7-9).

ETIOLOGY

Excessive abdominal weight and mass cause the individual to compensate to maintain balance when standing. Lordosis frequently is noted in prepubescent girls. A possible cause is rapid skeletal growth that occurs without the necessary natural stretching of the posterior soft tissues. Osteoporosis, with resulting loss of bone mass, may be the causative factor in the older population.

DIAGNOSIS

Observation of the spine in various postural positions and an examination of the lower spine are the primary steps in diagnosis. When the

condition results from pregnancy, no additional information usually is required to make the diagnosis. Further investigation includes radiographic studies to determine the extent of lordosis, along with a thorough history and physical examination to discover the underlying cause of the condition.

TREATMENT

When lordosis is caused by pregnancy, delivery of the infant usually resolves the condition. When obesity is the cause, weight loss and exercises to strengthen abdominal muscles are beneficial. Performing pelvic tilt exercises and maintaining good posture help to correct the condition. Progressive untreated lordosis can lead to degenerative lumbar disk disease or ruptured lumbar disks. Additional treatment of the condition can include the use of a brace, spinal fusion, and displacement osteotomy. This latter procedure requires the surgical division of a vertebra with shifting of the bone segments to change the alignment of, or alter weight-bearing stress on, the spine.

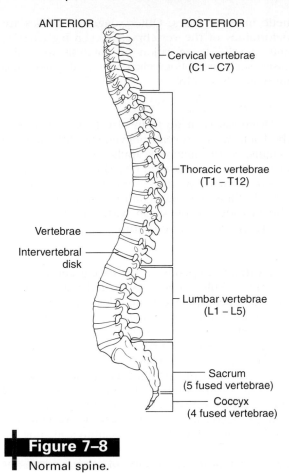

ANTERIOR   POSTERIOR

Cervical vertebrae
(C1 – C7)

Thoracic vertebrae
(T1 – T12)

Vertebrae

Intervertebral
disk

Lumbar vertebrae
(L1 – L5)

Sacrum
(5 fused vertebrae)

Coccyx
(4 fused vertebrae)

Figure 7–8
Normal spine.

KYPHOSIS

SYMPTOMS AND SIGNS

Kyphosis, an excessive posterior curve of the thoracic spine, often has an **insidious** onset and is **asymptomatic** until the hump becomes obvious. As the curve progresses, the patient begins to experience mild pain, fatigue, tenderness along the spine, and decreasing mobility of the spine. The shoulders appear rounded, and there is a forward protrusion of the head (Fig. 7–10).

ETIOLOGY

Kyphosis occurring in very young children has no specific cause. Adolescent kyphosis usually is related to Scheuermann's disease, an inflammatory deformity of the lower thoracic vertebrae. Additional disease processes that contribute to the occurrence of kyphosis include tumors or tuberculosis of the vertebral bodies and ankylosing spondylitis. Osteoporosis is often responsible

for the hunchback that develops in the older person, particularly the postmenopausal woman. Wearing away of the anterior portion of the vertebrae in a wedge-type manner (anterior wedging) or deterioration of the vertebrae, from whatever cause, results in the excessive curvature.

DIAGNOSIS

Visual inspection of the spine discloses the excessive curve in the thoracic region. Radiographic films and bone scan confirm the concave curvature of the thoracic spine along with the wedging of the anterior aspect of the vertebral bodies. Older patients with osteoporosis have a loss of bone density.

TREATMENT

Exercises to strengthen the muscles and ligaments are prescribed. Back braces also are used to stabilize the condition. The underlying cause must be determined and treated. Spinal fusion with instrumentation and immobilization, until

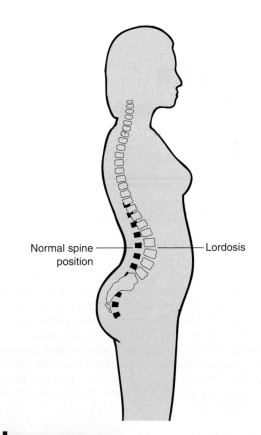

Normal spine
position

Lordosis

Figure 7–9
Lordosis.

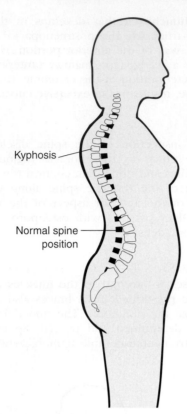

Figure 7–10

Kyphosis.

the graft is healed, is done when other measures fail to produce results and when the respiratory and cardiac systems are compromised.

SCOLIOSIS

SYMPTOMS AND SIGNS

Scoliosis, a lateral curvature of the spine, frequently has an insidious onset, with the first indication being unequal bra strap lengths. The patient, usually an adolescent female, reports back pain, fatigue, and **dyspnea.** Observation of the back reveals a lateral curve of the spine, one shoulder higher than the other, one scapula more prominent than the other, one hip higher than the other, and, when the patient bends over, an enlarged muscle mass on one side of the back (Fig. 7–11).

ETIOLOGY

Idiopathic scoliosis is the most common form; however, the cause is postulated to be ge-

netic in some cases. Other suggested causes are deformities of the vertebrae, uneven leg lengths, and muscle degeneration or paralysis from diseases such as poliomyelitis, cerebral palsy, and muscular dystrophy.

DIAGNOSIS

Diagnosis is made from visual examination of the back, which reveals uneven shoulder and hip heights, a prominent scapula on one side, an enlarged muscle mass on one side, and a definite torsional curve of the vertebral column. Radiographic films not only confirm the diagnosis but also provide the physician with a means of measuring the degree of curvature.

TREATMENT

Treatment depends on the extent and cause of the curve. Mild scoliosis is treated with exercise to strengthen the weak muscles. Bracing of the back with a Milwaukee brace or a molded plastic clamshell jacket along with an exercise program is the suggested course of treatment for the growing girl or boy. This bracing may take from 2 to 5 years to prevent further curvature. Curves that do not respond to the bracing or that are severe (greater than 40°) need surgical intervention to decrease the curve and to realign and stabilize the spine. These procedures include fusion of the vertebrae and internal fixation with instrumentation by means of rods, wires, or plates and pedicle screws. Some patients are placed in body casts or plastic jackets to main-

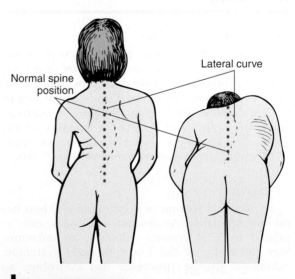

Figure 7–11

Scoliosis.

tain the integrity of the fixation until the fusion heals. The respiratory and cardiac systems may be compromised if the curvature is left untreated.

Osteoarthritis

SYMPTOMS AND SIGNS

Osteoarthritis, also known as degenerative joint disease, is the most common form of arthritis. It develops as a result of normal wear and tear on the joints and is more common in the elderly, being almost universal in those older than 75 years. Osteoarthritis occurs mainly in the large weight-bearing joints, especially the knees and hips (Figs. 7–12 and 7–13). To a lesser degree, involvement of the joints of the fingers—especially the proximal interphalangeal joints (Bouchard's nodes), wrists, elbows, and ankles—can occur. Degenerative changes in the spinal vertebrae and the joints of the pelvis also can occur. This chronic, progressive disease results in degeneration and loss of joint cartilage and the subsequent atrophy of the adjacent bone.

The onset of osteoartritis is usually insidious, and the symptoms vary with the severity of the disease. Joint soreness, aching, and stiffness, especially in the morning and with changes in the weather; edema; dull pain; and deformity are some common symptoms. Clicking or crackling sounds (crepitation) often are heard on joint movement. Decreased range of motion, joint instability, and an increase in pain with use of the joints are also common.

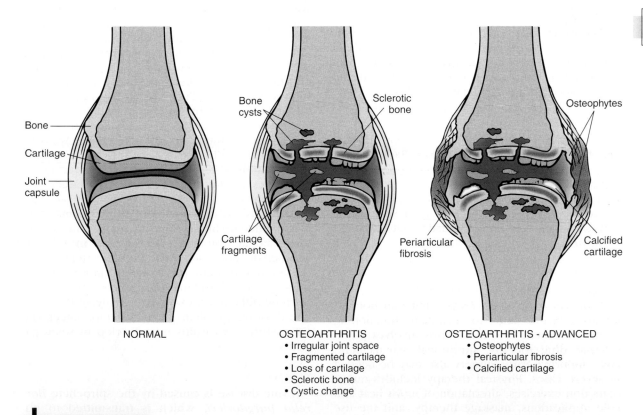

Figure 7–12

Schematic presentation of the pathologic changes in osteoarthritis. Fragmentation and loss of cartilage denude the subchondral bone, which undergoes sclerosis and cystic change. Osteophytes form on the lateral sides and protrude into the adjacent soft tissues, causing irritation, inflammation, and fibrosis. (From Damjanov I: Pathology for the Health-Related Professions. Philadelphia: WB Saunders, 1996, p 468. Used with permission.)

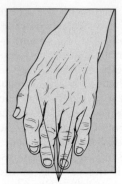 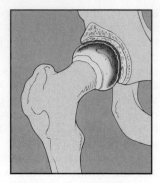

Bouchard's nodes

Degenerative process—
worn cartilage
and roughened bone

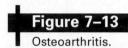
Figure 7–13
Osteoarthritis.

ETIOLOGY

The exact cause of osteoarthritis is unknown; however, **autoimmune** factors and a defective gene in the joint cartilage may contribute to its development. In some persons, osteoarthritis may be secondary to traumatic arthritis.

DIAGNOSIS

A physical examination and patient history may be sufficient for the diagnosis. Radiographic films, **computed tomography (CT)** scans, and **magnetic resonance imaging (MRI)** scans confirm the presence of **osteophytes.** They also indicate the narrowing or absent joint spaces and may show stenosis of the spinal canal or neural **foramina.**

TREATMENT

Because osteoarthritis cannot be cured, the goal of treatment is to reduce inflammation, to minimize pain, and to maintain functioning joints. Treatment of osteoarthritis involves physical and drug therapy, nutritional management, and supportive care. Surgery also may be needed in severe cases. Physical therapy includes range-of-motion exercises, alternation of moist heat and cold applications, massage therapy, and the use of elastic bandages and splints for limb support. Drug therapy can include the use of analgesics, muscle relaxants, and NSAIDs. Intraarticular steroid injections may be used for specific or individual joints. A diet high in vitamins A and C and low in fat and calories is needed for nutritional management. For supportive care, it may be nec-

essary to use a cane, walker, or crutches to lessen the strain on some joints. Restricting physical activity or resting affected joints also may be necessary. Surgery for osteoarthritis may involve total joint replacement. Joints commonly replaced are the hip and the knee. Ankle, wrist, elbow, and shoulder joint also are replaced, but less commonly. Joint fusion may be done to increase stability, as for the cervical and lumbar vertebrae.

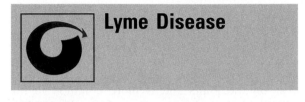

Lyme Disease

SYMPTOMS AND SIGNS

Lyme disease, also known as Lyme arthritis, was first discovered in 1975 in Lyme, Connecticut. It has become one of the fastest growing infectious diseases in the United States. Lyme disease is more prevalent in the northeast part of the country, especially New York, New Jersey, and Connecticut, where there are large areas of forests and fields. The disease has been found, however, in 43 states and on 5 continents.

Lyme disease can occur in any age group, and no one is immune to the infection. Approximately half of all patients with Lyme disease have a characteristic red, itchy rash with a red circle center resembling the bull's eye on a target (target lesion) (Fig. 7–14 A). Lyme disease can masquerade as arthritis (without joint edema) and cause influenza-like symptoms such as headache, fever, fatigue, joint pain, and general **malaise.** If the person does not seek medical attention for the symptoms, complications of muscle weakness, paralysis, and neurologic conditions (e.g., learning difficulties, excessive fatigue, and muscle coordination problems) can develop. Encephalitis, gastritis, or carditis may develop in some patients.

ETIOLOGY

Lyme disease is caused by the spirochete *Borrelia burgdorferi,* which is transmitted to humans by a bite from a small tick (Fig. 7–14 B) that is carried by mice or deer. The disease is transmitted to humans while they are camping or hiking in woods, fields, or other areas that ticks inhabit. The bacterium can infect any organ in the body, causing a variety of symptoms, which often leads to delay in the diagnosis.

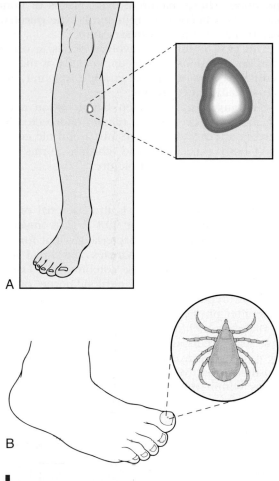

Recombinant Osp A) and ImuLyme are available in injection form and may be helpful in the prevention of Lyme disease.

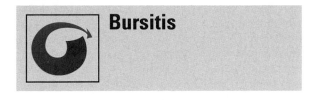

Bursitis

SYMPTOMS AND SIGNS

Bursitis is inflammation of a bursa, which is an enclosed sac of synovial fluid. Bursae are found between muscles and tendons and cover bony prominences, facilitating movement. They can become inflamed, infected, or traumatized; inflammation is the most common condition. The most frequently affected bursae are those of the shoulder (Fig. 7–15), elbow (commonly called tennis elbow), knee (referred to as housemaid's knee), and hip, and those between the tendons and muscles of the tibia.

The classic symptoms of bursitis are tenderness, pain when moving the affected part, flexion and extension limitation, and edema at the site of inflammation. Point tenderness may be present, in which case the patient actually can point to the spot of greatest tenderness. If bursae are continually or chronically irritated and inflamed, calcifications can develop. In addition,

Figure 7–14

A, Target lesion of Lyme disease. *B,* Tick that causes Lyme disease.

DIAGNOSIS

The diagnosis of Lyme disease can be based on physical examination (the discovery of a tick on the skin), the presence of the target lesion, and the patient history. Confirmation is made from a positive result from a blood test for the **antibodies.**

TREATMENT

Treatment of Lyme disease begins with removal of the tick, if it is found on skin or clothing. Early treatment with antibiotics is imperative. Antipyretics are given for headache and fever. Bed rest is necessary if neurologic symptoms are present, and physical therapy is prescribed for impaired musculoskeletal mobility.

The vaccines LYMErix (Lyme Disease Vaccine

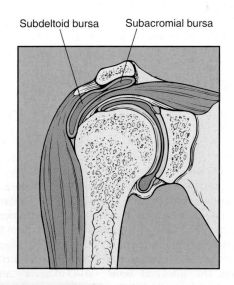

Subdeltoid bursa   Subacromial bursa

Figure 7–15

Bursae of the shoulder.

adhesions can occur around an affected bursa, which limits the movement of the tendons.

ETIOLOGY

Bursitis can result from continual or excessive friction between the bursae and the surrounding musculoskeletal tissues. Systemic diseases (e.g., gout and rheumatoid arthritis) and infection can lead to the development of bursitis. In addition, repeated trauma, from overuse of a limb or part, can cause bursitis (see Cumulative Trauma in Chapter 15).

DIAGNOSIS

The medical history of the patient and physical examination may be all that is needed for the diagnosis. Range of motion is impaired, and the pain is acute. MRI indicates an enlarged bursa, and radiographic films may show calcified deposits at the affected site.

TREATMENT

The treatment may include avoidance of activities until acute pain subsides, the application of moist heat, immobilization of the affected part, the use of aspirin or acetaminophen for pain, the administration of nonsteroidal antiinflammatory agents (e.g., ibuprofen and indomethacin), local injection of corticosteroid, and if infection is present, the use of antibiotics specific to the organism. Active range-of-motion exercises to prevent adhesions and to maintain or regain motion are needed after the acute pain subsides. Surgical excision of the bursal wall and calcified deposits, along with aspiration of the bursal fluid, also may be necessary.

Osteomyelitis

SYMPTOMS AND SIGNS

Osteomyelitis is an infection of the bone and its bone-forming tissue, the marrow. Inflammation, edema, localized heat, and erythema are characteristic signs of this infection. Symptoms of osteomyelitis include pain; the sudden onset of chills, fever, sweating, and tenderness on and around the affected bone; and malaise. As the infection progresses, a **purulent** material called a subperiosteal **abscess** may develop, causing pressure and eventual fracturing of small pieces of

the bone. These fractured, dead pieces of bone may in turn become surrounded by the purulent material and form a **sequestrum.**

The most commonly involved bones in osteomyelitic infections are the upper ends of the humerus and tibia, the lower end of the femur, and occasionally, the vertebrae.

Osteomyelitis most often begins as an acute infection; however, it can remain undetected for months or years and evolve into a chronic condition. Both the acute and chronic forms can present the same clinical picture.

ETIOLOGY

Staphylococcus aureus is the bacterial organism that is responsible for 90% of osteomyelitic infections. Streptococcal bacteria account for the second largest number. Viruses and fungi also have been known to cause osteomyelitis. Osteomyelitis can develop when blood-borne pathogens are deposited in the metaphyseal area of a bone after physical trauma or surgery.

Diabetes mellitus or peripheral vascular disease may predispose individuals to the development of osteomyelitis, as can the presence of prosthetic hardware (e.g., rods, screws, and plates within the bone) and total joint replacement. Osteomyelitis in infants and children develops as a secondary infection from streptococcal pharyngitis (strep throat). Persons with sickle cell disease or malignancies are also at increased risk for the development of osteomyelitis.

The development of osteomyelitis must be the concern of any person who has an open wound, sore (strep) throat, or a systemic infection that has the possibility of being transmitted to the bones.

DIAGNOSIS

Aspiration and culture of material taken from the site of the infection are essential to isolating the causative organisms. A blood culture, a white blood cell **(WBC)** count, and an erythrocyte sedimentation rate **(ESR)** are also helpful. MRI, CT, or bone scans aid in determining the site and extent of acute or chronic infection.

TREATMENT

Osteomyelitis usually requires extensive, long-term treatment with follow-up to prevent recurrent infections. Parenteral or locally administered antibiotics (e.g., aqueous penicillin, cephalosporin, erythromycin [for penicillin-allergic individuals], tetracycline, and ampicillin), at a dosage specific to the patient's age and the pathogenic organism, are needed. Additional measures include increased intake of proteins and vitamins A, B, and C to promote cell regeneration, bed rest as needed to conserve energy, control of chronic conditions (e.g., diabetes), immobilization of the affected part to prevent fracture of weakened bones, and analgesics. Surgical drainage to remove purulent material and sequestrum also may be necessary, along with bone grafting. Hyperbaric oxygen treatments may prove beneficial as well.

Gout

SYMPTOMS AND SIGNS

Gout is a chronic, hereditary disease of uric acid metabolism that occurs as an acute, episodic form of arthritis. It involves an overproduction or decreased excretion of uric acid and urate salts. This leads to high levels of uric acid in the blood and also in the synovial fluid of joints. Deposits of other urate compounds can be found in and around the joints of extremities, often leading to joint deformity and disability (Fig. 7-16 *A* and *B*).

Characteristically, gout affects the first metatarsal joint of the great toe, causing severe to excruciating pain with an attack. The joints of the metacarpal and carpal bones also can be affected. Pain usually peaks after several hours, then subsides gradually. An acute attack may be accompanied by a slight fever, chills, headache, or nausea. Between attacks, the person is characteristically free from any symptoms. Gout also is characterized by renal dysfunction, **hyperuricemia,** and renal calculi (kidney stones).

The disease is uncommon in children; gout generally appears after the age of 30 years. Men are affected more often than women. In women, gout often appears after menopause. Gout also can develop secondary to cell breakdown from drug therapy, especially with chemotherapy for malignant diseases (e.g., leukemia).

ETIOLOGY

The cause of this disease is thought to be metabolic or renal disorders. It may result from a lack of an enzyme needed to completely metabolize purines in foods for renal excretion. This incomplete metabolism leads to the buildup of uric acid, which is a breakdown product of pu-

rines. Renal gout is caused by some form of renal dysfunction. The body may produce levels of uric acid that are normal, but kidney function is insufficient to remove the product from the blood.

DIAGNOSIS

Microscopic examination of aspirated synovial joint fluid shows the presence of urate crystals (see. Fig. 7-16). Urinalysis and a serum uric acid test almost always indicate hyperuricemia. Radiographic films may be used to assess the amount of damage to affected joints.

TREATMENT

General treatment of an acute attack of gout could involve bed rest to lessen pressure on affected joints, immobilization of the affected limb, and the application of ice to the inflamed joints, if the patient is able to tolerate the pressure of an ice bag. An anti-inflammatory agent, aspirin for pain, and corticosteroids taken orally or injected into the gouty area may be prescribed. Dietary modifications include a low-purine diet and frequent fluid intake. The patient is given antihyperuricemic medications (e.g., probenecid and allopurinol). Another consideration involves weight loss, if the patient is obese.

Paget's Disease (Osteitis Deformans)

SYMPTOMS AND SIGNS

Paget's disease is a chronic disease of the normal bone maintenance system that keeps bones healthy and strong. New bone is produced faster than the old bone is broken down. The disease occurs characteristically in two stages. The initial stage is called the vascular stage. Bone tissue is broken down, but the spaces left are filled with blood vessels and fibrous tissue instead of new strong bone. In the second, or sclerotic, stage, the highly vascular fibrous tissue becomes hardened like bone but is fragile. This can lead to pathologic fractures.

This disease can occur in only a part of one bone, all of one bone, or many bones throughout the skeletal system. The most common sites of the disease are the pelvis and the tibia. Also frequently affected are the femur, spine, skull, and

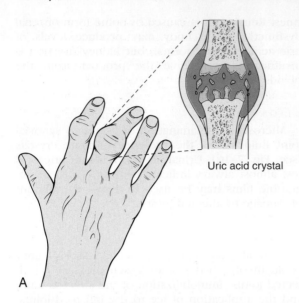

Uric acid crystal

A

194

Blood vessel

Chemotaxis
attracts
leukocytes

Inflammation

Phagocytosis
of crystals

Rupture of
leukocytes

Release of:
• Cytokines
• Enzymes

Deposits
of urate

Joint space

B   Uric acid crystals

Figure 7–16

A, Gout. *B,* Gouty arthritis. Deposits of uric acid crystals in the connective tissue have a chemotactic effect and cause exudation of leukocytes into the joint. The inflammation most often affects the metatarsophalangeal joint. (*B* from Damjanov I: Pathology for the Health-Related Professions. Philadelphia: WB Saunders, 1996, p 473. Used with permission.)

clavicle. Paget's disease usually affects individuals older than 40 years of age and becomes increasingly more common with advancing age.

Paget's disease can be asymptomatic. The symptoms usually include bone pain, the severity of which depends on the extent of the disease and the bones involved. The pain can become disabling. Aching is almost continuous and is often worse at night. Some patients may have edema or deformity in one of the bones or may notice that they need a larger hat size because the bones of the skull enlarge. If the ossicles of the ear are involved, hearing loss or deafness may occur. Other complications of Paget's disease can include frequent fractures, spinal cord injuries, hypercalcemia, renal calculi, and a deadly complication, bone sarcoma.

ETIOLOGY

Paget's disease is idiopathic.

DIAGNOSIS

A physical examination and a history of the patient's symptoms are needed. The physician then orders several tests and blood work to be done. Radiographic films, a bone scan, and possibly a bone marrow biopsy assist in the diagnosis. Blood analysis indicates an elevated serum concentration of alkaline phosphatase, and urinalysis reveals an elevated hydroxyproline concentration. Both these findings are produced by the high rate of bone production.

TREATMENT

An asymptomatic case of Paget's disease need not be treated. A more severe case may require treatment with analgesics, anti-inflammatory drugs, cytotoxic agents, or injections of a hormone called calcitonin. Calcitonin is produced naturally by the thyroid gland and works with parathyroid hormone (parathormone) and vitamin D to regulate the level of calcium in the blood. Increased amounts of calcitonin can reduce pain for some patients and prevent bone loss. A high-protein, high-calcium diet, with vitamin D supplementation, may be advised as well.

Marfan's Syndrome

SYMPTOMS AND SIGNS

Marfan's syndrome is a hereditary group of conditions of the connective tissue in which there is an abnormal length of the extremities. Additional deformities include **subluxation** of the lens of the eyes and cardiac and vascular anomalies. This condition may go undetected until harmful complications are precipitated. The person is tall and slender with long, narrow

digits. An asymmetry of the skull may be noted. Visual difficulties are encountered when lens involvement includes dissociation. Scoliosis is another manifestation. Mitral valve prolapse and thickening of the cardiac valves may be present but undetected (see Valvular Heart Disease in Chapter 10). Often, the first indication of the syndrome occurs during exercise, when an aortic aneurysm ruptures, with catastrophic results.

ETIOLOGY

This syndrome results from a genetic **autosomal** dominant disorder. It is thought that the long arm of chromosome 15 is responsible.

DIAGNOSIS

Diagnosis may be made in early childhood by the lens dissociation and mitral valve prolapse. The clinical picture of a rapid growth spurt and scoliosis, coupled with the visual disturbance and mitral valve prolapse, leads to further investigation. **Echocardiographic** measurements of the aortic diameter aid in detecting potential aortic dissection. Patients at risk for impending aortic dissection may be asymptomatic or may experience chest pain that is tearing in nature and radiates to the neck, back, and arms.

TREATMENT

Treatment involves controlling excessive height with hormones before puberty, preventing glaucoma, controlling blood pressure, and preventing aortic dissection. Ophthalmic examinations should be conducted on a routine basis to detect any problem at an early stage. Monitoring blood pressure and maintaining it at a normal level are essential. Close observation of aortic status is necessary, and surgical replacement of diseased portions may be indicated. Aortic and mitral valves may need to be replaced surgically. Echocardiography is used on a regular basis to assess the aortic status.

Musculoskeletal Tumors

SYMPTOMS AND SIGNS

The most frequent tumors of the musculoskeletal tissues are those affecting the bones. Muscles and cartilage also are involved, but synovial tumors are rare. Primary bone and cartilage tumors

195

are those that occur originally at a particular site, and most of them are benign (e.g., osteomas, osteochondromas, and chondromas). Secondary **metastasic** tumors are those that spread, or metastasize, from their original site to another (e.g., osteosarcomas, Ewing's sarcomas, and fibrosarcomas). Primary soft tissue cancers commonly metastasize to the bones from the breast, lungs, prostate, thyroid, and kidneys. The bones most frequently affected are the pelvis, vertebrae, ribs, hip, femur, and humerus. Metastatic, or secondary, tumors in bones occur more often than do primary tumors.

Radiographic studies of both types of tumors reveal osteonecrosis or increased ossification and calcification. The bone tumor weakens the bone and causes it to fracture under the slightest strain. This is called a pathologic fracture (see Fig. 7-19 *I*). A pathologic fracture is frequently one of the first indications of the presence of metastatic disease. Other symptoms are soreness and pain with limitation of movement. After cancer has metastasized to the bone, the outlook is poor.

Tumors in muscles are exceedingly rare. When they do occur, they are almost always benign and not life threatening (e.g., leiomyomas and rhabdomyomas). Malignant growths in a muscle are a serious, life-threatening matter because these tumors grow and metastasize rapidly and are difficult to treat (e.g., leiomyosarcomas and rhabdomyosarcomas). The first indication of a growth in a muscle is a detectable lump at the affected site, which may be tender or sore, and there are usually no further symptoms. If the growth is malignant, it enlarges rapidly and can become very painful.

ETIOLOGY

Tumors of the bones and muscles are idiopathic. Most bone tumors result from metastatic disease.

DIAGNOSIS

Many of the musculoskeletal tumors are composed of more than one type of cell, which makes their diagnosis more difficult. An accurate diagnosis is crucial because of the nature of the growth of malignant bone tumors and because of the variety of treatment options. The diagnosis is made from the patient history, physical examination, laboratory studies, and diagnostic procedures. Many diagnostic procedures, including radiographic studies, CT scan, MRI scan, and bone scan and biopsy, greatly aid in the diagnosis.

TREATMENT

The treatment of benign tumors can include just observation or surgical excision and bone grafts. Treatment of primary bone cancer can entail wide surgical excision, bone grafts when necessary, radiation therapy, cryosurgery, chemotherapy, hormone therapy, limb amputation, or a combination of these treatments. In all cases, the treatment is specific to the type of tumor, the stage of the disease, the age of the patient, and the patient's lifestyle and anticipated quality of life.

 Osteoporosis

SYMPTOMS AND SIGNS

Osteoporosis is a systemic condition in which there is wasting or deterioration of bone in mass and density. It occurs more frequently in women, especially postmenopausal women, at a 4:1 female:male ratio. Women who are small boned; who come from a northern European, especially Scandinavian, background; or, who have a family history of the disease are at the greatest risk for osteoporosis.

Unless it occurs in the vertebrae or weight-bearing bones, osteoporosis usually does not produce symptoms. Spontaneous fractures, especially in vertebrae at the mid thoracic level or at the thoracolumbar junction, and loss of height are the most common signs (Fig. 7-17).

ETIOLOGY

Osteoporosis is considered a metabolic musculoskeletal condition. It is caused by the imbalance between the breakdown of old bone tissue and the manufacture of new bone. Metabolic bone diseases primarily originate from endocrine or dietary factors or disuse, but trauma also may cause the development of this condition. Osteoporosis is the most common metabolic bone disease. **Senile** and postmenopausal osteoporosis, usually resulting from a lack of estrogen, are the most common forms.

DIAGNOSIS

The diagnosis of osteoporosis is based on the results of blood serum studies, radiographic films, urinalysis, CT scan, and bone scan. Serum

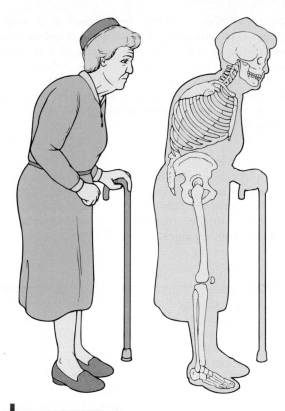

Figure 7-17

Typical posture in osteoporosis.

calcium levels are elevated. If more specific diagnostic data are needed, a bone biopsy may be ordered.

TREATMENT

Osteoporosis can cause permanent disability if not arrested, and treatment varies depending on the cause. Increased dietary intake of calcium, calcium carbonate, calcium carbonate with sodium fluoride, phosphate supplements, and vitamins, especially vitamin D, may be prescribed. Estrogen replacement therapy may be attempted for postmenopausal osteoporosis. For women not wishing to use estrogen replacement therapy, alendronate sodium (Fosamax) may be prescribed. Exercise can help to minimize osteoporosis by slowing the loss of calcium. Moderate exercise in the form of walking, swimming, or riding a stationary bicycle is best. Physical therapy exercises for persons who are immobilized or paralyzed are necessary. If, however, the bones have become brittle, exercise of any type may be prohibited. For pain and muscle spasms,

analgesics and muscle relaxants may be necessary.

Osteomalacia and Rickets

SYMPTOMS AND SIGNS

Osteomalacia is a disease characterized by loss of mineralization of the bones. This causes the bones to become increasingly soft, flexible, and deformed. When the disorder occurs in children, it is called rickets; in adults, it usually is referred to as osteomalacia.

Early symptoms may include general fatigue; progressive stiffness; tender, painful bones; backaches; muscle twitches and cramps; and difficulty in standing up. As the disease progresses, the patient may experience fractures and shortening of the spine, which leads to an overall reduction in height, and the development of a characteristic hump in the upper back.

ETIOLOGY

Osteomalacia is a metabolic bone disease resulting from a deficiency or ineffective use of vitamin D, which is essential to the process of bone formation. Without vitamin D, the body cannot absorb the bone-building minerals (calcium and phosphorus).

Other causes of this disorder may include an inadequate exposure to sunlight, which prevents the body from synthesizing its own vitamin D; intestinal malabsorption of vitamin D; and chronic renal diseases.

DIAGNOSIS

The diagnostic process may include a series of blood tests (e.g., serum calcium, serum alkaline phosphatase, and vitamin D levels) and ESR, radiographic studies, bone scan, and possibly a bone biopsy.

TREATMENT

Treatment involves taking vitamin D supplements and adding vitamin D, calcium, and calcitonin to the diet. Exposure to sunlight increases vitamin D metabolism and absorption, especially for elderly persons. Any underlying disorder causing the deficiency must be treated as well.

Hallux Valgus (Bunion)

SYMPTOMS AND SIGNS

A bunion is a bony protrusion from the lateral edge of the first **metatarsophalangeal** (MTP) joint of the great toe (Fig. 7–18). The condition is progressive, and if an inflamed bursa develops, secondary to pressure and inflammation at the joint, it can become painful. At times, the great toe may override or undercut the second toe. This causes crowding of the other toes and the possible development of hammer, claw, or mallet toe.

Bunion development is more common among women and adolescent girls.

ETIOLOGY

Bunion is usually the result of a foot disorder known as **hallux** valgus, in which the great toe is positioned toward the midline of the body.

The condition also has been associated with rheumatoid arthritis. A flatfoot also contributes to hallux valgus and the development of a bunion because of the fallen, or dropped, longitudinal arch of the foot. Hallux valgus is aggravated by the wearing of improperly fitting or high-heeled shoes. There is also a familial tendency for developing this condition.

DIAGNOSIS

A physical examination of the foot, along with the symptoms, may be sufficient for the diagnosis. Radiographic studies confirm the lateral displacement of the great toe and any degenerative arthritic joint changes.

TREATMENT

Management of a bunion can include wearing shoes with enlarged areas for the toes; wearing shoes with lower heels; using padding between the toes or around the bunion to relieve pressure; applying ice to the bunion to reduce the inflammation and lessen the pain; and resting the affected joints.

Analgesic-**antipyretic** medications (e.g., aspirin and acetaminophen) are given for pain. Intra-articular (joint) injections of corticosteroid may be helpful as well.

There are many different surgical procedures for the treatment or correction of hallux valgus. Bunionectomy, osteotomy, and arthroplasty are the more common procedures.

Hallux Rigidus

SYMPTOMS AND SIGNS

Hallux rigidus, a degenerative disorder of the MTP joint of the great toe, causes pain and loss of motion in the joint. The MTP joint becomes painful, stiff, and swollen. The onset may be insidious, with the limitation of movement being gradual.

ETIOLOGY

Over a period of time, constant wear and tear on the joint or repetitive minor trauma to the joint causes the articular cartilage of the joint to degenerate, resulting in raw bone surface rub-

Metatarsophalangeal joint

Figure 7–18

Bunion—hallux valgus.

bing against raw bone surface. This degenerative arthritic type process allows for the formation of bone spurs or osteophytes in the joint space, resulting in restriction of motion.

DIAGNOSIS

Diagnosis is made from the history of pain, either continuous or when walking, and restriction of motion of the MTP joint of the great toe. Physical examination usually reveals a straight hallux with an enlarged and tender joint with limited dorsiflexion (Fig. 7–19). Radiographic studies confirm the degenerative process, and the joint space is diminished. Advanced conditions may show chips of the cartilage in the joint space, which may eventually calcify.

TREATMENT

Conservative treatment includes drug therapy with anti-inflammatory agents and wearing of shoes with thick hard soles and low heels. When surgical intervention is indicated, a **cheilectomy** to remove bone spurs and degenerative changes of the joint is performed. A portion of the dorsal aspect of the metatarsal head also is removed. This procedure is followed by ROM exercises by the patient to ensure continued flexion and dorsiflexion of the joint. When the progression of the condition is extensive, **arthrodesis,** or fusion of the joint, may be the only method of pain relief. Some surgeons may perform an **arthroplasty** and replace the destroyed joint with a plastic prosthesis or an artifical joint. The problem with this procedure is that the lifetime of the joint usually is limited to 10 years, with additional procedures required to modify the joint in the future.

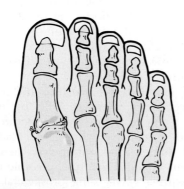
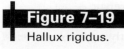

Figure 7–19
Hallux rigidus.

Hammer Toe

SYMPTOMS AND SIGNS

A hammer toe is an orthopedic condition of the toe in which the toe bends upward like a claw because of an abnormal flexion of the proximal interphalangeal (PIP) joint of one of the four lesser toes (Fig. 7–20 A). Usually occurring in the second toe, there is a hyperextension of the MTP joint. This deformity is painful and often causes a corn to develop on the top of the affected toe and callus formation on the sole of the foot.

ETIOLOGY

Many factors may contribute to the occurrence of hammer toe. Although a congenital tendency of a long second metatarsal bone may exist, often shoes that are too short and have pointed toes or high heels may be the contributing factor. Nerves supplying the muscles of the toe are subjected to repeated insult, resulting in muscle imbalance in the foot and the development of the hammer toe.

DIAGNOSIS

History of pain in the affected toe along with visual inspection is usually sufficient for diagnosis (Fig. 7–20 B). Imaging studies confirm the diagnosis.

TREATMENT

If the patient presents early in the onset of symptoms, often switching to shoes that fit properly and allowing for enough space for the second toe can reverse the process, and the toe will straighten. Splinting of the affected toe, along with exercises, is helpful. The more advanced conditions in which a contracture exists require surgical arthroplasty and possible fusion of the PIP joint (Fig. 7–20 C).

Traumatic and Sports Injuries

FRACTURES

Fractures, or broken bones, are caused by stress on the bone from a traumatic insult to the

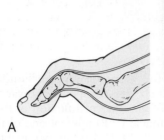

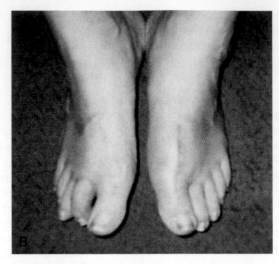

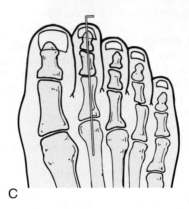

Figure 7–20

A, Hammer toe. *B,* Hammer toe second lesser toe, right foot. *C,* Pin in place after surgical arthroplasty and fusion of proximal interphalangeal (PIP) joint.

musculoskeletal system, severe muscle spasm, or bone disease. They can occur in any bone in the body and are classified by the nature of the fracture, which is the result of the mechanism of injury (Fig. 7–21).

Fractures of individual bones or in particular locations are described by specific names or by location:

• Colles' fracture is fracture of the distal head of the radius, with possible involvement of the ulnar styloid. Colles' fractures usually result from a fall when the person attempts to break the fall with an extended arm and open hand. Pain and swelling are experienced. Treatment includes **closed reduction** of the fracture and immobilization, including the elbow, with a cast.

• In fracture of the humerus, an obvious displacement of the bone of the upper arm is noted, along with shortening of the extremity and an abnormal mobility of the upper arm. Closed reduction of the fracture is followed by immobilization in a hanging arm cast and sling and swathe.

• Fracture of the pelvis is usually the result of a motor vehicle accident or a fall by an elderly person. Complications of this fracture include lacerated colon, paralytic ileus, bladder and urethral injury, and intrapelvic hemorrhage. Treatment includes bed rest, possible immobilization with a pelvic sling or skeletal traction, and **open reduction** and repair.

• A fractured hip is usually the result of a fall. This fracture most frequently occurs because of

Enrichment

AMPUTATION

Most limb amputations involve the legs and are necessary because of peripheral vascular disease and consequent gangrene. Trauma, malignancy, and congenital defects are additional reasons for amputation. Many upper extremity amputations are the sequelae of trauma including crushing injuries, open fractures, and thermal or electrical burns. Vascular disease, infection, or malignancy may also necessitate the amputation. The extent of the amputation can range from removal of a portion of a digit to a complete disarticulation at the hip or shoulder.

Rehabilitation is important and is attempted as soon as possible to afford the patient independence. Many prostheses are available for both upper and lower extremities and each is individualized to the patient.

osteoporosis in women older than 60 years of age. An outward rotation along with a shortening of the affected extremity is noted. Repair is surgical, with the insertion of a prosthesis or pins, or both.

- Fracture of the femoral shaft is more common in young adults as the result of a severe direct force from motor vehicle accidents or severe trauma. There is a marked angulation deformity and shortening of the affected leg. The patient is unable to move the knee or hip. The fracture is stabilized by **skeletal traction** or internal fixation with a rod or a plate and screws.
- Fracture of the tibia results from a strong force exerted on the lower leg that causes soft tissue damage in addition to the fracture. Open or closed reduction is employed, followed by immobilization with a cast.
- Vertebral fracture, usually occurring in the cervical region, is the result of acceleration-deceleration trauma. Immediate immobilization is imperative to prevent spinal cord damage and resulting paralysis. Thoracic and lumbar vertebrae also can be fractured. Immobilization may be followed by surgical repair for stabilization.

- Basilar skull fracture is fracture of the floor of the cranial vault (see Fig. 13-9 in Chapter 13). It is usually the result of massive trauma to the head from a motor vehicle accident.
- Le Fort's fracture, bilateral horizontal fracture of the maxilla, often results when the face is forced against the steering wheel in a motor vehicle accident.
- In Pott's fracture, the lower part of the fibula is fractured. The lower tibial articulation sustains serious injury.
- Clavicular fracture is fracture of the clavicle (collar bone). It is a common sports injury and occurs frequently in children of all ages.

SYMPTOMS AND SIGNS

Pain accompanies most fractures. Edema, tenderness, discoloration, and inability to move the affected part follow. In some instances, a deformity of the part is noted. The location of the fracture and the type of the fracture are determining factors in the symptoms and signs.

ETIOLOGY

Any force that disrupts the continuity of the bone causes a fracture. Diseases such as neoplasms, tuberculosis of the bone, and osteoporosis cause pathologic fractures.

Enrichment

PHANTOM LIMB AND PHANTOM LIMB PAIN

Phantom limb sensation is an unpleasant complication that sometimes follows an amputation, especially of a leg, and is difficult to treat. It is the feeling that the limb still is attached. Phantom limb pain of the leg can present as a burning sensation of the foot or as a feeling of having the toes stepped on when no limb exists.

Both conditions usually disappear with time and with the realization that the limb is gone. Phantom limb pain may necessitate injection or removal of troublesome nerve endings that are located in the stump.

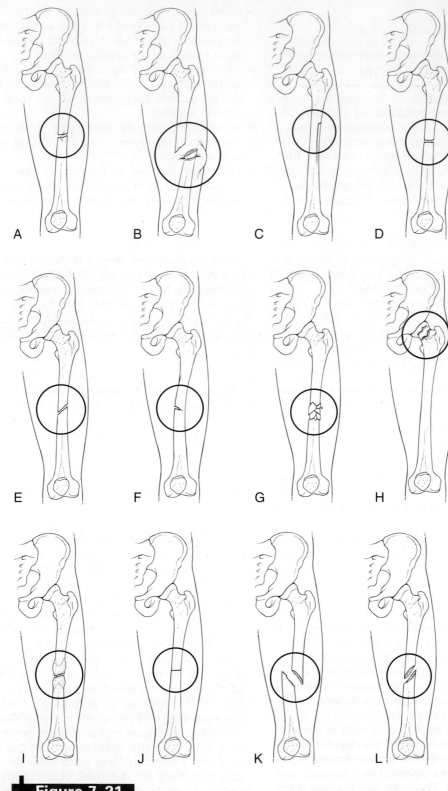

Figure 7–21

See legend on opposite page

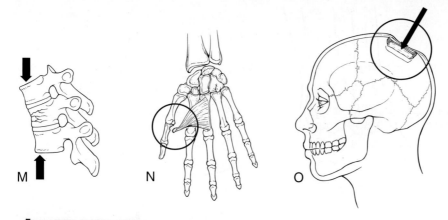

Figure 7–21

Types of fractures. *A,* Closed, or simple. The overlying skin is intact. *B,* Open, or compound. The skin overlying the bone ends is not intact. *C,* Longitudinal. The fracture extends along the length of the bone. *D,* Transverse. The fracture is at right angles to the axis of the bone. *E,* Oblique. The fracture extends in an oblique direction. *F,* Greenstick. The fracture is on one side of the bone; the other side is bent. *G,* Comminuted. The bone is splintered or crushed. *H,* Impacted. The fractured ends of the bone are driven into each other. *I,* Pathologic. The fracture results from weakening of the bone by disease. *J,* Nondisplaced. The bone ends remain in alignment. *K,* Displaced. The bone ends are out of alignment. *L,* Spiral. The fracture results from a twisting mechanism, causing the break to wind around the bone in a spiral. *M,* Compression. Excessive pressure causes the bone to collapse. *N,* Avulsion. Tearing away of a muscle or a ligament is accompanied by tearing away of a bone fragment. *O,* Depression. Bone fragments of the skull are driven inward.

DIAGNOSIS

A complete history and physical examination are followed by radiographic studies of the affected structure. Bone scans and MRI aid in diagnosis. Underlying pathologic change is investigated and determined.

TREATMENT

Treatment depends on the location, severity, type, and cause of the fracture. Simple fractures of long bones are reduced and immobilized. Compound fractures are cleaned, **débrided,** reduced, and immobilized. Immobilization is accomplished by splinting (including the use of posterior splints), casting, taping, and internal fixation. Internal fixation includes the use of surgically implanted pins, wires, rods, plates, screws, or other devices. Some fractures are placed in traction, to hold the ends of the bones in proper alignment, until healing takes place.

Complications of fractures include compartment syndrome, in which the circulation to the area is compromised because of edema; infec-tion; **necrosis;** fat emboli; and pulmonary emboli.

STRAINS AND SPRAINS

SYMPTOMS AND SIGNS

A strain is the result of overuse, overstretching, or excessive forcible stretching of a muscle beyond its functional capacity. It sometimes involves a tendon or a ligament. Strains can occur as an acute injury or can be the result of chronic overuse (cumulative trauma). They are classified as first, second, or third degree, or grade. Symptoms may include localized pain, weakness, numbness, and possibly edema in the area of the injury. The patient has difficulty in using, moving, or bearing weight on the affected limb or part. A strain is less serious than a sprain.

A sprain is an acute partial tear of a muscle, a tendon, or a ligament (Fig. 7–22). Sprains also may involve damage to blood vessels and nerves. With a sprain, edema, ecchymosis, and sharp,

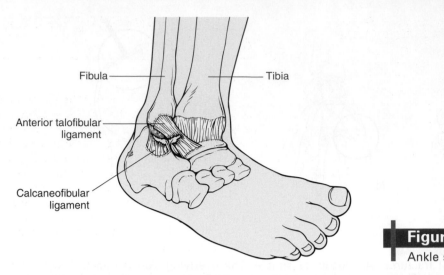

Fibula

Tibia

Anterior talofibular ligament

Calcaneofibular ligament

Figure 7–22
Ankle sprain.

transient pain may develop. Also, the patient may be unable to use, move, or bear weight on the injured joint. When sprains and strains are caused by chronic overuse, they typically cause stiffness, tenderness, and soreness.

ETIOLOGY

Strains and sprains can be caused by acute trauma (e.g., automobile accidents) or cumulative trauma (e.g., overuse, such as with some sports injuries).

DIAGNOSIS

A physical examination and medical history of a recent injury from physical activity, accident, or continued trauma may suggest the diagnosis. To rule out the possibility of a fracture, radiographic studies are needed.

TREATMENT

The treatment of strains and sprains is similar and depends on the degree, or grade, of the injury. The sprain, being the more serious injury, requires more intense treatment. Treatment of sprains and strains entails elevation and rest of the affected limb, along with the application of ice to control edema. Immobilization of the limb with an elastic bandage, soft cast, or splint may be necessary. Analgesics and possibly anti-inflammatory agents are used to control pain and inflammation. Surgery may be indicated if the injury is serious, as with a large tear, or if it heals improperly. Healing of a strain or sprain usually requires 2 to 4 weeks, longer with the more serious degrees of strain or sprain. Recognizing personal physical limitations, following safety

precautions, and taking time to warm up the muscles by slow, easy stretching before exercise or physical activity help to prevent these injuries.

DISLOCATIONS

SYMPTOMS AND SIGNS

A dislocation occurs when a bone that is normally in contact with a joint is separated from that joint and causes loss of the joint's function (Fig. 7–23). A joint that is dislocated appears misshapen, is extremely painful, and rapidly becomes edematous, ecchymotic, and immovable. Injury to the joint ligaments and joint capsule is present. Other symptoms that appear are related to, and dependent on, the extent of damage to the surrounding tissues, nerves, and blood vessels.

Dislocation of spinal vertebrae can result in damage to the entire spinal cord and cause paralysis below the injured area. A dislocation of a shoulder or hip can damage the nerve supply and cause paralysis of the limb. Some joints that have been dislocated tend to be susceptible to developing osteoarthritis in later years.

ETIOLOGY

The cause of a dislocation is usually a severe injury (e.g., a fall, automobile accident, or sports trauma) that exerts force great enough to tear the joint ligaments. Occasionally, the injury that causes the dislocation also causes a fracture.

Dislocations not caused by injury may be congenital or may result from a complication of

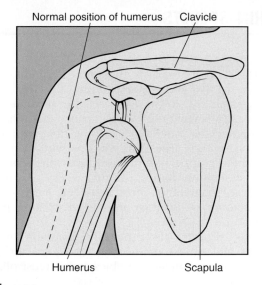

Normal position of humerus   Clavicle

Humerus   Scapula

Figure 7–23
Dislocation of the shoulder.

rheumatoid arthritis. They can happen repeatedly, without apparent cause, to a joint already weakened by an earlier injury. The jaw and shoulder joints are especially susceptible to recurring dislocation.

DIAGNOSIS

The obvious appearance of the affected joint, the history of the injury, and the physical examination may be all that is necessary for the diagnosis. A radiographic study determines whether a dislocation has occurred and if any fractures are present.

TREATMENT

An untrained individual never should attempt to reduce a dislocation; to do so may cause extensive damage. A physician should be seen within 15 to 30 minutes for proper repositioning. After that time, a dislocated joint normally becomes so edematous and painful that reduction may have to be done using general anesthesia. If dislocation is a recurring problem, patients may be taught how to reposition the joint themselves.

Surgery is sometimes necessary to achieve satisfactory reduction. If a joint has become weakened from repeated dislocation, surgery to tighten the ligaments that hold the adjoining bones may be recommended.

ADHESIVE CAPSULITIS (FROZEN SHOULDER)

SYMPTOMS AND SIGNS

A frozen shoulder means that the shoulder becomes stiff and painful, making normal movement impossible. The pain either can be localized in the shoulder itself or can spread to the upper arm or neck. It is often severe enough to disrupt sleep. Symptoms become worse during several months, then remain the same for a couple of months, and finally begin a gradual period of improvement. With time the pain subsides, but the mobility of the shoulder often remains permanently impaired, or frozen.

ETIOLOGY

Frozen shoulder is caused by disuse of the shoulder. It usually begins after a slight injury or minor problem, such as bursitis and **tendinitis,** which prevents normal use of the joint. This disuse leads to more and more stiffness, pain, and additional disuse.

DIAGNOSIS

The symptoms are usually enough to suggest this condition. However, a review of the patient history may indicate a recent injury from which bursitis or tendinitis developed.

TREATMENT

A stiff shoulder must be kept in motion, as much as possible, to prevent permanent immobility. A physical or occupational therapist may be needed to teach and assist the patient with ROM exercises. Analgesics and anti-inflammatory agents are needed, and possibly an injection of a steroid into the joint. If the condition is severe and persistent, the physician may suggest shoulder manipulation, under general anesthesia, to increase mobility.

SEVERED TENDON

SYMPTOMS AND SIGNS

Tendons are long, fibrous cords that connect muscles to bones (e.g., the ones that move the thumb, fingers, and toes). The muscles that move these parts are located in the forearms and the calves of the legs. A severed tendon produces immediate, severe pain, inflammation, and immobility of the affected parts (Fig. 7-24).

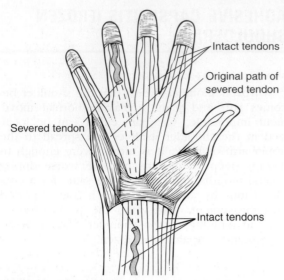

Figure 7–24

Severed tendon of the hand.

ETIOLOGY

The cause of a severed tendon is an injury or laceration. It involves the forearm, hand, calf of the leg, or foot. The injury may extend partially or completely through one or more tendons.

DIAGNOSIS

Physical examination of the injured site and the patient's inability to move the affected parts are usually sufficient for the diagnosis. A radiographic study rules out a fracture as the cause of the immobility.

TREATMENT

Tendons are under tension, so if they become severed, the two ends snap away from each other and are difficult to retrieve. A surgeon may attempt to suture the two ends of the tendon together (tenorrhaphy) immediately or may wait for the injury to heal, depending on the extent of the injury. A larger incision may be necessary to locate the ends of the tendon, before the tenorrhaphy can be attempted. To repair the damaged tendon, a piece of tendon from elsewhere in the body may need to be used.

The outcome of a tenoplasty is usually satisfactory. However, in some cases, the affected parts may be stiff and have less mobility than before the injury. Physical therapy ensures as much mobility as possible.

SHIN SPLINTS

SYMPTOMS AND SIGNS

The term shin splints applies to a painful condition involving the **periosteum,** the extensor muscles in the lower leg, and the surrounding tissues. Inflammation, edema, pain, and tenderness along the inner aspect of the tibia are common symptoms. The pain worsens with exercise and then disappears with rest. Shin splints occur most commonly during the first weeks of a new exercise program or after a sudden increase in the amount of exercise during an existing program.

This disorder is especially common with sports and fitness enthusiasts who jog, run, or engage in high-impact aerobics and is most often bilateral.

ETIOLOGY

Overuse and overpronation are the most common factors that predispose an individual to shin splints. Pronation of the foot is an inward rotation of the ankle that causes the inner arch of the foot to sag and the ankle joint to tip upward (Fig. 7-25). All people pronate to some degree;

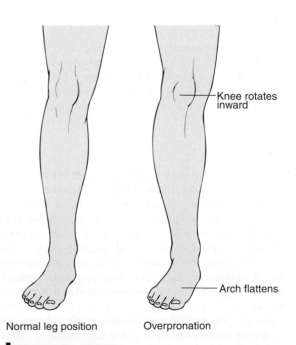

Figure 7–25

Excessive pronation of the foot.

however, excessive pronation places abnormal stress on the calf muscles. This leads to the development of shin splints and tendon and ligament strain around the ankles and knees.

Improper conditioning and running on hard surfaces also can contribute to the development of shin splints.

DIAGNOSIS

The diagnosis is based on physical examination and history of pain that worsens with exercise and disappears after rest. Radiographic films of the tibia or a bone scan may be ordered to rule out the possibility of a stress fracture.

TREATMENT

The key to successful treatment is rest. Applications of ice or heat, or both alternately, are essential in the treatment. Aspirin or stronger NSAIDs may be ordered to relieve the pain and to reduce inflammation. Specially designed shoes to correct overpronation or the use of an orthotic device in existing shoes may be recommended.

Proper conditioning and gradual stretching of the legs before exercise, jogging or running on grass or other soft surfaces, performing aerobic exercises on mats, and ensuring that exercise shoes are well padded for support can help to prevent this condition. Shin splints are painful but not dangerous, unless they are ignored and result in stress fractures.

PLANTAR FASCIITIS (CALCANEAL SPUR)

SYMPTOMS AND SIGNS

Plantar fasciitis, also known as calcaneal, or heel, spur syndrome, is an inflammatory response at the heel bone (calcaneus). It is a common problem among people who are active in sports, especially runners. The problem begins as a dull, intermittent pain in the heel, which can progress to a sharp persistent pain. Characteristically, the pain is worse on getting out of bed and taking the first few steps in the morning, after sitting for a time, after standing or walking, and when beginning a sporting activity. Plantar fascia injury also can occur at mid sole or near the toes.

The plantar fascia is a thick fibrous material on the bottom of the foot. It is attached to the calcaneus, fans forward toward the toes, and acts like a bowstring to maintain the arch of the foot.

ETIOLOGY

The problem usually occurs when part of the inflexible fascia is repeatedly placed under tension (e.g., when running). This constant tension causes an inflammatory response, usually at the point where the fascia is attached to the calcaneus. The result is pain and the development of the spur.

Contributing factors to the development of plantar fasciitis include:

- Flat (pronated) feet
- High-arched, rigid feet
- Toe running or hill running
- Running on soft terrain (e.g., sand)
- Poor shoe support
- Sudden increase in activity level
- Sudden weight increase
- Increasing age
- Familial tendency

The inflammatory response at the calcaneus can produce spike-like projections of new bone called calcaneal (heel) spurs (Fig. 7-26 *A*). They do not cause the initial pain, nor do they cause the initial problem; they are a result of the problem.

DIAGNOSIS

Physical examination and the patient history of symptoms usually provide sufficient information for diagnosis. Radiographic films sometimes show the spur (Fig. 7-26 *B*).

TREATMENT

The initial treatment of heel spurs consists of resting, applying ice to the sore area, taking anti-inflammatory or analgesic medication, using heel pads (doughnut-shaped pads that equalize and absorb the shock on the heel and ease pressure on the plantar fascia), and wearing a shoe with good support. In addition, the physician may tape the foot to maintain the arch and to help to take some of the tension off the plantar fascia. Shoe inserts called orthotics also may be prescribed.

After the inflammation has subsided, physical therapy to strengthen the small muscles of the foot can begin. If done regularly, this helps to prevent reinjury. Surgery rarely is required for the correction of heel spurs. It is considered only if all forms of more conservative treatment fail and the pain still is incapacitating after several months of treatment. When performed, surgery involves removing the bone spur and releasing the plantar fascia.

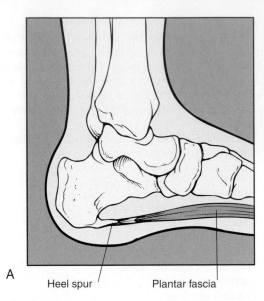

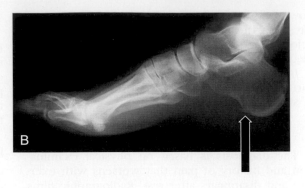

Figure 7–26

A, Calcaneal (heel) spur. *B,* Radiographic appearance.

GANGLION

SYMPTOMS AND SIGNS

A ganglion is a benign growth or tumor that is filled with a colorless, jelly-like substance. A ganglion most commonly develops on the back of the wrist as a single, smooth lump, just under the surface of the skin (Fig. 7–27). It can, however, develop around the ankle joint and on the fingers. Also, ganglia may appear as multiples or in clusters. Most are about the size of a pea, but others may grow as large as an inch or more in diameter. Ganglia may be soft to the touch or firm, and they are usually either painless or only somewhat bothersome. There may be occasional pain when moving the wrist, especially if the growth is large or inflamed.

ETIOLOGY

Although some physicians believe that ganglia are caused by repetitive minor injuries, the underlying cause remains unknown. Whatever triggers the growth's development, it usually arises either in the joint capsule or in a tendon sheath.

DIAGNOSIS

A ganglion usually can be diagnosed by palpation and by observation of the appearance of the lump and the characteristic site. If in doubt, the physician can perform a needle aspiration to withdraw some of the fluid for laboratory analysis.

TREATMENT

If the ganglion does not cause pain and is not large enough to cause disfigurement or to interfere with wrist function, treatment is unnecessary. However, if the ganglion is causing pain, disfigurement, or impairment of the ROM, several options are available. The physician may try to rupture the ganglion by applying firm pressure. Needle aspiration may be used to remove as much fluid as possible, followed by instillation of a steroid, such as cortisone, or a **sclerosing** solution that helps to prevent recurrences. The physician may recommend a surgical procedure called a ganglionectomy to remove the ganglion.

Ganglia that originate in the wrist joint may be difficult to remove completely and therefore tend to recur. Even after surgical excision, approximately 10% recur. During a period of months, ganglia often disappear on their own.

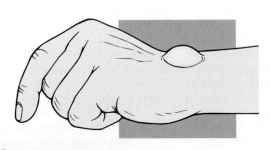

Figure 7–27

Ganglion.

TORN MENISCUS

SYMPTOMS AND SIGNS

The menisci are semilunar cartilages found in the knee joint. There are two menisci within the joint, a medial and a lateral (Fig. 7–28). The medial **meniscus** is larger and more restricted in movement than is the lateral meniscus and therefore is injured more frequently, or torn. Anterior and posterior cruciate ligament tears may accompany meniscal tears because the menisci are attached to the ligaments.

A person with a torn meniscus has acute pain when putting full weight on the affected leg and knee. The person may report that the knee "locks" or "gives way." Snapping or clicking sounds (crepitus) may be heard on flexion or extension. Full flexion of the affected knee may be difficult, and pain increases with full extension.

ETIOLOGY

Most torn menisci are related to sports injuries. Participants in football, baseball, and soccer are especially susceptible to this type of injury. Tears in the meniscus usually result from sudden twisting or external rotation of the leg while the knee is flexed.

DIAGNOSIS

Physical examination of the knee indicates the limitation of movement. Radiographic studies and MRI, which is the preferred procedure, are ordered; MRI may show the exact injury to the meniscus and, if any, to the ligaments.

TREATMENT

The injured knee should be immobilized immediately and elevated, with ice applied to slow bleeding and edema. No weight-bearing should be allowed, and the physician should be seen as soon as possible. The physician orders anti-inflammatory or analgesic medications as needed. An antibiotic also may be ordered.

The treatment of a torn meniscus usually can be done arthroscopically under anesthesia, unless there also has been injury to the cruciate ligaments. Ligament tears require more extensive surgery to expose and repair them. Total excision or partial excision of the torn meniscus is called a meniscectomy. A total meniscectomy usually is not done because it predisposes the knee to degenerative changes and instability.

An extensive exercise program, which varies depending on the injury, begins after the initial postoperative period and continues during the subsequent few months.

ROTATOR CUFF TEARS

SYMPTOMS AND SIGNS

The rotator cuff muscles of the shoulder partially surround the head of the humerus and sta-

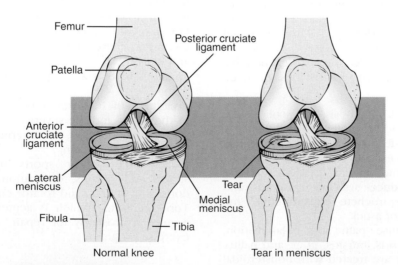

Femur

Posterior cruciate ligament

Patella

Anterior cruciate ligament

Lateral meniscus

Tear

Medial meniscus

Fibula

Tibia

Normal knee

Tear in meniscus

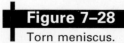

Figure 7–28

Torn meniscus.

bilize it in the **glenoid** cavity or socket. The infraspinatus muscle rotates the humerus externally, and the subscapularis muscle rotates the humerus internally. Other muscles involved in the rotator cuff are the supraspinatus and the teres minor.

Tears in the tendons of the rotator cuff muscles produce an immediate snapping sound and acute pain and leave the person unable to **abduct** the arm.

ETIOLOGY

Tears can result from acute trauma (most common) or from degenerative changes with age. Calcium deposits may develop in the insertion sites because of the degenerative changes and may predispose the tendons to tears or rupture. Also, steroid injections into the tendon areas can predispose them to tears or rupture.

DIAGNOSIS

Diagnosis is based on physical examination and the patient history. Confirmation is made by the results of an arthrogram or CT scan and arthroscopic views.

TREATMENT

Acute pain is managed with narcotic medication (e.g., codeine). Acetaminophen is given for moderate pain, and anti-inflammatory medication is given for the inflammation.

Acute tendon tears are repaired immediately to preserve strength of the muscles and to restore motion of the shoulder. After surgery, the affected arm is placed in a shoulder immobilizer or abduction splint for approximately 3 weeks. Extensive, active exercises are begun when the cast is removed.

Summary

Components of the musculoskeletal system support and protect the body, provide metabolic functions, and are designed to allow practical and functional, as well as recreational and artistic, forms of mobility. With normal function of all the elements (muscles, bones, ligaments, tendons, and cartilage) of the system, the body not only presents a superb image, but it is able to accomplish motion tasks from lifting a finger to climbing Mt. Everest. However, with congenital conditions, the onset of disease caused by trauma, inflammation, infection, or degenerative conditions, even rudimentary activities are compromised.

- Lordosis (swayback), kyphosis, and scoliosis are spinal disorders and postural abnormalities.
- Osteoarthritis, a degenerative disease of joints associated with wear and tear, causes pain, decreased range of motion, and disability.
- Lyme disease produces systemic symptoms and is caused by a spirochete transmitted to humans by the bite of a tick.
- Diseases that cause pain and inflammation, such as osteoarthritis, bursitis, gout, and hallux valgus, commonly are treated with nonsteroidal anti-inflammatory drugs (NSAIDs) or corticosteroids and supportive care to rest the joint(s).

- Osteomalacia results from vitamin D deficiency that impairs calcium absorption and calcification.
- Osteomyelitis, a bacterial infection of the bone, requires extensive long-term antibiotic therapy.
- Fibromyalgia and polymyositis are painful inflammatory muscle diseases usually accompanied by systemic symptoms.
- Osteoporosis, commonly a postmenopausal condition, causes deterioration of bone in mass and density.
- Phantom limb is a complication of limb amputation.
- Treatment of fractures depends on the nature of the break and the severity of trauma. Reduction, immobilization, or internal fixation may be required for healing.
- Other traumatic or sports injuries include strains and sprains, dislocations, severed tendons, shin splints, and rotator cuff tears.
- Torn meniscus, which is acutely painful, may require arthroscopy for repair, followed by an exercise program.

Review Challenge

REVIEW QUESTIONS

1. What are the functions of the normal skeletal system?
2. What procedures are employed in diagnosing scoliosis?
3. What pathology is characteristic of osteoarthritis?
4. The symptoms of Lyme disease mimic which disease?
5. Are there any preventive measures recommended for Lyme disease?
6. What is the clinical picture of a patient with osteomyelitis?
7. What causes joint deformity in gout?
8. Which disease is characterized by a high rate of bone production?
9. What would the treatment plan for an individual with osteoporosis include?
10. How is vitamin D deficiency related to osteomalacia?
11. What specific findings from a physical examination are typical of fibromyalgia?
12. What causative factors contribute to hallux valgus (bunion)? Hallux rigidus? Hammer toe?
13. How are fractures classified?
14. How would you describe Colles' fracture?
15. What is meant by phantom limb?
16. By what methods are fractures immobilized?
17. Why is a sprain considered more serious than a strain?
18. What joints are more susceptible to dislocation?
19. What conditions result in a "frozen shoulder"?
20. What is the relationship of overpronation to shin splints?
21. Under what conditions might plantar fasciitis (spur syndrome) develop?
22. What acute symptoms is a person with torn meniscus likely to describe? A person with rotator cuff tear?

Osteoporosis

A 72-year-old woman recently experienced midthoracic back pain after a minor fall. Imaging studies confirm fractures of T-7 and T-8. Measurement of this small-boned woman revealed a loss of 1 inch in height, 5 feet 1 inch now compared with 5 feet 2 inches at last physical examination 14 months ago. Serum calcium level is elevated. The CT scan is indicative of osteoporosis.

According to history, the patient does not include many dairy products in her diet and takes no dietary supplements. Additionally, she has never been on any form of estrogen replacement and does not exercise on a regular basis.

Questions

1. In what type of individual would you expect to find the greatest incidence of osteoporosis?
2. What bones other than vertebrae are prone to fracture in osteoporosis?
3. Why would serum calcium level be elevated in osteoporosis?
4. What is meant by osteoporosis being a metabolic bone disease?
5. What should be included in a diet to prevent or slow the onset of osteoporosis?
6. Why is daily exercise important in the prevention of osteoporosis?
7. What type of drug therapy may be prescribed for the patient?

Lyme Disease

A 27-year-old man has been experiencing flu-like symptoms for 4 days. He reports headache, fatigue, joint pain, and "just not feeling well." Vital signs are T 102.2°F, P—96, R—20, BP—132/86. Physical examination reveals two areas on the left lower leg that have a fading red rash in a circle-type pattern. The center of each circle is pale and it appears as if there could be a spot in the center of each.

Questioning discloses that the patient was deer hunting 5 days ago, walking through tall grass. He remembers experiencing itching on the lower left leg. Lyme disease is suspected. A blood test to detect antibodies to the spirochete *Borrelia burgdorferi* is ordered. Antibiotics are prescribed, as is acetaminophen for the fever, pain, and aches. Patient is encouraged to rest and return for recheck in a few days.

Questions

1. In what region of the country would you expect this patient to live?
2. What precautions should be taken by individuals who will be out walking in tall grass?
3. What should individuals who think that they have been bitten by a tick do as soon as they discover the bite?
4. If Lyme disease is not diagnosed in its early stages, what complications may develop?
5. What is the causative agent of Lyme disease?
6. Discuss prevention of Lyme disease, including vaccines.

RESOURCES

National Arthritis and Musculoskeletal and Skin Diseases Information Clearinghouse
1 AMS Circle
Bethesda, MD 20892-3675
301-495-4484
(http://www.nih.gov/niams)

Ankylosing Spondylitis Association
800-777-8189

Amyotrophic Lateral Sclerosis Association
27001 Agoura Rd, Ste 150
Calabasas Hills, CA 91301-5104
1-800-782-4747
(http://www.alsa-national.org)

Arthritis Foundation
27001 West Peachtree St
Atlanta, GA 30309
1-800-238-7800
(http://www.arthritis.org)

National Osteoporosis Foundation
1150 17th St, NW, Ste 500
Washington, DC 20036-4603
202-223-2226
(http://www.nof.org)
(http://www.orbdnrc@nof.org)

National Scoliosis Foundation, Inc.
3 Cabot Place
Stoughton, MA 02072
617-341-6333
(scoliosis@aol.com)

National Information Center for Children and Youth with Disabilities
PO Box 1492
Washington, DC 20013-1492
(nichey@aed.org)

Lyme Disease Foundation
One Financial Plaza, 18th Floor
Hartford, CT 06103
860-525-2000, 24-hr hotline 1-800-886-LYME
(http://www.lymenet.org)

National Fibromyalgia Research Association
PO Box 500
Salem, OR 97302

Myositis Association of America
755 Cantrell Ave, Suite C
Harrisonburg, VA 22801
540-433-7686
(http://maa@myositis.org)

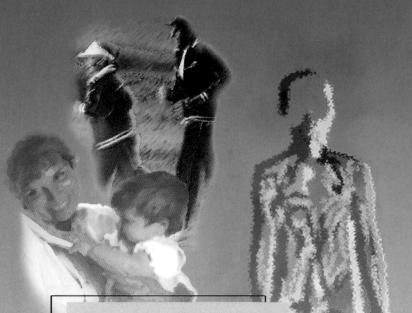

Chapter Outline

Diseases and Conditions of the Digestive System

Learning Objectives

After studying Chapter 8, you should be able to:

1. Trace the process of normal digestion and absorption.
2. Discuss the importance of normal teeth and a normal bite.
3. Describe the presenting symptoms of temporomandibular joint syndrome.
4. Compare the etiology of herpes simplex to the etiology of thrush.
5. Name a serious complication of esophageal varices.
6. Describe the pathology of peptic ulcers, and identify the etiology.
7. Explain the diagnosis of gastric cancer.
8. Describe a hiatal hernia.
9. Distinguish between the types of abdominal hernias.
10. Explain the differences between the pathology involved in Crohn's disease and ulcerative colitis.
11. Describe the etiology of gastroenteritis.
12. Explain the difference between a functional and a mechanical obstruction of the bowel.
13. Discuss the pathologic conditions that may result in intestinal obstruction.
14. Distinguish between diverticulosis and diverticulitis.
15. Discuss the treatment of colorectal cancer.
16. Explain the relationship between broad-spectrum antibiotics and pseudomembranous enterocolitis.
17. List the causes of inflammation of the peritoneum.
18. Explain the pathologic symptoms and signs of cirrhosis of the liver.
19. Contrast hepatitis A to hepatitis C in cause and prevention measures.
20. Describe the clinical picture of an individual with (1) biliary colic and (2) acute pancreatitis.
21. State the prognosis of pancreatic cancer.
22. Describe the clinical manifestations of malnutrition and malabsorption.
23. Explain the diagnostic criteria for celiac disease.
24. Distinguish between the clinical picture of the patient with anorexia and the patient with bulimia.
25. State the components of a successful weight loss program.

Key Terms

adenocarcinoma	(**ad**–ih–no–**kar**–sin–**OH**–ma)	hypokalemia	(**high**–poh–ka–**LEE**–me–ah)
anastomosis	(ah–**nas**–toh–**MOH**–sis)	inguinal	(**ING**–gwih–nal)
antiemetic	(**an**–tih–ee–**MET**–ik)	intussusception	(in–tah–sus–**SEP**–shun)
aphthous	(**AF**–thus)	periodontitis	(**per**–ee–oh–don–**TIE**–tis)
ascites	(ah–**SIGH**–teez)		
cholinergic	(**ko**–lin–**ER**–jik)	peritonitis	(**per**–ih–toh–**NIE**–tis)
endoscopy	(en–**DOS**–ko–pee)	proctoscopy	(prock–**TAHS**–ko–pee)
fistula	(**FIS**–tew–lah)		
fulminant	(**FUL**–mih–nant)	pseudomembranous	(**soo**–doe–**MEM**–brah–nus)
gastroscopy	(gas–**TROS**–koh–pee)		
gingivitis	(jin–jih–**VIE**–tis)	sigmoidoscopy	(**sig**–moy–**DOS**–ko–pee)
hematemesis	(hem–ah–**TEM**–eh–sis)	temporomandibular	(**tem**–poh–roh–man–**DIHB**–you–lar)
hepatomegaly	(**hep**–ah–toh–**MEG**–ah–lee)	varices	(**VAR**–ih–seez)

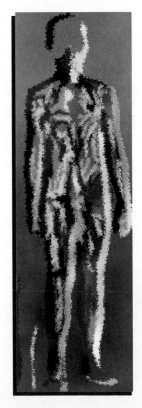

Orderly Function of the Digestive System

The digestive system comprises the alimentary canal and the accessory organs of digestion (Fig. 8-1). Each unit of the system must be normal in structure and function to regulate the ingestion, digestion, and absorption of nutrients. The alimentary canal processes and transports the products of digestion. The accessory organs, located outside the gastrointestinal (GI) tract, manufacture and secrete endocrine and exocrine enzymes; these secretions are essential to the digestion and absorption of nutrients.

Diseases of the GI tract affect health and threaten life because they interfere with the critical functions of ingestion and digestion of food, absorption of nutrients for metabolism, and elimination of wastes. General categories of diseases and conditions of the digestive system include erosion of tissue, inflammation, infection, benign and malignant tumors, obstruction, interference with blood or nerve supply, malnutrition, and malabsorption syndromes.

ACCESSORY ORGANS

MAIN ORGANS

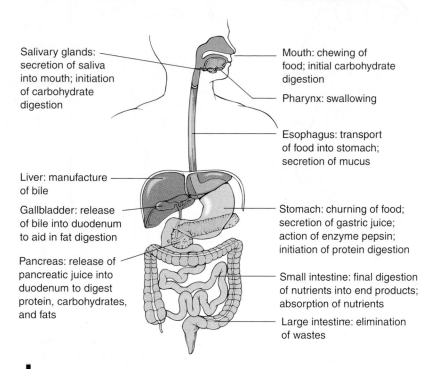

Salivary glands: secretion of saliva into mouth; initiation of carbohydrate digestion

Mouth: chewing of food; initial carbohydrate digestion

Pharynx: swallowing

Esophagus: transport of food into stomach; secretion of mucus

Liver: manufacture of bile

Gallbladder: release of bile into duodenum to aid in fat digestion

Pancreas: release of pancreatic juice into duodenum to digest protein, carbohydrates, and fats

Stomach: churning of food; secretion of gastric juice; action of enzyme pepsin; initiation of protein digestion

Small intestine: final digestion of nutrients into end products; absorption of nutrients

Large intestine: elimination of wastes

Figure 8–1

Main and accessory organs of the normal digestive system. (Redrawn from Miller M: Pathophysiology: Principles of Disease. Philadelphia: WB Saunders, 1983. Used with permission.)

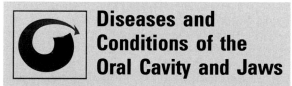

Diseases and Conditions of the Oral Cavity and Jaws

The function of the teeth is mastication (chewing) to break down food into pieces that can be swallowed and digested easily (Fig. 8-2 *A* and *B*). Hindrance of the chewing function by decay, infection of the teeth or gums, **malocclusion,** or missing teeth can interfere with this phase of the digestive process.

Most disorders affecting the mouth or the tongue are not serious, and treatment is simple and effective. Because malignant tumors are possible, any lump or change in the mouth or on the tongue that persists for longer than 10 days should be seen by a dentist or a physician.

MISSING TEETH

SYMPTOMS AND SIGNS

Missing permanent teeth, after the loss of primary teeth, can cause serious dental problems later in life (Fig. 8–3). Missing teeth can alter the bite, that is, how the teeth come together (occlusion). Malocclusion eventually leads to jaw pain, called temporomandibular joint disease (see Temporomandibular Joint Syndrome), if not corrected.

ETIOLOGY

There are three reasons for missing permanent teeth. The most common is loss from decay or accident. Teeth may be congenitally missing, or they may be impacted and prevented from erupting by the root of an adjacent tooth.

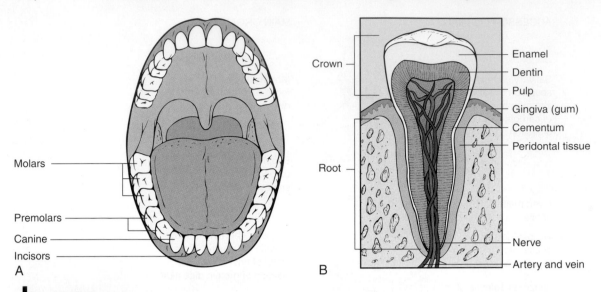

Figure 8–2

A, Thirty-two permanent teeth. *B,* Structure of a tooth.

DIAGNOSIS

The diagnosis of missing teeth may be as simple as performing an oral examination and obtaining radiographic films to determine whether the tooth is absent or impacted.

TREATMENT

Treatment is aimed at restoring the occlusion. This is accomplished by placement of a permanent or removable prosthesis (false tooth), by **orthodontics** or by use of a surgical implant.

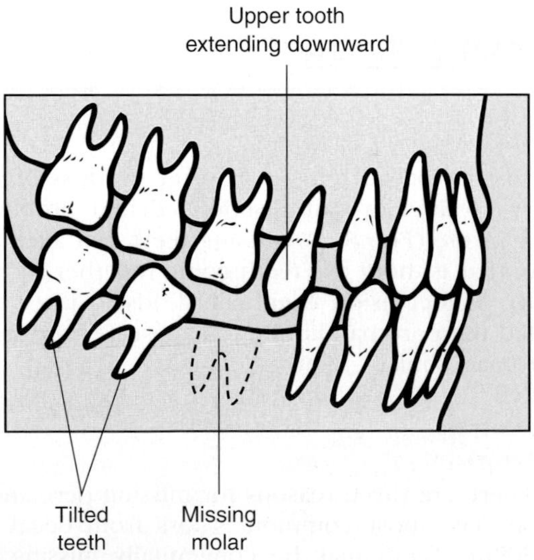

IMPACTED THIRD MOLARS

SYMPTOMS AND SIGNS

Third molars, also known as wisdom teeth, are the last teeth in the back of the mouth. They begin developing between the ages of 8 and 10 years and erupt between the ages of 17 and 21 years. In some people, one or more of these teeth never erupt. There are usually no symptoms until these teeth begin to emerge. Even when wisdom teeth develop in a normal manner, they are difficult to clean because of their position at the back of the mouth. Because of this, they decay much more often than other teeth, and pain results.

ETIOLOGY

Impaction occurs when these molars do not have enough room to erupt because of bone structure or when eruption is blocked by adjacent teeth (Fig. 8-4). Sometimes they erupt at an angle, creating a space in which food can become trapped. This can lead to **pericoronitis** around the tooth, which in turn causes pain when biting and a foul taste in the mouth. The gum around the tooth becomes red and swollen.

Figure 8–3

Missing molar.

Site of impaction

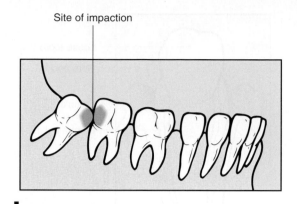

Figure 8–4

Impacted wisdom tooth.

DIAGNOSIS

Radiographic studies are needed to determine the position of the tooth if it is not completely erupted. An examination for the presence of infection also is performed.

TREATMENT

The dentist likely prescribes an antibiotic to clear up any infection that is present and an analgesic to relieve pain temporarily. After the infection clears up and pain has lessened, extraction of the impacted tooth is necessary to prevent recurrence.

DENTAL CARIES

SYMPTOMS AND SIGNS

The main symptom in the early stage of dental caries, also known as tooth decay, is a mild toothache, with hypersensitivity to sweets and temperature extremes in food or beverages. If caries is left untreated, an unpleasant taste in the mouth results from the accumulation of food and bacteria in the cavity. Eventually, the pulp becomes inflamed, and the pain may become persistent or feel like stabbing pains in the jaw. As the tooth continues to die, an **abscess** may form (see Tooth Abscesses).

ETIOLOGY

Dental caries occurs when bacteria in **plaque** break down the sugar found in food. This process forms acid, and this acid erodes the calcium in the tooth's enamel, causing the formation of a cavity (Fig. 8–5).

DIAGNOSIS

The dentist examines the teeth for signs of cavity formation and may obtain radiographic films to determine the extent of the decay.

TREATMENT

Early treatment consists of removing the diseased portion of the tooth enamel and pulp and filling the cavity to prevent more decay. If the decay has advanced into the pulp, the dentist may do a root canal procedure. This involves removing the infected pulp tissue and then filling and sealing the canals in the roots of the tooth. Tooth extraction may be necessary if root canal therapy fails or if the tooth is beyond saving.

Prevention of caries with good oral hygiene and regular cleaning of the teeth is recommended.

DISCOLORED TEETH

SYMPTOMS AND SIGNS

Symptoms of discolored teeth are obvious, and colors may range from a slight yellow to brown and gray. Some teeth may have brown spots, patches, and dark lines in or on them.

Dental caries (tooth decay)

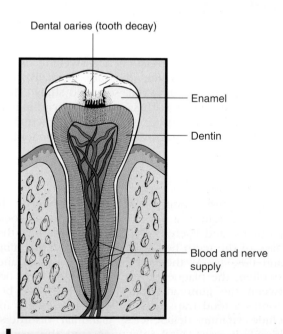

Enamel

Dentin

Blood and nerve supply

Figure 8–5

Dental caries (tooth decay).

ETIOLOGY

There are many causes of discolored teeth. Age alone causes a slight yellowing of the teeth. Smoking turns teeth surfaces brown, and a dead tooth often turns gray. Certain drugs (e.g., tetracyclines) taken in large quantities during childhood can cause the formation of defective, discolored enamel. Severe attacks of pertussis (whooping cough) and measles in children can cause discolored patches to form on the teeth. Naturally occurring fluoride can, in excessive amounts, produce white or brown spots in the teeth.

DIAGNOSIS

The dentist performs an oral examination. Pertinent history would include recent illness, medications, and trauma to the teeth. Hereditary factors also are considered.

TREATMENT

The extent of treatment varies and depends on whether the discoloration is superficial or deep within the enamel. Superficial discoloration can be removed or diminished by polishing with a rotary polisher. Deeper discolorations can be treated by capping or crowning and by bonding a synthetic veneer to the tooth.

GINGIVITIS

SYMPTOMS AND SIGNS

Gingivitis is inflammation and swelling of the gums (Fig. 8-6). Gums that are normally pale pink and firm become red, soft, and shiny. They bleed easily, even with gentle toothbrushing. If gingivitis is not treated, it leads to destruction of the gums and bone disease, called periodontitis (see Periodontitis).

ETIOLOGY

The most common cause of gingivitis is plaque. Plaque is a sticky deposit of mucus, food particles, and bacteria that builds up around the base of the teeth because of inadequate brushing and flossing. As the gums become inflamed and swollen, the plaque causes a pocket to form between the gum and the teeth; that space becomes a food trap. Other causes of gingivitis include vitamin deficiencies, glandular disorders, blood diseases, viral infections, and the use of certain medications. Pregnant women and diabetics are particularly susceptible to gingivitis.

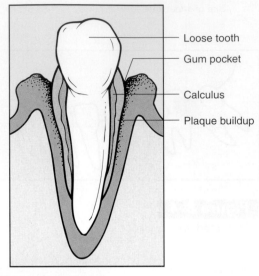

Loose tooth
Gum pocket
Calculus
Plaque buildup

Figure 8–6

Gingivitis.

DIAGNOSIS

If symptoms develop, a dentist should be seen as soon as possible to receive confirmation of gingivitis and to begin treatment to prevent complications.

TREATMENT

Treatment entails removal of the plaque and **calculus** by professional cleaning and then education by the dentist or dental hygienist as to the proper care of the teeth. In advanced cases of gingivitis, the dentist may prescribe an antibacterial mouthwash to help to clear up the infection.

PERIODONTITIS

SYMPTOMS AND SIGNS

Periodontitis, also called periodontal disease, is destructive gum and bone disease around one or more of the teeth. It is the end result of gingivitis (see Gingivitis) that was treated too late or not at all. The pockets that form between the teeth and gums in gingivitis gradually deepen, exposing the root. The plaque that develops there causes unpleasant tastes in the mouth and offensive breath odor (halitosis). As more and more root is exposed, the tooth or teeth become extremely sensitive to temperature extremes in food and painful during chewing. Abscesses can form (see Tooth Abscesses), and eventually a tooth or several teeth become loose and possibly fall out.

ETIOLOGY

The cause of periodontitis is unchecked gingivitis. Over a period of years, the bacteria in plaque destroy the bone surrounding and supporting the teeth.

DIAGNOSIS

To determine how advanced the periodontal disease is, the dentist measures the depth of the pockets and obtains radiographic films. Radiographic films reveal the condition of the underlying bone, and this knowledge aids the dentist in deciding how to treat the disease.

TREATMENT

Periodontal surgery may be required if the pockets have become deep. The procedure, called a gingivectomy, requires the dentist to trim the gums to reduce the depth of the pockets and to remove any damaged bone as well.

ORAL TUMORS

SYMPTOMS AND SIGNS

Tumors can develop anywhere in or on the surface of the mouth, gums, cheeks, or palate, but not on the teeth. They begin as single, small, pale lumps, in or on the mouth, that bleed easily. There are two types of tumors: benign, or noncancerous, and malignant, or cancerous. Benign tumors grow slowly over several years, do not **metastasize,** and are not life threatening. Malignant tumors are generally not painful until they reach advanced stages. They develop rapidly and metastasize within a few months; this is typical for tumors of the tongue. The malignant tumor develops into an **ulcer** that has a hard, raised rim and a fragile center. It erodes into the surrounding areas of the mouth. Carcinoma of the lip, generally affecting the lower lip, is a common malignant tumor. It occurs more often in men and rarely before the age of 40 years.

ETIOLOGY

The cause of benign and malignant oral tumors is unknown, although certain factors, such as tobacco use, seem to affect a tumor's development into a malignancy. Carcinoma of the lip may first appear as a chronic lesion, such as a sore or a crack that does not heal. Malignant tumors of the tongue may result from chronic irritation from a rough tooth or a poorly fitting denture.

DIAGNOSIS

An oral surgeon or a physician should be consulted if there is a lump, an ulcer, or a color change in or on the surface of the mouth that does not clear up within 10 days. If a tumor is discovered, a **biopsy** is necessary to confirm whether it is benign or malignant.

TREATMENT

If the tumor has been determined to be benign, it should be observed periodically to ensure that it has not become malignant. Benign tumors need to be excised if they interfere with the fit of a denture. The treatment of malignant tumors, and its success, depends on the stage of the disease. Tumors diagnosed at an early stage, before they metastasize, usually are cured by surgical excision. If the tumor has metastasized, the treatment is more aggressive, with surgical removal or radiation therapy, or both.

MALOCCLUSION

SYMPTOMS AND SIGNS

The relationship of the upper and lower teeth when the mouth is closed is called occlusion, or bite; a faulty bite is called malocclusion (Fig. 8–7). Signs of malocclusion include either a protrusion or a recession of the jaw, and teeth may be turned or twisted out of position because of crowding.

DIAGNOSIS

A visual examination and radiographic studies clearly identify the malocclusion.

ETIOLOGY

The cause of malocclusion stems from the characteristics inherited from each parent. Few people have perfectly aligned teeth. Heredity is not the only determining factor in malocclusion; crowding can be the result of early loss of primary teeth. This loss of teeth causes the loss of a space for the permanent tooth to erupt because other teeth shift position.

TREATMENT

Several treatments are used to correct this problem. They include the application of braces for a minor problem, extraction of one or more teeth, and surgical removal of portions of the jaw. The last approach is used for problems of

221

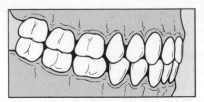

NORMAL TEETH

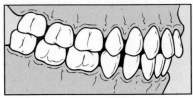

PROTRUDING UPPER TEETH

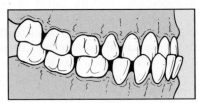

RECEDING UPPER TEETH

Figure 8–7
Malocclusion.

protrusion and recession of the jaw. Another possible treatment is combining crowns or bridges to replace the missing teeth.

TEMPOROMANDIBULAR JOINT (TMJ) SYNDROME

SYMPTOMS AND SIGNS

The **synovial** joints between the condyles of the mandible and the temporal bones of the skull are known as the temporomandibular joints. When these joints are inflamed or diseased, there is marked limitation of jaw movement. The patient reports hearing clicking sounds during chewing or experiencing severe pain or aching that is made worse by chewing. This pain and limitation of movement is usually unilateral. **Tinnitus** and even deafness may be present. A reduced ability to open the jaw not only interferes with chewing but also prevents adequate cleaning of the teeth and restoration of cavities. It also may prevent the making of dentures because of the inability to take impressions of the teeth.

ETIOLOGY

Temporomandibular disorders can be caused by a number of conditions, including malocclusion; poorly fitting dentures; rheumatoid, degenerative, or traumatic arthritis; and **neoplastic** diseases. Emotional stress, with accompanying clenching and grinding of the teeth, is also a contributing factor.

DIAGNOSIS

The diagnosis of temporomandibular joint syndrome is made by oral examination, the patient history, and radiographic studies. In the case of a neoplasm, a biopsy may be necessary to rule out a malignancy.

TREATMENT

Treatment is aimed at the cause of the condition or disease. Symptoms of rheumatoid or traumatic arthritis often subside after 3 to 5 days of immobilization of the mandible. Some patients wear special appliances to prevent them from grinding their teeth. Intra-articular injections of hydrocortisone may be necessary in more severe cases of rheumatoid or degenerative arthritis. When premature contacts exist between the teeth, the dentist adjusts the occlusion by grinding the surfaces of the teeth.

TOOTH ABSCESSES

SYMPTOMS AND SIGNS

A tooth abscess is a pus-filled sac that develops in the tissue surrounding the base of the root. An abscessed tooth aches or throbs persistently and can be extremely painful when biting and chewing food. Glands in the neck and face on the affected side may become swollen and tender. Fever also can develop, along with a feeling of general **malaise.**

ETIOLOGY

An abscess forms when a tooth is decayed or dying or if the gums have severely receded, exposing the root. The dead pulp, along with invading bacteria, can infect the surrounding tissues, even after a root canal procedure, and cause the formation of an abscess.

DIAGNOSIS

If any of the symptoms or signs are present, the dentist should be seen as soon as possible. Swelling in the neck or face must be dealt with immediately to prevent the infection from spreading further.

TREATMENT

Antibiotic therapy is prescribed, and if this does not correct the problem, an apicectomy may be necessary. In this procedure, the dentist or oral surgeon makes an incision into the gum and removes the bone that covers the tip of the root, and the infected tissue as well. If this fails to clear up the infection, the tooth needs to be extracted.

MOUTH ULCERS

SYMPTOMS AND SIGNS

An ulcer in the mouth is a lesion on the mucous membrane; it exposes the underlying sensitive tissue. Mouth ulcers are common and look alike but vary considerably in their cause and seriousness. The two most common types of ulcers are **aphthous ulcers,** which occur during stress or illness, and traumatic ulcers, which result from injury and are caused by a hot food burn, a rough denture, or even a toothbrush. Ulcers appear as pale yellow spots with red borders. Aphthous ulcers usually occur in clusters and last for 3 or 4 days. Traumatic ulcers are usually single and larger and last for a week or longer.

ETIOLOGY

A viral cause has not been established for aphthous ulcers. Acute ulcerations are usually the result of mechanical trauma, viral and bacterial infections, stress, or illness. In rare instances, an ulcer may be the first sign of a tumor in the mouth, anemia, or leukemia.

DIAGNOSIS

If an ulcer does not heal within 10 days, or keeps returning, a dentist or physician should be consulted. Blood tests and possibly a biopsy of the ulcer are necessary to determine whether there is some underlying condition or disease causing the ulcer. When the ulcer results from trauma, it does not heal until the cause is found and corrected.

TREATMENT

Self-help for treatment of ulcers includes using antiseptic mouthwashes, rinsing with warm salt water, and avoiding spicy or acidic foods and hot food or drinks. The dentist or physician may prescribe a steroid mouthwash or topical cream to speed the healing process.

HERPES SIMPLEX (COLD SORES)

SYMPTOMS AND SIGNS

Herpes simplex (cold sore) blisters can develop on the lips and inside the mouth, producing painful ulcers that last a few hours or days. These ulcers also can form on the gums, causing them to become red and swollen. Tingling and numbness around the mouth may precede or follow their appearance.

ETIOLOGY

Cold sores are caused by the herpes simplex virus type 1 (HSV-1) and are common. They tend to recur because of the ability of the virus to lie dormant. Exposure to sunshine or wind or the presence of another infection, such as a common cold, can reactivate the virus.

DIAGNOSIS

An oral examination is usually sufficient for the diagnosis. Isolation of the HSV-1 from local lesions can confirm the cause of the infection. A similar lesion in the oral cavity can be caused by the herpes simplex virus type 2 (HSV-2).

TREATMENT

Generally, cold sores clear up uneventfully. If the infection is mild, no treatment is necessary, although severe cases necessitate medical attention. Generally, a herpes simplex infection does not cause serious risks to health, but rubbing the eyes after touching the ulcer could cause the formation of a herpetic corneal ulcer; the infection can produce severe illness in an **immuno-compromised** patient. The dentist or physician may advise resting, taking aspirin, and using an **anesthetic** mouthwash and a topical cream to relieve the pain and to heal the sores.

THRUSH

SYMPTOMS AND SIGNS

Thrush is a fungal infection of relatively short duration that produces sore, slightly raised, pale yellow patches in the mouth and sometimes the throat. These lesions become painful when rubbed by dentures, toothbrushes, or food when eating. Thrush most frequently develops in young children and the elderly but can occur at any age.

ETIOLOGY

The fungus *Candida albicans* causes thrush. Normally present in the mouth in small numbers, the fungus can multiply out of control. This may occur with lowered resistance or as a result of prolonged treatment with antibiotics, which upsets the normal number of protective microbes. This same fungus can cause vaginitis.

DIAGNOSIS

Diagnosis is made by the dentist or physician with an oral examination and laboratory analysis of a sample taken from a lesion. Blood tests also may be needed to rule out a serious underlying disease, such as iron deficiency anemia.

TREATMENT

Thrush is treated successfully with an antifungal medication for 14 days, but the infection tends to recur.

ACUTE NECROTIZING ULCERATIVE GINGIVITIS (TRENCH MOUTH)

SYMPTOMS AND SIGNS

Trench mouth is a rare, painful ulceration and disease of the gums, particularly between the teeth; it sometimes is called Vincent's angina. The major symptom is painful, red, swollen gums with ulcers that bleed. The patient also may report a metallic taste in the mouth and bad breath.

ETIOLOGY

Trench mouth results from poor oral hygiene and bacterial infection secondary to gingivitis (see Gingivitis). Stress, poor nutrition, throat infections, smoking, and serious illness, such as leukemia, are also contributing factors.

DIAGNOSIS

An oral examination by a dentist or physician is needed as soon as possible. Throat cultures and blood work may be necessary to rule out any serious illness.

TREATMENT

The patient is given antibiotics, along with a hydrogen peroxide mouthwash, to relieve pain and inflammation. After the disease has been halted, a professional cleaning of the teeth and gums is necessary. A minor surgery on the gums, called a gingivectomy, also may be advised.

ORAL LEUKOPLAKIA

SYMPTOMS AND SIGNS

Leukoplakia or white plaque, is a thickening and hardening of a part of the mucous membrane in the mouth. It develops over several weeks and can vary in size. At first, there are no symptoms, but as it progresses, the mucous membrane becomes rough, hard, and whitish gray and is sensitive to hot or highly seasoned foods.

ETIOLOGY

Leukoplakia may develop at any age, but it is more common in the elderly. It usually results from friction caused by a denture or a rough tooth that rubs an area raw. Leukoplakia also may be a reaction to the heat from tobacco smoke.

DIAGNOSIS

An oral examination is necessary. If the condition has not cleared up in 2 or 3 weeks, a biopsy is advised because approximately 3% of oral leukoplakias develop into oral cancers.

TREATMENT

The treatment of leukoplakia consists of finding the source of the irritation. A rough tooth or denture may be smoothed, and giving up smoking may be advised. These measures are usually all that is needed to correct the condition.

Diseases of the Gastrointestinal Tract

The alimentary canal, or GI tract, is a hollow continuous tube that extends from the mouth to the anus. It propels the products of digestion by peristalsis. It is also the site of the processes of mechanical and chemical breakdown of food. As the food passes through the tract, it is broken down into molecules that can be absorbed through the intestinal wall for distribution to body cells for metabolism.

Absorption of water and electrolytes takes place in the proximal colon; storage of waste material occurs in the rectum, followed by voluntary evacuation of nondigestible wastes through the anus.

Enrichment

DIGESTIVE DISTRESS SIGNALS

- ⊃ Hiccup is an involuntary spasmodic contraction of the diaphragm causing a beginning inspiration that is suddenly checked by closure of the glottis, resulting in the characteristic sound. It is usually transient.
- ⊃ Indigestion is failure of digestion. The term frequently is used to denote vague abdominal discomfort after meals. Indigestion is a common symptom of upper GI tract disease.
- ⊃ Heartburn is a sensation of retrosternal warmth or burning occurring in waves and tending to rise upward toward the neck; it may be accompanied by a reflux of fluid into the mouth (regurgitation).
- ⊃ Nausea is an unpleasant sensation in the epigastrium. It often culminates in vomiting.
- ⊃ Vomiting is the forcible expulsion of the contents of the stomach through the mouth.
- ⊃ Colic is acute abdominal pain caused by spasms of the colon.
- ⊃ Flatulence is the presence of extensive amounts of air or gases in the stomach or intestines, leading to distention of the organs.
- ⊃ Diarrhea is abnormally frequent passage of loose stool.
- ⊃ Constipation refers to infrequency of bowel evacuation. It may be functional or organic.
- ⊃ Fecal incontinence is an inability to control defecation.

GASTROESOPHAGEAL REFLUX DISEASE

SYMPTOMS AND SIGNS

Gastroesophageal reflux disease (GERD), refers to clinical manifestations of regurgitation of stomach and duodenal contents into the esophagus, frequently occurring at night. Mild episodes may be described as heartburn by the patient. Typically, the patient experiences belching that expresses vomitus into the mouth, with a burning sensation in the chest and mouth. A coughing spell and wheezing from irritation to the oropharynx or respiratory tree may follow. Chronic and frequent GERD may lead to dysphagia and erosive esophagitis with bleeding. Erosion of tooth enamel leading to caries may develop. Other complications include esophageal stricture caused by scar tissue, ulceration of the mucosa, and pulmonary aspiration.

ETIOLOGY

Normal reflux can result from overeating, pregnancy, or weight gain. GERD that causes pathology frequently is associated with relaxation of the lower esophageal sphincter. Patients with hiatal hernia frequently experience GERD. Certain medications can contribute to GERD, including theophylline, calcium channel blockers, and meperidine. Some foods, coffee, and alcohol can irritate the condition.

DIAGNOSIS

The history and clinical evidence of GERD are most important in establishing a diagnosis. Barium swallow detects gross changes, erosion, or other abnormalities of the esophagus. If abnormal, endoscopy with esophageal biopsy is next. Esophageal pH monitoring, and scanning tests are other probative measures of diagnosis.

TREATMENT

When symptoms are mild and of short duration, simple measures to eliminate episodes of reflux are indicated. They include elevating the head of the bed about 6 inches, a light evening meal taken 4 hours before bedtime, and the use of antacids. Weight loss is indicated if the person is obese. Limiting or eliminating alcohol ingestion, and cessation of cigarette smoking is advised. When these measures fail, systemic medical management is initiated. The use of an **H$_2$-receptor antagonist** or a **proton pump inhibitor** inhibits acid secretion and allows for healing of the esophagus. Antireflux surgery is used conservatively. Symptomatic complications of chronic GERD are treated as required.

ESOPHAGEAL VARICES

SYMPTOMS AND SIGNS

Esophageal varices are varicose veins of the esophagus. The superficial veins lining the esophagus become swollen and twisted at the distal end of the esophagus and can rupture, causing hemorrhage. With rupture, the patient experiences **hematemesis** and abdominal pain, and signs of **hypovolemic shock** may develop.

ETIOLOGY

Varices result from pressure within the veins. This pressure develops when the venous return to the liver is obstructed. Esophageal varices are a frequent complication of cirrhosis of the liver because destruction of hepatic tissue interferes with emptying of the portal vein.

DIAGNOSIS

Diagnosis is made by the clinical picture and history of hepatic disease, specifically cirrhosis. Radiographic examination is indicated to study obstruction of blood flow that causes backpressure in the esophageal vessels. Esophageal varices can be noted during endoscopic examination.

TREATMENT

The treatment of a patient with bleeding esophageal varices is the same as that for any patient with gross GI bleeding. Attempts are made to control or stop the bleeding by ice water **lavage** or epigastric **tamponade** with an epigastric balloon. **Hemostasis** is restored by replacing the blood volume and maintaining the fluid and electrolyte balance.

ESOPHAGITIS

SYMPTOMS AND SIGNS

Esophagitis is inflammation of the esophagus. The main symptom that the patient experiences is burning chest pain (heartburn), which can make the patient believe that he or she is having a heart attack. Typically, the onset of pain follows eating or drinking. The patient even may have some vomiting of blood (hematemesis).

ETIOLOGY

The cause of esophagitis is **reflux** of the acid contents of the stomach resulting from a defect of the **cardiac sphincter.** High acidity in the stomach is irritating to the esophageal lining, and this causes the inflammatory response. Erosive esophagitis can occur after taking antibiotics such as tetracycline without adequate amounts of water. Esophagitis can appear as a GI manifestation of human immunodeficiency virus (HIV) infection.

DIAGNOSIS

The patient history, an upper GI tract radiographic film to rule out an ulcer or hiatal hernia, and possibly an **esophagoscopy** help the physician to make the diagnosis.

TREATMENT

Treatment of esophagitis includes several weeks of a bland diet to calm the inflammation and the use of strong antacids. Underlying causes of reflux, such as hiatal hernia, are addressed in the treatment plan. Sucralfate (Carafate) suspension sometimes is prescribed to relieve discomfort and to promote healing. Meals should be small and frequent, and alcohol must be avoided. The prognosis for esophagitis is good if the treatment that the physician prescribes is followed. There is no known prevention for esophagitis; however, the avoidance of alcohol, spicy foods, and caffeine helps to relieve the symptoms.

GASTRIC AND DUODENAL PEPTIC ULCERS

SYMPTOMS AND SIGNS

When the protective mucous membrane of the stomach or upper intestinal tract breaks down, the lining is prone to ulceration. These internal surface sores, or lesions, can be acute or chronic, clustered or singular, and shallow or deep, involving the deep muscle layer of tissue (Fig. 8–8).

When the peptic ulcer occurs in the stomach (gastric ulcer), the patient reports heartburn, or indigestion, and **epigastric** pain. Some patients experience pain or a feeling of uncomfortable fullness after eating, which can cause them to avoid eating and lose weight.

The most common peptic ulcer is the duodenal ulcer (an ulcer of the first part of the small intestine), which causes symptoms that vary from subtle midepigastric pain and heartburn to intense pain in the upper abdomen with nausea and vomiting. The patient can be observed guarding the painful area by clutching the stomach, assuming a crouching position, or sitting with the knees drawn up to the chest. Some patients state that frequent eating helps to relieve discomfort; the attacks of most intense pain come about 2 hours after a meal.

If these ulcers bleed internally, occult or frank blood is found in the vomitus or stool. The situation is more serious if the lesion invades deeply and perforates, causing hemorrhage and leakage

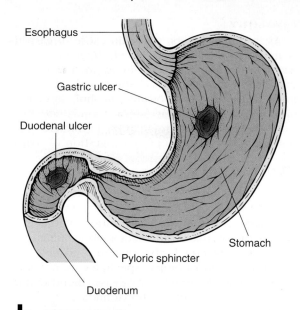

Figure 8–8

Peptic ulcer disease.

of the contents of the stomach or intestine into the abdominal cavity.

ETIOLOGY

Although the reason is not always clear, an area of breakdown of mucous membrane precipitates ulceration of the epithelial lining of the stomach or intestine. A crucial causal factor of peptic ulcers is *Helicobacter pylori* infection, thought to be the most common worldwide human bacterial infection. When present, it produces inflammation in the mucous membrane of the GI tract. The second most common form of ulcer is related to use of nonsteroidal antiinflammatory drugs (NSAIDs). Ulcers related to stress are the next most common form. The less common gastric ulcers follow chronic gastritis, with a change in the ability of the gastric mucosa to defend itself against erosion. Some of the known contributing catalysts are the ingestion of gastric irritants; the use of ulcerogenic drugs, such as alcohol, aspirin, and other antiinflammatory agents; psychogenic stress; smoking; and the presence of a bacterial infection. Gastric ulcers are most common in middle-aged men.

Duodenal ulcers, which usually occur from 45 to 70 years of age, are associated with an increase of acid and gastric juice (pepsin). Predisposing factors include the presence of sustained anxiety and emotional stress, coupled with certain genetic factors.

DIAGNOSIS

The way in which a patient describes her or his illness can help to distinguish between a gastric and a duodenal ulcer. The diagnosis of peptic ulcer can be suspected based on the patient's history and physical examination. To confirm the diagnosis, upper GI tract **barium** radiographic films are obtained to study the upper GI tract for abnormal appearance and function. The visualization of the ulcer is possible through upper GI tract **endoscopy** (Fig. 8–9). Diagnostic studies are available to determine *H. pylori*. Gastric contents are collected and analyzed for the level of acidity or the presence of blood in the secretions. The patient's stool also is checked for evidence of blood. When the ulcer is complicated by bleeding that causes anemia, blood tests show a reduced hemoglobin (Hb) concentration and decreased **hematocrit** (Hct). A biopsy, with microscopic study of the tissue, rules out or confirms the presence of cancer. Serum albumin and **transferrin** levels may be decreased if there is weight loss and malnutrition. Abdominal radiographic studies to investigate the possibility of perforation or other abdominal conditions are performed.

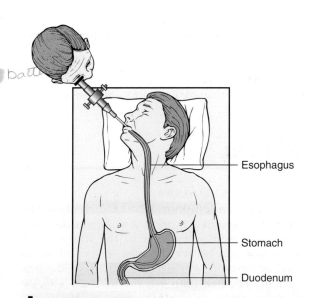

Figure 8–9

Upper gastrointestinal tract endoscopy. A flexible lighted fiberoptic tube (endoscope) is inserted through the mouth to allow the direct visualization of the upper gastrointestinal tract. When indicated, a biopsy may be taken during the procedure.

227

228

TREATMENT

The management of peptic ulcers necessitates rest, the administration of medication, changes in the diet, and adjustments in lifestyle. In severe cases, surgery may be indicated. If the cause is certain (e.g., the use of an ulcerogenic drug), it must be eliminated. Decreasing stress and physical activity promotes healing; if necessary, sedatives and tranquilizers are prescribed. Drug therapy includes one or more of the following: histamine$_2$ (H$_2$) receptor blocking agents to control gastric secretion (e.g., nizatidine [Axid], famotidine [Pepcid], cimetidine [Tagamet], and ranitidine [Zantac]), antacids (e.g., magnesium hydroxide–aluminum hydroxide [Maalox]) to reduce gastric acidity, and coating agents (e.g., sucralfate) to protect the mucosa, and proton pump inhibitors (e.g, omeprazole [Prilosec] and lansoprazole [Prevacid]) to suppress secretion of gastric acid. When *H. pylori* is a causative factor, antibiotic therapy with clarithromycin (Biaxin) or azithromycin (Zithromax), combined with a proton pump inhibitor, may be prescribed.

Small, frequent meals of soft, bland foods are better tolerated. All these measures attempt to relieve symptoms and to encourage the healing process. Significant bleeding or perforation of the ulcer calls for more aggressive measures, such as surgical intervention, the administration of intravenous fluids, and blood replacement.

Peptic ulcers can heal. Still, patients are instructed to observe ongoing preventive measures because peptic ulcer disease tends to recur. Any nonhealing ulcer, especially a gastric ulcer, should be evaluated by endoscopy to rule out cancer.

GASTRITIS

SYMPTOMS AND SIGNS

Gastritis is an inflammation of the lining of the stomach; the acute form is a common disorder. Normally, the mucous layer of the stomach creates a physical barrier to resist injury, inflammation, or erosion. When the stomach lining becomes inflamed, the patient experiences epigastric pain, indigestion, and the feeling of fullness after meals. Other discomforts, such as nausea, belching, and fatty food intolerance, cause the patient to lose the appetite. When the gastric mucosa is inflamed and swollen, it can bleed, and the blood can be seen and detected in the patient's vomitus and stool.

ETIOLOGY

As in peptic ulcers, the main cause of gastritis is inflammation associated with *H. pylori.* Many agents damage the gastric lining, including common medications such as aspirin and other anti-inflammatory drugs, poisons, alcohol, infectious diseases, stress, and mechanical injury resulting from swallowing a foreign object. Allergic reaction to foods or the repeated ingestion of irritating foods causes the gastric mucosa to be irritated. The cause is not always certain.

DIAGNOSIS

Gastroscopy allows visualization of the interior of the stomach, and radiographic films rule out other structural abnormalities. Samples of gastric juices and a biopsy specimen are obtained to determine the extent of disease. Blood counts and serum tests offer additional findings.

TREATMENT

Frequently, curing *H. pylori* infection with antibiotic therapy rapidly resolves superficial gastritis. If any other source of irritation is known, it is eliminated or controlled. Gastric discomfort is relieved with the use of antacids and medications, such as cimetidine and ranitidine hydrochloride to reduce the secretion of gastric acid. If there is bleeding, it is monitored and treated with medicine that constricts blood vessels. Antibiotics are given for infection; antiemetics help to control nausea and vomiting. The patient is given a bland diet as tolerated, with vitamin and mineral supplements as needed.

When a patient has been under extreme stress because of a serious illness or emotional tension, counseling is part of the treatment plan. Teaching the patient about the relationship between his or her gastritis and contributing lifestyle factors can promote healing and prevent recurrences.

GASTRIC CANCER

SYMPTOMS AND SIGNS

Most gastric neoplasms are malignant. The patient with early carcinoma of the stomach is frequently **asymptomatic;** there are no specific symptoms, and pain is absent. The first symptoms are vague indigestion, gastric discomfort, and occasional vomiting, combined with a loss of appetite **(anorexia).** Anorexia occurs far more often with gastric cancer than with ulcers. Symptoms that appear in the later stages of the disease include severe boring pain in the upper abdomen, weight loss, frequent vomiting, bloody bowel movements, bloody emesis, and anemia.

ETIOLOGY

Cancer of the stomach usually begins as an ulcer in the lining of the stomach (Fig. 8–10). However, not all ulcers become malignant. Why a small number of ulcers become cancerous is not understood. Worldwide epidemiology of gastric cancer seems to suggest that environment and diet are significant causative factors, although this remains unproven.

Gastric cancer can be manifested in various ways (see Fig. 8–10).

DIAGNOSIS

The physician should be contacted if indigestion or anorexia persists for longer than 3 days. He or she may order barium swallow studies and gastric endoscopy with biopsy and cytology of tissue sample. An analysis of the gastric secretions (gastric analysis) also may be done. Computed tomography (CT) or standard ultrasonography defines the extent of the tumor.

TREATMENT

A partial or total removal of the stomach (gastrectomy) may be necessary. To slow the development of the cancer, radiation therapy may be used. Chemotherapy may be advised when surgery is not feasible. The 5-year survival rate depends on whether there is adjacent lymph node involvement.

ACUTE APPENDICITIS

SYMPTOMS AND SIGNS

Appendicitis is inflammation of the appendix, a narrow pouch about 3½ inches long that extends from the first part of the large intestine (cecum) (Fig. 8–11). The appendix has no known function in humans, and its only importance seems to be, unfortunately, that it can become inflamed. Classic symptoms include abdominal pain that usually starts as vague discomfort around the navel and, within a few hours, localizes in the right lower quadrant. As the condition worsens, the patient becomes nauseated and may vomit, runs a fever, and has diarrhea or constipation.

ETIOLOGY

The reason the appendix becomes swollen, inflamed, and abscessed is not completely understood. It may be initiated by obstruction with fecal material, neoplasm, a foreign body, or worms. Whatever the cause, the pathophysiology of the disease is the same. As bacteria multiply, they invade the wall of the appendix, and eventually the circulation to the appendix is compro-

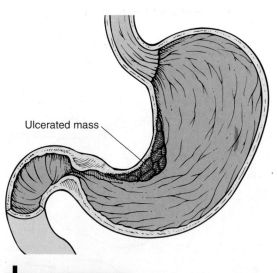
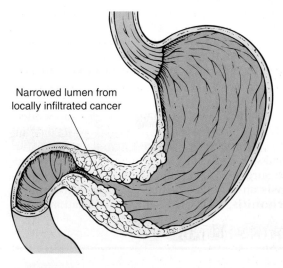

Ulcerated mass

Narrowed lumen from locally infiltrated cancer

Figure 8–10

Gastric cancer.

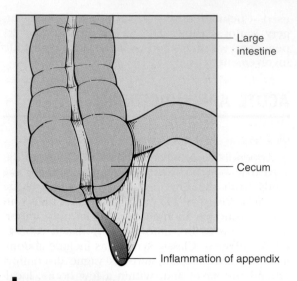

Figure 8–11

Acute appendicitis.

mised. The highest incidence of appendicitis occurs in the 20- to 40-year-old age bracket.

DIAGNOSIS

A differential diagnosis of appendicitis to rule out other causes of right lower abdominal pain and acute abdomen is undertaken. Diagnosis of appendicitis generally can be made from the physical examination and the symptoms described by the patient; one significant diagnostic indicator is maximal tenderness of the abdomen at **McBurney's point.** A complete blood count (CBC) and urinalysis are done and possibly repeated while hospital observation takes place. Laboratory findings indicate an elevation of the **white blood cell (WBC) count (leukocytosis).**

TREATMENT

Surgical removal of the appendix (appendectomy) is the best treatment and is performed as soon as confirmation of appendicitis is made. Broad-spectrum antibiotic therapy is initiated before surgery. If appendicitis is left untreated, **necrosis** and rupture of the appendix can result in **peritonitis,** a life-threatening complication.

HIATAL HERNIA

SYMPTOMS AND SIGNS

A hiatal hernia exists when the upper part of the stomach protrudes through the esophageal

opening of the diaphragm into the thoracic cavity (Fig. 8–12). The cardiac sphincter muscle at the top of the stomach malfunctions, allowing the contents of the stomach to regurgitate into the esophagus. This esophageal reflux (see Gastroesophageal Reflux Disease) can be irritating to the lining of the esophagus. The patient reports heartburn, which is usually worse when reclining. Symptoms of chest pain and difficulty in swallowing may suggest that a large portion of the stomach has slipped into the opening.

Some hiatal hernias are asymptomatic.

ETIOLOGY

Hiatal hernia, a common condition, can be caused by a congenital defect in the diaphragm or a weakness that develops in the diaphragm, allowing protrusion of part of the stomach into the thoracic cavity. The weakening of the muscle can result from obesity, old age, trauma, or intra-abdominal pressure; sometimes the exact cause is uncertain.

DIAGNOSIS

Large hiatal hernias may show on a radiographic chest film. A diagnosis is made by barium radiographic studies of the esophagus and stomach. Endoscopy confirms the diagnosis and differentiates the condition from other diseases, such as peptic ulcer and malignant tumor. Additional diagnostic studies include measurement of reflux pH and examination of the reflux contents for the presence of blood.

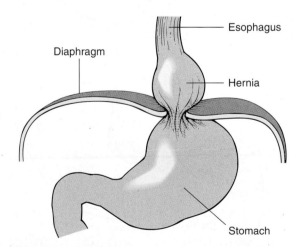

Figure 8–12

Hiatal hernia.

TREATMENT

Conservative treatment that relieves the symptoms and prevents complications is the first course. This includes dietary modification (smaller, more frequent meals of bland food). The person is advised to minimize activities that increase intra-abdominal pressure, such as straining and coughing. The obese patient is advised to lose weight.

Antacids and medications that control the acid secretions in the stomach are given. Drug therapy may include a **cholinergic** agent, which helps to control the episodes of reflux by strengthening the lower esophageal sphincter. Smoking is discouraged because it aggravates the heartburn. Because gravity plays a role in hiatal hernia, the patient is advised to avoid lying down for 2 hours after a meal; elevating the head of the bed on blocks also helps.

If these measures do not work or if the hernia becomes strangulated, surgical repair of the hiatus is the treatment of choice.

ABDOMINAL HERNIA

SYMPTOMS AND SIGNS

An abdominal hernia can occur when there is a weak spot in the muscles and membranes of the abdominal wall that allows an organ or part of an organ to break through (herniate) or protrude.

The inguinal canal is a common site for hernias; a loop of bowel protrudes into the inguinal canal and, in a male, fills the scrotal sac (Fig. 8–13 A). The patient notices a lump or bulge in the inguinal area and may discover that it can be reduced by pressing on the hernia to push it back into the abdomen. A sharp pain in the groin is continuous or made worse when standing or straining.

If there is severe pain, the hernia may be trapped or strangulated (Fig. 8–13 B). This means that the blood flow to the herniated organ or bowel has been stopped, and **gangrene,** a serious situation, can set in.

The signs and symptoms of abdominal hernias vary with the site and the size of the hernia.

ETIOLOGY

An abdominal hernia begins when an abnormal opening develops in a weak area or when a congenital malformation exists in the containing structures of the abdominal cavity. Trauma or increased intra-abdominal pressure due to heavy lifting or pregnancy also can cause a hernia.

The site of the hernia and the various organs that might protrude into the sac-like bulge can vary. The umbilicus is another common site of herniation (Fig. 8–13 C). Occasionally, a hernia develops near the weakened site of a previous surgical scar.

DIAGNOSIS

A visible hernia can be palpated for size and inspected with the patient standing and then lying down. The physician listens for bowel sounds. An inguinal hernia can be detected in the male by asking him to perform **Valsalva's maneuver.** The medical assessment also might include radiographic studies of the abdomen and a white blood cell count.

TREATMENT

Therapeutic measures vary with the type of hernia as well as with the age and physical condition of the patient. If the hernia is uncomplicated and the hernial sac can be pushed back into the abdominal cavity, the patient can wear a device called a **truss.** If this measure keeps the patient comfortable and there are no signs of strangulation, surgical intervention may not be required. Most often, surgical repair of the hernia (herniorrhaphy) is the treatment of choice in children and healthy adults.

CROHN'S DISEASE (REGIONAL ENTERITIS)

SYMPTOMS AND SIGNS

Crohn's disease is a fairly common chronic inflammatory disease of the alimentary canal in which all layers of the bowel wall are edematous and inflamed. Any portion of the GI tract from mouth to anus can be affected. Patients with Crohn's disease have chronic diarrhea along with cramping abdominal pain, frequently in the right lower quadrant of the abdomen. They also may experience weight loss, anorexia, fever, and abdominal fullness. If obstruction develops, patients have symptoms of an **acute abdomen.** The abdomen is tender and distended, and patients may experience vomiting and blood in the stools. If the condition is chronic, signs and symptoms of malnutrition begin to materialize; perianal **fissures** and **fistulas** commonly develop. Complications associated with the chronic inflammation include symptoms of bowel obstruction.

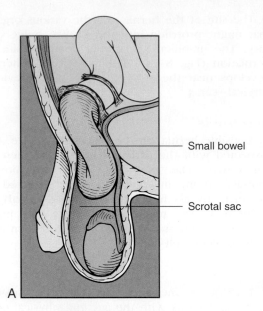

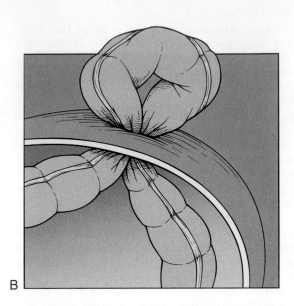

Small bowel

Scrotal sac

A

B

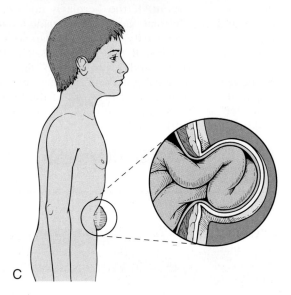

C

Figure 8–13

Abdominal hernia. *A,* Inguinal hernia. *B,* Strangulated hernia. *C,* Umbilical hernia.

ETIOLOGY

There has been much research into the etiology of Crohn's disease, yet the cause is not known. Immunologic factors, infectious agents, psychosomatic illness, and dietary factors play a role; autoimmune factors, allergies, and genetic causes also have been investigated.

DIAGNOSIS

Diagnosis is made from symptoms, air-contrast barium enema radiographic studies, and flat plate studies of the abdomen. The radiographic films reveal the diseased segments (strictures) sepa-

rated by normal bowel. Anemia, leukocytosis, and **hypoalbuminemia** may be detected in blood tests. Electrolyte abnormalities reflect the severity of diarrhea. **Colonoscopy** (Fig. 8–14) and biopsy confirm the diagnosis.

TREATMENT

Crohn's disease is considered a medically incurable condition. The general medical management includes nutritional support and control of symptoms. The patient may require dietary supplements of vitamins, minerals, protein, and calories. Drug therapy with anticholinergics and nar-

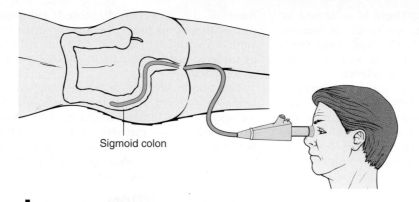

Figure 8–14

Colonoscopy. A lighted fiberoptic endoscope is inserted through the anus to allow direct examination of the colon. This method is useful in differential diagnosis of bowel disease, to obtain biopsy, and in minor surgery such as polypectomy.

Sigmoid colon

cotic agents relieves the cramping and diarrhea. If there is bacterial involvement, antibacterial agents, such as sulfasalazine, are prescribed. Corticosteroid therapy and **immunosuppressive** drugs also are used. If bowel obstruction, an abscess, or perforation develops, surgery to remove the affected portion of the intestine is indicated. Because of the chronic nature of this disease, patients may benefit from counseling, participation in a support group, and physical rest.

ULCERATIVE COLITIS

SYMPTOMS AND SIGNS

Ulcerative colitis, a common cause of serious bowel disease, can affect any age group. The symptoms result from a chronic, diffuse, continuous inflammation of the mucosa of the rectum and colon. The patient reports intermittent episodes of bloody diarrhea, abdominal cramping, urgency to defecate, and mucoid stools. As the disease progresses, the stools become looser and more frequent (10-20 per day), with cramping and rectal pressure; weight loss, fever, and malaise are also present. Some patients report diarrhea alternating with constipation. The watery stools contain blood, mucus, and pus because of mucosal ulceration of the bowel. If the disease is **fulminant,** major complications develop from severe diarrhea, massive bleeding, and perforation.

ETIOLOGY

There is some familial tendency, but the cause is unknown.

DIAGNOSIS

The diagnosis is made from the clinical picture, examination of the stool for blood, and laboratory values. The findings could include decreased hemoglobin level and leukocytosis. Electrolyte abnormalities may be noted when diarrhea is severe. Plain films of the abdomen also are taken. Barium enema studies and colonoscopy are done at the physician's discretion. Stool cultures are necessary to rule out bacterial causes. Biopsy shows typical inflammatory changes in the mucosa.

TREATMENT

A well-balanced diet devoid of foods that the patient finds irritating is encouraged. Anticholinergic drugs and occasionally antidiarrheal agents are prescribed. Corticosteroid therapy is used in more severe cases. Surgical removal of the diseased colon is indicated for severe hemorrhage or perforation. The patient is examined annually because chronic ulcerative colitis is associated with an increased risk of colon cancer.

GASTROENTERITIS

SYMPTONS AND SIGNS

The stomach and intestines usually protect themselves from infections and irritations by the presence of normal bacterial flora and acid secretions and the healthy motility of the GI tract. When these mechanisms fail to rid the body of **toxins** or large numbers of disease-causing bacteria and viruses, the stomach and intestines become filled with the products of inflammation, and gastroenteritis results. There is increased intestinal motility, with the presence of mucus, pus, and blood in the stool. The body loses fluids too rapidly, causing dehydration with a disturbance in the body's electrolyte balance.

The common syndrome of gastroenteritis called traveler's diarrhea is characterized by varying degrees of anorexia, abdominal cramping, frequent loose stools, and nausea and profuse vomiting. If the infection is severe enough, fever and weakness follow. The same symptoms are present in intestinal influenza, food or chemical poisoning, allergic reactions to food, and some drug reactions.

ETIOLOGY

Transmission of disease-causing bacteria or parasites from contaminated food or water is the major cause of traveler's diarrhea, whereas intestinal influenza is usually the result of a virus. Some bacteria produce toxins in food that result in food poisoning when ingested (see Food Poisoning). Ingestion of poison in certain foods (e.g., poisonous mushrooms) or chemicals (e.g., arsenic) causes gastroenteritis. In some people, gastroenteritis is stress induced.

DIAGNOSIS

Consideration of the medical history is the first important step in identifying the cause. Laboratory analysis and culture of the stool reveal the signs as well as the actual causes of infection or poisoning. The stool is inspected for leukocytes, erythrocytes, pus, abnormal bacteria, and viruses by electron microscopy. The clinical evaluation includes blood studies for causative organisms, the presence of antibodies, abnormal blood cell counts, and serum electrolyte values. Endoscopy also may be performed.

TREATMENT

The treatment varies with the cause, the severity of the disease, and the age and general health of the patient. Often, gastroenteritis is self-limiting, although it can become severe and life threatening, with complications such as ulceration of the stomach or intestine. There is danger of perforation and hemorrhage of these lesions. The very young, the elderly, and the chronically ill are most vulnerable to electrolyte imbalance from dehydration, which can lead to death in a short time.

The goal of treatment is to control symptoms and to maintain a normal fluid and electrolyte balance. This is accomplished by direct management of the cause as diagnosed; subsequently, the treatment includes the use of **antiemetics,** antibiotics, and rehydration solutions either orally or intravenously. The patient should rest and eat as tolerated.

Education directed at eliminating the cause helps to prevent recurrences. Infection control techniques, including frequent and thorough hand washing and the avoidance of food that has not been well refrigerated and well cooked, are excellent preventive measures for the most common causes of gastroenteritis.

INTUSSUSCEPTION

SYMPTOMS AND SIGNS

Intussusception, a telescoping of one portion of the bowel into an adjacent part, occurs mainly in infants and children. The child usually cries and draws up her or his legs, which is indicative of severe abdominal pain. A fever may develop, and the child experiences vomiting and initially loose bloody stools (sometimes described as currant jelly stools) followed by constipation.

ETIOLOGY

The prolapse of one portion of the bowel into another is most likely to occur in the area of the ileocecal valve (Fig. 8–15). This results in an obstruction of the bowel with interruption of the

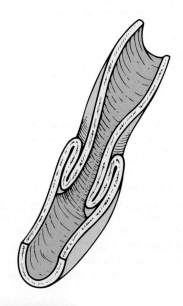

Figure 8–15

Intussusception.

blood flow to the affected portions. Prompt treatment of **infarction** of the affected bowel is indicated to prevent gangrene, perforation, and peritonitis.

In adults, intussusception is linked to tumors, polyps, and other intestinal alterations. In infants, the cause may be unknown.

DIAGNOSIS

Diagnosis is made from the clinical picture, the medical history, and radiographic studies of the abdomen. In the laboratory, occult blood usually is detected in the stool. Often, the diagnostic technique used for barium enema studies reduces the intussusception.

TREATMENT

Treatment usually necessitates surgical intervention to relieve the obstruction and to prevent complications such as strangulation and peritonitis. Fluid and electrolyte levels and **hemodynamic** balance need to be monitored and restored.

VOLVULUS

SYMPTOMS AND SIGNS

Volvulus is a twisting of the bowel on itself, causing intestinal blockage (Fig. 8–16). The patient, commonly a neonate, experiences abdominal pain, nausea, and vomiting. The infant fails to

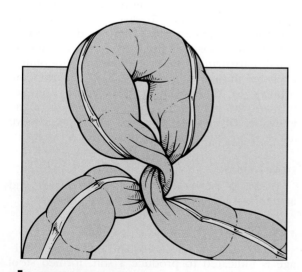

Figure 8–16

Volvulus.

pass any **meconium.** The abdomen is tender and distended, and the volvulus may be palpated.

ETIOLOGY

Volvulus results from abnormal embryonic development in which the colon does not rotate correctly or the mesentery does not attach correctly; this allows the intestine to twist on itself, resulting in an intestinal obstruction. Necrosis of the tissue results if the condition is not resolved quickly.

DIAGNOSIS

Diagnosis is made from the clinical picture and radiographic examination (upper GI radiographic studies and barium enema studies).

TREATMENT

Surgical intervention to relieve the twisting and obstruction is necessary.

INTESTINAL OBSTRUCTION

SYMPTOMS AND SIGNS

Intestinal obstruction exists when the contents of the intestine cannot move forward because of a partial or complete blockage of the bowel. Although the cause and nature of the obstruction can vary, the patient's discomfort and the signs of blockage are characteristic: nausea and vomiting and a bloated and painful abdomen without passage of stool or gas. Electrolyte imbalances and an elevated WBC count are present. The bowel sounds can be hyperactive or missing, depending on the nature of the obstruction. This condition of the bowel can occur at any age but is more common in middle-aged and elderly people.

ETIOLOGY

Mechanical blockage of the bowel narrows the normal lumen and prevents the flow of waste products. Mechanical causes of intestinal obstruction are many:

- Neoplasm (benign or malignant) (see Fig. 8–18)
- Foreign bodies
- Fecal impaction
- Strictures
- Compression of the bowel
- Volvulus (a twisting of the bowel on itself) (see Fig. 8–16)
- Intussusception (when the bowel telescopes into itself) (see Fig. 8–15)

- Strangulated hernia (see Fig. 8–13 *B*)
- Adhesions that form tight bands of scar tissue on the bowel (see Fig. 8–20)

In some cases of mechanical obstruction, there is interference with the blood supply to the affected area of intestine, which results in the death of tissue; this leads to the threat of perforation, with spillage of the contents of the intestine into the abdominal cavity. This becomes a toxic condition that endangers the patient.

If the obstruction is nonmechanical (functional), it is called ileus, a paralytic condition of the small bowel; ileus can occur postoperatively, when peristalsis and bowel sounds are absent after abdominal surgery. Normal peristalsis also can be inhibited by the use of certain medications or disease conditions such as peritonitis. Often, the motility of the bowel returns spontaneously. If it does not return within 48 hours, a syndrome of continuous pain, abdominal distention, vomiting of fecal material, and shock can be dangerous and life threatening.

DIAGNOSIS

Barium swallow films of the abdomen show the point of obstruction of the bowel. A CBC shows an elevated WBC count; there are also electrolyte imbalances and acid–base disturbances.

TREATMENT

When the obstruction is mechanical, surgery to remove the lesion or whatever is causing the blockage is done as soon as possible. If necessary, the diseased bowel is removed and the colon is reconstructed; an **ostomy** may be necessary. A second surgical procedure is required to perform takedown of the ostomy and to rejoin the bowel.

In a nonmechanical or functional obstruction (ileus), the patient is not given anything by mouth and is fed intravenously until peristalsis has returned. A stomach tube is inserted to relieve distention and vomiting. Surgery is not usually indicated for functional obstruction.

DIVERTICULOSIS

SYMPTOMS AND SIGNS

Diverticulosis is a condition in which outpouches (diverticula) of the mucosa penetrate weak points in the muscular layer of the large intestine. Diverticulosis occurs particularly in the distal part of the colon, the sigmoid colon (Fig.

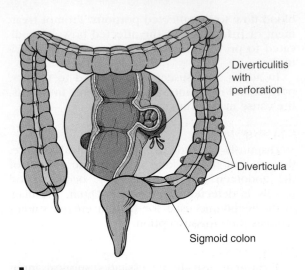

Figure 8–17
Diverticulosis and diverticulitis.

8-17). Diverticulosis usually causes no symptoms, and there is no inflammation. Occasionally, the patient reports nonspecific abdominal distress, such as pain and flatulence, and difficulty in defecation. The patient may experience alternating constipation and diarrhea and even blood in the stool.

ETIOLOGY

A diet that contains inadequate roughage and excessive amounts of highly refined foods is thought to contribute to diverticulosis. Lack of roughage produces small-caliber, drier stools, which fail to distend the bowel lumen. This luminal narrowing causes higher intra-abdominal pressure during defecation, which in turn contributes to the small herniations or pouches through the mucosa of the muscular wall of the intestine. Diverticular disease can be progressive and is more common after the age of 35 years.

DIAGNOSIS

Diagnosis is made by the clinical picture and air-contrast barium enema radiographic study.

TREATMENT

A diet that includes adequate fluids and roughage is indicated to produce a soft, formed stool daily; foods with kernels and seeds are omitted. Reduction of stress is encouraged, and treatment should include rest and the administration of anticholinergic drugs.

DIVERTICULITIS
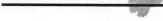

SYMPTOMS AND SIGNS

When fecal matter becomes trapped in one or more diverticula, inflammation and infection can ensue, causing diverticulitis (see Fig. 8–17). The patient then has fever, nausea, and abdominal pain in the left lower quadrant, with distention; a palpable mass may be felt, and the patient reports changes in bowel function. Occasionally, the pain may be in the right lower quadrant or in the suprapubic area. Blood in the stools is indicative of small hemorrhages. With perforation into the abdominal cavity, symptoms of peritonitis, intestinal obstruction, and sepsis can result. Chronic diverticulitis can cause complications, such as the formation of adhesions, abscesses, and fistulas.

ETIOLOGY

Diverticulitis, which is not nearly as common as diverticulosis, can develop when one or more diverticula become inflamed and perforate. Lack of dietary bulk, inadequate fluid intake, and constipation are thought to contribute. Fecal plugs in the diverticula can predispose individuals to infection by colonic bacteria.

DIAGNOSIS

The patient is assessed for constipation, fiber and fluid intake, abdominal pain, and blood in the stools. **Sigmoidoscopy** or colonoscopy is performed to visualize the area and to rule out carcinoma. Barium enema study (contraindicated if perforation exists) and flat plate radiographic examination of the abdomen may reveal the diverticular sacs and the narrowing of the colonic lumen. Blood tests may show leukocytosis and low hemoglobin level and low hematocrit.

TREATMENT

Treatment is similar to that for diverticulosis. Antibiotics are indicated until the inflammation has resolved; medication can be used to control hemorrhage. If the symptoms are severe or if the bowel perforates, surgical intervention to remove the diseased portion of the colon is indicated.

COLORECTAL CANCER

SYMPTOMS AND SIGNS

Colorectal cancer is a term for several forms of cancer that develop in either the colon or the rectum (Fig. 8-18). During early stages of the

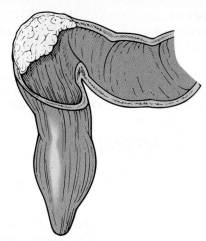

Figure 8–18

Colorectal cancer.

disease, symptoms are vague and depend on the site of neoplasia and the stage of the cancer. Many patients present with anemia or a positive result of the guaiac test for occult blood (**Hemoccult**) as the only sign of colorectal cancer. Changes in bowel movements, such as abnormal constipation and diarrhea, lasting longer than 7 to 10 days and bloody stools are early warning signs. Later symptoms include indigestion, pain with tenderness in the lower abdomen, pallor, ascites, **cachexia, lymphadenopathy,** and **hepatomegaly.** The patient may be asymptomatic until a cancerous mass causes an intestinal obstruction or the intestine ruptures and causes peritonitis.

ETIOLOGY

The cause of colorectal cancer is unknown, but predisposing factors include diets that are high in red meat and highly refined foods and low in fiber. Other factors include a history of irritable bowel syndrome, diseases of the digestive tract such as ulcerative colitis and Crohn's disease, and familial **polyposis.**

DIAGNOSIS

A careful history and physical examination, including a rectal examination, are done by the physician. The patient also needs to provide a stool sample to test for occult blood (guaiac test). If the physician suspects that a tumor might be present, he or she probably will order a barium enema study, sigmoidoscopy, or a colonoscopy. An abdominal CT scan also may be useful in detecting metastatic lesions.

TREATMENT

Surgery is the best treatment for colorectal cancer that has not metastasized. If the cancer is in the colon, a resection (removal) of the diseased bowel is done; some cases require a **colostomy** (Fig. 8–19). When the cancer has become too widespread for surgery, radiation and chemotherapy can be used.

PSEUDOMEMBRANOUS ENTEROCOLITIS

SYMPTOMS AND SIGNS

Enterocolitis in which bowel mucosa has a membranous appearance is a disease marked by mild to severe diarrhea. The patient may have a fever, feel weak, and report abdominal cramping and tenderness. Some patients feel nauseated and experience vomiting. If the diarrhea is severe enough, the patient has a dry mouth, is lightheaded and dizzy, and shows signs of dehydration and electrolyte imbalance. The urine is dark and concentrated, and there is decreased skin **turgor.** Irritation develops around the anal area from the frequent and watery stools; fecal incontinence can be a problem. Blood and mucus may be reported in the stools.

ETIOLOGY

Pseudomembranous enterocolitis is related to the use of broad-spectrum antibiotics; the patient either is taking the antibiotics or has been undergoing antibiotic therapy during the previous 6 weeks. Antibiotic therapy destroys the body's protective natural intestinal flora (along with the target pathogens) and allows a bacterial infection with *Clostridium difficile* to develop. This organism produces powerful toxins that cause the bowel wall to become inflamed, ulcerated, and necrotic. The products of inflammation and dead tissue form a coating that is referred to as a pseudomembrane.

This disease is more common in health-care facilities, where fecal contamination is more likely. Those who have had abdominal surgery are more susceptible.

DIAGNOSIS

A diagnosis is made when the causative bacteria are found in a stool culture or when *C. difficile* toxin is found in the stool; a rectal biopsy shows the pseudomembranous enterocolitis. The WBC count is elevated from the immune response to the infection. In severe cases, the blood protein (serum albumin) levels are lowered and the serum electrolyte levels are abnormal. Abdominal radiographic films show a distended colon.

TREATMENT

Treatment begins by discontinuing the broad-spectrum antibiotic and substituting vancomycin to fight the infection. In milder cases, cholestyramine resin (Questran) is given to bind the toxins produced by the causative bacteria. Drugs that slow bowel activity are not recommended because they boost the retention of the toxins, thereby increasing damage to the bowel.

The general management of the patient includes monitoring the fluid and electrolyte balance, with oral or intravenous supplement as needed. Surgery is rarely necessary. Careful hand washing and decontamination techniques are encouraged to prevent cross-infection.

SHORT-BOWEL SYNDROME

SYMPTOMS AND SIGNS

Short-bowel syndrome is the result of an insufficient amount of functioning small bowel to ab-

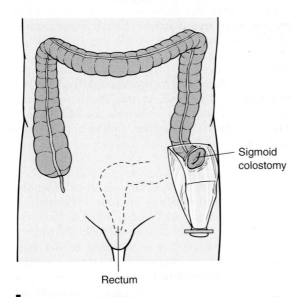

Sigmoid colostomy

Rectum

Figure 8–19

Colostomy. Colostomy is a surgical creation of an opening for feces to pass through the abdominal wall. The opening in the colon is brought to the surface of the skin to divert feces into an external pouch worn by the patient. The colostomy may be temporary to promote healing or permanent if the distal bowel has been removed because of malignancy or other disease.

sorb the nutrients, fluid, vitamins, and minerals that the body needs. Depending on the amount of missing or damaged bowel, significant signs of malnutrition are noted, including pathologic changes in other organs and body systems. Because there is not enough small bowel to digest and absorb food adequately, diarrhea and abnormal stools occur. The patient loses weight and feels weak, tired, and dizzy. As the malnutrition continues, the hair and nails become brittle and rashes develop.

ETIOLOGY

Short-bowel syndrome develops when the length of intact or functioning small bowel is altered significantly by disease or surgery. This loss of functioning small bowel interferes with the digestion and absorption of needed nutrients.

DIAGNOSIS

Initially, the patient history may indicate the presence of bowel disease, with or without surgical intervention, that has altered the length or function of part of the small bowel. In short-bowel syndrome, the results of blood tests reflect abnormal electrolyte levels, pH disturbance, and anemia. Stool studies show an increased amount of fat.

TREATMENT

The plan of treatment depends on the cause of the syndrome and what manifestations of malnutrition are noted. Medical management includes prescribing drugs for infection, diarrhea, vitamin and mineral deficiency, and pain as required. Food supplements are administered orally or intravenously as needed. Surgery may be performed to correct the underlying condition or to reconstruct the bowel.

PERITONITIS

SYMPTOMS AND SIGNS

Peritonitis, the inflammation of the peritoneum, can be acute or chronic and local or generalized. The large serous membrane that lines the abdominal cavity and folds over the visceral organs is normally transparent and sterile. When it is irritated or infected, the peritoneum becomes **hyperemic** and edematous, with fluid accumulation in the peritoneal space. The inflammatory process of peritonitis has the potential to cause abscesses and adhesions to form in the abdominal cavity (Fig. 8–20).

The patient reports abdominal pain, nausea

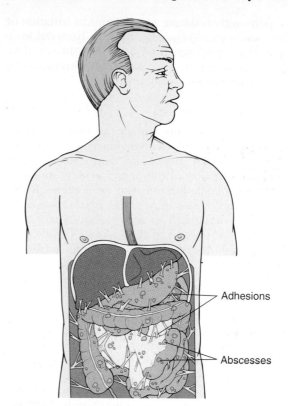

Adhesions

Abscesses

Figure 8–20
Peritonitis.

and vomiting, weakness, and profuse sweating. Abdominal pain may be so severe that the patient may prefer not to move. The clinician who examines the patient finds fever, a tender and distended abdomen, and possibly paralytic ileus. In a fulminating case of peritonitis, the toxic exudate is absorbed by the body, leading to septicemia, shock, and death.

ETIOLOGY

Peritonitis can occur as a primary infection from blood-borne organisms or organisms originating from the genital tract. It is considered secondary if the source of infection is contamination by GI secretions resulting from a perforation of the GI tract or intra-abdominal organs. For example, bacterial invasion could occur postoperatively owing to breakdown of **anastomoses,** allowing spillage of contaminated intestinal secretions into the abdominal cavity. A penetrating wound to the abdomen is another common cause.

Noninfective secretions, such as bile from a ruptured inflamed gallbladder, can cause an aseptic peritonitis resulting from chemical irritation of the membrane. Eventually, there is bacterial invasion. The organisms most commonly involved include *Escherichia coli,* anaerobic streptococci, and *Pseudomonas aeruginosa.*

DIAGNOSIS

Diagnostic findings include an elevated WBC, abnormal serum electrolyte levels (e.g., altered levels of sodium, potassium, and chloride), and gaseous distention of the bowel evident on radiographic examination of the abdomen. Radiographic studies also may reveal perforation of an abdominal organ and air in the abdominal cavity. Aspiration of peritoneal fluid shows cloudy peritoneal fluid and allows culture and sensitivity study to identify the causative organism.

TREATMENT

The clinical manifestations of peritonitis must be assessed and the source of the irritation or infection identified. Prompt and aggressive treatment with broad-spectrum antibiotics, analgesics, and antiemetics is provided. The patient is not given anything by mouth, and fluid and electrolyte losses are replaced parenterally. If there is a perforation, surgery is required to correct the source of infection and to drain the spilled contents. Continuous peritoneal lavage with a saline-antibiotic solution may be appropriate as part of the effort to eliminate the infection.

HEMORRHOIDS

SYMPTOMS AND SIGNS

Hemorrhoids are tumor-like lesions in the anal area caused by dilated veins; often, hemorrhoids are painless. If symptomatic, the patient experiences rectal pain, itching, protrusion, or bleeding, especially after defecation. The patient also may experience a mucous discharge from the rectum, a sensation of incomplete evacuation, and difficulty in cleaning the anal area.

ETIOLOGY

The veins in the rectal and anal area become varicose, swollen, and tender from blockage. If they are within the rectal wall, these swollen and twisted varicosities are considered internal hemorrhoids; varicosities in the anal area are considered external hemorrhoids (Fig. 8–21). A large, firm subcutaneous lump indicates thrombosis of the external hemorrhoids. Constipation, straining,

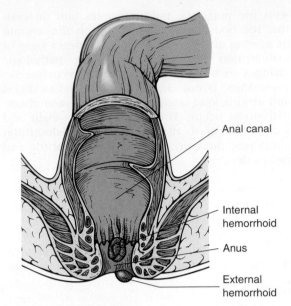

Figure 8–21
Hemorrhoids.

pregnancy, or any condition that increases pressure on the veins frequently causes an **exacerbation** of this condition.

DIAGNOSIS

Diagnosis is made by visual inspection of the anal area and **proctoscopy** to visualize internal hemorrhoids of the rectum. The patient's hemoglobin level and red blood cell (RBC) count may be below normal if there has been significant bleeding.

TREATMENT

Conservative treatment consists of measures to correct constipation and to prevent straining. Stool softeners and a diet high in fruits, vegetables, and whole-grain cereals are recommended. Warm sitz baths may be prescribed, along with a topical anesthetic ointment or witch hazel compresses. Products such as hydrocortisone acetate–pramoxine hydrochloride (ProctoCream-HC) may be applied locally to reduce inflammation. If these measures do not help, **sclerotherapy** injections to induce scar formation and to decrease prolapse are available. The hemorrhoids can be destroyed by ligation or by cryosurgery, a procedure that uses a probe to expose the hemorrhoids to extreme cold. When bleeding and other symptoms are severe, a hemorrhoidectomy is the best treatment.

Diseases of the Liver, Biliary Tract, and Pancreas

The liver, gallbladder, and pancreas are accessory organs of digestion that introduce digestive hormones and enzymes into the alimentary canal, ensuring that the nutrients critical to life can be absorbed selectively by the small intestines into the bloodstream.

CIRRHOSIS OF THE LIVER

SYMPTOMS AND SIGNS

Cirrhosis of the liver is a chronic degenerative disease that is irreversible. There is slow deterioration of the liver, resulting in the replacement of normal liver cells with hard, fibrous scar tissue, known as hobnail liver. Cirrhosis is twice as common in men as in women. As many as 40% of persons with cirrhosis of the liver are asymptomatic.

In the early stages of the disease, the symptoms are vague and mild. As the liver is destroyed, there is loss of appetite and weight, nausea and vomiting, indigestion, abdominal distention (due to ascites), and edema. There is a tendency to bleed and bruise more easily, and frequent nosebleeds are common. The skin appears **jaundiced** and is dry with **pruritus.** Small, red, spidery marks (spider nevi) may appear on the face and body. Changes in the endocrine system cause testicular **atrophy,** gynecomastia, and loss of chest hair in the male (Fig. 8–22).

As the cirrhosis advances, memory is impaired, and confusion and drowsiness occur and intensify. Eventually, if cirrhosis is left untreated, hepatic failure and death follow.

ETIOLOGY

The causes of cirrhosis are numerous, but the most common cause is chronic alcoholism. Malnutrition, hepatitis (see Hepatitis A and Hepatitis C), parasites, toxic (poisonous) chemicals, and congestive heart failure are other possible causes of this disease. Cirrhosis also may be **idiopathic.**

DIAGNOSIS

On physical examination, the liver feels enlarged and firm to hard with a palpable blunt edge; abdominal radiographic films show this en-

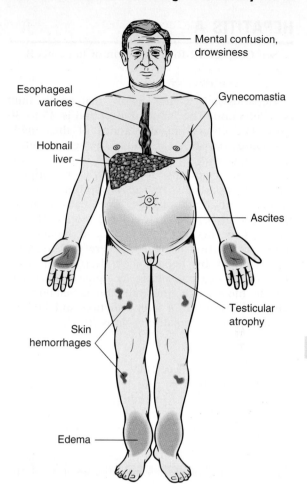

Figure 8–22

Cirrhosis of the liver (in the male).

largement. Blood studies may reveal an elevation of the liver enzyme and bilirubin levels. A liver scan and needle biopsy of the liver are essential to determine the type and extent of fibrosis.

TREATMENT

Treatment is directed at the cause of the disease, in an attempt to prevent further damage to the liver. Whatever the underlying cause may be, alcohol intake is prohibited. Malnutrition must be prevented, and adequate rest is essential. Vitamin and mineral supplements along with antacids are given. **Diuretics** reduce the excessive fluid (edema) that accumulates in the abdomen (ascites) and ankles. When there is progression to liver failure, liver transplantation is a viable option.

241

HEPATITIS A

See Chapter 12 for discussion of hepatitis B.

SYMPTOMS AND SIGNS

Hepatitis A is a viral disease that causes mild liver infection. The incubation period is 25 to 30 days. The clinical manifestations of this highly contagious hepatitis can be mild to severe; often, they begin with a sudden onset of nonspecific prodromal symptoms, followed by the appearance of jaundice. Typical symptoms include headache, anorexia, malaise, fever, nausea, **myalgia,** dark urine, and clay-colored stools. The inflamed liver becomes enlarged and tender and does not function normally. Severe viral hepatitis A is marked by hepatic cell destruction, with necrotic changes resulting in signs of liver failure. In most cases, the infection is self-limiting, with full recovery of liver function and lifelong immunity to the hepatitis A virus (HAV).

ETIOLOGY

The causative virus, HAV, is highly contagious and is transmitted by the fecal–oral route from contaminated food (including shellfish), water, and stools. This form of hepatitis is sometimes known as epidemic or infective hepatitis because it frequently occurs at schools, camps, or institutions. The administration of immune globulin after known exposure lessens the severity of the disease.

DIAGNOSIS

A hepatitis profile is performed to identify the causative virus by identifying **antibodies** specific to the virus. Liver function studies are used to support the diagnosis. Because the liver has many functions, there are many possible abnormal findings in laboratory tests. Blood tests show elevated serum levels of alanine transaminase (ALT) and aspartate transaminase (AST), usually found in the liver. The **prothrombin time** (PT) is prolonged, and the serum bilirubin level is elevated. Urine tests show **proteinuria** and **bilirubinuria.** The presence of antibody to hepatitis A in the serum confirms the diagnosis.

TREATMENT

General medical management includes rest and control of symptoms. The administration of immune globulin intramuscularly is recommended within 2 weeks of exposure. The patient is isolated, and care is taken to prevent cross-infection. Medications to control nausea and pain

are given as needed. Other measures taken while the liver heals are a low-fat, high-carbohydrate diet and restriction of physical activity.

A noninfectious vaccine called HAVRIX currently is recommended before travel into areas where hepatitis A is endemic or prevalent (e.g., Mexico). The vaccine should be received at least 2 weeks ahead of potential exposure. One dose is sufficient for primary immunization, with a booster dose between 6 and 12 months later. The duration of immunity has not been established.

HEPATITIS C

SYMPTOMS AND SIGNS

Hepatitis C is a viral liver disease also known as blood-borne non-A, non-B hepatitis (NANB hepatitis). Considered a widespread epidemic, it currently affects approximately 4 million people in the United States, causing a clinical syndrome of variable severity. Many persons infected with HCV are asymptomatic and may infect others unknowingly; the incubation period varies from 2 weeks to 6 months. About half of all persons who become infected do not know *how* they were infected with HCV. If present, symptoms resemble hepatitis A, but are typically less severe: fever, anorexia, vague abdominal pain, severe fatigue, jaundice, nausea, and vomiting.

Abnormal laboratory findings may include elevated serum levels of liver enzymes and bilirubin, although this evidence is inconclusive without a positive blood test for anti-HCV antibodies. Sometimes the liver is tender and enlarged on physical examination. Most infected patients recover completely. Some patients exhibit signs of chronic hepatitis and eventually, in approximately 20% of the cases, cirrhosis of the liver. There is increased incidence of liver cancer in chronic hepatitis. Some patients die of liver failure.

ETIOLOGY

Hepatitis C is caused by HCV, which is transmitted by blood and body fluids. Exposure may be traced to blood transfusions especially before 1992, kidney dialysis, an organ transplant before 1992, or behaviors involving contact with the blood of an infected person, including sexual contact. Other risk factors include working in the health-care environment, injecting illegal drugs, or sharing articles of personal hygiene with an infected individual. In many cases, the source of infection is not discovered.

DIAGNOSIS

A clinical history of possible exposure to HCV accompanied by symptoms of hepatitis may indicate the diagnosis. Laboratory findings include elevated serum levels of liver enzymes, elevated serum bilirubin, and bilirubinuria. A positive blood test result for the presence of anti-HCV antibodies is indicative of infection, past or present. Liver biopsy confirms hepatitis.

TREATMENT

There is no cure for hepatitis C. Treatment is aimed at controlling the symptoms and long-term improvement in liver function. Drug therapy may include gamma globulin, the antiviral agent *interferon-alpha,* and glucocorticoids to decrease inflammation. Supportive measures include rest and a well-balanced diet. The increase in HCV infections has contributed to a high demand for liver transplants in the United States.

There is no vaccine for hepatitis C. Proper precautions and avoidance of the aforementioned risk factors are recommended. HCV can exist in a carrier state, that is, without any active disease or in a low-grade infection. In the case of a known infection, every precaution must be taken to avoid transmission of the virus.

CANCER OF THE LIVER

SYMPTOMS AND SIGNS

Primary cancer of the liver is rare, as are benign tumors. Cancer of the liver usually is discovered after finding the disease in some other part of the body. Initially, the symptoms are those from the primary site, usually the breast, lung, or GI tract. As the liver cancer develops, it causes weight loss; anorexia; abdominal discomfort, especially in the right upper abdominal quadrant; and a general feeling of poor health. In the later stages of the disease, enlargement of the liver (hepatomegaly) is particularly prominent, and jaundice may appear.

ETIOLOGY

Cancer of the liver is usually secondary; it develops as a metastasis from another site in the body, reaching the liver via the blood stream.

DIAGNOSIS

The diagnosis is based on the results of abdominal radiographic studies, laboratory analysis of the blood, and techniques such as liver scan and needle biopsy of the liver. Diagnosis typi-

cally is delayed until an advanced stage because early symptoms are nonspecific.

TREATMENT

After cancer has invaded the liver, the prognosis is poor. Surgical removal is nearly impossible, and radiation and chemotherapy may not be effective in controlling the spread. Benign tumors, if discovered at all, usually can be surgically removed.

CHOLELITHIASIS (GALLSTONES)

SYMPTOMS AND SIGNS

The patient with cholelithiasis (gallstones) may be asymptomatic unless the bile ducts become obstructed by the stones (Fig. 8–23). Colicky pain, or biliary colic, signals the obstruction of the cystic duct or the common bile duct with one or more stones. The pain is in the epigastric region or the right upper quadrant of the abdomen, often radiating to the right upper back in the area of the scapula. Nausea and vomiting accompany the pain. If the obstruction is prolonged, jaundice may appear.

ETIOLOGY

Gallstones form in the gallbladder from insoluble cholesterol and bile salts; they vary in size and number. The reasons for formation are not always clear, although the occurrence is more frequent with increasing age, with the high-calorie, high-cholesterol diet associated with obesity, and in the female population. Other risk factors are oral contraceptive use, pancreatitis, and ileal disease.

DIAGNOSIS

The clinical picture and ultrasonography of the gallbladder and biliary ducts are highly accurate in confirming the presence of cholelithiasis. Other diagnostic studies that visualize gallstones include radioisotope scan, oral **cholecystogram,** and intravenous **cholangiogram.** The size and type of stones can be estimated with some accuracy in test results. The serum bilirubin level is elevated with obstruction of the common bile duct.

hydascan – No stones present on ultrasound

TREATMENT

Asymptomatic gallstones are usually left alone. Fatty intake should be controlled by diet. If the patient experiences pain on a recurring basis, surgery is indicated, with removal of the gallbladder (cholecystectomy) being performed. A surgi-

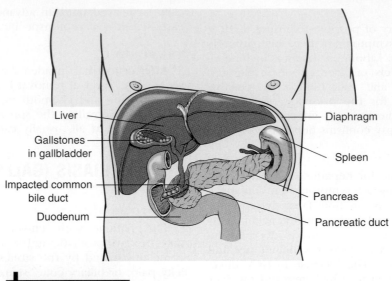

Liver
Gallstones in gallbladder
Impacted common bile duct
Duodenum
Diaphragm
Spleen
Pancreas
Pancreatic duct

Figure 8–23

Cholelithiasis.

cal procedure called laparoscopic cholecystectomy has shortened hospitalization and recovery time. The use of drugs to dissolve the gallstones may be attempted in some cases; it is most successful in patients with pure cholesterol gallstones. It is usually not successful with calcified stones. Extracorporeal shock wave **lithotripsy** (ESWL) is considered experimental therapy.

CHOLECYSTITIS

SYMPTOMS AND SIGNS

Cholecystitis, or inflammation of the gallbladder, commonly is associated with cholelithiasis; infection often follows the inflammation. The condition can become chronic.

The patient experiences acute colicky pain, which localizes in the right upper quadrant of the abdomen and becomes more severe while radiating around to the right lower scapular region. Additionally, the patient experiences nausea and vomiting followed by guarding of the right upper quadrant muscles and shallow respirations. A fever may ensue. In some cases, the acutely inflamed gallbladder ruptures, causing peritonitis. Otherwise, the cholecystitis may spontaneously subside, and the pain begins to abate in a few days.

ETIOLOGY

Most cholecystitis results from an obstructed biliary duct caused by gallstones. Occasionally,

trauma or other insults to the gallbladder, including infection, may be the cause.

DIAGNOSIS

Diagnosis is made by the clinical picture and an ultrasonogram of the gallbladder and biliary ducts. Radiographic gallbladder studies that indicate a *nonvisualized* gallbladder are indicative of gallbladder disease. Other findings include an elevated WBC count and an increased serum bilirubin level.

TREATMENT

Treatment in uncomplicated cases consists of dietary modification with elimination of fatty foods. The acutely ill patient with persistent vomiting is given nothing by mouth and has a nasogastric tube inserted. Intravenous feeding is given for fluid and electrolyte replacement. When the patient is stabilized, surgical intervention to remove the gallbladder (cholecystectomy) is indicated. Medical management may include the administration of antibiotics, analgesics, and antiemetics.

ACUTE AND CHRONIC PANCREATITIS

SYMPTOMS AND SIGNS

Pancreatitis is inflammation of the pancreas (Fig. 8-24). It can occur as a mild and self-limiting disease or as chronic and fatal destruction of

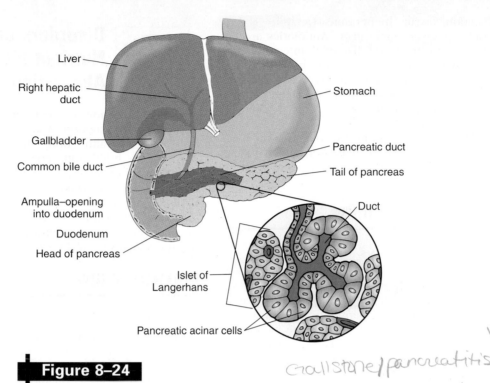

Figure 8–24

Location and structure of the pancreas.

[handwritten margin notes: treat first; Gallstone/pancreatitis; Inflammation of pancreas due to gallstone 3-5 days hosp.]

pancreatic tissue. In pancreatitis, the pancreas, which functions as both an endocrine and an exocrine organ, becomes inflamed, edematous, hemorrhagic, and necrotic. The patient with acute pancreatitis has a sudden onset of severe abdominal pain, which radiates to the back, along with nausea and vomiting. The patient is acutely ill, **diaphoretic,** and **tachycardic** and experiences shallow, rapid respirations. Blood pressure falls and the temperature is elevated. Abdominal tenderness is present, especially in the upper abdomen radiating to the lower abdomen. Bowel sounds are decreased. There are numerous possible local and systemic complications (e.g., pancreatic abscess and pneumonia).

Chronic pancreatitis can present a more vague clinical picture. The patient may report constant pain in the back, with repeated mild episodes of the symptoms of acute pancreatitis. As pancreatic function deteriorates and the organ becomes fibrotic, signs of malabsorption and diabetes mellitus appear.

ETIOLOGY

The pancreas becomes damaged from autodigestion by the exocrine secretions that it usually releases into the duodenum. Pancreatitis may be caused by alcoholism, biliary tract disease,

trauma, infection, structural anomalies, hemorrhage, **hyperlipidemia,** or drugs. Gallstones are frequently responsible for pancreatitis in the nonalcoholic individual. Less commonly, the cause is a metabolic or endocrine disorder.

DIAGNOSIS

Diagnosis is made by the clinical picture, with dramatically elevated serum amylase and lipase levels on the first day of the attack. Serum amylase and lipase levels usually return to normal by the third day. The WBC count and hematocrit are elevated. Glucose levels may be high, indicating hyperglycemia. Radiographic films and ultrasonograms may demonstrate stones in the biliary tract or dilation of the common bile duct; the bilirubin level may be elevated. CT scan, with oral or intravenous contrast material, identifies pancreatic changes and complications.

TREATMENT

Acute pancreatitis may necessitate emergency treatment consisting of intravenous fluid and electrolyte replacement. The patient is not given anything by mouth. The placement of a nasogastric suction tube with intermittent suction may be indicated for approximately 1 week. Pain medication, usually meperidine (Demerol) hydrochloride, is given generously. Antibiotics are administered to treat the bacterial infection, and anticholinergics are given to slow bowel motility and to decrease the pancreatic secretions; laboratory blood values of electrolytes, serum amylase and lipase, hematocrit, glucose, and serum calcium are monitored.

In chronic pancreatitis, the patient also must be monitored closely for malabsorption, **steatorrhea,** and impaired glucose tolerance indicating diabetes mellitus.

PANCREATIC CANCER

SYMPTOMS AND SIGNS

Cancer of the pancreas is a neoplasm, usually an **adenocarcinoma,** which occurs more frequently in the head of the pancreas. The classic symptoms are loss of appetite and weight; upper abdominal pain, which radiates to the back; nausea and vomiting; and jaundice. As pancreatic tissue is infiltrated and destroyed, the patient experiences glucose intolerence, increasing weakness, fatigue, and diarrhea.

ETIOLOGY

The cause of pancreatic cancer is unknown. Smoking cigarettes, drinking large amounts of coffee, ingesting a high-fat diet, and being exposed to chemicals in the workplace all have been associated with an increased frequency of the disease.

DIAGNOSIS

If cancer is suspected, the physician orders a hemoglobin and hematocrit determination, which may be lowered if there is bleeding. An upper gastrointestinal tract radiographic series may show evidence of compression of the small intestine from the neoplasm. Other tests that are useful in the diagnosis include an ultrasonogram, a CT scan, and an endoscopic retrograde cholangiopancreatogram (ERCP).

TREATMENT

Because most pancreatic cancers are discovered after they already have metastasized, treatment is usually **palliative** and the prognosis is poor. If the cancer is detected in its early stages, surgical removal of localized tumors is possible and may even provide a cure. Radiation treatments and chemotherapy also may be employed.

Disorders of Nutrient Intake and Absorption

Proper nutrition is necessary to enable the regulation and function of all body processes and to ensure a healthy body that has energy and nutrients to build and repair tissue. Nutritional deficiencies, excesses, or imbalances can affect the body's **homeostasis.** Any inability of the GI tract to digest or absorb nutrients can cause forms of malnutrition, even with adequate intake of food. Prolonged malnutrition or malabsorption results in anatomic lesions or disease entities.

MALNUTRITION

SYMPTOMS AND SIGNS

Disturbances in nutrition can result from eating too much or too little food or from having an imbalanced diet. However, even when diet is sufficient, if the body is unable to absorb or to use food properly, malnutrition results. Malnutrition disrupts the body's metabolic processes, disturbing normal physical structure and biologic function.

Malnourishment can cause many specific disease conditions, such as abnormal growth, with physical and intellectual impairment. The body deprived of adequate nutrition begins to manifest the loss of well-being externally and internally. The appetite may decrease or increase, resulting in emaciation or obesity. Signs and symptoms of malnutrition include loss of energy, diarrhea, drastic weight change, skin lesions, loss of hair, poor nails, generalized edema, and delayed healing. Some more advanced signs may include muscle wasting, enlarged glands, and **hepatomegaly.** There are many possible abnormal findings of blood and urine tests.

ETIOLOGY

Various conditions and circumstances cause malnutrition, including famine, eating disorders, chronic illnesses, fad diets, poverty, biochemical disorders, certain medications, and various malabsorption syndromes. Without a special diet, a burn patient or a patient with severe trauma easily could have inadequate nutrition.

When the body experiences prolonged deprivation of calories and nutrients, it begins to break down its own tissue to meet its caloric

Enrichment

HYPERVITAMINOSIS

- Hypervitaminosis is toxicity from any vitamin, but especially the fat-soluble vitamins A and D.
- The four fat (lipid) soluble vitamins A, D, E, and K are stored in fat tissue.
- Symptoms of vitamin A toxicity include irritability, loss of hair, anorexia, enlargement of the liver and spleen, jaundice, skin changes, and psychiatric disorders. Vitamin A excess can be toxic to a developing fetus. Chronic toxicity in infants and children can cause increased pressure in the brain, tinnitus, pruritus, swelling of the optic nerve, and abnormal bone growth.
- Vitamin D is considered highly toxic, especially in infants and children. It can cause calcification of soft tissue, kidney damage, excessive thirst and urination, and mental changes.
- Very high doses of vitamin E may interfere with the blood-clotting action of vitamin K.
- Vitamin K toxicity is not common. Rapid infusion causes dyspnea, flushing, cardiovascular complications, red blood cell hemolysis, jaundice, and brain damage.
- Water-soluble vitamin C taken in excess causes nausea, diarrhea, and acidification of urine; Niacin (B_3) may cause flushing, hyperglycemia, and liver damage; vitamin B_6 may cause photosensitivity and peripheral nerve damage.
- Overload of nutritional trace elements also produces toxicity.

needs. Another syndrome results if caloric intake is adequate, but protein intake is low: the patient may not appear malnourished, but there is loss of important proteins.

DIAGNOSIS

Clinical evaluation of the patient includes a complete physical examination with special attention to weight and measurements of body fat and muscle mass. Laboratory diagnostic findings differ depending on the cause and type of malnutrition. Laboratory testing includes blood protein levels, complete blood counts, and a 24-hour urine test for urea nitrogen. The tests may show evidence of mineral deficiency, anemia, abnormal protein metabolism, and other changes in metabolism related to malnourishment.

TREATMENT

The treatment of malnutrition is based on the underlying cause. After the patient's nutritional needs are assessed, nutritional supplements and replacement begin with appropriate oral and intravenous feedings. Certain pathologic conditions may necessitate feedings through a nasogastric tube. Treatment may entail a combination of dietary modifications, including appropriate supplements of proteins, vitamins, and minerals. Diarrhea and infections are controlled with medications.

Surgery may be indicated when lesions of the GI tract cause the malnutrition. Patients with eating disorders require special counseling with medical treatment. The poor and elderly may require community services to make good nutrition available on a daily basis.

MALABSORPTION SYNDROME

SYMPTOMS AND SIGNS

A person with malabsorption syndrome is unable to absorb fat or certain other elements of diet. Symptoms include abdominal discomfort, bloating with gas, chronic diarrhea, and abnormal bowel movements. Stools may appear yellowish gray and may be greasy looking. The stools tend to float because of their high fat content. Over time, untreated malabsorption leads to weight loss, shortness of breath, and symptoms of vitamin and mineral deficiencies.

ETIOLOGY

The main cause of malabsorption syndrome is defective mucosal cells in the small intestine. Ab-

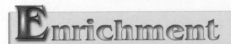

FACTS ABOUT OBESITY

- About 34 million adult Americans are overweight despite the prevalence of fad diets and sugar- and fat-free products in plenty.
- More women are afflicted with obesity than men, especially as they age.
- Obesity is measured objectively by height–weight tables, and defined as being 20% or more overweight.
- The causes of obesity are many and complex, but it frequently is associated with greater energy intake than output.
- There is a strong genetic component to fatness and to the regional distribution of fat.
- Factors that may contribute to obesity include overeating (sometimes linked to psychological stress or environment), a low rate of energy expenditure, inactivity, and more rarely, endocrine disorders.
- Obesity can lead to severe health problems, such as diabetes mellitus, hypertension, cardiovascular disease, sleep apnea, blood lipid abnormalities, and skin problems. It is more dangerous to be overweight when younger than 45 years of age.
- Obesity can make a person feel self-conscious and impair social relationships; sometimes overweight people experience prejudice and discrimination.
- Treatment goals are (1) to lose as much nonessential fat as possible while minimizing the loss of lean body mass and (2) to maintain a balance between energy intake and energy expenditure.
- Important elements of success in weight loss are active patient self-control, a supportive physician, a reduced-calorie, nutritionally adequate diet, and increased physical activity.
- Other controversial treatment modalities that have known risks, or lack proven long-term success, include extremely low-calorie diets, anorectic drugs, and surgical procedures.
- Many individuals have great difficulty maintaining reduced body weight. Exercise and control of food intake through behavior modification remain consequential.
- Consultation with a physician is recommended before starting a substantial weight loss program.

---

sorption also is hindered if the intestinal enzymes and chemicals are not properly assisting the digestive process. Secondary malabsorption syndrome may be caused by a diseased pancreas or a blocked pancreatic duct, which deprives the small intestine of **lipase.** Reduced secretion of bile, caused by hepatic disease or a bile duct obstruction, also prevents lipid (fat) digestion. Metabolic or endocrine disorders such as **hyperparathyroidism** and diabetes mellitus are other possible causes of the syndrome.

DIAGNOSIS

The physician probably orders several blood tests to determine the levels of proteins, fats, and minerals in the patient's blood stream. A laboratory analysis of a stool sample also may be done.

TREATMENT

The main task for the physician is to discover the underlying cause and to decide on the course of treatment. Diet is controlled carefully. A high-protein, high-calorie diet with vitamin and mineral supplements, such as the fat-soluble vitamins A, D, E, and K, which are not being absorbed, aids the recovery.

CELIAC DISEASE (GLUTEN ENTEROPATHY)

SYMPTOMS AND SIGNS

Celiac disease (celiac sprue) is a disease of the small intestine that is characterized by malabsorption, gluten intolerance, and damage to the lining of the intestine.

Symptoms include weight loss, anorexia, diarrhea, flatulence (gas), abdominal distention, intestinal bleeding, dermatitis, and the characteristically large, pale, greasy, foul-smelling stools.

ETIOLOGY

The cause of this disease may be either a toxic or an immunologic reaction to gluten (a protein that is found in wheat and wheat products). Celiac disease may be inherited because the occurrence is higher in siblings; females are affected twice as often as males.

DIAGNOSIS

Celiac disease is often difficult to diagnose and differentiate from other intestinal diseases and disorders. For a positive diagnosis, two criteria are needed: (1) a biopsy of the small intestine showing changes or destruction in the mucosal lining and (2) improvement while on a gluten-free diet. Laboratory tests that may be ordered include blood tests for WBC count, platelet count, albumin level, PT, and a glucose tolerance test. An upper GI and a small bowel radiographic series demonstrate characteristic abnormal patterns of barium passage.

TREATMENT

A gluten-free diet must be adhered to strictly. If improvement is not experienced while on the diet, corticosteroid drugs may be used.

There is no known prevention for celiac disease; however, with the proper treatment, the prognosis is favorable. Patients with this disease more frequently have abdominal lymphoma and cancer that develop later in life, and they should be examined if GI symptoms develop.

FOOD POISONING

SYMPTOMS AND SIGNS

Food poisoning is an illness resulting from eating foods that contain bacterial or toxic substances. Symptoms of food poisoning are determined, in part, by the cause. The onset is sudden, with rumbling stomach sounds, nausea, vomiting, diarrhea with abdominal pain and cramps, malaise, and fever. Usually, the symptoms disappear within 24 to 48 hours. If an extreme case of food poisoning persists, the patient becomes disabled and the situation becomes life threatening.

ETIOLOGY

True food poisoning includes poisoning from mushrooms, shellfish, foods contaminated with poisonous insecticides, and toxic substances such as lead and mercury. Also, poisoning occurs from eating foods that have undergone putrefaction or decomposition and foods contaminated with bacteria or their toxins (Table 8-1).

DIAGNOSIS

The patient's history is important to diagnosis and can point to the cause. Endoscopy may be performed by the physician. A stool or blood culture identifies the presence of any parasites or bacteria. Culturing of the actual contaminated food also may be done.

TREATMENT

Most treatment is symptomatic. Bed rest is desirable. To prevent or minimize fluid and electrolyte imbalances, nutritional support and fluid replacement are essential. These may have to be given intravenously if the patient becomes dehydrated. Antidiarrheal and antiemetic agents may be prescribed by the physician.

The prognosis for this condition varies with the cause; generally, it is good if the cause has been determined and the treatment has begun. The earlier the diagnosis is made and treatment is begun, the better the chances are for a successful recovery.

ANOREXIA NERVOSA

SYMPTOMS AND SIGNS

Anorexia nervosa is linked to a psychological disturbance in which hunger is denied by self-imposed starvation, resulting from a distorted body image and a compulsion to be thin (Fig. 8-25). The typical anorectic patient is a female adolescent who is meticulous, is a high achiever, and is refusing food intake; she is preoccupied with obesity and obsessed with her weight. Although she experiences continued weight loss, she does not believe that there is anything wrong. Usually, concerned family members are the ones who bring forth the problem to the physician when the girl loses weight and body mass. She may have amenorrhea, constipation, bloating, or abdominal distress. This girl is usually hyperactive, exercises a great deal, is hypotensive, and experiences bradycardia and hypothermia. Without medical intervention, life-threatening complications, such as cardiac arrest, are possible.

TABLE 8-1 ➤ Bacterial Causes of Food Poisoning

ORGANISM	MAJOR FOOD SOURCE(S)	PATHOPHYSIOLOGIC MECHANISM	
		Toxin in Food	Ingestion of Bacteria
Staphylococcus aureus	Cooked meat, cheese, pasta, cream buns, custard pies	Yes	No
Clostridium perfringens type A	Cooked meat, vegetable soup (prepared in bulk)	No	Yes (bacteria release enterotoxin in intestine)
Clostridium botulinum	Uneviscerated cured fish, preserved or fermented meat, home-preserved vegetables	Yes	No
Salmonella enteritidis/Salmonella typhimurium	Raw eggs, mayonnaise, incompletely cooked meat and poultry	No	Yes
Salmonella dublin	Raw milk, unpasteurized cheese	No	Yes
Salmonella typhi/Salmonella paratyphi	Food contamination by infected food handlers	No	Yes
Vibrio cholerae O1	Raw seafood	No	Yes
Vibrio cholerae non-O1	Raw oysters	No	Yes
Vibrio parahaemolyticus	Raw seafood	No	Yes
Vibrio vulnificus	Raw seafood (especially oysters)	No	Yes
Listeria monocytogenes	Soft cheese	No	Yes
Shigella species	Food contamination during preparation	No	Yes
Escherichia coli O157 : H7	Ground beef	No	Yes
Campylobacter jejuni/Campylobacter coli	Incompletely cooked poultry and other meats, raw milk	No	Yes
Bacillus cereus			
Heat-stable toxin	Fried rice	Yes	No
Enterotoxin	Meat products	Yes	No
Yersinia enterocolitica	Pork, raw milk	No	Yes

From: Bennett JC, Plum F: Cecil Textbook of Medicine, 20th ed, Vol. 1. Philadelphia: WB Saunders, 1996, p 739. Used with permission.

ETIOLOGY

Anorexia nervosa afflicts predominately younger, affluent females. The etiology is unknown, although it is believed that family and social factors may precipitate the condition. Current social and cultural factors promote thinness, which maintains anorectic behavior. It is possible that there is a genetic predisposition. Frequently, the patient is intelligent with a compulsive personality driven to achieve.

DIAGNOSIS

Diagnosis is made by the clinical picture and history; the patient has lost significant weight and may appear emaciated, has intense fear of weight gain, and if female, has absent or irregular menstruation. The nutritional status and the electrolyte balance are evaluated by laboratory tests, including blood tests, urinalysis, and an **electrocardiogram.**

TREATMENT

The goal of treatment is to promote normal weight and to restore nutrition. Often the patient is hospitalized to provide fluid and electrolyte replacement, to remove the patient from the home environment, and to place the patient in a controlled environment. Long-term emotional support is necessary, and often psychiatric counseling is indicated to correct any underlying dysfunction.

BULIMIA

SYMPTOMS AND SIGNS

Bulimia is a behavioral disorder characterized by recurring episodes of binge eating followed by self-induced vomiting or purging, usually in secret. This binge–purge eating pattern is fueled by a morbid fear of becoming fat. The frequent presence of vomitus in the mouth causes erosion of the teeth. The patients also abuse laxatives and diuretics by using them excessively. Other signs are compulsive exercise, swollen salivary glands, and broken blood vessels in the eye. These patients, generally females, are usually more obese than anorectic patients and experience a wide fluctuation in weight.

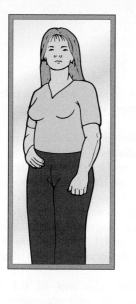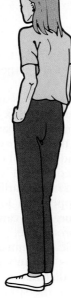

Figure 8–25

Anorexia nervosa. Persons with anorexia overestimate their body width, insisting that they are too fat despite profound weight loss.

ETIOLOGY

Although the etiologic factors are similar to those for anorexia nervosa, the exact cause is not certain. Psychosocial factors, depression, control issues, and conflict frequently are identified. A typical disordered eating pattern, with self-induced vomiting, is reported by the patient, although frequently this ritual is denied and kept secret. Characteristic perfectionist personality traits are identified, as in anorexia nervosa.

DIAGNOSIS

The diagnostic approach is similar to that for anorexia nervosa. Increased loss of electrolytes and metabolic acidosis are noted in laboratory testing. The patient exhibits loss of muscle mass, cardiac irregularities, and dehydration. Anger and denial are part of the emotional state. Sudden death can occur because of **hypokalemia** and resulting cardiac arrhythmias.

TREATMENT

Treatment is similar to that of anorexia nervosa, with a multidimensional approach, including the administration of antidepressant drugs and participation in a support group.

MOTION SICKNESS

SYMPTOMS AND SIGNS

During an episode of motion sickness, the patient experiences nausea and vomiting when riding in a motor vehicle, boat, airplane, or other means of transportation. The nausea and vomiting may be preceded by air hunger, excessive salivation, pallor, sweating, dizziness, or headache.

ETIOLOGY

Motion sickness results from a disturbance in the sense of balance. The fluid in the semicircular canals of the ears becomes dislocated because of the motion. Additionally, excessive stimulation of the vestibular apparatus in the inner ear is caused by repetitive acceleration and deceleration as well as by angular and linear motion.

DIAGNOSIS

Diagnosis is made from the clinical picture.

TREATMENT

Prevention of this condition is easier than the treatment. The person is encouraged to sit in the vehicle in the position where there is the least amount of motion and where he or she is able to view the horizon. Avoidance of foods and liquids before travel is recommended. If the individual must eat, only small amounts of food should be eaten. Prophylaxis with dermal patches of scopolamine often is employed. Dimenhydrinate (Dramamine) is another drug that helps to prevent, and also treats, motion sickness.

Summary

Chapter 8 addresses the various conditions that can afflict the alimentary canal and the accessory organs of the digestive system. Gastrointestinal (GT) problems are common and usually are cause for considerable anxiety because of the way in which they interfere with a sense of well-being. The "gut" often is associated with emotional responses ("butterflies in the stomach," "a gut feeling"). Some conditions are straightforward and easily treatable (such as dental caries and hemorrhoids), whereas others can be life threatening and more difficult to pinpoint (such as peritonitis and gastric cancer).

- The process of ingestion, digestion, and absorption of food and the elimination of waste products can be hampered by a variety of diseases and conditions.
- Teeth that are missing, impacted, decayed, or maloccluded can cause pain and interfere with mastication.
- Untreated gingivitis can lead to periodontal disease.
- Periodontitis can cause halitosis, extreme temperature sensitivity, and tooth abscess; eventually the surrounding bone is compromised.
- Oral tumors are diagnosed as benign or malignant, and treated accordingly.
- Malocclusion is at least one possible cause of temporomandibular joint (TMJ) syndrome, causing pain and limitation of the jaw.
- Lesions in the mouth (ulcers, cold sores, thrush, trench mouth, and leukoplakia) are common but have different causative mechanisms and organisms.
- Diseases of the esophagus involve inflammation and pain and may interfere with swallowing; hematemesis or hemorrhage of varices may take place.
- A crucial causal factor of peptic ulcer and superficial gastritis is *Helicobactor pylori*.
- Gastric cancer and colorectal cancer have only vague symptoms during early stages; Hemoccult testing is used to screen for colorectal cancer.
- Appendicitis, most common in the 20- to 40-year age bracket, is treated with appendectomy and antibiotic therapy to avoid serious complications.
- Hiatal hernia is one possible cause of gastroesophageal reflux disease (GERD).
- Abdominal hernias are treated according to the type, the severity of the protrusion, and the age and physical condition of the patient.
- Endoscopy and colonoscopy allow for direct visualization during diagnostic investigation of the upper and lower GI tract; biopsy and minor surgeries can be accomplished during either procedure.
- Chronic inflammatory diseases of the bowel, such as Crohn's disease and ulcerative colitis, cause diarrhea with episodes of cramping and blood in the stools.
- Gastroenteritis, sometimes called traveler's diarrhea, has numerous possible causes and varies greatly in severity.
- Mechanical obstructions of the bowel include tumors, strictures, hernias, volvulus, intussusception, and other obstructive conditions; ileus causes a functional obstruction.
- Outpouches (diverticula) of the intestines can become infected (diverticulitis); rarely the condition causes perforation of the intestinal wall, requiring emergency surgical intervention.
- A temporary or permanent colostomy may be necessary after bowel resection surgery.
- Pseudomembranous enterocolitis is related directly to the use of broad-spectrum antibiotics.
- Peritonitis can be a primary infection or secondary to contamination by gastrointestinal secretions or pelvic inflammatory disease.
- A vaccine called HAVRIX is available for hepatitis A; no protective vaccine is available for hepatitis C.
- Cirrhosis of the liver is irreversible liver damage resulting from various causes such as toxins, severe viral hepatitis, and chronic alcoholism; cirrhosis also may be idiopathic.
- Cancer of the liver is usually secondary; the cause of pancreatic cancer is uncertain.

- Colicky pain is experienced in cholecystitis and cholelithiasis; in the latter condition, diagnostic tests reveal stones in the gallbladder or the ducts.
- Chronic pancreatitis causes signs of malabsorption and diabetes mellitus resulting from destruction of pancreatic tissue.
- Malabsorption syndrome, celiac disease, severe food poisoning, and eating disorders can result in the signs and symptoms of malnutrition.
- Successful treatment of obesity relies on patient self-control and proven safe methods of balancing energy intake and energy output.
- Hypervitaminosis toxicity results from any vitamins and nutritional trace elements, but especially the fat-soluble vitamins A and D.

Review Challenge

REVIEW QUESTIONS

1. What are the accessory organs of digestion and their functions?
2. How does malocclusion lead to complications?
3. What problem may result from untreated gingivitis?
4. How would you describe the symptoms of temporomandibular joint (TMJ) disease?
5. What is the difference between an aphthous mouth ulcer and a "cold sore"?
6. What causes gastroesophageal reflux disease? How is it treated?
7. How does *Helicobacter pylori* relate to peptic ulcers and gastritis?
8. What is a serious possible complication of esophageal varices?
9. How are peptic ulcers treated?
10. What is the diagnostic value in (1) an endoscopy and (2) a colonoscopy?
11. Is pain usually the initial symptom of gastric cancer?
12. What is the diagnostic significance of McBurney's point?
13. What is meant by a strangulated hernia?
14. What is the difference between ulcerative colitis and Crohn's disease?
15. What is the goal in treatment of gastroenteritis?
16. What is the difference between a functional and a mechanical intestinal obstruction? Give an example of each.
17. How would you compare the pathology of diverticulosis to diverticulitis?
18. How is colorectal cancer detected?
19. What causes pseudomembranous enterocolitis?
20. If a person has peritonitis, what serious complications may occur?
21. What are the signs and symptoms of cirrhosis of the liver?
22. How do hepatitis A and hepatitis C compare in etiology? What are the prevention measures for each disease?
23. What are the presenting symptoms of a patient with (1) biliary colic and (2) acute pancreatitis?
24. What are the causes of pancreatitis?
25. What are some of examples of disorders of nutrition caused by deficiencies and excesses?
26. In what ways do pathogens cause food poisoning?
27. What are two diagnostic criteria for celiac disease?
28. What are the similarities and differences between anorexia nervosa and bulimia?

REAL-LIFE CHALLENGE

Cholelithiasis

A 43-year-old woman is experiencing intermittent colicky-type pain in the right upper quadrant of the abdomen, radiating to the right scapular region. The onset was approximately 1 week ago. In the past few days, she has had nausea and vomiting, increasing in the past 24 hours. The pain is more severe today, and the emesis is bile colored. Vital signs are T — 99.6°, P — 96, R — 26, BP — 144/92. Her skin is warm and dry, slightly jaundiced. The patient is somewhat obese and has been on oral contraceptives for 15 years.

Cholelithiasis is suspected. A CT scan of the gallbladder confirms the presence of stones in the gallbladder and also in the common bile duct. Serum bilirubin is elevated. The patient is scheduled for laparoscopic surgery.

Questions

1. When would a patient with gallstones be asymptomatic?
2. How do gallstones develop?
3. Which type of individual would be most likely to develop gallstones?
4. Which diagnostic imaging studies would be ordered when gallstones are suspected?
5. Which blood studies would be ordered when gallstones are suspected?
6. What is the usual treatment for asymptomatic gallstones?
7. What is the treatment for symptomatic gallstones?
8. What is the difference between cholelithiasis and cholecystitis?

REAL-LIFE CHALLENGE

Ulcers

A 50-year-old man is experiencing midepigastric pain and heartburn along with nausea and vomiting, onset approximately 1 week ago. Patient states that the pain is better immediately after eating but more severe 2 hours after eating. The patient is observed sitting slightly bent over with knees drawn up. Vital signs are T — 99.8°, P — 104, R — 24, BP — 136/88. His skin is warm, dry, and pale. The physician suspects a duodenal ulcer. The abdomen is slightly distended, tender to palpation.

Diagnostic investigation includes Hb, Hct, gastric analysis, stool examination for occult blood, upper GI series, and a gastroscopy. Drug therapy includes antacid, histamine$_2$ blockers, and an antibiotic. The patient is instructed to adhere to a bland diet, including small and more frequent meals.

Questions

1. What population is most prone to develop ulcers?
2. Compare gastric, duodenal, and peptic ulcers.
3. Why would symptoms of gastric and duodenal ulcer vary?
4. Discuss theories of cause of ulcers. Include stress versus ulcerogenic drugs versus bacterial origin.
5. What warnings should be given to patients taking NSAIDs?
6. Explain the complications of perforation.
7. Discuss the various forms of drug therapy available to treat ulcers.
8. What side effects might a patient on histamine$_2$ blockers experience?
9. What would a positive guaiac test result indicate?

RESOURCES

American Celiac Society
cdf@celiac.org
(http://www.primenet.com/cdf)

American Anorexia/Bulimia Association
16J W 46th St, Suite 1108
New York, NY 10036
973-325-8837
(http://www.4woman/org)

National Association of Anorexia Nervosa and Associated Diseases
Box 7
Highland Park, IL 60035
847-831-3438

American Dental Association
211 E Chicago Ave
Chicago, IL 60611
312-440-2500
(http://www.ada.org)

American Liver Foundation
75 Maiden L, Ste 603
New York, NY 10038
1-800-GO-LIVER (465-4837)
(http://www.gi.ucsf.edu/alf)

American Society for Gastrointestinal Endoscopy
13 Elm St
Manchester, MA 01944-1314
978-526-8330
asge@shore.net

National Institute of Dental Craniofacial Research
9000 Rockville Pike, 31 Center Dr MSC
Building 31, 2C39
Bethesda, MD 20892-2290
(http://www.nidcr.nih.gov)

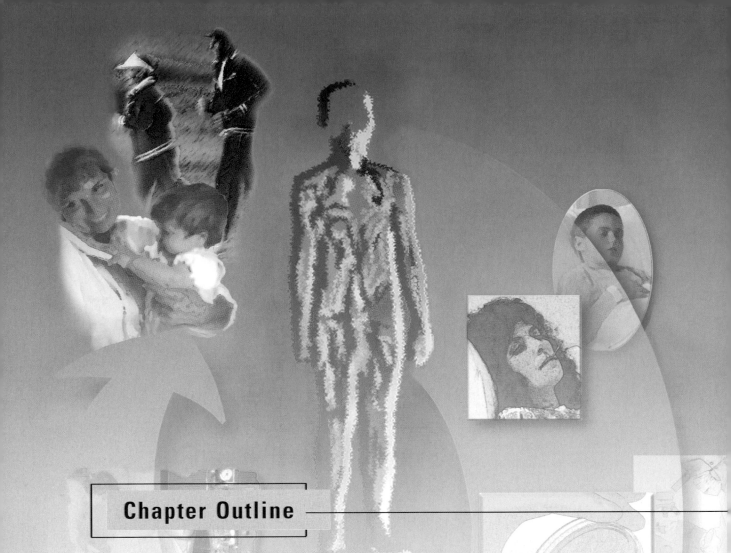

Chapter Outline

Diseases and Conditions of the Respiratory System

1. Explain the process of respiration.
2. Discuss the causes and medical treatment for (a) the common cold, (b) sinusitis, and (c) pharyngitis.
3. Name the treatment of choice for nasal polyps.
4. Comment on the prognosis of cancer of the larynx.
5. Define atelectasis and discuss some possible causes.
6. Name some systemic disorders that might cause epistaxis.
7. Compare the clinical picture of a patient with (a) pulmonary embolism and one with (b) pneumonia.
8. List some possible causes of pulmonary abscess.
9. Compare legionellosis with Pontiac fever.
10. Explain who is at greatest risk for (a) respiratory syncytial virus pneumonia and (b) histoplasmosis.
11. List the groups recommended for prophylactic use of influenza vaccines.
12. Contrast the pathologic course of acute bronchitis with that of chronic bronchitis.
13. Compare the pathology involved in bronchiectasis with that of pulmonary emphysema.
14. Name and describe three causes of pneumoconiosis.
15. Explain the difference between pneumothorax and hemothorax.
16. Describe the presenting symptoms of pleurisy.
17. Discuss contributing factors to and concern about the rising prevalence of pulmonary tuberculosis.
18. Describe the clinical course of infectious mononucleosis.
19. Explain the pathologic changes of the lungs in adult respiratory distress syndrome (ARDS).
20. Name the leading cause of cancer deaths in the United States.

Key Terms

anosmia	(an–**OZ**–me–ah)	lymphadenitis	(limf–**ad**–eh–**NIGH**–tis)
anthracosis	(an–thrah–**KOE**–sis)		
aphonia	(ah–**FOE**–nee–ah)	lymphadenopathy	(limf–**ad**–eh–**NOP**–ah–thee)
asbestosis	(as–beh–**STOH**–sis)		
aspiration	(as–pih–**RAY**–shun)	pneumoconiosis	(**nu**–moh–koh–nee–**OH**–sis)
circumoral cyanosis	(sir–kum–**OH**–ral sigh–an–**OH**–sis)	rhonchi	(**RONG**–ki)
dysphonia	(dis–**FOE**–nee–ah)	silicosis	(sill–ih–**KO**–sis)
epistaxis	(**ep**–ih–**STAK**–sis)	sinusotomy	(sigh–nus–**OT**–oh–me)
exsanguination	(eck–**sang**–win–**AY**–shun)	stridor	(**STRY**–dor)
		syncytial virus	(sin–**SIGH**–shal virus)
hemoptysis	(he–**MOP**–tih–sis)	tachypnea	(**tach**–ip–**NEE**–ah)
laryngectomy	(lar–in–**JECK**–toh–me)	thoracentesis	(**tho**–rah–sen–**TEE**–sis)

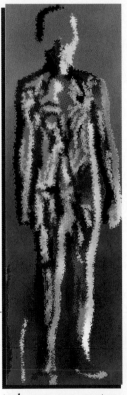

Orderly Function of the Respiratory System

The primary function of the lungs is respiration (Fig. 9-1). Respiration maintains life by supplying oxygen to cells and allowing for the removal of carbon dioxide (a waste product of metabolism). This process is dependent on ventilation (the bellows-like action of the chest) and healthy pulmonary tissue that is adequately perfused with blood. The central nervous system controls breathing in the medulla oblongata and pons. Pulmonary circulation is composed of pulmonary arteries that carry venous blood from the heart; pulmonary capillaries in which gas exchange occurs; and pulmonary veins, which return the freshly oxygenated blood to the heart for systemic circulation. Lung tissue itself is supplied with oxygen and nutrients by blood supply from the bronchial arteries.

The lungs also have a major metabolic function: the maintenance of acid–base (pH) balance of the blood. Lack of oxygen with hypercapnia (increased carbon dioxide in the blood) causes respiratory acidosis; hyperventilation may produce hypocapnia (a decreased amount of carbon dioxide in the blood), causing respiratory alkalosis. In both conditions, arterial blood gases are abnormal.

In the lungs, oxygen inhaled from the air is exchanged with carbon dioxide from the blood; this process is called external respiration. Internal respiration refers to the exchange of gases between the blood and tissue cells. Carbon dioxide then is exhaled as a waste product. Inhaled and exhaled air passes through the respiratory tract, which includes the nose, pharynx, larynx, and trachea (Fig. 9-2).

In the chest, the trachea **bifurcates** into the

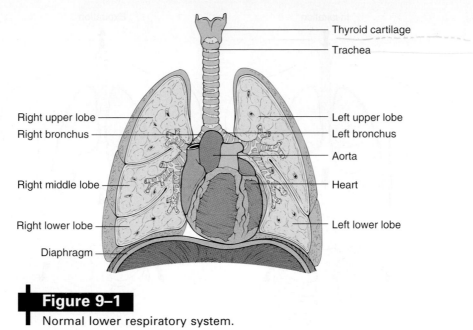

	Thyroid cartilage
	Trachea
Right upper lobe	Left upper lobe
Right bronchus	Left bronchus
	Aorta
Right middle lobe	Heart
Right lower lobe	Left lower lobe
Diaphragm	

Figure 9–1

Normal lower respiratory system.

bronchi. Each bronchus enters a lung, where it further divides into increasingly smaller air passages called bronchioles. At the end of each bronchiole is a sac-like cavity called an alveolus. There are approximately 300 million alveoli in each lung. The vital exchange of carbon dioxide for oxygen takes place through minute blood vessels in each alveolus.

A muscular, dome-shaped partition called the diaphragm attaches to the lower ribs and sepa-

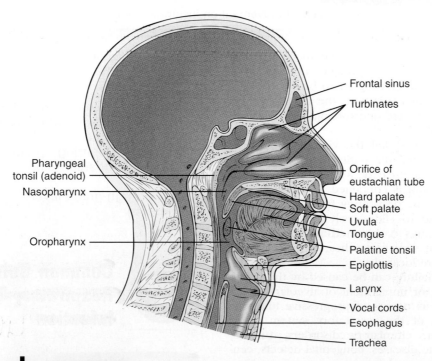

	Frontal sinus
	Turbinates
Pharyngeal tonsil (adenoid)	Orifice of eustachian tube
Nasopharynx	Hard palate
	Soft palate
	Uvula
	Tongue
Oropharynx	Palatine tonsil
	Epiglottis
	Larynx
	Vocal cords
	Esophagus
	Trachea

Figure 9–2

Normal upper respiratory system.

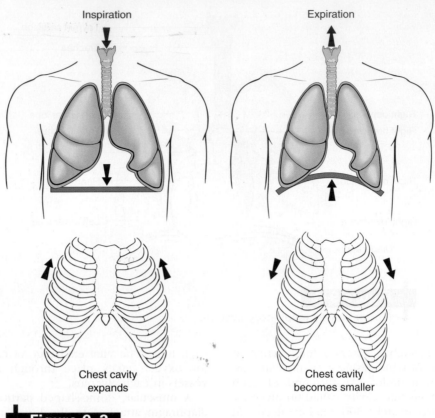

Inspiration

Expiration

Chest cavity
expands

Chest cavity
becomes smaller

Figure 9–3

Diaphragm and chest movement on inspiration and expiration.

rates the thoracic cavity from the abdominal cavity. On inspiration, the diaphragm contracts, pulling downward and causing air to be sucked into the lungs. During expiration, the diaphragm relaxes, pushing upward and forcing air out of the lungs (Fig. 9-3).

The membrane called the visceral pleura encases the lungs, and the parietal pleura lines the inside of the pleural cavity. Approximately 5 to 6 ml of pleural fluid is contained in the space between the pleurae, preventing friction and allowing the pleurae to slide easily on each other. Between the lungs is the **mediastinum,** where the heart, great vessels, trachea, esophagus, and lymph nodes are located.

Respiratory failure can be caused by the inability to ventilate or impairment of alveolar–arterial gas exchange, as occurs in progressive lung disease. Diseases of the respiratory system result from infection, circulatory disorders, tumors, trauma, immune diseases, congenital defects, central nervous system damage or diseases, or environmental conditions.

Chief symptoms indicating respiratory tract disorders that should receive medical attention include:

➲ Chest pain
➲ Dyspnea (difficulty in breathing)
➲ Productive or nonproductive cough that is acute or chronic
➲ Hemoptysis (spitting up blood)
➲ Dysphonia (hoarseness)
➲ Chills
➲ Low- or high-grade fever
➲ Wheezing
➲ Fatigue

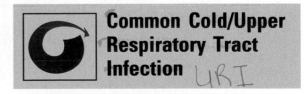

Common Cold/Upper Respiratory Tract Infection URI

SYMPTOMS AND SIGNS

The common cold, also referred to as an upper respiratory tract infection (URI), is an acute inflammatory process affecting the mucous membrane that lines the upper respiratory tract. Although the common, or "head," cold is confined to the nose and pharynx, the same viruses can infect the larynx (see Laryngitis) and the lungs (see Acute and Chronic Bronchitis). The symptoms of a cold, to some extent, depend on which virus is responsible and include nasal congestion and discharge, sneezing, watering eyes, sore throat, hoarseness of the voice, and coughing. When this highly contagious inflammatory process first begins, the nasal discharge is usually clear and thin. As the cold progresses, the discharge becomes greenish yellow and thick. **Cephalalgia,** a slight fever, and chills often accompany a cold. A high fever and **malaise,** however, are more likely to be symptoms of influenza (see Influenza).

ETIOLOGY

The common cold is a group of minor illnesses that can be caused by almost 200 different viruses. Rhinoviruses cause about one half of colds in adults. (Some colds may result from **mycoplasma,** also transmitted by airborne respiratory droplets.) These viral infections sometimes are followed by bacterial infections of the pharynx, middle ear (see Otitis Media in Chapter 5), sinuses, larynx, or lungs.

DIAGNOSIS

Diagnosis is made from the symptoms described by the patient. To rule out more serious disease, cultures of the nasal discharge and sputum, along with a complete blood count (CBC), may be needed.

TREATMENT

An ordinary cold should clear up in 3 or 4 days, and a bacterial infection should resolve in no longer than a week. Nasal congestion may persist for an indefinite period. There is no cure for a cold. Resting, drinking plenty of fluids, using a vaporizer, and taking over-the-counter cold tablets, cough syrups, and aspirin can give temporary relief. The advantage of oral antihistamines in colds is controversial. Antibiotics are of little value in viral infections; however, patients with recurring attacks of bronchitis (see Acute and Chronic Bronchitis) or frequent middle ear infections may receive some protection against these bacteria-caused complications.

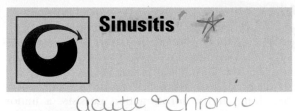

Sinusitis

Acute & Chronic

SYMPTOMS AND SIGNS

The sinuses, cavities in the bones lying behind the nose, are normally air filled. Sinusitis is inflammation of the mucous membranes of the paranasal sinuses. The frontal sinuses (located in the forehead above the eyes) and the maxillary sinuses (located under the maxillary bones in the face) are the most commonly involved sinuses. When the frontal sinuses are affected, headache is common over one or both eyes, especially on waking up in the morning. Pain and tenderness, presenting just above the eyes and occurring when bending over, are also common symptoms. Pain in the cheeks and upper teeth is a symptom of sinusitis affecting the maxillary sinuses. If drainage is present, it is a thick and greenish yellow mucopurulent discharge. The course of acute sinusitis is 3 to 4 weeks.

ETIOLOGY

Sinusitis can be caused by either viral or, more commonly, bacterial infections that travel to the sinuses from the nose, often after a common cold. This occurs easily because the mucous membranes of the nasal cavity extend into and line the sinuses. One is predisposed to sinusitis by any condition that blocks sinus drainage and ventilation (e.g., a deviated nasal septum). Sinusitis also may result from swimming or diving, tooth extractions, or tooth **abscess,** as well as nasal allergies. The cause of chronic sinusitis may never be determined; however, common variable immunodeficiency disease may be involved (see Chapter 3).

DIAGNOSIS

The diagnosis of sinusitis is made by a physical examination, the patient history, sinus radiographic studies and endoscopic sinuscopy. Sinuses that are air filled appear as dark patches on a radiographic film, whereas fluid-filled sinuses appear as white areas. Bedside transillumination can suggest the presence of sinusitis. Additionally, a specimen of nasal secretions may be taken for culture to identify or rule out bacterial agents.

261

TREATMENT

Treatment consists of the use of a broad-spectrum antibiotic, decongestants, and antihistamines. Decongestants work by shrinking the swollen mucous membranes and drying up the drainage. This widens the airway and eases breathing. If the inflammation persists, a minor surgery called sinusotomy may be advised by the physician. With the patient under local anesthesia, the physician pierces the maxillary sinus, allowing drainage and relief of pressure. The physician often instills sterile water into the sinus to flush out any residual material. Analgesics usually are given for pain relief.

Pharyngitis

SYMPTOMS AND SIGNS

Pharyngitis, inflammation of the pharynx, may be acute or chronic. A sore throat with dryness, a burning sensation, or the sensation of a lump in the throat is common. Chills, fever, **dysphonia, dysphagia,** and cervical **lymphadenopathy** are frequent. The mucosa of the pharynx is red and swollen.

ETIOLOGY

The most frequent cause of pharyngitis is a viral infection. In children, it is often an extension of a bacterial streptococcal infection from the tonsils, adenoids, nose, or sinuses. Persistent infection, or chronic pharyngitis, occurs when an infection (respiratory, sinus, or oral disease) spreads to the pharynx and remains. Acute pharyngitis may be secondary to systemic viral infections, such as chickenpox and measles, whereas chronic pharyngitis may accompany diseases such as syphilis and tuberculosis. Pharyngitis also can be caused by irritation and inflammation without infection. Occasionally, inhalation or swallowing of irritating substances, such as tobacco smoke and alcohol, is responsible for trauma to the mucous membranes of the pharynx, as are heat, chemical irritants, and sharp objects.

DIAGNOSIS

Physical examination usually shows red, swollen mucous membranes. This, along with the patient history, is usually sufficient for the diagnosis of acute pharyngitis. For chronic pharyngitis, the physician needs to identify and locate the primary source of the infection or irritation. Further examination of the nasopharyngeal area, a CBC, and sinus radiographic films may be necessary.

TREATMENT

Home treatment using lozenges, mouthwashes, salt water gargles, an ice collar, and aspirin may be helpful for viral infections. If symptoms persist for longer than a few days, a physician should be consulted. Acute bacterial infections necessitate systemic administration of antibiotics or sulfonamides. Chronic tonsillitis, adenoiditis, and adenoid **hypertrophy** may be treated by surgical excision. Bed rest and copious amounts of fluids may be advised.

Laryngitis

SYMPTOMS AND SIGNS

Inflammation of the larynx, including the vocal cords, is called laryngitis. Because the opening of the larynx is narrow, the inflammation sometimes interferes with breathing. Symptoms vary with the severity of the inflammation, but the main symptom of laryngitis is hoarseness, which causes **aphonia.** Fever, malaise, a painful throat, dysphagia, and other symptoms associated with influenza occur in more severe infections.

ETIOLOGY

The cause of laryngitis can be either viral or bacterial infection, and the condition can be either chronic or acute. URIs such as the common cold, tonsillitis, pharyngitis, and sinusitis are the most frequent causes of inflammation of the larynx. Laryngitis also occurs with bronchitis, pertussis, influenza, pneumonia, measles, mononucleosis, diphtheria, syphilis, and tuberculosis. Occasionally, laryngitis is caused by irritation without infection. Inclement weather, tobacco smoke, drinking alcohol, inhalation of irritating materials, and excessive use of the voice are all predisposing factors, especially in chronic laryngitis.

DIAGNOSIS

Laryngoscopic examination reveals mildly or highly inflamed mucosa, and vocal cord movement may be limited. If there is no inflammation, laryngitis is not the cause, and further diagnostic tests are needed to determine the underlying condition.

TREATMENT

Treatment of viral laryngitis includes the following palliative measures: absolute voice rest, bed rest in a well-humidified room, liberal fluid intake, no tobacco or alcohol consumption, and the use of lozenges and cough syrup. Improvement should be seen in 4 or 5 days. Antibiotic administration gives good results when laryngitis occurs in the course of another disease. When hoarseness persists for longer than 1 week, the condition may be chronic. Treatment of chronic laryngitis is based on elimination, as much as possible, of the causative factors.

Deviated Septum

SYMPTOMS AND SIGNS

A crooked nasal septum, the cartilage partition between the nostrils, is called a deviated septum. Deviated septum causes narrowing and obstruction of the air passage, making breathing somewhat difficult. Other than mild breathing problems or a slightly increased tendency to develop sinusitis, there are no significant symptoms associated with a deviated septum. The nose can appear normal on the exterior, with the deviation visible only on examination with a nasal speculum.

ETIOLOGY

Congenital anomaly is usually the cause of minor deviation of the septum. Substantial septal deviation is uncommon and is usually the result of trauma to the nose.

DIAGNOSIS

A deviated septum may or may not be visible without the aid of a nasal speculum. The patient history and the amount of obstruction aid the physician in the diagnosis and treatment of this condition.

TREATMENT

Treatment is not usually necessary unless compromise of the air passage is noted. The septum can be straightened surgically for significant obstruction or for cosmetic reasons. Straightening a deviated septum involves removing the cartilage.

Once removed, the cartilage can be reshaped and repositioned in the nose, if needed, to maintain the nasal structure.

Nasal Polyps

SYMPTOMS AND SIGNS

Nasal polyps are growths that form from distended mucous membranes protruding into the nasal cavity. They are not harmful but can be large enough to obstruct the nasal airway, making breathing difficult. Polyps often affect or impair the sense of smell (see Anosmia). When polyps obstruct one of the sinuses, symptoms of sinusitis (see Sinusitis) are present.

ETIOLOGY

Polyps are caused by the overproduction of fluid in the cells of the mucous membrane. This overproduction is frequently the result of a condition called allergic rhinitis. Some aspirin-sensitive persons have the triad of nasal polyps, asthma, and urticaria (hives).

DIAGNOSIS

The physician examines the inside of the nose using an instrument called a nasal speculum. Polyps appear as pearly gray lumps along the nasal passage.

TREATMENT

Surgical removal is the treatment of choice; however, considerable relief may be obtained through the injection of a steroid directly into the polyps. This procedure is repeated at 5- to 7-day intervals until relief is obtained. Removal of polyps is a minor procedure necessitating a local **anesthetic.** When the lining of the sinus also must be removed, a general anesthetic is used.

Anosmia

SYMPTOMS AND SIGNS

The loss of smell that continues without an obvious cause is termed anosmia. The ability to taste liquids and food also is impaired or lost.

ETIOLOGY

A chronic condition, such as nasal polyps and allergic rhinitis, is the most common cause of anosmia. It may, however, be the result of damage to the olfactory nerves from head injury or, rarely, a symptom of a brain tumor.

DIAGNOSIS

If on examination the physician does not find any physical abnormality, or the patient history does not reveal recent head trauma or an allergic condition, a neurologist may be consulted for diagnostic tests.

TREATMENT

Treatment is aimed at the cause of the condition. When polyps are found, they are removed. Damage to the nerves may or may not be able to be corrected. For allergic rhinitis, a series of injections containing increasingly stronger concentrations of the **allergen** is used to desensitize the patient.

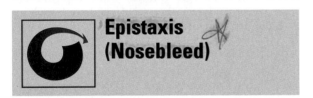

Epistaxis (Nosebleed)

SYMPTOMS AND SIGNS

Hemorrhage from the nose, known as **epistaxis,** is a common, sudden emergency. It usually occurs from only one nostril, and there is no apparent explanation for the bleeding. Nosebleeds are seldom cause for concern. They are unlikely to be a symptom of any other disorders, unless injury has occurred or associated serious systemic conditions are present. Epistaxis is more common in children than in adults.

ETIOLOGY

Common causes of epistaxis are colds and infections such as rhinitis, sinusitis, and nasopharyngitis, which cause crusting that damages the mucous membrane lining the nose. Direct trauma to the nose and the presence of a foreign body are the most frequent causes of epistaxis. Nasal hemorrhage has been encountered in many systemic disorders, such as measles, scarlet fever, pertussis, rheumatic fever, hypertension, conges-

tive heart failure, and chronic renal disease. Epistaxis may be the foremost symptom of conditions such as hemophilia, **thrombocytopenia, agranulocytosis,** and leukemia. An infrequent cause of epistaxis is extensive hepatic disease.

DIAGNOSIS

The diagnosis of epistaxis is made on the patient history of how frequent the nosebleeds are, whether an injury has occurred, or whether the symptoms indicate that systemic disease may be present.

TREATMENT

Specific treatment of the underlying disease, if present, is of prime importance. Mild hemorrhage may be controlled by applying direct pressure on either side of the bridge of the nose for 5 to 10 minutes. If bleeding continues, a posterior nasal packing may be necessary. The packing should be removed within 24 hours to prevent infection. A mild sclerosing agent also may be injected into a bleeding vessel if it can be visualized by the physician.

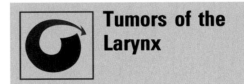

Tumors of the Larynx

SYMPTOMS AND SIGNS

Growths or tumors on the larynx may be either benign or malignant. Dysphonia is usually the only symptom of a tumor on the larynx. There are no influenza-like symptoms as with laryngitis (see Laryngitis), but when the tumor is malignant, dysphagia may be experienced. In children with tumors, a high-pitched crowing sound called **stridor** is present because of their small airway. Hoarseness caused by a benign tumor is usually intermittent, whereas that due to cancer is continuous and gradually becomes worse. Neither type of laryngeal tumor is common, but malignant tumors are slightly more common and affect men more often than women.

ETIOLOGY

There are two types of benign tumors: papillomas, which usually appear as multiples, and polyps, which usually appear singly (Fig. 9–4). These tumors are caused by misuse or overuse of

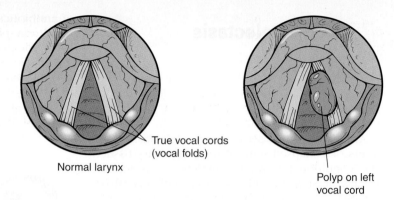

True vocal cords
(vocal folds)

Normal larynx

Polyp on left
vocal cord

Figure 9–4
Vocal cord polyp.

the vocal cords. Malignant tumors occur more often in heavy tobacco users.

DIAGNOSIS

The physician or otolaryngologist thoroughly examines the larynx and vocal cords. When a tumor or tumors are found, a **biopsy** is done to determine whether a malignancy is present. Cancer of the larynx almost always can be cured if it is diagnosed early.

TREATMENT

Benign growths, whether papillomas or polyps, usually are excised under local anesthesia. Malignant tumors, if discovered early, often are treated and cured by radiation therapy. When the cancer has **metastasized,** a laryngectomy may be needed. After a laryngectomy, the patient needs extensive speech therapy to learn a substitute form of speech.

Hemoptysis

SYMPTOMS AND SIGNS

Hemoptysis, the coughing or spitting up of blood from the respiratory tract, can be slight or it can indicate a serious underlying condition. The patient coughs up bright or dark blood–streaked sputum from the pulmonary or bronchial circulation.

ETIOLOGY

Trauma, erosion of a vessel, calcification, or tumors can cause bronchial bleeding, as can bronchitis or bronchiectasis. Venous hypertension and left-sided heart failure precipitate bleeding from pulmonary vessels. Additional origins of the bleeding are fungal infections, pulmonary **infarcts,** tumors or **ulcerations** of the larynx or pharynx, and **coagulation** (clotting) defects. Figures may vary; however, in approximately 75% of cases, hemoptysis is not a sign of serious disease.

DIAGNOSIS

Of primary importance is the determination of the source of the bleeding. This is accomplished by visual examination of the mouth and nasopharynx; visualization of the larynx, trachea, and bronchi by **endoscopy;** and inspection of the lung fields by radiographic studies. Coagulation studies of the blood ascertain whether the problem is a clotting deficiency. A lung scan and a pulmonary angiogram may be indicated if previously mentioned investigations are inconclusive.

TREATMENT

After the location and the cause of the bleeding are determined, the source is treated. When the bleeding is severe, ligation or surgical removal or repair of the involved vessels is indicated. Measures are implemented to prevent asphyxiation by clotted blood in the air passages; to prevent obstruction of the bronchial tree by clots, with resulting lung collapse; and to prevent **exsanguination** of the patient. Steps are taken to allay fear and anxiety that the patient might experience. Patients are encouraged to cough to remove blood from the lungs. Postural drainage and inhalation of warm, moist air are beneficial. When bleeding results from an infection (e.g., tuberculosis), the infection is treated with antimicrobial agents.

Atelectasis

SYMPTOMS AND SIGNS

Although not a disease entity, atelectasis is an airless or collapsed state of the pulmonary tissue. The condition follows incomplete expansion of lobules or segments of the lung, with partial or complete collapse of the lung. Atelectasis results in **hypoxia,** causing the patient to experience dyspnea. When only a small segment of the lung is involved, dyspnea may be the only clinical symptom. When a large area of the pulmonary tissue is involved, there is a decreased area for gas exchange and the dyspnea becomes severe. Additionally, the patient experiences anxiety, **diaphoresis, tachycardia, substernal retraction,** and **cyanosis.** Atelectasis also can occur with incomplete expansion of the lungs at birth.

ETIOLOGY

Atelectasis is caused by an obstruction in the bronchial tree by a mucous plug, foreign body, bronchogenic cancer, or inflammatory pulmonary disease. Any condition that makes deep breathing difficult can lead to atelectasis. Failure to deep breathe postoperatively or prolonged inactivity also can induce the collapse of pulmonary tissue. In the newborn, causes include prematurity, **hyaline membrane** disease, decreased stimulus to breathe, narcotics that cross the placental barrier during labor, and obstruction of the bronchus by a mucous plug.

DIAGNOSIS

Radiographic chest films, a thorough history, and physical examination play important roles in the diagnosis. Lung scans may be necessary to detect subtle changes. Breath sounds are diminished over the affected area, and percussion is dull. **Bronchoscopy** may be indicated to evaluate obstruction by a foreign body or a neoplasm.

TREATMENT

Because postoperative patients are at high risk for atelectasis, they are encouraged to deep breathe and cough periodically. Other therapeutic measures include suctioning of the airway to remove any obstruction, spirometry, and the use

of antibiotics to treat accompanying infection. Intermittent positive pressure breathing (IPPB) ensures adequate lung expansion. When atelectasis is chronic, surgical removal of the affected area may be necessary. Suctioning the trachea of the newborn is indicated to remove mucus and to facilitate a patent airway. Suctioning usually is followed by the administration of oxygen.

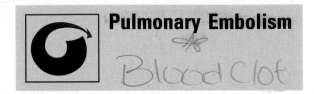

Pulmonary Embolism

SYMPTOMS AND SIGNS

A pulmonary embolism occurs when a clot of foreign material lodges in and occludes an artery in the pulmonary circulation (Fig. 9–5). The size and location of the embolism, coupled with the general physical condition of the patient, determine the consequences of the interruption of blood supply to the area and the resulting symptoms and signs. The symptoms do not appear until the embolism has lodged in an artery and interrupts the blood flow. Apprehension is common. The patient with a small, uncomplicated embolism experiences a cough, chest pain, and a low-grade fever. The patient with a more extensive infarction experiences dyspnea, **tachypnea**

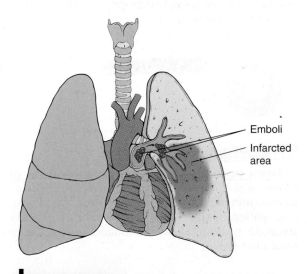

Figure 9–5
Pulmonary embolism.

266

(with a respiratory rate of at least 20 breaths per minute), chest pain, and occasionally hemoptysis. Massive embolism leads to the sudden onset of cyanosis, shock, and death.

ETIOLOGY

Although most **emboli** are thrombi (blood clots) that have broken loose from a deep vein in the legs or pelvis, other emboli may be composed of air, fat globules, a small piece of tissue, or a cluster of bacteria. The mass moves through the venous circulation and is pumped by the right side of the heart to the pulmonary circulation, where it becomes lodged in a vessel, usually at a division of an artery where it narrows.

Stasis of blood flow from immobility, injury to a vessel, predisposition to clot formation, cardiovascular disease, or pulmonary disease increases the risk of embolism formation. In pregnancy, multiple factors predispose individuals to venous thrombosis.

DIAGNOSIS

The clinical picture, along with a history of immobility or other risk factors, leads to further investigation of respiratory status. Radiographic chest films, lung scans, and **magnetic resonance imaging (MRI)** scans are used to image the lung fields. Pulmonary angiography is the definitive method of making the diagnosis. **Auscultation** often reveals **rales** and pleural rub in the area of the embolism. Arterial blood gas determination shows reduced partial pressure of oxygen and carbon dioxide. Studies to find residual thrombi in the veins of the lower extremities are helpful in deciding whether to use anticoagulants.

TREATMENT

Primary treatment is aimed at preventing a potentially fatal episode and maintaining cardiopulmonary integrity and adequate ventilation and **perfusion.** Oxygen therapy and **anticoagulant** administration are used to meet these goals. Heparin is the anticoagulant drug of choice in most cases. Additionally, thrombolytic drugs sometimes are administered to dissolve a clot.

Prevention is important; therefore, persons with cardiovascular disease and those who are immobile should be observed for early signs of any clot formation. Early ambulation and the use of thromboembolic disease (TED) stockings, or antiembolism stockings, are employed as preventive measures for patients who have had surgery.

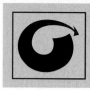

Pneumonia

SYMPTOMS AND SIGNS

Pneumonia is not only a condition but also a general term for several types of inflammation of the lungs. The inflammation may be either unilateral or bilateral and involve all or only a portion of an infected lung (Fig. 9-6). The symptoms of pneumonia vary. The patient may have a cough, fever, shortness of breath while at rest, chills, sweating, chest pains, cyanosis, and blood in the sputum. The larger the area of lung affected, the more severe the symptoms are. How quickly the symptoms develop and which symptoms are most evident vary with the cause.

Aspiration pneumonia results from aspiration of liquids, or other material, into the tracheobronchial tree. It tends to occur in patients who have serious problems with swallowing; among these are people afflicted with cancer or stroke. *Older people -gereactrics*

ETIOLOGY

Pneumonia usually is caused by viral or bacterial infections. Organisms commonly causing bacterial pneumonia are pneumococci, staphylococci, group A **hemolytic** streptococci, *Klebsiella pneumoniae* types 1 and 2, and other gram-negative organisms or *Legionella* (legionnaires' disease organism), *Haemophilus influen-*

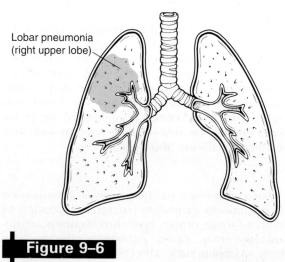

Lobar pneumonia
(right upper lobe)

Figure 9-6
Pneumonia.

zae type B, and *Francisella tularensis.* Viruses such as adenoviruses, influenza viruses, and respiratory syncytial viruses also can produce pneumonia. It also may be caused by damage to the lungs from inhalation of a poisonous gas such as chlorine or by aspiration of foreign matter. The pneumonia can range from a mild complication of URI to a life-threatening illness. Bacterial pneumonia can be community acquired (nosocomial). The severely or chronically ill are more predisposed. Pneumonia is the fifth leading cause of death in the United States.

DIAGNOSIS

Physical examination, the patient history, and a determination of smoking and drinking habits may be all that is necessary for the diagnosis. Further tests such as radiographic chest studies and sputum and blood cultures also are done.

TREATMENT

Treatment is based on the underlying cause of the pneumonia. Organism-specific antibiotics are prescribed for bacterial pneumonia. Penicillin is the drug of choice for a pneumococcal pneumonia. Tetracycline drugs, erythromycin, and sulfonamides may be administered. The use of **analgesics** such as aspirin helps to relieve chest pain, and oxygen therapy may be necessary for shortness of breath. Bed rest, increased fluid intake, a high-calorie diet, and postural drainage also prove beneficial.

PULMONARY ABSCESS

SYMPTOMS AND SIGNS

An area of contained infectious material in the lung is known as a pulmonary abscess (Fig. 9–7). Abscesses are more common in the lower portions of the lungs and in the right lung because of its more vertical bronchus. The main symptoms are alternating chills and fever. Chest pain and a productive cough accompanied by **purulent,** bloody, or foul-smelling sputum and foul-smelling breath are also present.

ETIOLOGY

Lung abscesses are frequently a complication of pneumonia caused by bacteria. Aspiration of food, a foreign object, bronchial **stenosis,** or **neoplasms** may cause pulmonary abscesses to form. A pulmonary abscess also may develop when a septic embolism is carried to the lung via the pulmonary circulation.

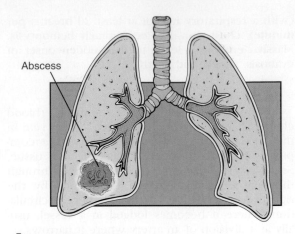

Figure 9–7
Pulmonary abscess.

DIAGNOSIS

Decreased breath sounds are revealed on chest auscultation. The patient history may indicate recent aspiration. A radiographic chest film is necessary to locate the site of the affected portion of the lung. Blood and sputum cultures are used to detect the causative organism.

TREATMENT

The treatment of choice for an abscess is the use of antibiotics for a fairly long duration or until the abscess is gone. Surgical resection of the abscess and a portion of the affected lung may be required if the antibiotic therapy is not successful.

LEGIONELLOSIS (LEGIONNAIRES' DISEASE AND PONTIAC FEVER)

SYMPTOMS AND SIGNS

Legionellosis, an infection caused by the bacterium *Legionella pneumophila,* can evolve in two different forms, the more severe legionnaires' disease and the milder form, Pontiac fever. Legionnaires' disease, an acute respiratory tract infection producing severe pneumonia-like symptoms or possibly fatal pneumonia, was named after an epidemic outbreak at an American Legion convention in Philadelphia in July 1976. More than 200 people became ill, and 34 died of the disease.

Typical symptoms include general malaise, headache, and cough. These are followed rapidly by the onset of chills, fever, chest pain, dyspnea, **myalgia,** vomiting, diarrhea, and **anorexia.** The symptoms often mimic those of pneumonia. The incubation period for legionnaires' disease is 2 to 10 days, usually about 1 week. Pontiac fever's symptoms are less severe and include a high fever and muscle aches, with a duration of 2 to 5 days. The incubation period of Pontiac fever is much shorter, a few hours to 2 days.

ETIOLOGY

Both disorders are caused by *L. pneumophila* and are not contagious. These bacteria thrive in warm aquatic environments and are inhaled from contaminated aerosolized water droplets. Air conditioning systems, cooling towers, whirlpool spas, showers, and the hot water plumbing of buildings in which the temperature of the water is between 95° and 115°F permit the reproduction of the bacterium. Predisposing factors include smoking, physical debilitation, especially among patients with chronic obstructive pulmonary disease (COPD), immunosuppression, and alcoholism. Pontiac fever usually occurs in otherwise healthy individuals.

DIAGNOSIS

A complete physical examination, along with radiographic chest studies and testing of blood samples, is done. Laboratory analysis of the blood indicates an elevation of the **white blood cell (WBC) count,** liver enzyme level, and **erythrocyte sedimentation rate (ESR).** A culture from the sputum to isolate the legionella bacterium is necessary for confirmation of legionnaires' disease. The detection of the presence of bacteria in a urine sample indicates the disease. Convalescent serum samples to detect antibodies are the best diagnostic tool.

TREATMENT

Typically, antibiotic therapy is initiated before there is a confirmation of the diagnosis because the response to treatment is usually slow. Erythromycin is the antibiotic most frequently used for treatment. Rifampin may be prescribed when the response to erythromycin is not as desired. Oxygen may be used for the dyspnea; **antipyretics, antiemetics,** and analgesics are also helpful.

Pontiac fever usually resolves itself in a few days, requiring no specific treatment.

Legionellosis occurs worldwide. The National Center for Infectious Diseases monitors the incidence of legionellosis in the United States. Attempts are made to identify the sources of the disease transmission, as are recommendations for prevention and control measures. Prevention can be accomplished by appropriate design of facilities in which water may become stagnant. The temperature of the water in cooling towers and air conditioning units must be maintained either below 95°F or above 115°F, or it must have adequate chlorination to kill the legionella bacillus. Monitoring of chlorine content of whirlpool baths and spas is a necessary obligation of the owner.

RESPIRATORY SYNCYTIAL VIRUS PNEUMONIA

SYMPTOMS AND SIGNS

Respiratory syncytial virus (RSV) pneumonia, an inflammatory and infectious condition of the lungs, is most common in infants, young children, and the elderly. RSV causes cold-like symptoms, including nasal congestion, **otitis media,** and coughing, in the mild upper respiratory tract form of infection. As the virus progresses downward to the lower respiratory tract, the patient experiences fever, malaise, lethargy, more frequent coughing, and dyspnea.

ETIOLOGY

Respiratory syncytial virus is the causative agent of RSV pneumonia. The greatest occurrence of these infections is during the winter months, December to March, and they most seriously affect children younger than 3 years of age and the elderly, especially patients whose respiratory systems already are compromised by underlying disease or predisposing factors. At greatest risk are infants who were premature or who have a congenital cardiac defect or a pre-existing pulmonary disorder. Most people have experienced several RSV upper respiratory tract infections in their lifetimes, and most cases of mild RSV infection are self-limiting.

RSV is spread by contact with secretions of an infected person. Thorough hand washing and the use of disposable tissues for nasal secretions can prevent the spread of this disease.

DIAGNOSIS

The clinical picture, a thorough physical examination, and **lavage** of the nasal pharynx aid in the diagnosis of RSV pneumonia. The secretions obtained from the lavage are examined for the presence of RSV. When grown in tissue culture, RSV produces giant syncytial cells. Laboratory confirmation of RSV is helpful for antiviral therapy.

TREATMENT

Most cases of RSV infection involving the upper respiratory tract are self-limiting. Antipyretics are prescribed for fever, and antibiotics are given for otitis media. When the infection invades the lower respiratory tract of an infant or a young child, treatment may involve inhalation therapy. Hospitalization may be required for oxygen therapy and hydration.

HISTOPLASMOSIS

SYMPTOMS AND SIGNS

Histoplasmosis is a fungal disease originating in the lungs that is caused by inhalation of dust containing *Histoplasma capsulatum*. It may cause pneumonia or may become systemic. Many patients with histoplasmosis are **asymptomatic** at onset. As the fungus disseminates throughout the pulmonary tissue, the patient reports dyspnea and loss of energy to the point of incapacitation. The patient becomes febrile. The spleen and lymph nodes become enlarged. In patients with acquired immunodeficiency syndrome (AIDS), histoplasmosis may occur as an opportunistic infection.

ETIOLOGY

Histoplasmosis is caused by the fungus *H. capsulatum*, which is carried by dust and is inhaled. The greatest occurrence of histoplasmosis is in the midwestern United States. Often, the fungus is found in soil contaminated by bird droppings specific to this area, which may be a source of the airborne fungus.

DIAGNOSIS

Diagnosis is made by the clinical picture, a positive skin test result, blood **serologic** findings specific for the fungus, or the identification of the fungus in pus, sputum, or tissue specimens. Radiographic chest films may be normal or may reveal patchy infiltrates and diffuse opacities.

TREATMENT

If the disease is self-limiting, no antifungal therapy is necessary. The antifungal drug amphotericin B is used to treat severe or progressive histoplasmosis.

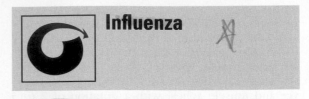

Influenza

SYMPTOMS AND SIGNS

Influenza is a generalized, highly contagious, acute viral disease that occurs in annual outbreaks. It is characterized by inflammation of the upper and lower respiratory tract mucous membranes, a severe protracted cough, fever, headache, sore throat, and generalized malaise. The onset is usually sudden, marked by chills and a feverish feeling. In mild cases, the temperature may reach 101 to 102°F and the fever may last for 2 or 3 days. In severe cases, a 103 to 104°F temperature is possible, lasting 4 or 5 days. Acute symptoms usually subside rapidly with decreasing fever. The weakness, sweating, and fatigue may continue for a few days to a few weeks; malaise may persist several days before full recovery.

Fever, cough, and other respiratory symptoms persisting for longer than 5 days may indicate a secondary bacterial pneumonia. Possible complications of influenza are bronchitis, sinusitis, otitis media, and cervical **lymphadenitis.**

Epidemics can be responsible for substantial morbidity, financial loss, and even death.

ETIOLOGY

Known viruses that cause influenza are designated as types A, B, and C. However, many mutant strains also reproduce in both humans and animals. Acute uncomplicated influenza with recovery is the most frequently encountered type of this disease. Secondary bacterial pneumonia after influenza most often is caused by hemolytic streptococcus, staphylococcus, or pneumococcus.

Influenza may be sporadic or epidemic. Epidemics occur every 1 to 4 years and spread rapidly because the incubation period is only 1 to 3 days. Transmission is by inhalation of the virus in airborne mucus discharge. Fatalities can occur in as short a time as 48 hours after the onset of symptoms.

DIAGNOSIS

Clinically, influenza may be indistinguishable from the common cold. When differentiating influenza from other respiratory tract infections, consideration should be given to the length of onset, the presence of an epidemic, and the severity of the symptoms. Frequent recurrences of influenza-like syndromes may make the physician suspect tuberculosis (see Pulmonary Tuberculosis). A complicating pneumonia may be present if the patient has dyspnea, cyanosis, hemoptysis, or rales in the lungs. A WBC count may indicate **leukopenia** with relative **lymphocytosis.** Confirmation of the influenza diagnosis is made by isolation of the virus from a throat culture. A sputum culture isolates bacteria in secondary infections.

TREATMENT

The **prophylactic** use of vaccines against influenza is effective in reducing the occurrence of the disease, especially for the elderly or infirm (Table 9-1). Because immunity from vaccination lasts only 1 year, annual booster doses are needed for optimal protection. After vaccination, about 2 to 4 weeks is required for immunity to develop. Because vaccines are useless after the disease is established, treatment is symptomatic.

TABLE 9-1 ➤ Target Groups for Influenza Immunization

GROUPS AT INCREASED RISK OF COMPLICATIONS

Persons aged 65 years and older
Residents of nursing homes and other chronic care facilities
Patients with chronic pulmonary (including asthma) or cardiac disorder
Patients with chronic metabolic disease (including diabetes), renal dysfunction, hemoglobinopathies, or immunosuppression
Children and teens receiving long-term aspirin

GROUPS IN CONTACT WITH HIGH-RISK PERSONS

Physicians, nurses, and other health care providers
Employees of nursing homes and chronic care facilities
Providers of home care to high-risk persons
Household members (including children) of high-risk persons

OTHER GROUPS

Providers of essential community services (e.g., police, fire)
International travelers
Students, dormitory residents
Anyone wishing to reduce risk of influenza

Adapted from Advisory Committee on Immunization Practices, Centers for Disease Control and Prevention. MMWR 43(No RR-9):1, 1994. From: Bennett JC, Plum F: Cecil Textbook of Medicine, 20th ed, Vol 1. Philadelphia: WB Saunders, 1996, p 1756. Used with permission.

Bed rest, increased fluid intake, a light diet, and the use of antipyretic and analgesic drugs when needed are helpful. Amantadine, an antiviral agent, sometimes may help to treat influenza. In less severe cases, treatment of respiratory tract symptoms may not be necessary; however, warm salt water gargles, steam inhalation, and the use of cough syrups may be comforting. Antibiotics are effective against bacterial pneumonia and other less serious complications such as sinusitis, otitis media, and lymphadenitis.

Chronic Obstructive Pulmonary Disease

Chronic obstructive pulmonary disease (COPD), or chronic obstructive lung disease (COLD), encompasses several obstructive diseases of the lungs, including chronic bronchitis, bronchiectasis, asthma, emphysema, cystic fibrosis, and pneumoconiosis. Although the mechanism of the obstruction varies, the patient with COPD is unable to ventilate the lungs freely, resulting in an ineffective exchange of respiratory gases. This causes the patient's normal respiratory response to elevated carbon dioxide levels to become diminished.

ACUTE AND CHRONIC BRONCHITIS

SYMPTOMS AND SIGNS

Bronchitis is inflammation of the mucous membrane lining the bronchi. A deep, productive cough is the main symptom. The patient has thick yellow to gray sputum. Other symptoms include shortness of breath, wheezing, a slightly elevated temperature, and pain in the upper chest, which is aggravated by the cough. Acute symptoms subside within a week, but the cough may continue for 2 to 3 weeks. Physical signs within the lungs are few or absent if the bronchitis is uncomplicated. Scattered or occasional rales often are heard on ausculation.

Chronic bronchitis is similar to acute bronchitis, except that the inflammation persists and becomes worse. Mild forms may exist for many years, with only a slight cough in the mornings, and then become aggravated after acute upper respiratory tract infections. As the condition progresses, obstructive and asthmatic symptoms appear, along with dyspnea. Chest expansion becomes diminished, and frequently, scattered rales and wheezing are heard. In the beginning stages of the disease, flare-ups of chronic bronchitis are likely to occur after severe colds or influenza. In later stages, a minor head cold can cause a severe attack. During the final stages, the coughing, shortness of breath, and wheezing occur nearly continuously. Prolonged, recurrent attacks cause gradual deterioration of the lungs.

For both acute and chronic bronchitis, the symptoms appear more troublesome during the winter months. Living or working in a cold, damp environment or in a polluted atmosphere can aggravate the condition.

ETIOLOGY

Acute bronchitis is part of a general URI. It begins after a common cold or other viral infections of the nasopharynx and pharynx or occurs as a complication of bacterial infections. Recurring attacks in adults may indicate a focus of infection, such as chronic sinusitis (see Sinusitis), bronchiectasis (see Bronchiectasis), and pneumonia (see Pneumonia). In children, hypertrophied tonsils and adenoids may be the source of acute bronchitis. Allergens are also frequently predisposing factors.

No single or specific bacterium is responsible for chronic bronchitis; however, in many cases of recurrent infections, *Pneumococcus* or *H. influenzae* has been the main organism. Chronic bronchitis frequently accompanies chronic asthma, pulmonary **fibrosis,** obstructive emphysema, pulmonary tuberculosis, or congestive heart failure. Chronic bronchitis often is associated with the cause of some forms of emphysema.

DIAGNOSIS

Acute or chronic bronchitis can be suspected on the basis of the patient's symptoms and history. The presence of other diseases or their complications must be ruled out, especially if the symptoms are serious or prolonged. Diagnostic tests include radiographic chest studies, pulmonary function tests, and blood and sputum analysis.

TREATMENT

Because acute bronchitis usually is caused by a viral infection, there is no specific treatment, except to relieve the symptoms. Aspirin may be used to control fever. Increased fluid intake, along with the use of a vaporizer and humidifier, helps to clear the nasal passages and bronchi.

The physician may prescribe the use of a bronchodilator aerosol inhaler for wheezing and shortness of breath and a cough suppressant if the chest is sore from coughing. If a secondary bacterial infection is suspected, an antibiotic is prescribed.

The treatment of chronic bronchitis is based on the stage of the disease before consulting professional help. Prompt treatment of acute infections, when they occur, is of primary importance. The patient is advised to give up smoking, to avoid smoke-filled rooms, to stay away from people with colds, and to live in a warm, dry climate.

BRONCHIECTASIS

SYMPTOMS AND SIGNS

Bronchiectasis is the permanent, irreversible dilation or distortion of one or more of the bronchi, resulting from destruction of muscular and elastic portions of the bronchial walls. The condition, which takes many years to develop, is usually bilateral and involves the lower lobes of the lungs. A chronic cough producing large quantities of a purulent, foul-smelling sputum is the main symptom of bronchiectasis. Hemoptysis, dyspnea, wheezing, fever, and general malaise develop as the condition progresses. The patient also may experience chronic halitosis.

ETIOLOGY

Bronchiectasis may be caused by repeated damage to the bronchial wall from heavy smoking. It also can result from pneumonia, tuberculosis, bronchial obstruction, or inhalation of a corrosive gas. This condition is also a frequent life-threatening complication of cystic fibrosis or other childhood infections, such as measles and pertussis (whooping cough). It also may be the result of immune deficiency (e.g., hypogammaglobulinemia).

DIAGNOSIS

Initially, when symptoms are vague, the diagnosis of bronchiectasis may be difficult. Physical examination, history of symptoms, radiographic chest films, a high-resolution computed tomographic (CT) scan of the chest, bronchoscopy, sputum culture, and pulmonary function tests are most valuable in the diagnosis.

TREATMENT

Antibiotics and bronchodilators are prescribed, and postural drainage is encouraged. Avoiding environmental irritants such as smoke, fumes, and large amounts of dust is important. If there is a great deal of hemoptysis, surgery to remove the affected part of the lung may be advised.

ASTHMA

See Chapter 2 for a discussion of asthma.

PULMONARY EMPHYSEMA

SYMPTOMS AND SIGNS

Pulmonary emphysema, a destructive disease of the alveolar septa, interferes with both the breathing process and gas exchange in the lungs. There is an enlargement of the alveoli, which is accompanied by destruction of the alveolar walls and damage to the adjacent capillary walls. As a result of the decreased area for gas exchange and the trapped air, the patient experiences dyspnea. The onset of symptoms is **insidious,** with a gradual difficulty in breathing; dyspnea, tachypnea, wheezing, and moist, persistent cough are the first indications of the disease. The inability to exhale carbon dioxide in a normal manner requires the patient with emphysema to use accessory muscles to force out air trapped in the alveoli, and subsequently to produce the characteristic barrel chest (Fig. 9–8). Shortness of breath and dyspnea increase, and the patient purses the lips to assist in exhaling. As the disease progresses, the patient develops **circumoral cyanosis,** symptoms of right ventricular heart failure (see Cor Pulmonale in Chapter 10), and digital clubbing.

ETIOLOGY

Although the etiology of pulmonary emphysema is not completely understood, long-term cigarette smoking appears to be a contributing factor. Repeated respiratory tract infections from childhood on throughout life also may contribute to the increased occurrence of the disease. Additionally, irritants such as ozone, sulfur dioxide, and nitrogen oxides are thought to play a role in the etiology. The possibility of familial tendency is supported by the increased frequency of the disease in families who experience an **antitrypsin** deficiency.

DIAGNOSIS

Diagnosis incorporates a clinical examination and a thorough patient history, usually showing a prolonged exposure to possible respiratory irritants, especially cigarette smoking. Pulmonary function studies indicate increased tidal volume and residual volume, along with decreased vital capacity and expiratory maneuver volumes. Radiographic chest studies show translucent-appearing lungs, a depressed or flattened diaphragm, and **cardiomegaly.** The patient exhibits tachypnea, tachycardia, hypertension, polycythemia, diminished breath sounds, and wheezing or **rhonchi.** Anteroposterior chest diameter is increased—a typical barrel chest (see Fig. 9–8). Individuals with extensive progressive disease

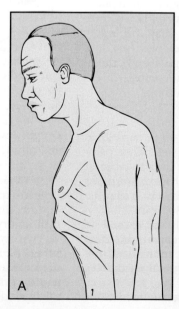
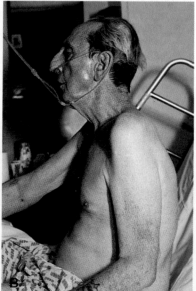

Figure 9–8

A, Note barrel chest of emphysema and bluish discoloration around mouth. *B,* Note bolt upright position and pursed lip breathing. (*B* from Henry MC, Stapleton ER: EMT Prehospital Care, 2nd ed. Philadelphia: WB Saunders, 1997, p 289. Used with permission.)

present with distended neck veins, **hepatomegaly,** peripheral edema, clubbed fingers, and cyanosis. **Blood gas** determinations in the advanced stages indicate decreased arterial oxygen tension and increased carbon dioxide.

TREATMENT

The patient is instructed and encouraged to avoid the inhalation of irritating substances, particularly cigarette smoke. Patients with pulmonary emphysema should take care to avoid exposure to possible respiratory tract infections and should receive influenza virus vaccination annually. A high-protein diet in small portions along with supplemental vitamins is recommended. Supplemental low concentrations of oxygen may help.

Drug therapy includes beta$_2$-adrenergic sympathomimetic drugs, such as albuterol (Ventolin and Proventil), terbutaline sulfate (Brethine), and metaproterenol sulfate (Alupent), for bronchodilation and antispasmodic activity; theophylline; expectorants; and antibiotics.

PNEUMOCONIOSIS

SYMPTOMS AND SIGNS

Pneumoconiosis means dust in the lungs. It refers to a number of occupational diseases that cause progressive, chronic inflammation and infection in the lungs. Dyspnea on exertion is usually the first symptom. In all types of dust disease, a dry cough, which later turns productive and is similar to the cough of chronic bronchitis, is typical. Pulmonary hypertension, tachypnea, general malaise, and recurrent respiratory tract infections are common. There may be other symptoms associated with tuberculosis (see Pulmonary Tuberculosis) of the lungs. Family members are also at risk for pneumoconiosis if exposed to dusts in the worker's clothing.

ETIOLOGY

Pneumoconiosis is considered an occupational disease caused by inhaling inorganic dust particles over a prolonged period. It usually takes at least 10 years of continual daily exposure for pneumoconiosis to develop; however, it may be as short as 2 years or as long as 30 years.

Asbestosis is a form of dust disease caused by exposure to asbestos fibers. It is characterized by a slow and progressively diffuse fibrosis of the lungs. Asbestosis is the most frequently occurring type of pneumoconiosis.

Another form of pneumoconiosis is anthra-

cosis, also known as black lung or coal-miner's lung. Anthracosis is caused by the accumulation of carbon deposits in the lungs from inhaling smoke or coal dust.

Silicosis, another type of dust disease, affects workers who are stone masons or metal grinders or who work in quarries. Silicosis develops from inhaling silica (quartz) dust and causes a dense fibrosis of the lungs and emphysema with respiratory impairment.

Other workers who are also susceptible to dust diseases are those who work with aluminum, beryllium, iron, cotton, sugar cane, and a number of synthetic fibers.

DIAGNOSIS

A thorough patient history and a complete physical examination are essential. Radiographic chest studies, pulmonary function tests, and arterial blood gas determination confirm the diagnosis.

TREATMENT

The treatment of all pneumoconioses is symptomatic and supportive. Typically, this includes the administration of bronchodilators, oxygen therapy, and chest physical therapy to help to remove secretions, and the use of corticosteroid drugs. A common complication, tuberculosis, must be treated aggressively.

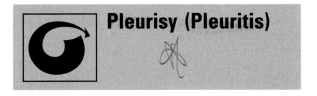

Pleurisy (Pleuritis)

SYMPTOMS AND SIGNS

Pleurisy is an inflammation of the membranes surrounding the lungs and lining the pleural cavity (Fig. 9-9). The patient reports sharp, needle-like pain, which increases with inspiration and coughing. Additionally, this patient experiences a cough, fever, and chills. Inspirations are shallow and rapid.

ETIOLOGY

Pleurisy is usually secondary to other diseases or infections. The inflammation also may result from injury or the presence of a tumor.

Two types of pleurisy exist, wet and dry. When pleural fluid is present, the increased volume causes compression of the pulmonary tissue and dyspnea. Dry pleurisy occurs when the pleural fluid decreases in volume, resulting in a dry-

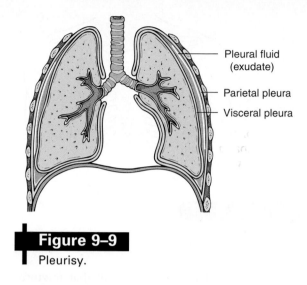

Figure 9–9

Pleurisy.

ness between the pleura; the layers rub together and become congested and edematous.

DIAGNOSIS

Diagnosis is made from the symptoms, history, and physical examination. A pleural rub can be heard on auscultation of the lungs. Radiographic films indicate the presence of underlying pulmonary disease.

TREATMENT

Treatment is directed at the underlying cause. Antibiotic therapy and analgesics to control the pain may be given.

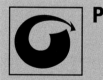

Pneumothorax

SYMPTOMS AND SIGNS

Pneumothorax is a collection of air or gas in the pleural cavity, resulting in a collapsed or partially collapsed lung (Fig. 9–10). Collapse of a lung causes severe shortness of breath, sudden sharp chest pain, falling blood pressure, rapid weak pulse, and shallow and weak respirations. Increased air pressure on the affected side causes a mediastinal shift to the unaffected side.

ETIOLOGY

Pneumothorax can be spontaneous or traumatic. Spontaneous pneumothorax occurs when there is an opening on the surface of a lung.

Causative factors can be erosion of alveoli from tumor or disease, increased pressure from within the respiratory system (too great a force with artificial ventilation), or a spontaneous tear in the tissue. Traumatic pneumothorax occurs when the integrity of the pleural cavity is breached from without as the result of trauma, such as gunshot wound, stab wound, or crushing-type wound to the chest. The object (possibly the patient's own rib) penetrates the chest cavity, allowing air to enter from the atmosphere.

DIAGNOSIS

Diagnosis is made from the history, the clinical picture, and radiographic studies. Radiographic films show the air in the pleural cavity, the collapsed portion of the lung, and mediastinal shift. Breath sounds are diminished, and sucking air sounds are heard at the wound. The patient is in acute distress.

TREATMENT

The patient is more comfortable in a **Fowler** or a semi-Fowler position and may require oxygen. An occlusive dressing is placed over any sucking wound to seal the portal of entry and to prevent additional air from entering the chest

275

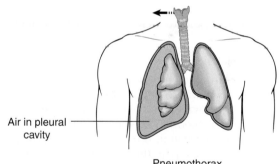

Air in pleural cavity

Pneumothorax

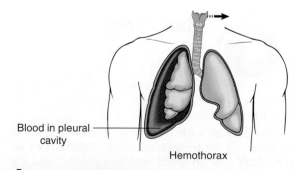

Blood in pleural cavity

Hemothorax

Figure 9–10

Pneumothorax and hemothorax.

cavity. A **thoracentesis** is performed to withdraw air from the cavity. A closed drainage system is established if air continues to leak into the pleural space. This allows reexpansion and healing of the lung.

Hemothorax

SYMPTOMS AND SIGNS

Hemothorax is blood in the pleural cavity (see Fig. 9-10). The patient experiences symptoms similar to those of pneumothorax. Signs of hemorrhage include pale and clammy skin, a weak and thready pulse, and falling blood pressure. Respirations are labored and shallow.

ETIOLOGY

Blood enters the pleural space as the result of trauma or the erosion of a pulmonary vessel. This causes the lung to collapse.

DIAGNOSIS

Breath sounds are diminished or absent on the affected side, as is chest wall movement. Radiographic films show blood in the pleural space. Blood tests indicate hemorrhage. The patient is in acute distress.

TREATMENT

The treatment employed is similar to that for pneumothorax. The lung must be re-expanded, usually by thoracentesis with closed drainage to evacuate the blood. The underlying cause, once discovered, is treated, often necessitating surgical intervention to repair the wound. Vital signs are monitored, and blood loss is replaced.

Flail Chest

SYMPTOMS AND SIGNS

The patient with flail chest, a double fracture of three or more adjacent ribs, experiences severe pain and dyspnea and is cyanotic and extremely anxious. The segment of the chest involved moves inward during inspiration and outward during expiration.

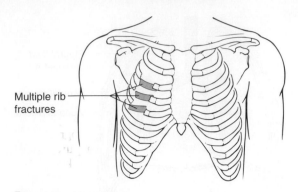

Multiple rib fractures

Figure 9–11
Flail chest.

ETIOLOGY

Direct trauma to the chest wall that fractures three or more adjacent ribs is the cause of flail chest. This trauma may be from direct compression by a heavy object, a motor vehicle accident (especially injury by the steering wheel), a hard fall onto a solid object, or an industrial accident. The paradoxical movement and instability of the chest wall occur when three or more adjacent ribs are broken in two places or break loose from the sternum while also being broken at another site (Fig. 9-11).

DIAGNOSIS

Diagnosis is made by history of chest trauma and the observation of the paradoxical movement of the chest wall. Radiographic chest films confirm the suggested diagnosis.

TREATMENT

The treatment of flail chest involves allowing the rib fractures to heal while maintaining respiratory integrity. This may entail mechanical ventilation and sedation of the patient with an endotracheal tube in place. Pain medications such as morphine and meperidine hydrochloride (Demerol) are administered to keep the patient comfortable. Additionally, supplemental oxygen is administered.

Pulmonary Tuberculosis

SYMPTOMS AND SIGNS

Pulmonary tuberculosis, an infectious and inflammatory disease of the lungs, is acquired by

276

the inhalation of a dried droplet nucleus that contains the tubercle bacillus. These droplet nuclei may remain suspended in room air for many hours. The patient with a primary tuberculosis infection is often asymptomatic. When the infection is secondary, the patient experiences vague symptoms such as weight loss, reduced appetite, listlessness, vague chest pain, dry cough, loss of energy, and fever. As the disease progresses, the patient has productive cough with purulent sputum, the appearance of blood streaking or hemoptysis, fever, and night sweats.

ETIOLOGY

The tubercle bacillus *Mycobacterium tuberculosis* causes tuberculosis and is spread by droplet nuclei. The primary lesion usually is located in the lungs. The bacteria can survive in the dried form for months if not exposed to sunlight. Any tissue of the body can be affected; however, the lung is the typical site (Fig. 9–12).

The infection begins with a primary lesion in the lower area of the lung. As the body's defense mechanisms respond to the bacterial invasion, antigens are produced, which cause **necrosis** followed by fibrosis and calcification of the affected tissue. The infection then may be arrested and the disease becomes inactive, remaining so for years. If the infection is not arrested, the patient experiences progressive primary tuberculosis.

The patient's resistance to secondary tuberculosis depends on general health and environment. Malnutrition, poor health, an unsanitary and crowded living environment, and other illnesses tend to lower resistance to reinfection

with the disease. The source of a secondary **exacerbation** of tuberculosis can be a reactivation of the previous primary infection or another infected person.

Human immunodeficiency virus (HIV) infection and the AIDS epidemic have contributed to an increase of tuberculosis in the United States.

DIAGNOSIS

The Mantoux test is a standard intradermal test used to detect the presence of tuberculin antibodies. The test is interpreted in 48 to 72 hours; an induration of 8 to 10 mm indicates a sensitivity to the bacillus and is considered positive. The positive test result is followed by radiographic chest studies, examination of gastric washings, and sputum cultures. The typical walled-off lesions (tubercles) can be seen in chest radiographic film. Apical pulmonary infiltrates with cavities are present in patients with tuberculosis. Final confirmation is positive culture of the sputum for the tubercle bacillus.

TREATMENT

Persons with communicable tuberculosis must either be treated or quarantined. Recently, there is concern over the increasing prevalence of drug-resistant tuberculosis.

Treatment of uncomplicated tuberculosis consists of drug therapy using multiple antituberculosis agents. Isoniazid (INH) is the drug of choice and is administered with rifampin, ethambutol, aminosalicylic acid, or cycloserine. Early and complete treatment offers an excellent prognosis.

Tuberculosis is considered infectious; therefore, good hand-washing techniques and respiratory precautions must be practiced. Patient and family education about sources of contagion is indicated. A nutritious diet and sanitary living conditions are important for recovery.

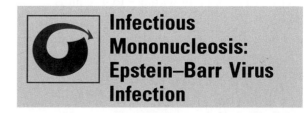

Infectious Mononucleosis: Epstein–Barr Virus Infection

SYMPTOMS AND SIGNS

Infectious mononucleosis, also known as glandular fever, is an acute URI. The two main symptoms of this infection are lymphadenopathy and fever. Initially, symptoms are vague. They include

Fibrinous pleurisy

Tubercle

Figure 9–12
Tuberculosis.

general malaise, anorexia, and chills. As the infection progresses, symptoms include sore throat, fever, headache, fatigue, and cervical and generalized lymphadenopathy. The syndrome causes a mild transient hepatitis and atypical lymphocytosis. The incubation period is from 5 to 15 days. This disease affects primarily adolescents and young adults. Infection is rare after the age of 35 years.

ETIOLOGY

Mononucleosis is caused by the Epstein–Barr virus (EBV), a herpes virus. The virus is carried in the saliva of previously infected individuals and may be transmitted through the oral pharyngeal route (e.g., during kissing) or through blood transfusions. After it is inside the body, the virus infects a type of white blood cell found in lymph, blood, and connective tissue.

DIAGNOSIS

A thorough patient history and physical examination are essential to rule out **hepatitis** and other lymphomatous disorders, such as leukemia, Hodgkin's disease, and lymphosarcoma. Two procedures of prime diagnostic importance are examination of a blood smear and immunologic study of the blood serum. Laboratory findings include lymphocytosis.

TREATMENT

The treatment is based almost entirely on the symptoms. During the acute phase of fever and malaise, bed rest should be enforced. Fluid intake should be forced orally, or if needed for high fever, intravenous fluids are indicated. Antipyretic medications such as acetaminophen are needed when the temperature becomes high (103°F in adults and 104°F in children). Secondary bacterial infections respond to treatment with sulfonamide or penicillin. Barring complications, recovery is complete within 3 to 4 months.

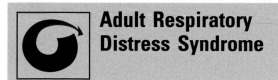

Adult Respiratory Distress Syndrome

SYMPTOMS AND SIGNS

The sudden onset of severe hypoxemia, progressive **hypercapnia,** and **acidemia** in the patient who recently has experienced trauma, **septicemia,** shock, or insult to the lungs or the rest of the body is termed adult respiratory distress syndrome (ARDS), or shock lung. The lungs are hemorrhagic, wet, boggy, congested, and unable to diffuse oxygen. The onset of symptoms is usually 24 to 48 hours after medical or surgical insult to the body. Primary symptoms include sudden and severe dyspnea with rapid and shallow respirations. Inspiratory intercostal and suprasternal retractions are noted, along with cyanosis or mottled skin. During the Vietnam War, this condition was referred to as Da Nang lung. No improvement in the respiratory status is noted with the administration of supplemental oxygen. Rales, rhonchi, and wheezes may be present.

ETIOLOGY

Pulmonary edema and resulting respiratory failure follow the increased capillary permeability in the lungs. Injury to the cells activates leukocytes and platelets in the capillaries to release products that cause additional injury. The alveoli fill with exudate 12 to 48 hours after the insult. The fluid-filled alveoli tend to collapse at the end of expiration, leaving less pulmonary tissue available for gas exchange. Consequently, low pulmonary compliance, pulmonary hypertension, decreased functional residual capacity, and hypoxemia result.

DIAGNOSIS

Patients with ARDS have an underlying cause, such as severe trauma, pneumonia, aspiration of gastric contents, **hypovolemic shock,** a near-drowning episode, fat embolism, or cardiopulmonary bypass. Most patients appear to be doing well when they experience dyspnea, and arterial blood gas determinations indicate reduced perfusion and increased pH. Radiographic chest films show diffuse bilateral alveolar infiltration with a normal cardiac silhouette.

TREATMENT

Oxygenation must be maintained; if necessary, ventilation is accomplished by **positive end-expiratory pressure (PEEP).** Attempts are made to correct the underlying cause. Nutritional status and cautious hydration are maintained intravenously, and the oxygen toxicity is treated. The patient is observed for signs of renal failure and superinfection, with intervention undertaken if necessary. Arterial blood gases, blood pressure, and urine output are monitored.

Lung Cancer

SYMPTOMS AND SIGNS

Of the various malignant neoplasms that may appear in the trachea, bronchi, or alveoli, carcinoma of the lung is the most common (Fig. 9–13). Lung or bronchial carcinoma is the leading cause of cancer deaths in the United States. In its early stages, lung cancer is asymptomatic. When symptoms appear, they may include a smoker's cough, wheezing, dyspnea, blood-streaked sputum, and hemoptysis. The patient has dull and persistent chest pain or sharp chest pain that is worse on inspiration. Often, the first symptoms of bronchial cancer are recognized in other organs, and then the symptoms depend on which organ is affected. Metastasis to the brain, liver, bone, and skin are common.

ETIOLOGY

Although the exact triggering mechanism is unknown, 80% of lung cancers are linked either directly or indirectly (passive exposure) to smoking. Tobacco smoke contains chemicals known to be **carcinogenic.** Long-term exposure to pollution from the atmosphere or to pulmonary irritants is associated with the increased occurrence of bronchial cancer. Asbestos is an important environmental carcinogen.

DIAGNOSIS

Advanced lesions of lung cancer can be seen on radiographic chest films. Sputum **cytologic** analysis that is positive for malignant cells is useful for diagnosis. A tissue biopsy specimen, taken during the bronchoscopy, is required for a definitive diagnosis.

TREATMENT

Treatment of lung cancer usually involves a combination of surgery, radiation, and chemotherapy. If the cancer is discovered early, the affected portion of the lung often can be surgically removed. Most people who have lung cancer, however, do not seek professional help until the cancer has metastasized beyond the point where surgery can be effective; therefore, the prognosis is poor.

Prevention includes public education that deters smoking, especially starting at a young age.

279

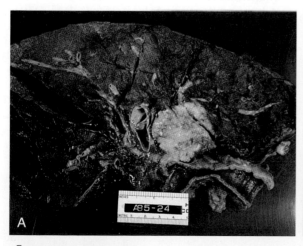 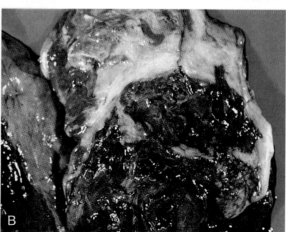

Figure 9–13

Examples of lung carcinomas. *A,* Centrally located tumor attached to bronchus. *B,* Mesothelioma on pleural surface. (From Damjanov I: Pathology for the Health-Related Professions. Philadelphia, WB Saunders Co., 1996. Used with permission.)

Summary

The respiratory and circulatory systems work together to (1) provide and circulate oxygen, (2) nourish tissue cells for metabolism, and (3) regulate the pH of blood. Acute and chronic disease conditions of the respiratory system cause conditions ranging from mild transient distress (as in a common cold) to life-threatening illness (as in lung cancer).

- Inflammatory conditions of the upper respiratory tract include the common cold, sinusitis, pharyngitis, and laryngitis.
- A crooked or deviated nasal septum and growths that protrude into the nasal cavity are noninfectious, obstructive conditions of the upper respiratory tract that impede breathing and can cause other complications.
- Tumors of the larynx are biopsied and excised; if malignant, radiation therapy or laryngectomy, or both, may be indicated.
- Deep breathing and coughing exercises are recommended after anesthesia and surgery to help prevent respiratory complications such as atelectasis, pulmonary embolism, or pneumonia.
- Bacterial pneumonia is treated with organism-specific antibiotics and supportive therapy.
- Legionellosis, or the milder form, Pontiac fever, can be contracted from bacteria that thrives in warm water, especially in water heaters, hot water plumbing, and cooling towers.
- The fungus that causes histoplasmosis is found in dust particles that, when inhaled, may cause pneumonia or systemic disease.
- Epidemic influenza immunization is recommended for certain target groups.
- Respiratory syncytial virus pneumonia most commonly afflicts infants, children, and the elderly.
- Chronic obstructive pulmonary disease (COPD) refers to several destructive lung diseases that can hinder breathing and therefore inhibit the exchange of respiratory gases. Those described in this chapter include bronchitis, bronchiectasis, emphysema, and pneumoconiosis.
- Inflammation of the plural membranes is termed pleurisy; pneumothorax refers to air in the pleural cavity; hemothorax is blood in the pleural cavity. The latter two conditions may result in a collapsed or partially collapsed lung.
- Flail chest, pneumothorax, and hemothorax are conditions that may result from chest trauma.
- Recently, there has been an increased incidence of tuberculosis in the United States and some concern over the rising prevalence of drug-resistant tuberculosis.
- Infectious mononucleosis, caused by the Epstein–Barr virus (EBV), is transmitted through the oral–pharyngeal route or through blood transfusions.
- Adult respiratory distress syndrome (ARDS), also referred to as "shock lung," often is associated with traumatic insult to the body.
- Eighty percent of lung cancer is linked directly or indirectly to smoking.

Review Challenge

REVIEW QUESTIONS

1. What are the physical and chemical dynamics of normal respiration?
2. Why is the common cold so common?
3. How is sinusitis treated?
4. What are the possible causes of nasal polyps?
5. How is severe epistaxis treated?
6. What is the prognosis of malignant tumors of the larynx?
7. What are some causes of and risk factors for (a) atelectasis and (b) pulmonary embolism?
8. What determines the treatment of pneumonia?
9. Why does the patient with pulmonary abscess exhibit foul-smelling sputum?
10. Where does the causative organism of legionnaires' disease thrive?
11. What is the profile of individuals vulnerable to respiratory syncytial virus pneumonia?
12. How is histoplasmosis contracted?
13. Who would benefit from influenza immunization?
14. Why is influenza considered a serious infection?
15. To what does COPD refer?
16. How is chronic bronchitis associated with other pulmonary conditions?
17. Are emphysema and bronchiectasis reversible? What are some causes of both conditions?
18. Why is pneumoconiosis considered an occupational disease?
19. What is the treatment of hemothorax and pneumothorax?
20. Why is pulmonary tuberculosis more prevalent and difficult to treat today?
21. How would you describe the pathology in a patient with ARDS?
22. What is recommended to prevent lung cancer? How may the prognosis be improved?

REAL-LIFE CHALLENGE

Sinusitis

A 45-year-old man is experiencing headache over both eyes on awakening. The patient states that he also experiences pain above the eyes when bending over. Tenderness above the eyes in the frontal area of the forehead and also in both cheeks is noted on palpation. A thick greenish-yellow mucous drainage is present. Sinus radiographs show a cloudiness in the region of the maxillary and frontal sinuses.

Vital signs are T—99.8°, P—90, R—26, BP—136/88. Mouth breathing is noted.

Questions

1. Compare symptoms and signs of sinusitis and upper respiratory tract infection.
2. What are the causes of sinusitis?
3. Discuss the correlation between allergies and sinusitis.
4. What drug therapy might be prescribed for treatment of sinusitis.
5. What is the principle behind the use of decongestants for sinusitis?
6. How would radiographic films of air-filled sinuses appear?

REAL-LIFE CHALLENGE

Acute Bronchitis

A 39-year-old woman is experiencing a deep cough that produces a thick yellow sputum. She reports shortness of breath and pain in the upper chest. Audible wheezing is heard without a stethoscope. Vital signs are T—100.2°, P—102, R—32, BP—134/88. Auscultation of the chest confirms the presence of bilateral wheezing and scattered rales.

The patient has a history of an upper respiratory infection 2 weeks before the onset of coughing 3 days ago. Her husband is a cigarette smoker. Diagnostic studies ordered include chest radiographs, pulmonary studies, sputum analysis, CBC, and ESR. The patient is diagnosed with acute bacterial bronchitis.

Questions

1. Why would it be safe for the patient to take aspirin for control of the fever?
2. Why would increased fluid intake be recommended?
3. Which treatment would be recommended to relieve the wheezing?
4. Which treatment would be recommended to relieve the coughing?
5. Compare the symptoms and signs of chronic bronchitis versus acute bronchitis.
6. Compare the etiology of chronic versus acute bronchitis.
7. How significant is the exposure to primary or secondary smoke to both acute and chronic bronchitis patients?
8. What would this patient's chances be for developing chronic bronchitis?

RESOURCES

Asthma Information Line
   800-822-ASMA

Asthma and Allergy Foundation of America (AAFA)
   1125 15th St NW
   Washington, DC 20005
   800-7-ASTHMA
   (http://www.aafa.com)

American Academy of Allergy and Asthma Immunology
   611 E. Wells St
   Milwaukee, WI 53202
   (http://www.aaaai.org)

Lung Line National Asthma Center
   National Jewish Center for Immunology and Respiratory
   Medicine
   1400 Jackson St
   Denver, CO 80206
   1-800-222-LUNG
   303-355-LUNG in Denver

American Lung Association
   1740 Broadway
   New York, NY 10019
   1-800-586-4872 1-800-LUNG-USA
   (http://www.lungusa.org)

American Cancer Society
   1-800-ACS-2345

National Institute of Allergies and Infectious Diseases
   National Institutes of Health
   (http://www.niaid.nih.gov)

Cancer Information Line and Antismoking Helpline
   1-800-4-CANCER
   1-800-638-6070—Alaska
   1-800-524-1234—Hawaii

Chapter Outline

Diseases and Conditions of the Circulatory System

Learning Objectives

After studying Chapter 10, you should be able to:

1. Name the common presenting symptoms in patients with cardiovascular disease.
2. Describe the pathology of coronary artery disease.
3. Name the contributing factors for coronary heart disease.
4. Explain what causes the pain of angina pectoris.
5. Explain the difference between myocardial infarction and angina pectoris.
6. Describe the treatment of myocardial infarction.
7. Name and describe the symptoms of the most prevalent cardiovascular disorder in the United States.
8. Explain what happens when the pumping action of the heart fails.
9. Compare right-sided heart failure with left-sided heart failure.
10. Name some causes of cardiomyopathy.
11. Distinguish among pericarditis, myocarditis, and endocarditis.
12. Explain why rheumatic fever is considered a systemic disease.
13. Recall the cardiac manifestations of rheumatic heart disease.
14. Explain the pathophysiology of valvular heart disease.
15. Name the causes of cardiac arrhythmias.
16. Describe the signs and symptoms of shock.
17. Explain the possible consequences of emboli.
18. Compare arteriosclerosis with atherosclerosis.
19. Describe an aneurysm and explain how it is diagnosed.
20. Explain the treatment for a) thrombophlebitis and b) varicose veins.
21. Describe the vascular pathology of Raynaud's disease.
22. Define anemia and list the presenting symptoms.
23. Describe how anemias are classified and state some examples.
24. State the causes of agranulocytosis.
25. Describe the typical symptoms in all types of leukemias.
26. Distinguish between lymphedema and lymphangitis.
27. Explain the diagnostic significance of Reed-Sternberg cells in lymphoma.
28. Name the signs and symptoms of transfusion incompatibility reaction.
29. Explain the cause of classic hemophilia.

Key Terms

agglutination	(ah–**glue**–tih–**NAY**–shun)	hematopoiesis	(**hem**–ah–toh–poy–**EE**–sis)
aggregation	(**ag**–reh–**GAY**–shun)	hemolytic	(**hem**–oh–**LIT**–ik)
angioplasty	(**AN**–jee–oh–**plas**–tee)	hypovolemia	(**high**–poh–voh–**LEE**–mee–ah)
arteriosclerosis	(ar–**tee**–ree–oh–skleh–**ROW**–sis)	hypoxia	(high–**POX**–see–ah)
asystole	(a–**SIS**–toh–lee)	ischemia	(is–**KEY**–mee–ah)
atherosclerosis	(**ath**–er–**oh**–skleh–**ROW**–sis)	orthopnea	(**or**–**THOP**–nee–ah)
		perfusion	(per–**FYOU**–zhun)
bradycardia	(brady–**KAR**–dee–ah)	petechiae	(pee–**TEE**–kee–ee)
bruit	(**BREW**–ee)	phlebotomy	(phleh–**BOT**–oh–mee)
cardiomegaly	(**car**–dee–oh–**MEG**–ah–lee)	plaque	(**PLACK**)
		purpura	(**PUR**–pu–rah)
cardiomyopathy	(**car**–dee–oh–my–**OP**–ah–thee)	syncope	(**SIN**–ko–pee)
		tachycardia	(**tack**–ee–**CAR**–dee–ah)
cellulitis	(sell–u–**LIE**–tis)		
dyscrasia	(dis–**CRAY**–zee–ah)	tamponade	(**tam**–pon–**ADE**)
ecchymosis	(ech–ih–**MO**–sis)	thrombus	(**THROM**–bus)
embolism	(**EM**–boh–lizm)		

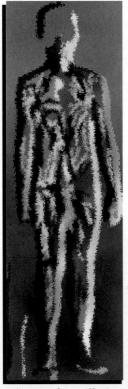

Orderly Function of the Circulatory System

Circulation of blood is the primary function of the circulatory system. The heart is at the center of the circulatory system. Its steady beating pumps 5 quarts of blood through a complete vascular circuit of the body every minute in an adult; this is called the cardiac cycle. This circuit is accomplished through a network of vessels: the arteries, veins, and capillaries (Fig. 10–1).

The heart consists of two side-by-side pumps divided into four chambers: two upper chambers called atria, and two lower chambers called ventricles. As blood returns to the heart from the body, it enters the right atrium, passes through the tricuspid valve, and with atrial contraction, enters the right ventricle. Heart valves keep the blood flowing in the correct direction. From the ventricle, blood is pumped through the pulmonary valve and, with ventricular contraction, into the pulmonary arteries and on to the lungs. In the lungs, carbon dioxide is removed and oxygen is added to the blood. Freshly oxygenated blood then returns to the heart via the pulmonary veins. It enters the left atrium, moves through

The heart is enclosed by the double-layered pericardium composed of an inner serous layer (visceral pericardium or epicardium) and an outer fibrous layer (parietal pericardium). Between these layers in the pericardial cavity is a small amount of serous fluid that reduces friction during cardiac movements. Cardiac muscle tissue or myocardium is composed of striated muscle cells that can contract rhythmically on their own. Inside the cavities of the heart, there is a smooth serous lining called endocardium (Fig. 10-3). The entire conduction system of the heart coordinates the contraction and relaxation (cardiac cycle) of the heart by initiating and distributing impulses throughout the myocardium (see Fig. 10-12). Coronary arteries and a network of vessels continuously supply cardiac muscle tissue with oxygen (Fig. 10-4).

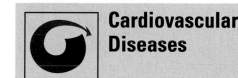

Cardiovascular Diseases

There are many and varied disorders of the heart and circulatory system. In some disorders, the rhythm of the heartbeats may become irregular, abnormally fast (**tachycardia**), or abnormally slow (bradycardia). Disorders of cardiac rhythm are called **arrhythmias** or **dysrhythmias.**

Almost one third of all deaths in Western countries are attributed to heart disease. Most of these deaths are caused by coronary artery disease and hypertension. Cardiovascular disorders

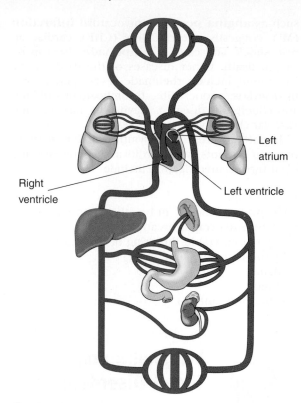

Figure 10–1
Circulation through the body.

the mitral (bicuspid) valve with atrial contraction, and enters the left ventricle. As the ventricle contracts again, the blood is forced out of the ventricle through the aortic valve into the aorta and on to the rest of the body (Fig. 10-2).

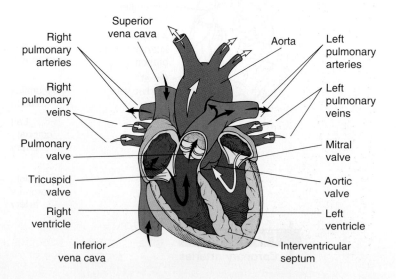

Figure 10–2
Circulation through the heart.

such as **angina pectoris,** myocardial **infarction** (MI), congestive heart failure (CHF), cardiac arrest, shock, and cardiac **tamponade** also can result in death. Other diseases of the cardiovascular system include rheumatic fever, pericarditis, myocarditis, endocarditis, thromboangiitis obliterans (Buerger's disease), Raynaud's disease, and vascular (blood vessel) diseases.

Important presenting symptoms that tend to recur in patients with cardiovascular disease and need further investigation include

- Chest pain
- **Dyspnea** (difficulty in breathing) on exertion
- **Tachypnea** (rapid breathing)
- Palpitations (rapid fluttering of the heart)
- **Cyanosis** (slight blue color)
- Edema
- Fatigue
- **Syncope** (fainting)

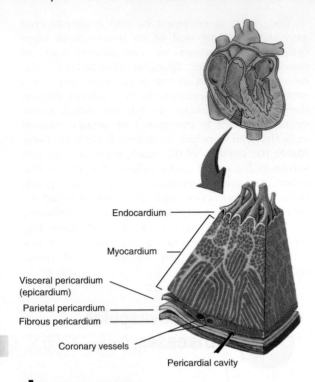

Endocardium

Myocardium

Visceral pericardium (epicardium)

Parietal pericardium

Fibrous pericardium

Coronary vessels

Pericardial cavity

Figure 10–3

Layers of the heart wall. (From Applegate EJ: The Anatomy and Physiology Learning System: Textbook. Philadelphia: WB Saunders, 1995, p 247. Used with permission.)

Lymphatic and Blood Disorders

See under discussion of specific diseases.

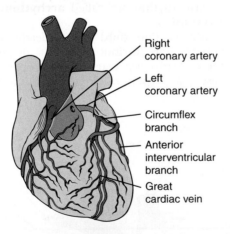

Right coronary artery

Left coronary artery

Circumflex branch

Anterior interventricular branch

Great cardiac vein

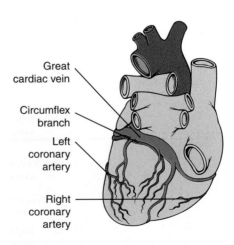

Great cardiac vein

Circumflex branch

Left coronary artery

Right coronary artery

Figure 10–4

Coronary arteries.

Coronary Artery Disease

SYMPTOMS AND SIGNS

Coronary artery disease (CAD) is a condition involving the arteries supplying the myocardium (heart muscle) (see Fig. 10–4). The arteries become narrowed by atherosclerotic deposits over time, causing temporary cardiac **ischemia** and eventually MI (heart attack). Patients are **asymptomatic** initially, with the first symptom being the pain of angina pectoris (see Angina Pectoris). In advanced disease, the severe pain of MI is described as burning, squeezing, crushing, and radiating to the arm, neck, or jaw (see Myocardial Infarction). Nausea, vomiting, and weakness also can be experienced. Changes in the **electrocardiogram (ECG)** are recognized.

ETIOLOGY

Deposits of fat-containing substances called **plaque** on the lumen (opening) of the coronary arteries result in *atherosclerosis* and subsequent narrowing of the lumen of the arteries. The myocardium must have an adequate blood supply to function. The coronary arteries supply the cardiac muscle with blood but become constricted by atherosclerosis.

Arteriosclerosis, commonly referred to as "hardening of the arteries," is associated with the elderly or diabetics. Eventually, the arteries lose elasticity and become hard and narrow, resulting in cardiac ischemia; gradually, the cells in the myocardium weaken and die. Replacement scar tissue forms, interfering with the heart's ability to pump, resulting in heart failure.

Persons at higher risk for CAD are those who have a genetic predisposition to the disease, those older than 40 years of age, men (slightly more than women), postmenopausal women, and white persons. Other factors contributing to increased risk of the disease include history of smoking; residence in an urban society; the presence of hypertension, diabetes, or obesity; and a history of elevated serum cholesterol or decreased serum high-density lipoprotein (HDL) levels. Lack of exercise (a sedentary lifestyle) and stress are additional risk factors.

DIAGNOSIS

The patient usually does not experience chest pain from atherosclerosis until the coronary arteries are approximately 75% occluded. Often, **collateral** circulation develops to supply the tissue with needed oxygen and nutrients. An ECG shows ischemia (lack of blood supply) and possi-

289

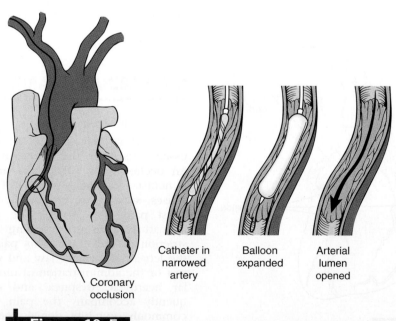

Coronary occlusion

Catheter in narrowed artery

Balloon expanded

Arterial lumen opened

Figure 10–5

Angioplasty.

bly arrhythmias. Treadmill testing, **thallium scan,** cardiac catheterization, and angiograms are other tools of cardiac status evaluation used to detect insufficient oxygen supply and to confirm the diagnosis.

TREATMENT

Treatment consists of restoring adequate blood flow to the myocardium. Vasodilators are prescribed. **Angioplasty** is attempted in some instances to open the constricted arteries (Fig. 10–5). Claims of reduction of the plaque buildup with hypolipidemic drugs are being confirmed in some cases. When the blockage is severe or does not respond to drug therapy or angioplasty, coronary artery bypass surgery may be indicated to restore circulation to the affected myocardium (Fig. 10-6).

Experimental gene therapy uses injections of DNA directly into cardiac muscle to stimulate new growth of blood vessels.

Prevention of CAD includes a diet that is low in salt, fat, and cholesterol combined with exercise. Patients are encouraged to reduce stress and, if smokers, to stop or reduce smoking.

ANGINA PECTORIS

SYMPTOMS AND SIGNS

Angina pectoris, chest pain after exertion, is the result of decreased oxygen supply to the my-

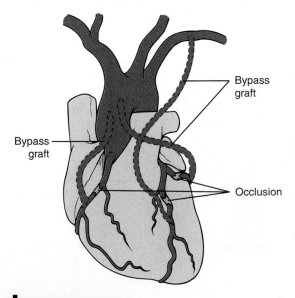

Bypass graft

Bypass graft

Occlusion

Figure 10–6

Coronary artery bypass.

ocardium. The patient has sudden onset of left-sided chest pain after exertion. The pain may radiate to the left arm or back (Fig. 10-7). Additionally, the patient may experience dyspnea. The pain usually is relieved by ceasing the strenuous activity and placing nitroglycerin tablets sublingually (under the tongue). The blood pressure may increase during the attack, and arrhythmias may occur.

ETIOLOGY

Atherosclerosis causes a narrowing of the coronary arteries, compromising the blood flow to the myocardium. Exertion necessitates increased blood flow for more oxygen, but the vessels cannot supply it. Spasms of the coronary arteries also may be a causative factor. Severe prolonged tachycardia, anemias, and respiratory disease also can cause cardiac ischemia.

DIAGNOSIS

The patient history reveals a previous exertional chest pain. An ECG taken during the anginal episode may show ischemia. Other diagnostic measures, such as those described for CAD, are performed.

TREATMENT

Treatment consists of stopping the strenuous activity and placing nitroglycerin tablets under the tongue. Transdermal nitroglycerin is helpful in preventing angina. When angina persists after treatment or for more than 20 minutes, immediate medical attention is indicated.

MYOCARDIAL INFARCTION

SYMPTOMS AND SIGNS

Myocardial infarction is death of myocardial tissue caused by the development of ischemia. An occlusion of a coronary artery resulting in ischemia and infarct (death) of the myocardium causes sudden, severe substernal or left-sided chest pain (Fig. 10-8). The pain is crushing in nature, causing a feeling of massive constriction of the chest. This pain may radiate to the left arm, back, or jaw and is not relieved by rest or the administration of nitroglycerin. Irregular heartbeat, dyspnea, and **diaphoresis** frequently accompany the pain, and the patient commonly exhibits denial and usually experiences severe anxiety. Occasionally, MI may be clinically silent.

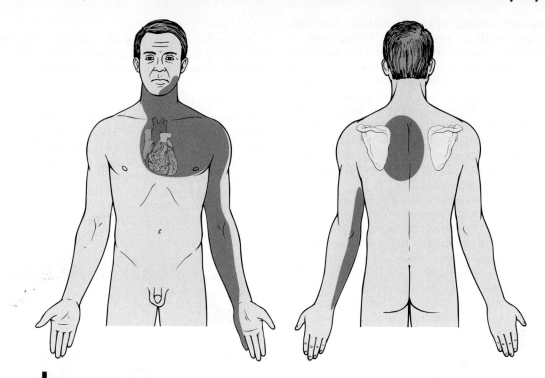

Figure 10–7

Common sites of pain in angina pectoris.

ETIOLOGY

MI results from insufficient oxygen supply, as when a coronary artery is occluded by atherosclerotic plaque, thrombus, or myocardial muscle spasm. The pain is caused by ischemia, and if ischemia is not reversed in about 6 hours, the cardiac muscle dies. Coronary thrombosis is the most common cause of MI.

DIAGNOSIS

Diagnosis includes a thorough history, ECG, chest radiographic studies, and laboratory tests for cardiac enzyme levels. Changes in enzyme levels indicate the death of cardiac tissue and include (1) creatine phosphokinase (CPK), which is elevated in the first 6 to 24 hours after MI, (2) lactic dehydrogenase (LDH), which peaks at 48 hours, and (3) aspartate aminotransferase (AST). When an elevation of these enzymes is detected, cardiac isoenzymes are ordered to confirm the diagnosis. ECG changes in the PR and QRS complexes and in the ST segment correspond to the ischemic areas. Diagnostic confirmation is assisted by elevated cardiac enzyme levels and altered isoenzyme levels identified with blood tests.

TREATMENT

Early and immediate intervention enhances the chance for survival and minimizes irreversible injury to the myocardium. Recent recommenda-

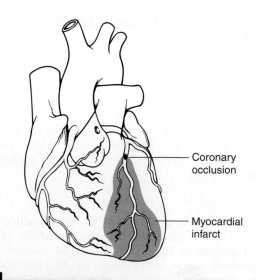

Coronary occlusion

Myocardial infarct

Figure 10–8

Myocardial infarction.

tions include calling 911 for entrance into the emergency medical system and taking one 5 grain/325 mg aspirin tablet. Immediate hospitalization is important to initiate treatment aimed at controlling pain, stabilizing heart rhythm, and minimizing damage to the heart muscle. Most death caused by MI is the result of primary ventricular fibrillation. Thus, immediate ECG monitoring and implementing defibrillation is of primary concern. The American Heart Association currently recommends defibrillation training for all certified first responders.

Oxygen is administered, and morphine is given for pain. Vasodilation is attempted by nitroglycerin drip. Lidocaine given by an intravenous drip, after a loading bolus, helps to control arrhythmias. Thrombolytic drugs, including tissue plasminogen activator (TPA), streptokinase, or alteplase (Activase) may be administered as soon as possible after the diagnosis, unless there are contraindications. Within the 6-hour window before permanent damage, an attempt may be made to open the occlusion and to restore blood flow to the area by angioplasty (see Fig. 10-5), the administration of thrombolytic drugs, or coronary artery bypass surgery (see Fig. 10-6).

Approximately 65% of deaths caused by MI occur in the first hour. Prognosis is determined by immediate defibrillation for ventricular fibrillation. Late mortality depends on the extent of damage to the heart muscle and the occurrence of complications. Most late cardiac death is sudden, caused by the onset of fatal arrhythmia.

Cardiac Arrest

SYMPTOMS AND SIGNS

Cardiac arrest is the sudden unexpected cessation of cardiac activity. The patient is unresponsive, with no respiratory effort and no palpable pulse.

ETIOLOGY

Cardiac arrest results from anoxia (absence of oxygen to the tissue) or interruption of the electrical stimuli to the heart. It can be caused by respiratory arrest, arrhythmia, or MI. Electrocution, drowning, severe trauma, massive hemorrhage, or drug overdose also can be responsible for cardiac arrest.

DIAGNOSIS

Diagnosis is made by the absence of respiratory effort and lack of palpable pulse. The ECG shows ventricular fibrillation or **asystole.**

TREATMENT

Cardiopulmonary resuscitation (CPR) must be instituted within 4 to 6 minutes of the cardiac arrest. Cardiac defibrillation is attempted by trained advanced life support personnel. Cardiac drugs, including epinephrine (Adrenalin) and isoproterenol (Isuprel), to stimulate the heart are administered. Antiarrhythmic drugs, including lidocaine and bretylium, also may be administered.

Hypertensive Heart Disease

Hypertensive heart disease, the most prevalent cardiovascular disorder in the United States, is the result of chronically elevated pressure throughout the vascular system. Atherosclerosis, arteriosclerosis, renal disease, and any condition that creates increased vascular pressure cause the heart to work harder as it pumps against increased resistance.

ESSENTIAL HYPERTENSION

SYMPTOMS AND SIGNS

Essential, or primary, hypertension, a condition of abnormally high blood pressure in the arterial system, has an **insidious** onset, with the patient exhibiting few, if any, symptoms until permanent damage is done. The patient may experience headaches, **epistaxis,** lightheadedness, or **syncope.** The hypertension generally is detected when blood pressure is taken during a physical examination or screening process. Hypertension is more prevalent with increased age in all groups. If hypertension is accompanied by hyperlipidemia, it may lead to atherosclerosis.

ETIOLOGY

The etiology is unknown, although many factors are thought to contribute to the condition. Stress is considered a major factor in hypertension. Age, heredity, smoking, obesity, and hyperactive personality or type A personality are possible causative factors in essential hypertension.

DIAGNOSIS

Elevated blood pressure readings are the first indication of hypertension. A systolic reading of greater than 140 mm Hg and a diastolic reading of greater than 90 mm Hg indicate hypertension. The diagnosis is based on a series of blood pressure readings, with elevated values being obtained several times. A careful complete medical history, physical examination, and laboratory evaluation should be performed before diagnosis is confirmed and therapy is initiated.

TREATMENT

Drug therapy used in the treatment of hypertension includes **diuretics** (to reduce circulating blood volume), beta-adrenergic blockers (to slow the heartbeat and to dilate vessels), vasodilators (to dilate vessels), calcium channel blockers (to slow the heartbeat, to reduce conduction irritability, and to dilate vessels), and **angiotensin-converting enzyme** (ACE) inhibitors (to produce vasodilation and to increase renal blood flow). These drugs may be prescribed singly or in combination. A program of drug therapy is designed to fit each patient's needs and response. Additional modes of therapy include limitation of sodium intake, dietary management, weight reduction, exercise, reduction of stressful situations, and cessation of smoking.

Teaching the patient that this condition is not cured but only controlled by drug therapy is essential. Education reinforces the necessity of monitoring the blood pressure on a regular basis and the need to continue drug therapy for life.

MALIGNANT HYPERTENSION

SYMPTOMS AND SIGNS

Malignant hypertension is a severe form of hypertension and is life threatening. Severe headache, blurred vision, and dyspnea are symptoms that suggest the condition. The symptoms may have sudden onset.

ETIOLOGY

The etiology of this severe form of essential hypertension is unknown, although extreme stress is thought to be a contributing factor.

DIAGNOSIS

Marked blood pressure elevation is considered malignant hypertension. In severe cases, the systolic pressure reading may be greater than 200 mm Hg and the diastolic pressure reading greater than 120 mm Hg. These patients are at risk for a cerebrovascular accident (CVA), or stroke, and irreversible renal damage.

TREATMENT

Aggressive intervention is indicated in severe malignant hypertension. Intravenous vasodilators such as diazoxide (Hyperstat) and sodium nitroprusside (Nipride) should be administered. After the condition is under control, blood pressure should be monitored on a regular basis and drug therapy continued for life.

Congestive Heart Failure

SYMPTOMS AND SIGNS

Congestive heart failure is the inadequacy of the heart to pump enough blood throughout the body to meet demands. It usually has an insidious onset. The patient experiences gradually increasing dyspnea. Cardiac and respiratory rates increase, and the patient becomes anxious. As the condition progresses, the neck veins distend and edema is noted in the ankles. When the right side of the heart fails, the liver and spleen enlarge and the peripheral edema is more prominent. Left-sided CHF causes increased pulmonary congestion and more pronounced respiratory difficulties (Fig. 10-9).

ETIOLOGY

The pumping action of the heart is not able to meet the body's demand for blood, resulting in inadequate **perfusion.** Some of the causes of the heart failure are hypertension, CAD, MI, chronic obstructive pulmonary disease (COPD), cardiac valve damage, arrhythmias (dysrhythmias), and cardiomyopathy.

DIAGNOSIS

Diagnosis is made after a thorough history and physical examination. Breath sounds are diminished and radiographic film indicates the presence of fluid in the lungs. An ECG is used to discover the underlying causes. An **echocardiogram** helps in evaluating cardiac chamber size, ventricular function, and disease of the myocardium, valves, cardiac structures (walls, septum, and papillary muscles), and pericardium (the covering of the heart).

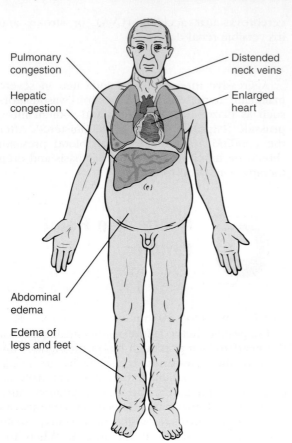

Pulmonary congestion

Hepatic congestion

Distended neck veins

Enlarged heart

Abdominal edema

Edema of legs and feet

294

Figure 10–9
Signs of congestive heart failure.

TREATMENT

Treatment is directed at reducing the workload of the heart and increasing its efficiency. Digitalis preparations are administered to strengthen and slow the heartbeat. Diuretics help to reduce the volume of fluid in the body, and vasodilators help to reduce vascular pressure. Intake of fluid and sodium is restricted.

Cor Pulmonale

SYMPTOMS AND SIGNS

Cor pulmonale, or right-sided heart failure, causes the patient to experience dyspnea, distended neck veins, and edema of the extremities. The liver is enlarged and tender.

ETIOLOGY

Right-sided heart failure is an outcome of acute or chronic pulmonary disease and pulmonary hypertension. The diseased pulmonary blood vessels impair the blood flow to pulmonary tissue. The increased pulmonary blood pressure escalates the workload of the right side of the heart, causing the right ventricle to **hypertrophy** and thus to become less effective in pumping blood to the lungs. Chronic conditions causing cor pulmonale include emphysema and **fibrotic** pulmonary lesions, whereas pulmonary **emboli** are the primary acute causative factor. Chronic hypoxemia stimulates the bone marrow in an adaptive mechanism to produce an increased number of red blood cells (RBCs) to carry additional oxygen. This condition of above-normal levels of RBCs (polycythemia) increases the blood viscosity.

DIAGNOSIS

Diagnosis is based on a history of pulmonary disease and hypoxia. The patient's respiratory and cardiac status are assessed for neck vein distention and peripheral edema. Radiographic chest studies and echocardiography reveal pulmonary congestion and right-sided heart enlargement, and the ECG frequently shows arrhythmias. If polycythemia is present, the RBC count is elevated.

TREATMENT

Treatment entails relieving the causative factors in the pulmonary system and reducing hypoxemia. Bronchodilators are administered. Supplemental oxygen provides additional comfort to the patient. Bed rest is encouraged, and digitalis preparations are administered to strengthen and slow the heartbeat. **Phlebotomy** may be used when polycythemia is a problem.

Pulmonary Edema

SYMPTOMS AND SIGNS

Pulmonary edema is a condition of fluid shift into the extravascular spaces of the lungs. Patients experience dyspnea and coughing, **orthopnea,** and increased cardiac and respiratory rates and often have bloody, frothy sputum.

Blood pressure may fall, and the skin becomes cold and clammy. Frequently, the symptoms occur at night after the patient has lain down.

ETIOLOGY

Pulmonary edema is caused by left-sided heart failure, mitral valve disease, pulmonary embolus, systemic hypertension, arrhythmias, and renal failure. There is an excessive accumulation of fluid in the lungs (pulmonary tissue and air spaces). The pulmonary circulation is overloaded with an excessive volume of blood.

DIAGNOSIS

The clinical picture of dyspnea, orthopnea, and bloody, frothy sputum leads to further investigation. Breath sounds are diminished, with the presence of **rales, rhonchi,** and wheezing. Arterial **blood gas** measurement shows reduced oxygen saturation, increased carbon dioxide retention, increased bicarbonate levels, and decreased pH of the blood. Radiographic chest films show increased **opacity** of the pulmonary tissue, an enlarged heart, and prominent pulmonary vessels.

TREATMENT

The patient is placed in **Fowler's position** (sitting), and oxygen therapy is administered. Drug therapy includes diuretics to improve fluid excretion, digitalis preparations to increase the efficiency of the heart, morphine sulfate to induce venous dilation, and beta$_2$-adrenergic drugs to dilate bronchioles and to control bronchial spasms. Severe cases may require mechanical ventilation. Pulmonary edema is a life-threatening condition and is considered a medical emergency.

 Cardiomyopathy

SYMPTOMS AND SIGNS

Cardiomyopathy is a noninflammatory disease of the cardiac muscle resulting in enlargement of the myocardium and ventricular dysfunction. It causes the patient to experience symptoms of CHF, including dyspnea, fatigue, tachycardia, palpitations, and occasionally chest pain. Peripheral edema and hepatic congestion also may be present. Syncope and cardiac murmurs may occur. The symptoms and signs vary with the type and cause of this condition.

ETIOLOGY

Primary causes are mostly unknown. Cardiomyopathies are divided into three groups: dilated, hypertrophic, and restrictive. Dilated cardiomyopathy can be the result of chronic alcoholism, an autoimmune process, or viral infections. Regardless of the cause, dilated cardiomyopathies result in a diffuse degeneration of the myocardial fibers. This is followed by a decrease in contractile effort.

Hypertrophic cardiomyopathies are thought to be genetic and are considered **idiopathic.** The left ventricular wall hypertrophies, as does the interventricular septum, resulting in a small and elongated left ventricle and possible obstruction of the aortic valve.

Restrictive cardiomyopathies occur when any infiltrative process of the heart causes fibrosis and thickening of the myocardium.

DIAGNOSIS

Diagnosis includes a careful patient history and a complete physical examination. **Cardiomegaly** at various stages is present, along with assorted cardiac murmurs. The radiographic chest film confirms the presence of cardiomegaly, and the ECG reveals rate and rhythm abnormalities. Echocardiograms and cardiac catheterization may help to identify the type of cardiomyopathy and the extent of the condition. **Biopsy** may be required.

TREATMENT

Treatment is determined by the type of cardiomyopathy. Therapy for dilated cardiomyopathies is aimed at appropriate control of the CHF, with measures as previously mentioned for treatment of CHF. Antiarrhythmic agents and **anticoagulant** drugs are prescribed. Activities are limited, with some patients being restricted to bed rest. The condition is often fatal, with the only hope for survival being heart transplantation.

Treatment of hypertrophic cardiomyopathies also is aimed at reducing the workload of the heart. Beta-adrenergic blockers such as propranolol hydrochloride (Inderal) decrease the myocardial contractility and reduce the heart rate and the conductivity, thus preventing arrhythmias. Medication improves the survival rate of these patients.

Treatment of restrictive cardiomyopathies also includes reducing the workload of the heart. The changes in the cardiac muscle caused by the infiltrates are irreversible, making the prognosis for these patients poor.

Pericarditis

SYMPTOMS AND SIGNS

Pericarditis is an acute or chronic inflammation of the pericardium (serosa), the sac enclosing and protecting the heart. The space between the outer parietal layer of pericardium and the inner visceral layer of epicardium (heart wall) normally is filled with a small amount of thin, lubricating serous fluid (see Fig. 10-3). When blood or inflammatory exudate is released into the pericardial sac, or pericardial space, friction and irritation between the layers result in pericarditis. Associated manifestations include fever, **malaise,** chest pain that fluctuates with inspiration or heartbeat, dyspnea, and chills. The patient may feel anxious and report a "pounding heart." A detectable friction rub, or grating sound, in phase with the heartbeat can be heard on **auscultation** with a stethoscope. Tachycardia may be present. Pericarditis can occur in different forms. It can be a benign or isolated process or can be secondary to infection elsewhere in the body; thus, the clinical signs vary.

ETIOLOGY

Pericarditis is idiopathic or a consequence of inflammation or infection elsewhere in the body. Other causative agents are viruses, bacteria (producing a suppurative pericarditis), trauma, rheumatic fever, and malignant **neoplastic** disease. The condition may occur secondary to myocardial infarction. Acute inflammation of the pericardium can cause adhesions (scarring) to form between it and the heart or a loss of elasticity to occur, producing a constrictive pericarditis. Conversely, chronic pericarditis can incite fibrous calcification of the visceral membrane, which comes in direct contact with the myocardium. A scarred and rigid pericardium interferes with the heart's ability to contract normally, with a subsequent drop in cardiac output.

DIAGNOSIS

Blood studies may lead to the identification of a causative organism. They also may reveal elevated **white blood cell (WBC) count, erythrocyte sedimentation rate (ESR),** and cardiac enzyme levels. Changes are noted on ECG. Echocardiogram confirms the presence of pericardial fluid and reveals a thickened pericardium. In constrictive pericarditis, cardiac catheterization shows elevated pressures in the cardiac chambers.

TREATMENT

Treatment is directed at managing the underlying systemic disease and at reducing inflammation and pain. Therapy for infectious pericarditis necessitates antibiotic drugs and possibly surgical drainage or aspiration. Complete bed rest and the administration of **analgesics, antipyretics,** and nonsteroidal anti-inflammatory drugs (NSAIDs) are prescribed. Acute pericarditis usually resolves with complete recovery. Extensive adhesions or calcification from chronic pericarditis may necessitate resection of pericardium.

Myocarditis

SYMPTOMS AND SIGNS

Myocarditis is inflammation of the muscular walls of the heart. It involves damage to the myocardium by pathogenic invasion or **toxic** insult. The condition may be acute or chronic, may involve a small part of the endocardium (the lining of the heart) or be diffuse, and can occur at any age. The patient may report palpitations, fatigue, and dyspnea. Physical examination may reveal fever, arrhythmia, and tenderness in the chest.

ETIOLOGY

Myocarditis is frequently a viral, bacterial, fungal, or protozoal infection or a complication of other diseases such as influenza, diphtheria, mumps, and most significantly, rheumatic fever; occasionally, it is idiopathic. Exposure to certain toxic agents, through lithium use, chronic use of cocaine, chronic alcoholism, radiation, and chemical poisoning, can cause inflammation of the myocardium.

DIAGNOSIS

Diagnostic findings may include an elevated WBC count, increased ESR, elevated cardiac enzyme levels, ventricular enlargement noted on radiographic chest film, and an abnormal ECG. Myocardial biopsy confirms the inflammation of cardiac muscle tissue and may identify the cause.

TREATMENT

When infection is the underlying cause, appropriate anti-infective agents are given. The patient is advised to rest and to reduce the heart's workload. Medications such as quinidine and procainamide may be required to stabilize arrhythmia. The prognosis for complete recovery is favorable, unless the condition is chronic and causes damage to the cardiac muscle.

Endocarditis

SYMPTOMS AND SIGNS

Endocarditis is inflammation of the lining and the valves of the heart. It is usually secondary to infection elsewhere in the body (Fig. 10–10), the result of preexisting heart disease, or the consequence of an abnormal immunologic reaction.

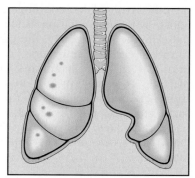

Respiratory tract infection

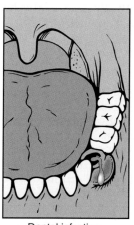

Dental infection

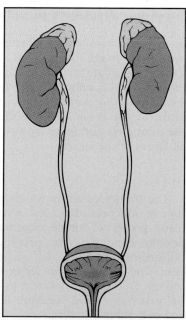

Urinary tract infection

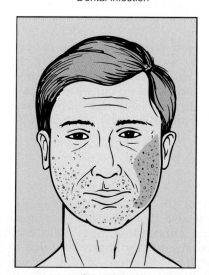

Skin infection

Figure 10–10

Causative factors in endocarditis.

The patient may have vague to pronounced symptoms of infection: fever, chills, weakness, **anorexia,** and fatigue.

The condition is characterized by vegetative growths on the cardiac valves that may be released into the blood stream in the form of emboli. These emboli can lodge in vessels and cause symptoms of ischemia. The sites of ischemia may be the heart, lungs, kidneys, brain, or extremities. Dysfunction of the valves, which may not close effectively, disrupts or obstructs blood flow through the chambers of the heart; the dysfunction of the valves usually produces a cardiac murmur heard on auscultation. Serious obstruction or regurgitation of blood flow through the heart affects the pumping effectiveness of the heart and causes complications.

ETIOLOGY

Bacteremia, or the presence of infectious agents in the blood stream, can lead to endocarditis. Common infecting organisms include *Staphylococcus aureus,* group A beta-hemolytic streptococci, and *Escherichia coli.* Intravenous drug users are at high risk for fungal endocarditis. Patients with damaged cardiac valves from rheumatic disease are more prone to endocarditis.

DIAGNOSIS

A complete blood count (CBC) may indicate leukocytosis, and an elevated ESR may be present. Blood cultures may reveal the causative organism. Echocardiogram shows valve involvement with vegetation or **abscesses.** ECG may indicate arrhythmia and conduction defects.

TREATMENT

Identification of the causative organism dictates the anti-infective therapy, which continues for several weeks. Other medications include antipyretics, anticoagulants, and drugs indicated to treat any complications. Bed rest is recommended during the acute phase. Damaged cardiac valves may necessitate surgical repair or replacement. After recovery, the patient needs to understand the importance of taking **prophylactic** antibiotics before dental work, childbirth, or any invasive procedures associated with transient bacteremia.

Rheumatic Fever

SYMPTOMS AND SIGNS

Rheumatic fever is a systemic inflammatory and **autoimmune** disease involving the joints and cardiac tissue. It follows a sore throat caused by group A beta-hemolytic streptococcus. The patient, usually a child, experiences a fever and polyarthritis, including joint pain, edema, redness, and limited range of motion. Joints frequently involved include finger, knee, and ankle joints, with inflammation being transient among these joints. Additionally, the patient experiences carditis, cardiac murmurs, cardiomegaly, and even CHF. Other symptoms include weakness, malaise, anorexia, weight loss, a rash on the trunk, abdominal pain, and the development of small nodules on the tendon sheaths in the knees, knuckles, and elbows. The symptoms occur 1 to 5 weeks after the upper respiratory tract infection.

ETIOLOGY

After a sore throat caused by group A beta-hemolytic streptococcus, **antibodies** develop against the bacteria and cross-react with normal tissue. This autoimmune disease causes the antibodies to attack the body's own cells and to initiate an inflammatory reaction. The antibodies migrate to the endocardium and the mitral and sometimes the aortic valves, where vegetations form on the tissue. The carditis usually follows the joint pain and fever by a week and can affect all layers of the heart.

DIAGNOSIS

The history of an upper respiratory tract infection in the preceding few weeks suggests rheumatic fever. No single diagnostic feature identifies the condition. The presence of carditis and polyarthritis adds to the suggestion of the disease. The streptococcal antibody level, antistreptolysin O titer, is elevated in a series of tests. Increases in cardiac enzyme levels, WBC count, and ESR aid in the diagnosis.

TREATMENT

After the diagnosis of streptococcal pharyngitis (strep throat), which precedes rheumatic fever, treatment with a *complete* course of antibiotics prevents the onset of the fever and subsequent rheumatic heart disease. The administration of antibiotics (penicillin) is necessary to eradicate the streptococcal infection. Antipyretics are given for fever and anti-inflammatory agents for relief of the arthritic symptoms. Bed rest is indicated, as is prophylactic administration of antibiotics.

RHEUMATIC HEART DISEASE

SYMPTOMS AND SIGNS

Rheumatic heart disease refers to cardiac manifestations that follow rheumatic fever. The acute endocarditis, which leads to chronic cardiac involvement, includes valvular damage because the vegetations cause stenosis of the valves, particularly the mitral and aortic valves (Fig. 10-11). Congestive heart failure causes dyspnea, tachycardia, edema, a nonproductive cough, and cardiac murmurs.

ETIOLOGY

After rheumatic fever, the vegetations may become enlarged or the valves may scar, causing stenosis of the openings. The frequency of rheumatic heart disease is decreasing as a result of diagnosis and aggressive antibiotic treatment of streptococcal pharyngitis (strep throat). Patients who experienced rheumatic fever and rheumatic heart disease before the advent of penicillin may have damaged cardiac valves.

DIAGNOSIS

Diagnosis is made from the history of rheumatic fever and cardiac murmurs. An echocardiogram shows the vegetations or resulting damage to the valves.

TREATMENT

Treatment is aimed at reducing the stenosis of the valves and preventing further damage. Surgery to relieve the stenosis or to replace the valve may be necessary. Good dental hygiene is important to prevent gingival infection, which would cause further bloodborne infection and

299

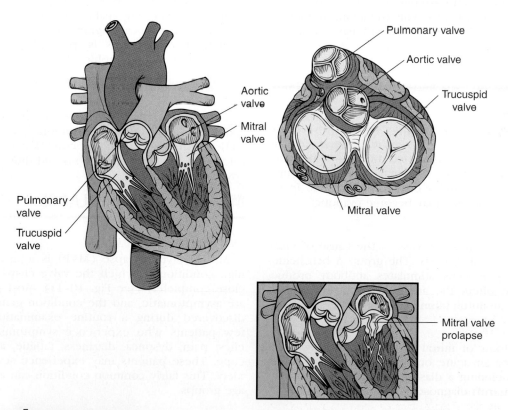

Aortic valve
Mitral valve
Pulmonary valve
Trucuspid valve

Pulmonary valve
Aortic valve
Trucuspid valve
Mitral valve

Mitral valve prolapse

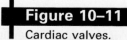
Figure 10-11
Cardiac valves.

damage the valves. Prophylactic antibiotics are given to the patient before any dental procedures.

Valvular Heart Disease

Valvular heart disease is an acquired or congenital disorder that can involve any of the four valves of the heart (see Fig. 10–11). This condition can occur in the form of either insufficiency or stenosis. Insufficiency, the failure of the valves to close completely, allows blood to be forced back into the previous chamber as the heart contracts. This exerts added pressure on that chamber and increases the heart's workload. Stenosis, a hardening of the cusps of the valves that prevents complete opening of the valves, impedes the blood flow into the next chamber. The mitral valve is involved most frequently. Diagnosis of valvular heart disease includes ECG, radiographic chest studies, echocardiogram, and cardiac catheterization. Treatment entails the administration of digitalis or quinidine for arrhythmias and antibiotic prophylaxis.

MITRAL STENOSIS

SYMPTOMS AND SIGNS

The mitral, or bicuspid, valve lies between the left atrium and the left ventricle. Mitral stenosis causes patients to have exertional dyspnea and fatigue. Additionally, they may experience cough and palpitations followed by **hemoptysis.** In severe cases, patients may become cyanotic.

ETIOLOGY

Rheumatic heart disease is the cause of most cases of mitral stenosis. The group A beta-hemolytic streptococcus stimulates antibody production, and often, the antibodies attack the body tissue in an autoimmune response.

DIAGNOSIS

Symptoms of mitral stenosis may have an insidious or an acute onset. A cardiac murmur is heard, including a diastolic murmur. Echocardiogram confirms diagnostic suspicions.

TREATMENT

Limitation of sodium intake, along with the administration of diuretics, is helpful in reducing the workload of the heart. Anticoagulants prevent the formation of thrombi. Surgical intervention in the form of a **commissurotomy** may be necessary to free up the valve and to allow adequate blood flow. Valve replacement is a final option.

MITRAL INSUFFICIENCY

SYMPTOMS AND SIGNS

In mitral insufficiency, the mitral valve fails to close completely. The patient experiences dyspnea and fatigue. A heart murmur can be heard as the blood leaks back into the left atrium as a result of the valve's not closing completely.

ETIOLOGY

Often the valve fails to close because of scar from inflammation and vegetations, a consequence of rheumatic fever. Mitral valve prolapse also may be the culprit.

DIAGNOSIS

Diagnosis is made from a thorough patient history, especially a history of a sore throat or rheumatic fever. Physical examination reveals a murmur, and echocardiogram discloses the insufficiency. Cardiac status is assessed additionally with an ECG, radiographic chest film, and cardiac catheterization.

TREATMENT

Treatment includes bed rest, oxygen therapy, and the administration of antibiotics for any infectious process. When the condition is complicated by CHF, fluid restrictions and diuretic therapy are implemented.

MITRAL VALVE PROLAPSE

SYMPTOMS AND SIGNS

Mitral valve prolapse (MVP) is a usually benign condition in which the valve cusps do not close completely (see Fig. 10–11). Most patients are asymptomatic, and the condition generally is discovered during a routine examination. The few patients who experience symptoms report chest pain, dyspnea, dizziness, fatigue, and syncope. These patients may experience severe anxiety. This fairly common condition can affect all age groups.

ETIOLOGY

Abnormally long or short chordae tendineae may be the cause of the valve's inability to close properly. Malfunctioning papillary muscles may add to the severity of the condition. Regurgitation of blood occurs during left ventricular systole and results in the rushing, gurgling cardiac murmur characteristic of the prolapse.

DIAGNOSIS

The typical click-murmur syndrome is heard on auscultation of the heart. Echocardiogram confirms the failure of the valve to close. The premature ventricular contractions (PVCs) that are detected on ECG are not considered harmful and are not an indication of insult to the myocardium.

TREATMENT

Treatment generally is not required for asymptomatic patients. Those who experience discomfort and anxiety often are treated with beta-blockers, and they are advised to avoid caffeine and large, heavy meals.

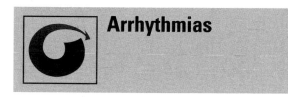

Arrhythmias

SYMPTOMS AND SIGNS

Arrhythmias occur when there is interference with the conduction system of the heart, resulting in an abnormality of the heartbeat. Symptoms include palpitations, rapid heartbeat (tachycardia), skipped heartbeats, slow heart rate (bradycardia), syncope, and fatigue.

ETIOLOGY

Arrhythmias can arise from disturbances in the normal conduction system of the heart, including the pacemaker (the sinoatrial [SA] node), the atrioventricular (AV) node, the bundle branches, and the Purkinje fibers (Fig. 10–12). Ischemia and drugs are responsible for many arrhythmias. Failure of the SA node may be responsible. Table 10-1 lists the causes of arrhythmias.

DIAGNOSIS

Diagnosis is made from a 12-lead ECG. Various arrhythmias are evident to the physician. Echocardiography may aid in the confirmation of a particular arrhythmia. A Holter monitor (ambulatory ECG) may be worn by the patient to capture any arrhythmic event.

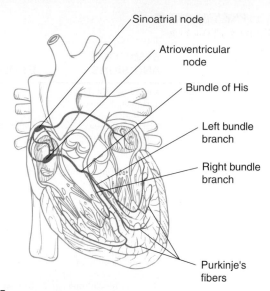

Figure 10–12

Conduction system of the heart.

TREATMENT

Treatment depends on the cause (see Table 10-1). Drug-induced arrhythmias usually resolve with cessation of the drug administration. Ischemia should respond to oxygen administration and increased blood flow to the tissue. Occasionally, the heart rhythm does not stabilize and the arrhythmia can be fatal.

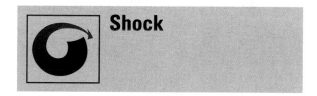

Shock

SYMPTOMS AND SIGNS

Shock is the collapse (vasodilation and fluid shift accompanied by inefficient cardiac output) of the cardiovascular system. It causes inadequate perfusion of organs and tissues. The patient has pale, cold, and clammy skin; a rapid, weak, and thready pulse; rapid breathing; and an altered level of consciousness. The blood pressure drops, and the patient may be anxious, irritable, or restless and often expresses a feeling of impending doom. There may be dizziness, extreme thirst, and profuse sweating. In late stages, the pupils dilate, the eyes become dull and lusterless, and the patient experiences shaking and trembling.

TABLE 10–1 ➤ Arrhythmias

TYPES	SYMPTOMS AND SIGNS	ETIOLOGY	DIAGNOSIS	TREATMENT
Normal sinus rhythm	Rate of 60–100 bpm, regular, P wave uniform	Impulse originates in SA node, conduction normal	Normal	None indicated
Sinus tachycardia	Rate >100 bpm, regular, P wave uniform	Rapid impulse originates in SA node, conduction normal	Rapid rate	Beta blockers, calcium channel blockers
Sinus bradycardia	Rate <60 bpm, regular, P wave uniform	Slow impulse originates in SA node, conduction normal	Slow rate	Atropine
Premature atrial contraction	Rate depends on underlying rhythm, usually normal P wave, different morphology from other P waves	Irritable atrium, single ectopic beat that arises prematurely, conduction through ventricle normal	Irregular heartbeat, diagnosis by ECG	Treatment usually unnecessary; if needed, antiarrhythmic drugs
Atrial tachycardia	Rate of 150–250 bpm, rhythm normal, sudden onset	Irritable atrium, firing at rapid rates, normal conduction	Rapid rate with atrial and ventricular rates identical, diagnosis by ECG	Reflex vagal stimulation, calcium channel–blocking drugs (verapamil), cardioversion
Atrial fibrillation	Atrial rate >350 bpm, ventricular rate <100 bpm (controlled) or >100 bpm (rapid ventricular response)	Atrial ectopic foci discharging at too rapid and chaotic rate for muscles to respond and contract, resulting in quivering of atrium—AV node blocks some impulses and ventricle responds irregularly	ECG shows no P waves, grossly irregular ventricular rate	IV verapamil; if unsuccessful, procainamide; if unsuccessful, cardioversion
First-degree heart block	Rate depends on rate of underlying rhythm, PR interval >0.20 second	Delay at AV node, impulse eventually conducted	ECG shows PR interval >0.20 second	Atropine; if unsuccessful, artificial pacemaker insertion
Second-degree heart block, Wenckebach block	Intermittent block with progressively longer delay in conduction until one beat is blocked—atrial rate normal, ventricular rate slower than normal, rhythm irregular	SA node initiates impulse, conduction through AV node is blocked intermittently	ECG shows normal P waves, some P waves not followed by QRS complex; PR interval progressively longer, followed by block of impulse	Mild forms, no treatment; severe, insertion of artificial pacemaker
Classic second-degree heart block	Ventricular rate slow (½, ⅓, or ¼ of atrial rate)—rhythm, regular—P waves normal, QRS complex dropped every 2nd, 3rd, or 4th beat	SA node initiates impulse, conduction through AV node is blocked	ECG shows P waves present, QRS complex blocked every 2nd, 3rd, or 4th impulse	Artificial pacemaker is inserted
Third-degree heart block	Atrial rate normal, ventricular rate 20–40 or 40–60 bpm—no relationship between P wave and QRS complex	SA node initiates impulse, which is completely blocked from conduction, causing atria and ventricles to beat independently	ECG shows P waves and QRS complexes with no relationship to each other, rhythms are regular but independent of each other	Insertion of artificial pacemaker is necessary

302

TABLE 10–1 ➤ Arrhythmias *Continued*

TYPES	SYMPTOMS AND SIGNS	ETIOLOGY	DIAGNOSIS	TREATMENT
Premature ventricular contraction (single focus)	Single ectopic beat, arising from ventricle, followed by compensatory pause	Ectopic beat originates in irritable ventricle	ECG shows a wide, bizarre QRS complex >0.12 second usually followed by a compensatory pause	Usually no treatment if <6 per minute and single focus
Multifocal arrhythmia Coupling, 2 in a row Bigeminy, every other beat Trigeminy, every 3rd beat Quadrigeminy, every 4th beat	Rate dependent on underlying rhythm—rhythm regular or irregular—P wave absent before ectopic beat	Same as single focus (above)	Same as single focus (above)	Same as single focus (above)
Ventricular tachycardia	Rate of 150–250 bpm, rhythm usually regular—focus of pacemaker normally single, patient experiences palpitations, dyspnea, and anxiety followed by chest pain	4 or more consecutive PVCs at a rapid rate due to advanced irritability of myocardium, indicating ventricular command of heart rate	ECG shows runs of 4 or more PVCs, P wave buried in QRS complex	Often forerunner of ventricular fibrillation—immediate intervention necessary—IV lidocaine; if unsuccessful, follow by cardioversion—procainamide or bretylium may be used
Ventricular fibrillation (a lethal arrhythmia)	Patient loses consciousness immediately after onset—no peripheral pulses palpable, no heart sounds, no blood pressure	Ventricular fibers twitch rather than contract, reason unknown	Pulseless, unconscious patient—ECG shows rapid, repetitive, chaotic waves originating in ventricle	Recognize and terminate rhythm—precordial shock (defibrillation)

AV, atrioventricular; bpm, beats per minute; ECG, electrocardiogram; IV, intravenous; PR, pulse rate; PVCs, premature ventricular contractions; SA, sinoatrial.

ETIOLOGY

This life-threatening emergency can be caused by **anaphylaxis,** hemorrhage, sepsis, respiratory distress, heart failure, neurologic failure, emotional catastrophe, or severe metabolic insult. Regardless of the cause, there is a decrease in the amount of blood that is effectively circulating in the body. The final effect is that the vital organs (heart, brain, lungs, and kidneys) do not receive the oxygen and nutrients needed to sustain life. Rapid blood loss or significant fluid loss with subsequent hypovolemia precipitates shock. Failure of the heart to pump adequately is another cause of shock. Vascular collapse with subsequent massive dilation or constriction of the vessels can cause blood to pool away from vital areas. Insufficient oxygen supply to the circulating system can generate shock.

DIAGNOSIS

The clinical picture, along with history of a precipitating event, leads to the diagnosis of shock due to inadequate cellular perfusion. The altered level of consciousness and respiratory distress suggest shock. Immediate intervention must take place to halt the progression of the condition.

TREATMENT

Because of the severity and rapid progression of the condition, aggressive intervention is undertaken at the earliest possible opportunity. The ABCs (airway, breathing, and circulation) of emergency care indicate maintaining an open airway and establishing ventilation to supply the vital organs with oxygen. Any visible bleeding is controlled, and surgical intervention may be necessary to halt internal bleeding. The patient should be placed in a **supine** position, with the feet and legs elevated, and should be kept warm but not overheated. If the patient is not in an inpatient facility, contact with the emergency medical service (EMS) for immediate transport to an emergency facility is indicated. Vital signs are monitored, and volume replacement is instituted with intravenous fluids. When supplemental oxygen is available, it is administered.

CARDIOGENIC SHOCK

SYMPTOMS AND SIGNS

In cardiogenic shock (inadequate cardiac output), the myocardium fails to pump effectively. The patient exhibits the previously mentioned symptoms and signs of shock. The event usually is preceded by MI or severe heart failure, certain arrhythmias, or acute valve failure.

ETIOLOGY

Any insult that disturbs the heart's ability to pump blood can cause cardiogenic shock. MI, severe heart failure, certain arrhythmias, or valve failure can lead to cardiogenic shock.

DIAGNOSIS

The clinical picture and a history of a major cardiac insult lead to the suspicion of cardiogenic shock. An ECG is another diagnostic tool, as are radiographic chest studies. A hypotensive state that continues to worsen also indicates the diagnosis.

TREATMENT

Treatment consists of general measures for shock, along with the administration of medications that increase the efficiency of the myocardium. Blood supply to vital organs must be improved, and myocardial tissue oxygen demands need to be reduced. Blood volume assessment determines whether drugs are given to dilate or constrict cardiac vessels.

Cardiac Tamponade

SYMPTOMS AND SIGNS

Cardiac tamponade occurs when a coronary, epicardial, or pericardial vessel breaks and blood is trapped in the pericardial sac. Additionally, the myocardium may rupture, also sending blood into the pericardial sac. The blood constricts heart movement, and less blood can enter the heart chambers per beat. The patient with cardiac tamponade experiences sudden severe dyspnea and rapidly falling blood pressure. The pulse becomes weak, thready, and rapid. The patient is in shock and becomes cyanotic above the nipple line. The level of consciousness falls.

ETIOLOGY

Cardiac tamponade occurs when there is an insult to the integrity of a vessel in the pericardium, allowing blood to fill the pericardial space. The pressure of the blood causes the heart to beat inappropriately, leading to cardiac arrest.

DIAGNOSIS

Diagnosis is made from the clinical picture and a history of a traumatic event. Heart sounds become muffled or distant, whereas breath sounds remain normal.

TREATMENT

Treatment consists of inserting a needle into the pericardial space and withdrawing the offending blood. Surgery usually is indicated to repair the leak.

Vascular Conditions

The vascular system, a closed transport system composed of arteries, arterioles, capillaries, venules, and veins, is responsible for supplying blood tissues with blood containing oxygen and nutrients. Waste products and carbon dioxide also are conveyed to the appropriate organs for excretion by this system. Arteries carry blood away from the heart (Fig. 10-13A), veins transport blood back to the heart (Fig. 10-13B), whereas capillaries are the point of exchange at the cellular level (Fig. 10-13C).

Blood vessel walls, other than one-cell–walled capillaries, are composed of three coats: the tunica intima, the tunica media, and the tunica externa (Fig. 10-14). The lining of the vessel lumen, the tunica intima, is composed of smooth,

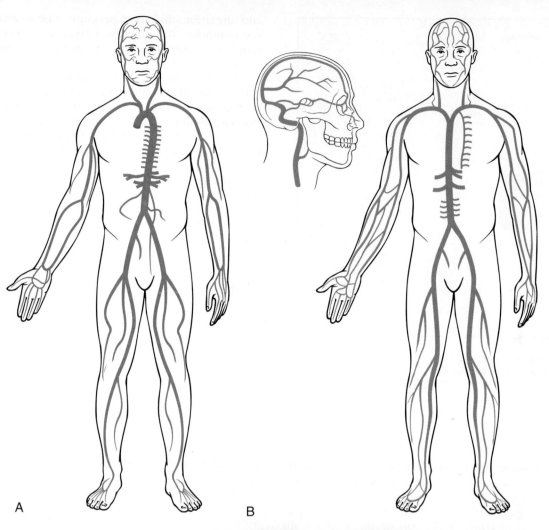

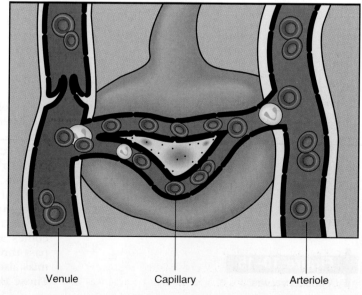

A

B

Figure 10–13

Vascular system. *A,* Arteries. *B,* Veins. *C,* Capillary exchange.

C   Venule   Capillary   Arteriole

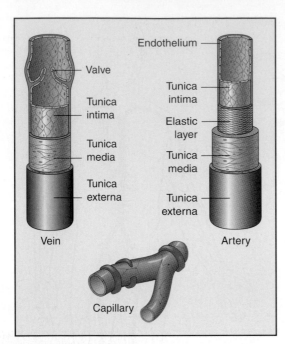

Figure 10–14

Vessel wall structure.

thin endothelium, allowing decreased friction of the flowing blood. The middle portion, the tunica media, is composed of smooth muscle and elastic tissue, which is under the control of the sympathetic nervous system. This innervation allows constriction or dilation of the vessel walls

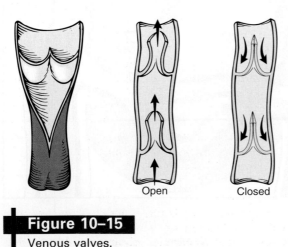

Figure 10–15

Venous valves.

and alterations in blood pressure. Connective tissue composes the outermost layer, the tunica externa, providing support and protection for the vessels.

Arterial walls are much thicker than venous walls, with the tunica media being heavier in arteries to compensate for the stronger blood pressure under which the arteries must function. Veins, with their lower blood pressure, contain valves to prevent backflow and to assist the return of blood to the heart (Fig. 10-15).

Vascular conditions include emboli, arteriosclerosis, atherosclerosis, aneurysms, phlebitis, thrombophlebitis, varicose veins, thromboangiitis obliterans (Buerger's disease), and Raynaud's disease.

EMBOLI

SYMPTOMS AND SIGNS

Emboli are clots of **aggregated** material (usually blood). They can lodge in a blood vessel and inhibit the blood flow. Symptoms depend on the location of the vessel that is occluded and the magnitude of the area of tissue served by the blood supply. The initial symptom is severe pain in the area of the embolus. Emboli lodging in arteries of the extremities cause the area to become pale, numb, and cold to the touch. Additionally, arterial pulses are absent below the occlusion if it is arterial. When a large artery is involved, the patient also experiences nausea, vomiting, fainting, and eventually shock. Pulmonary obstructions are discussed in Chapter 9. Cerebral obstructions and CVAs are discussed in Chapter 13.

ETIOLOGY

Emboli are most often blood clots; however, the offending embolus may be composed of air bubbles, fat globules, bacterial clumps, or pieces of tissue, including placenta. The most common offender is a venous thrombosis, a blood clot that has formed in the deep veins of the legs as a result of venous stasis (Fig. 10-16). A portion of the thrombus breaks loose from the clot and travels through the venous system until it becomes lodged in a vessel that is too narrow to pass through, often in the lungs. Cardiac arrhythmias also can cause thrombi to form in the heart. Those that travel from the left ventricle can en-

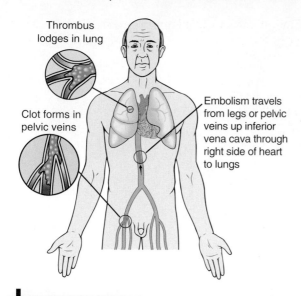

Thrombus lodges in lung

Clot forms in pelvic veins

Embolism travels from legs or pelvic veins up inferior vena cava through right side of heart to lungs

Figure 10–16
Venous thrombosis.

ter the coronary arteries, resulting in an MI, or the carotid and cerebral arteries, compromising blood supply and resulting in CVAs.

DIAGNOSIS

The clinical picture and a history of bed rest, physical inactivity, heart failure, arrhythmias, and any condition that has put pressure on or decreased flow in the veins of the legs or pelvis alert the physician to the possibility of an embolus. Pain in the calf of the leg in a patient who has any of the aforementioned predispositions is another clue.

TREATMENT

Treatment depends on the area of involvement. Treatment of pulmonary embolism (see Chapter 9), myocardial infarction, and CVA (see Chapter 13) is aggressive and immediate if the patient is to survive. The treatment of a patient with an arterial embolus in an extremity is also aggressive and immediate to prevent the death of tissue and eventual **gangrene.** Blood flow is reestablished to the affected part by lowering the limb and wrapping it to maintain warmth to the area and by treating any constriction of blood vessels. Heparin is administered to deter further clot formation, and antispasmodic drugs are given for vascular spasms. If this therapy is not successful, surgical intervention may be indicated to remove the obstruction and to restore circulation.

ARTERIOSCLEROSIS

Arteriosclerosis is a group of diseases characterized by hardening of the arteries. It has three forms: atherosclerosis, Mönckeberg's arteriosclerosis, and arteriolosclerosis. Atherosclerosis occurs when plaques of fatty deposits form within the arterial tunica intima. Mönckeberg's arteriosclerosis, medial calcific sclerosis, involves the arterial tunica media; there is destruction of muscle and elastic fibers along with calcium deposits. Arteriosclerosis occurs when there is a thickening of the walls of the arterioles, with loss of elasticity and contractility.

Atherosclerosis

SYMPTOMS AND SIGNS

Atherosclerosis, a thickening and hardening of the arteries, occurs when plaques of cholesterol and lipids are formed in the arterial tunica intima. Atherosclerosis is responsible for most myocardial and cerebral infarctions. Often, the patient with atherosclerosis is asymptomatic. The first symptoms may be angina pectoris, dizziness, elevated blood pressure, and shortness of breath.

ETIOLOGY

The etiology of atherosclerosis is multifactorial and complicated; however, there are risk factors that appear to increase the probability of the condition developing. Heredity seems to play a role in increased frequency, as do a sedentary lifestyle, a diet rich in lipids and cholesterol-producing foods, cigarette smoking, diabetes mellitus, hypertension, and obesity. The lipids and cholesterol in the blood form thick, stiff, and hardened lesions in the medium-sized and large arteries. The lesions are eccentric and expand to occlude the artery eventually (Fig. 10–17). A fatty streak forms in the arterial wall, migrating to the tunica intima. Plaque forms and thickens the arterial wall. A sequela is an **ulceration,** crack, or fissure in the plaque where platelets can aggregate and form a thrombosis. Ischemia results from decreased blood supply to the dependent tissue, with resulting pain. Infarct occurs with advanced occlusion of the artery and is followed by tissue **necrosis.**

DIAGNOSIS

Diagnosis often is made during a routine physical examination or screening process. Blood studies indicate elevated cholesterol, triglyceride, and lipid levels. Hypertension may be noted.

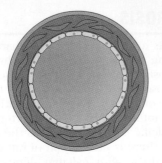
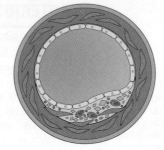
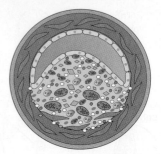

Normal arterial
lumen

Atherosclerotic
plaque deposit

Advanced arterial
atherosclerotic
disease

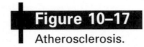

Figure 10–17
Atherosclerosis.

Doppler studies of major vessels show reduced blood flow.

TREATMENT

Treatment consists of dietary alterations to reduce saturated fats and foods high in cholesterol and lipids. Cigarette smokers are encouraged to stop smoking. Hypertension and diabetes mellitus are treated and controlled. Hyperlipidemic drugs such as lovastatin (Mevacor) and simvastatin (Zocor) are prescribed. Research is being conducted to confirm claims that hyperlipidemic drug therapy can bring about regression of the condition and actually reverse the plaque buildup.

Prevention is important, as is education about risk factors and alterations in lifestyle.

ANEURYSMS

SYMPTOMS AND SIGNS

An aneurysm is a weakening and resulting local dilation of the wall of an artery (Fig. 10–18). The symptoms may have either an insidious or a sudden, acute onset. Symptoms depend on the location and size of the aneurysm and the extent of the dilation. Abdominal aortic aneurysm is the most common form. An asymptomatic aneurysm of the aorta frequently is discovered during a routine physical examination when the abdomen is being palpated or as the result of an abdominal radiographic study for another reason. As the aortic aneurysm enlarges, the patient may experience abdominal or back pain, and a pulsating mass is observed in the abdomen. A complication of any aneurysm is leakage from the wall of the artery or sudden rupture of the weak area.

When this occurs, the patient exhibits symptoms and signs of hemorrhagic shock. Rupture of a cerebral aneurysm mimics signs of a CVA, with unilateral neurologic deficits being noted.

ETIOLOGY

A common cause of aneurysms is a buildup of atherosclerotic plaque, which weakens the vessel

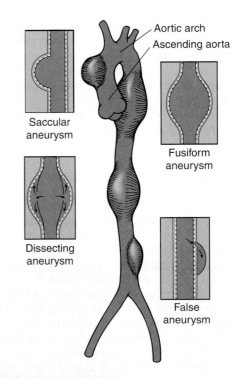

Aortic arch
Ascending aorta

Saccular
aneurysm

Fusiform
aneurysm

Dissecting
aneurysm

False
aneurysm

Figure 10–18
Types of aortic aneurysms.

wall. Trauma, infection or inflammation, and congenital tendencies are additional causative factors.

DIAGNOSIS

The aortic mass is noted mid abdomen, and pulsation is observed. A **bruit** heard on auscultation is another sign of the existing arterial dilation. Cerebral aneurysms usually are discovered when they rupture with catastrophic consequences. Radiographic studies, ultrasonography, computed tomography (CT), and magnetic resonance imaging (MRI) all help to confirm the diagnosis. The ruptured aneurysm precipitates symptoms and signs of shock.

TREATMENT

Treatment depends on the size, location, and likelihood of rupture of the defect. Most diagnosed aortic aneurysms should have surgical repair before leakage or rupture. After the aorta wall's integrity has been breached, immediate surgical intervention is required to repair the rupture, usually with a synthetic graft, if the patient is to survive. Watchful waiting often is employed when the aneurysm is small itself or is in a small vessel.

PHLEBITIS

SYMPTOMS AND SIGNS

Phlebitis, an inflammation of a vein, occurs most commonly in the lower legs; however, any vein, including cranial veins, may be affected. Superficial vein involvement results in pain and tenderness in the affected area and becomes more severe as the condition progresses. Swelling, redness, and warmth are noted, followed by the development of a tender cord-like mass under the skin.

Deep venous inflammation affects the tunica intima, allowing the formation of clots (thrombophlebitis).

ETIOLOGY

The cause is uncertain, and the condition may appear for no apparent reason; however, venous stasis, obesity, blood disorders, injury, or surgery may be the origin.

DIAGNOSIS

The clinical picture and history of a preceding event are helpful in establishing the diagnosis.

TREATMENT

Treatment of superficial phlebitis is symptomatic, with analgesics given for pain. Caution must be taken not to massage the affected tender area because this manipulation may cause stimulation of clot formation or the release of formed clots as emboli.

THROMBOPHLEBITIS

SYMPTOMS AND SIGNS

Thrombophlebitis is the result of inflammation of a vein with the formation of a thrombus on the vessel wall. It causes an interference with blood flow and resulting edema. As with phlebitis, the patient experiences pain, swelling, heaviness, and warmth in the affected area along with chills and fever. The involved area is tender to palpation.

ETIOLOGY

Venous stasis, blood disorders that cause a **hypercoagulable** state, and injury to the venous wall play important roles in the occurrence of thrombophlebitis. The deep venous inflammation of phlebitis affects the tunica intima, allowing the formation of clots (thrombophlebitis).

DIAGNOSIS

The clinical picture of gross edema in one leg, resulting in a measurable difference in the circumference of the legs, suggests thrombophlebitis. The affected area is tender to palpation. Imaging of the vessel with radiographic venography and ultrasonography confirms the diagnosis.

TREATMENT

Immediate intervention is necessary. The affected part is immobilized to prevent the thrombus from spreading and dislodging to become an embolus. Heparin is administered to prevent the clot from enlarging, and antibiotics are given to prevent infection. Generally, the condition resolves and no further treatment is indicated. If the condition does not resolve, surgical intervention may be needed to ligate the affected vessel. Collateral circulation develops.

VARICOSE VEINS

SYMPTOMS AND SIGNS

Varicose veins are swollen, tortuous, and knotted veins that usually occur in the lower legs

(Fig. 10-19). Symptoms develop gradually, with a feeling of fatigue in the legs, followed by a continuous dull ache. Leg cramps may be experienced at night, and the ankles may swell. As the condition progresses, the veins thicken and feel hard to the touch. Pain worsens and can have a dull or stabbing quality.

ETIOLOGY

There is no clearly identifiable cause of varicose veins. However, defective or absent valves may be suspected. Prolonged standing or sitting causes pressure on the valves in the superficial veins of the lower legs. Normal movement of the legs causes the muscles to contract and relax, thus "milking" the blood upward. When the person stands or sits for extended periods, gravity pushes the blood downward, with resulting pressure on the valves. Without the normal muscular contractions, the venous walls distend, reaching a point at which they and the valves are no longer competent. Stasis of blood follows, causing the swelling of the veins. The enlarging uterus during pregnancy increases the pressure on the leg veins and pelvic veins, compromising the free flow of the venous blood.

DIAGNOSIS

The presence of the twisted, swollen, knotted veins of the lower legs on clinical inspection and a history of prolonged standing, prolonged sitting, or pregnancy are usually all that is needed to make the diagnosis. Advanced varicosities cause the skin around the affected areas to take on a brown discoloration.

TREATMENT

Rest periods throughout the day, with the patient lying down and elevating the feet higher than the heart, afford relief in mild cases. Engaging in exercise and submerging the legs in warm water increase the flow of blood. Support stockings that encourage the return flow of blood may be worn. Those who have to stand for extended periods are instructed to move the legs at frequent intervals to stimulate the muscular milking of the veins.

Painful, twisted, and swollen veins that have progressed beyond treatment by rest and exercise usually necessitate surgical intervention in the form of a vein ligation and stripping or injection of **sclerosing** solutions that harden and eventually **atrophy** the affected veins. Collateral circulation develops to augment the blood return to the heart.

THROMBOANGIITIS OBLITERANS (BUERGER'S DISEASE)

SYMPTOMS AND SIGNS

Thromboangiitis obliterans (Buerger's disease) is an inflammation of the peripheral arteries and veins of the extremities with clot formation. The patient experiences intense pain in the affected area, usually the legs or the instep of the foot, which is aggravated by exercise and relieved by rest. If the condition is not resolved and circulation is not restored to the affected area, atrophy, ulcers, and even gangrene can develop.

ETIOLOGY

The primary cause of Buerger's disease is a long duration of smoking tobacco. The inflammation and resulting clot formation in the vessels continue to advance until the entire vessel is obliterated and circulation is completely compromised to the area. The ischemic tissue dies, and gangrene follows. This condition affects primarily males, most generally those of Jewish descent.

DIAGNOSIS

Diagnosis follows reports of intense pain, usually in the legs or the instep. An arteriogram and other studies such as an ultrasonogram identify

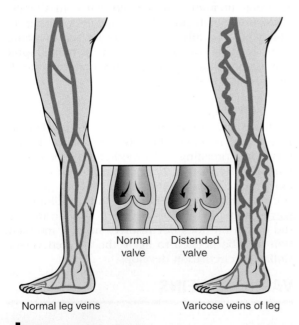

Normal valve   Distended valve

Normal leg veins   Varicose veins of leg

Figure 10–19

Varicose veins.

the site of the clot or obliteration. The ulcers on the skin are another indication of the disease and its severity. The history of a long duration of smoking tobacco products suggests the diagnosis.

TREATMENT

The first step in treatment is the immediate and complete cessation of smoking. This often reduces the inflammation and restores partial circulation to the area. Buerger-Allen exercises also help to improve circulation to the area. These exercises consist of elevating the feet and legs 45 to 90° until they blanch and then lowering them below the rest of the body until they redden. This is followed by having the patient rest in a supine position. When circulation is not restored, surgical intervention to establish detours or to bore a pathway through the clot itself may be necessary. Amputation of gangrenous tissue is imperative. Education of the patient includes information about the care of foot injuries and instructions about avoidance of constrictions around the affected limb.

RAYNAUD'S DISEASE

SYMPTOMS AND SIGNS

Raynaud's disease is a vasospastic condition of the fingers, hands, or feet. It causes pain, numbness, and sometimes discoloration in these areas. This bilateral condition is precipitated by cold and causes a blanching (white) discoloration, which is followed by blue as venous blood remains, and finally changes to red or purple when circulation is restored. Occasionally, the attacks are triggered by stressful events. Raynaud's disease is much more common in women than in men. When the disorder is primary, it is called Raynaud's disease; when it is secondary to another disease, it is referred to as Raynaud's phenomenon. In severe cases, the digits may ulcerate and become quite painful. In most cases, the prognosis is good.

ETIOLOGY

The small peripheral arteries and arterioles supplying the fingers, hands, and feet spasm and constrict, compromising the circulation to these appendages. The spasm follows exposure to cold or is possibly the result of a stressful occurrence. The episode usually resolves spontaneously after the application of warmth. The condition also is made worse by smoking tobacco.

DIAGNOSIS

Diagnosis is made by the clinical picture and a history of numbness and paleness of the areas. Normal arterial pulses are present. The condition most frequently affects women between puberty and the age of 40 years, especially those who smoke. In severe cases, the compromised circulation can lead to tissue necrosis and even amputation.

TREATMENT

Treatment of the episode involves the application of warmth to the areas. Patients are encouraged to stop smoking, to avoid exposure to cold, and to avoid stressful situations that bring on the attacks. Drug therapy to dilate vessels and to increase blood flow includes vasodilators, alpha-adrenergic blockers, and calcium channel blockers. Frequently, the side effects of the drug therapy are worse than the condition.

Blood Dyscrasias

311

Blood is composed of formed elements, red blood cells (erythrocytes), white blood cells (leukocytes), platelets (thrombocytes), and a liquid portion (plasma). It is responsible for transporting vital elements, including oxygen, nutrients, and hormones, to the body cells. It also plays a part in the removal of waste products, in the inflammatory response, and in the function of the immune system. Additionally, blood helps to maintain **hemostasis,** acid–base and fluid balance, and body temperature.

Blood is synthesized by the **hematopoietic** system in the bone marrow (myeloid) and lymphoid tissue found in the lymph nodes, spleen, thymus, bone marrow, and gastrointestinal tract (Fig. 10-20). The **reticuloendothelial** system is found in the spleen, liver, lymph nodes, and bone marrow. It is responsible for removing worn-out blood cells from the bloodstream and breaking down the blood cell components for recycling or elimination from the body.

Stem cells in the bone marrow form blast cells, including erythroblasts (rubriblasts), which eventually become erythrocytes, and myeloblasts, which eventually become leukocytes (Fig. 10-21).

Deviation or malfunctioning in this system results in various blood dyscrasias either by impair-

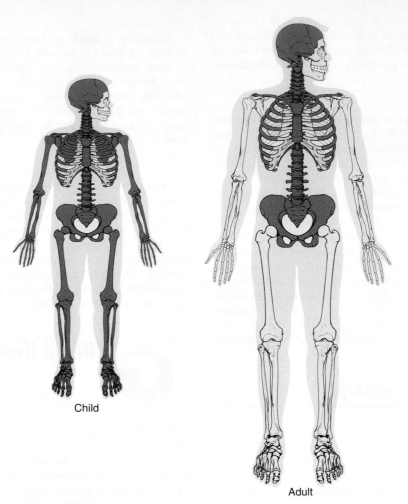

Child

Adult

Figure 10–20
Sites of blood cell formation.

ment in the formation of the blood components or by unusual destruction of the cells. Dyscrasias involving erythrocytes and platelets are anemias, thrombocytoses, thrombocytopenias, and polycythemias. Leukocyte dyscrasias include leukemias, lymphomas, and leukopenias. Bleeding and clotting problems arise from alterations affecting thrombocytes and plasma-clotting factors. Normal values of blood components are measured by specific laboratory testing.

Figure 10–21
Blood cell production (hematopoiesis). *Erythrocytes* transport oxygen. *Basophils* promote the inflammatory response and release histamine and the anticoagulant heparin; called mast cells in the tissues. *Eosinophils* counteract histamine in allergic reactions; destroy parasitic worms. *Neutrophils* are immune phagocytes. *Monocytes* are phagocytic cells (macrophages) that dispose of dead cells and other debris. *B cells* and *T cells* are lymphocytes that function in immunity. *Thrombocytes* help control blood loss by forming platelet plug and releasing blood-clotting factors.

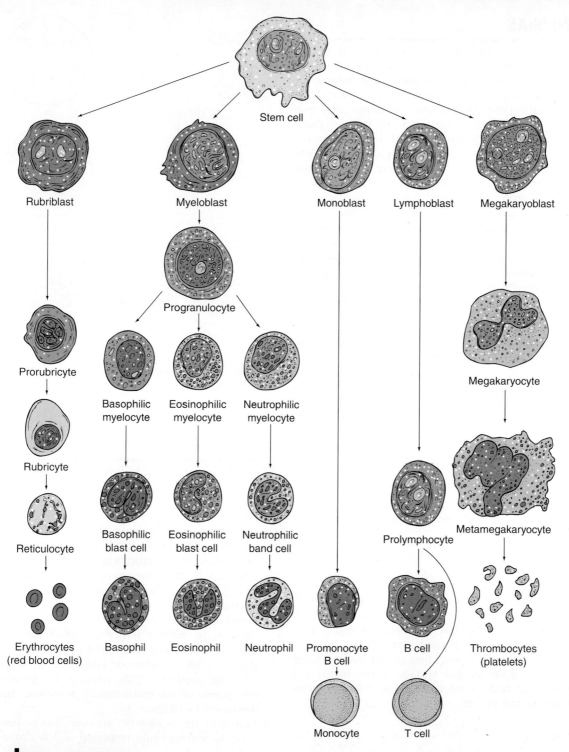

Stem cell

Rubriblast

Myeloblast

Monoblast

Lymphoblast

Megakaryoblast

Progranulocyte

Prorubricyte

Basophilic myelocyte

Eosinophilic myelocyte

Neutrophilic myelocyte

Megakaryocyte

Rubricyte

Basophilic blast cell

Eosinophilic blast cell

Neutrophilic band cell

Prolymphocyte

Metamegakaryocyte

Reticulocyte

Erythrocytes (red blood cells)

Basophil

Eosinophil

Neutrophil

Promonocyte B cell

B cell

Thrombocytes (platelets)

Monocyte

T cell

313

Figure 10–21

See legend on opposite page.

ANEMIAS

Anemia is defined as a condition in which there is a reduction in the quantity of either RBCs or hemoglobin in a measured volume of blood, reducing the blood's ability to carry oxygen to the cells. Depending on its severity, one or many symptoms occur: pallor, fatigue, dizziness, shortness of breath, and irregular heartbeats. The treatment varies with the cause. Several possible causes include acute or chronic blood loss, impaired production of RBCs (aplastic anemia, iron deficiency anemia, anemias of chronic disease, or megaloblastic anemia), inherited or acquired hemolytic conditions, and hemolytic–hemoglobin disorders. Hemoglobin in RBCs is necessary to transport oxygen to all cells, and any condition that reduces the amount of hemoglobin results in anemia. Iron and other components are necessary to synthesize the hemoglobin.

Types of anemias include iron deficiency, folic acid deficiency, pernicious, aplastic, sickle cell, hemorrhagic, and hemolytic.

Important presenting symptoms that tend to recur in patients with anemia and need further investigation include

- Fatigue
- Dyspnea (difficulty in breathing)
- Headache
- Loss of appetite
- Heartburn
- Edema, especially of the ankles
- Numbness and tingling sensations
- Syncope (fainting)
- Pallor

SYMPTOMS AND SIGNS

Regardless of the cause, anemic patients experience fatigue. Most appear pale. As the disease progresses, the symptoms become more pronounced, and the patient may have dyspnea, tachycardia, and a pounding of the heart. Pallor is noted on the palmar surface of the hands and in the nail beds, conjunctiva, and mucous membranes of the mouth.

ETIOLOGY

Anemias are classified by the color and size of the RBC as hypochromic, normochromic, or hyperchromic (spherocytosis) and as microcytic, normocytic, or macrocytic (Fig. 10–22), respectively. They also are classified by the causative factor, as previously mentioned.

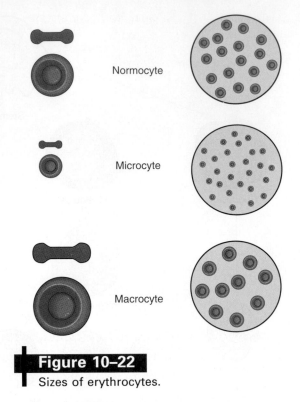

Normocyte

Microcyte

Macrocyte

Figure 10–22

Sizes of erythrocytes.

- Iron deficiency anemia may be secondary to blood loss through hemorrhage, a slow insidious bleed such as bleeding hemorrhoids and even heavy menstrual flow, or lack of sufficient dietary iron intake.
- Folic acid deficiency anemia results when there are insufficient amounts of folic acid available for DNA (deoxyribonucleic acid) synthesis, thus preventing the maturation of the blood cells. This can be the consequence of a dietary deficiency and is clinically similar to pernicious anemia.
- Pernicious anemia is considered a macrocytic anemia, in which immature RBCs are larger than normal. The hemoglobin volume is reduced, with subsequent reduction in oxygen-carrying capacity. This anemia is considered the result of an autoimmune response and is discussed in Chapter 3.
- Autoimmune hemolytic anemia also is considered an autoimmune response and is discussed in Chapter 3.
- Aplastic anemia occurs because of an insult to the hematopoietic cells (stem cells) in the bone marrow. Erythrocyte, leukocyte, and thrombocyte production all are decreased because of exposure to myelotoxins, such as benzene, al-

kylating agents, antimetabolites, certain drugs and insecticides, and radiation.

- Sickle cell anemia, a chronic hereditary **hemolytic** form of anemia, is found predominately in those of the black race. The presence of hemoglobin S along with hemoglobin A is noted in erythrocytes, causing them to acquire a sickle or elongated shape on deoxygenation (Fig. 10–23). These rigid misshapen cells obstruct capillary flow and lead to tissue hypoxia and further sickling; this in turn causes further obstruction and eventually infarction. When the sickled cells are reoxygenated, they resume the natural round disk shape of a normal erythrocyte. Additionally, hemoglobin S has reduced oxygen-carrying capacity.
- Hemorrhagic anemia results from the loss of large amounts of blood volume (hypovolemia) in a short time.
- Hemolytic anemia is caused by abnormal destruction of the RBCs. Heredity plays a role in some hemolytic anemias; however, exposure to chemical toxins and certain bacterial toxins or autoimmunity may be the cause.

DIAGNOSIS

Blood studies indicate reduced RBC numbers, reduced hemoglobin levels and **hematocrit,** and changes in the morphology of the corpuscles (Table 10–2). Bone marrow studies may be ordered to detect any aberrations.

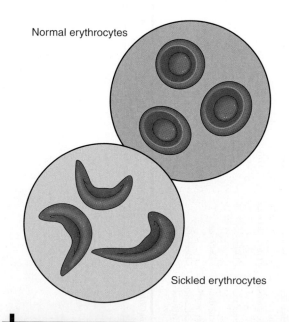

Normal erythrocytes

Sickled erythrocytes

Figure 10–23
Sickled erythrocytes.

TREATMENT

Treatment is directed at the cause of the anemia. Dietary or supplemental iron administration is beneficial in iron deficiency anemias. If anemia is the result of a slow insidious bleed, the underlying cause must be found and treated. Folic acid replacement is indicated in folic acid deficiency anemia. Vitamin B_{12} injections are the treatment of choice for pernicious anemia. The causative factor must be uncovered in hemolytic and aplastic anemias and, if possible, eliminated. There is no cure for sickle cell anemia, so treatment is symptomatic. Rest, increased fluid intake, and the administration of analgesics are helpful. When there is an exacerbation of the condition, the patient requires hospitalization for oxygen administration, intravenous therapy, the use of narcotic analgesics, and packed RBC transfusion. In all forms of anemia, blood replacement may be necessary when other measures fail to restore the RBC numbers and hemoglobin levels.

AGRANULOCYTOSIS

SYMPTOMS AND SIGNS

Agranulocytosis (also called neutropenia) is a blood dyscrasia in which leukocyte levels become extremely low. This condition can have a rapid onset. The patient experiences severe fatigue and weakness, which are followed by a sore throat, ulcerations on the oral mucosa, **dysphagia,** elevated body temperature, weak and rapid pulse, and chills.

ETIOLOGY

Agranulocytosis usually is caused by drug toxicity or hypersensitivity. Cancer chemotherapy with chemotoxic agents is an example. Benzene is another chemical agent that causes neutropenia. Agranulocytosis, or neutropenia, is an acute insult to the body's immune system and drastically reduces the body's response to bacterial infection. The infectious agents usually invade the body through the oral or pharyngeal mucosa and often are already present but are no longer held in check by the now-absent granulocytes. Occasionally, patients are sensitive to a particular drug, such as chlorpromazine, propylthiouracil, phenytoin, chloramphenicol, and phenylbutazone. Agranulocytosis also can accompany aplastic or megaloblastic anemia, tuberculosis, **uremia,** or malaria. This condition occurs most frequently in the female population.

315

TABLE 10-2 ▶ Blood Values in Anemia

	RBC (per mm³)	Hb (g/dl)	Hct (%)	MCV (per μm³)	MCH (pg)	MCHC (g/dl)	WBC (per mm³)	RETICULOCYTE COUNT (per mm³)	PLATELET COUNT (per mm³)
Normal	Male: 4.7–6.1, female: 4.2–5.4	Male: 14–18, female: 12–16	Male: 42–52, female: 37–47	80–90	27–31	32–36	5000–10,000	0.5–2	150,000–400,000
Acute hemorrhagic anemia	Initial increase, latent decrease	Initial decrease, latent decrease	Normal initially, latent decrease	Increase	Decrease	Normal	Increase	Increase	Decrease
Chronic hemorrhagic anemia	Decrease	Decrease	Decrease	Slight decrease	Slight decrease	Slight decrease	Normal	Decrease	Normal
Iron deficiency anemia	Decrease	Decrease	Decrease	Decrease	Decrease	Decrease	Normal	Decrease	Normal to increase
Aplastic anemia	Gross decrease	Gross decrease	Gross decrease	Moderate decrease	Gross decrease	Gross decrease	Gross decrease	Decrease	Gross decrease
Pernicious anemia	Decrease	Gross decrease	Gross decrease	Increase	Increase	Increase	Slight decrease	Decrease	Slight decrease
Folic acid deficiency anemia	Decrease	Gross decrease	Gross decrease	Increase	Increase	Increase	Slight decrease	Decrease	Slight decrease
Sickle cell anemia	Decrease	Decrease	Decrease	Decrease	Normal	Normal	Increase	Increase	Normal
Hemolytic anemia	Decrease	Decrease	Decrease	Increase	Slight decrease	Normal	Normal	Increase	Normal to increase

Hb, hemoglobin; Hct, hematocrit; MCH, mean corpuscular hemoglobin; MCHC, mean corpuscular hemoglobin concentration; MCV, mean corpuscular volume; RBC, red blood cell; WBC, white blood cell.

DIAGNOSIS

Blood studies show leukopenia, with a marked decrease in the number of polymorphonuclear cells. Bone marrow studies reveal a lack of granulocytes, and the developing WBCs lack maturation and are decreased in number. History may reveal exposure to the offending infectious agents; blood, urine, and oral cultures may be positive for bacteria, and toxins may be present.

TREATMENT

The primary thrust of treatment is to eliminate any offending microorganism with aggressive antimicrobial therapy. Cultures are repeated several times and are monitored for the growth of microbes. If it is determined that the toxicity was caused by a drug or chemical, exposure to the toxic agent must be halted. Aggressive therapy is indicated because the condition can be fatal within a week if left untreated.

POLYCYTHEMIA

SYMPTOMS AND SIGNS

Polycythemia is an abnormal increase in the amount of hemoglobin, the RBC count, or hematocrit, causing an absolute increase in RBC mass. Symptoms are related to the increased RBC mass and include headaches, dyspnea, irritability, mental sluggishness, dizziness, syncope, night sweats, and weight loss. Circulatory stagnation, thrombus, and increased blood viscosity may be noted. **Splenomegaly** and clubbing of the fingers along with cyanosis may be observed.

ETIOLOGY

It is not known why a sustained increase in the hematopoiesis of the bone marrow causes absolute, or primary, polycythemia. Relative polycythemia results when the plasma volume is decreased by dehydration, plasma loss, fluid and electrolyte imbalances, or burns. Decreased oxygen supply to the tissues results in a compensation by the body as it manufactures additional hemoglobin to carry additional oxygen. The body uses this compensatory process when patients have chronic pulmonary and cardiac diseases or live at high altitudes, where the oxygen concentration is reduced.

DIAGNOSIS

An abnormal increase in RBC numbers, hemoglobin levels, and hematocrit suggests the condition. Leukocyte and thrombocyte counts also are elevated, and the spleen may be enlarged. The clinical picture aids in the diagnosis. The total RBC mass evaluation is also diagnostic.

TREATMENT

Periodic **phlebotomy** is employed to reduce the blood volume. Myelosuppressive drugs and radiation also improve the blood count. Relative polycythemia usually subsides when the causative factors are resolved.

THROMBOCYTOPENIA

Idiopathic thrombocytopenic purpura is considered an autoimmune response. This dyscrasia involving decreased clotting capabilities of the blood is discussed in Chapter 3.

 Leukemias

Leukemias are malignant neoplasms of the hematopoietic tissue of the blood-forming organs: bone marrow, spleen, and lymph nodes. The abnormal proliferation of red or white blood cells is uncontrolled and usually involves one specific type of blood cell. These cells are immature and usually hypofunctional but sometimes hyperfunctional. Leukemic cells infiltrate numerous organs, such as the liver, brain, and spinal cord, causing them to become enlarged, soft, and pale. The numbers of erythrocytes and platelets may be reduced, with subsequent anemia and clotting problems.

Common types of leukemia include acute lymphocytic leukemia, chronic lymphocytic leukemia, acute myelocytic leukemia, and chronic myelocytic leukemia. Erythroleukemia, megakaryocytic leukemia, and plasma cell leukemia occur less frequently. Related cancers include lymphoma, multiple myeloma, and Hodgkin's disease. Acute forms have rapid progression and can be quickly fatal. In lymphocytic leukemias (cancer of the lymph nodes), lymphocytes are the only leukocytes that are increased in number. In myelocytic leukemias (cancer of the bone marrow), there is an increase in the primitive WBCs (myelocytes). Adult myelocytic leukemia patients younger than 60 years of age usually have a better prognosis.

Typical symptoms in all types of leukemia include joint and bone pain, fever, **hepatomegaly,** splenomegaly, and enlarged lymph glands. Although the cause is unknown, viral infections, immunologic defects, genetic aberrations, and exposure to certain chemicals and large doses of radiation are suspected.

Currently there is no known way to prevent most cases of leukemia and no special tests are recommended to detect acute leukemia early. Younger patients have a better prognosis.

ACUTE LYMPHOCYTIC LEUKEMIA

SYMPTOMS AND SIGNS

Acute lymphocytic leukemia has a rapid onset and has a tendency to affect children and those older than 65 years of age. The aberrant cells are lymphoblasts produced in the bone marrow and lymph nodes. The patient is susceptible to infections and has bleeding tendencies. As the leukocytes infiltrate the spleen, liver, lymph nodes, and nervous system, there is an interference with the normal functioning of these organs. The patient appears pale and reports bone pain, weight loss, sore throat, fatigue, night sweats, and weakness. Bleeding may be noted from the oral mucosa. There is a tendency for increased bruising and recurrent infections. Necrotic infective lesions of the mouth and throat are common.

ETIOLOGY

The exact cause is unknown. Prolonged exposure to radiation, certain chemicals and drugs, smoking, viruses, and genetic factors (inherited DNA mutations) are considered contributing factors.

DIAGNOSIS

Blood studies show increased numbers of immature lymphocytes and decreased numbers of erythrocytes and platelets. Cerebral spinal fluid (CSF) may be withdrawn and examined for leukemic cells. Imaging studies also are used. Bone marrow studies indicate a proliferation of similar leukemic cells; this confirms the presence of acute leukemia.

TREATMENT

Without treatment, 90% of patients with acute leukemia would die within a year. This cancer is the most common form in children and usually affects children from 2 to 9 years of age. It kills more children between 2 and 15 years of age than any other disease; it kills more adults than children. Treatment is aggressive, with systemic combination chemotherapy followed by bone marrow or stem cell transplantation. Treatment

usually induces remission, and with bone marrow transplantation, there is approximately a 50% survival rate. The increased susceptibility to infection necessitates diligent prevention of exposure to microbes and immediate antibiotic intervention when infections ensue.

CHRONIC LYMPHOCYTIC LEUKEMIA

SYMPTOMS AND SIGNS

Chronic lymphocytic leukemia is a chronic, slowly progressive disease marked by **lymphocytosis.** It is a disease of later life and has a gradual onset. Patients exhibit weight loss, possible fever, enlarged lymph nodes, and splenomegaly. There is secondary anemia, and the patients are susceptible to secondary infection.

ETIOLOGY

The cause is unknown, although research points to a hereditary factor.

DIAGNOSIS

Diagnosis is made from the clinical picture and blood and bone marrow studies. Blood tests reveal abnormal lymphocytes that are hypermature and increased in number. The lymphocytes are more mature and more differentiated than in the acute manifestation. The hemoglobin count is low.

TREATMENT

Treatment often is withheld until the patient is symptomatic. Treatment involves systemic combination chemotherapy and radiation to control symptoms caused by enlarged lymph nodes or a grossly enlarged spleen.

ACUTE MYELOCYTIC LEUKEMIA

SYMPTOMS AND SIGNS

Acute myelocytic leukemia (AML) is the most common adult leukemia; it also is known as myelogenous or granulocytic leukemia. Patients with AML have fatigue and weakness because of rapid accumulation of myeloblasts (myeloid precursors). They experience fever, have anemia, and are pale. Headache and bone and joint pain are common, along with abnormal bleeding and bruising. Lymph nodes, liver, and spleen are enlarged, and the patients are prone to recurrent infections.

ETIOLOGY

The etiology is unknown. Predisposing factors include certain viral infections, hereditary factors, and radiation exposure.

DIAGNOSIS

Diagnosis is made from the clinical picture and blood and bone marrow studies. An aberration in the growth of **megakaryocytes** may be noted. There also is a maturational arrest and proliferation of specific cell types in myeloblastic or monoblastic stages.

TREATMENT

Treatment consists of antineoplastic drugs as systemic combination chemotherapy. Bone marrow transplantation may be attempted. AML can be kept in remission for a long time and even cured in 20 to 30% of adults.

CHRONIC MYELOCYTIC LEUKEMIA

SYMPTOMS AND SIGNS

Chronic myelocytic leukemia manifests itself with loss of appetite, fatigue, weight loss, hepatomegaly, and splenomegaly. The patient experiences joint and bone pain, unusual bleeding and bruising, and fever. Lymph nodes may be enlarged.

ETIOLOGY

The etiology is unknown. Exposure to ionizing radiation increases the risk.

DIAGNOSIS

Diagnosis is made from the clinical picture and blood and bone marrow studies. Blood studies indicate leukocytosis and thrombocytosis. There is an increase in granulocyte production.

TREATMENT

Treatment consists of antineoplastic drugs as systemic combination chemotherapy. Bone marrow transplantation may be attempted. Median survival rate is greater than 5 years.

Lymphatic Diseases

The lymphatic system is composed of lymphatic vessels, lymphatic tissue (lymph nodes, tonsils, thymus, and spleen), and **lymph.** The lymphatic vessels originate at the capillary level and, along with the venous system, progress to empty into the right and left subclavian veins (Fig. 10–24). There is no pump for this system. Lymph nodes, collections of lymphatic tissue, filter foreign material such as bacteria and viruses from the lymphatic circulation (Fig. 10–25). Lymphocytes are produced mainly in the lymph nodes as part of the body's defense mechanism. The lymphatic vessels are thin walled, and valves are contained in the larger vessels. Similar to the case for the venous system, the muscles exert intermittent pressure on the vessels, causing the lymph to flow by a milking action. Vessel wall smooth muscle contracts to aid in the return of lymph to the cardiovascular system. Swollen lymph nodes or glands may indicate trapping of microbes during an infectious process.

LYMPHEDEMA

SYMPTOMS AND SIGNS

Lymphedema is an abnormal collection of lymph, usually in the extremities. It results in a swelling of the extremity. The patient experi-

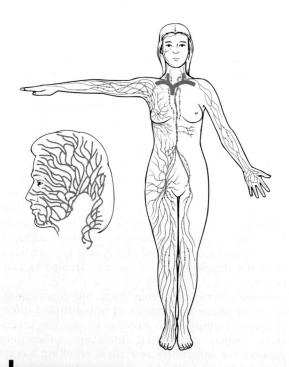

Figure 10–24

Lymphatic system.

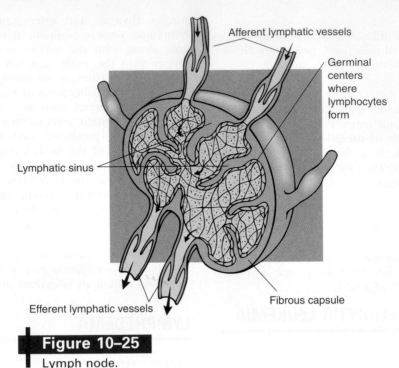

Afferent lymphatic vessels

Germinal centers where lymphocytes form

Lymphatic sinus

Fibrous capsule

Efferent lymphatic vessels

Figure 10–25
Lymph node.

ences no pain. The extremity becomes swollen and grossly distended (Fig. 10–26).

ETIOLOGY

The obstruction of the lymph vessel or node may be inflammatory or mechanical. If lymphedema is left untreated, the connective tissues lose their elasticity and the edema becomes permanent. The lymphatic circulation may be compromised by infections, neoplasms, or thrombus. Allergic reactions also may be implicated, along with trauma or surgery involving the affected part. Tight clothing that constricts the lymphatic vessels can cause temporary lymphedema. Removing the constriction usually resolves the swelling. Women who have had mastectomies may experience lymphedema in the adjacent arm. Prolonged lymphedema rarely is associated with the development of lymphosarcoma (a cancer).

Lymphedema is not in itself life threatening; however, there is a danger of uncontrolled infection developing in the affected tissue. The essentially stagnant interstitial fluids are a breeding ground for infections and their resulting toxins (poisons). Local defenses are overwhelmed, and the normal systemic defense system is not activated.

DIAGNOSIS

Painless swelling in an extremity suggests lymphedema. Imaging procedures, including lymphangiography and radioactive isotope studies, are means of confirming the diagnosis and ascertaining the site of obstruction.

TREATMENT

Treatment is aimed at reducing the swelling. The affected limb is elevated above the heart to encourage drainage of the lymph. Elastic bandages or stockings are applied when the affected part is elevated to compress the area, also encouraging improved lymph drainage. Diuretics may be administered to decrease fluid volume. Surgical intervention may be attempted to relieve a mechanical obstruction. Antibiotics are administered for any infection that may exist.

LYMPHANGITIS

SYMPTOMS AND SIGNS

Lymphangitis is an inflammation of the lymph vessels. It usually is manifested by a red streak at the site of entry of the infective organism. The redness extends to the regional lymph node, which is swollen and tender. Cellulitis may de-

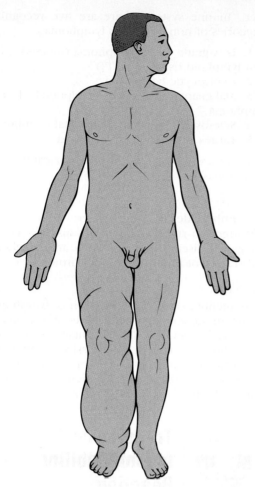

Figure 10–26
Lymphedema.

velop in surrounding tissue. Manifestations of generalized infection, including fever, chills, and malaise, are present.

ETIOLOGY

Bacterial invasion into the lymph vessels at the site of local trauma or ulceration is a frequent cause of lymphangitis. Occasionally, there is no detectable portal of entry. The bacteria travel to the regional lymph nodes and stimulate inflammation.

DIAGNOSIS

Visual inspection of the involved area and the recognition of typical systemic manifestations of bacterial invasion are usually sufficient for diagnosis. Blood studies indicate leukocytosis. Final

confirmation is made by cultures of the infected tissue.

TREATMENT

Treatment includes the administration of systemic antibiotics. The affected area is elevated and rested, and local warm and wet dressings are applied. Surgical drainage of **purulent** material is indicated.

LYMPHOMA

Lymphomas are malignant neoplasms (cancers) of lymph nodes and lymphoid tissue. They include Hodgkin's disease and other types grouped as non-Hodgkin's lymphoma. There is an uncontrolled proliferation of dysfunctional lymphocytes that replace normal cells. They may be B cells or T cells or rarely both. They may be well or poorly differentiated or plasmacytic.

Treatment selection is determined by the cell type and the stage of the disease.

Stage I—There is involvement of a single node or region.
Stage II—There is involvement of two or more nodular regions, with the involvement being on the same side of the diaphragm.
Stage III—There is involvement of nodular regions on both sides of the diaphragm.
Stage IV—There is widespread involvement of extranodal tissue above and below the diaphragm.

Stage I lymphomas are removed surgically, and localized irradiation is administered. Stage II lymphomas are removed surgically, and localized irradiation is applied to the extended field. Stage III lymphomas are treated by combination chemotherapy with or without extensive irradiation. Treatment of stage IV lymphomas is variable, depending on circumstances. Combination chemotherapy is employed, usually in conjunction with total-body irradiation. Severe cases are treated with massive chemotherapy, which is followed by bone marrow transplantation.

Hodgkin's Disease

SYMPTOMS AND SIGNS

The initial symptoms of Hodgkin's disease, a malignant neoplasm of the lymphatic system, are painless enlargement of the lymph nodes, lymphadenopathy, and severe itching. As the disease progresses, the patient experiences fever, night sweats, weight loss, and malaise. Splenomegaly and hepatomegaly follow, and along with the lymphadenopathy, there is coughing, breathlessness, and wheezing.

ETIOLOGY

The exact cause of Hodgkin's disease is uncertain, although an association with viral infections, especially Epstein–Barr virus infection, has been suggested. Reed-Sternberg cells, large malignant cells with a multilobed nucleus, are present in lymphatic tissue.

DIAGNOSIS

A history of painless lymphadenopathy and the typical clinical picture lead to lymph node biopsy. The node biopsy shows the presence of Reed-Sternberg cells. Blood studies indicate a mild normochromic, normocytic anemia; neutrophilic leukocytosis; lymphopenia; and eosinophilia. The ESR is elevated, as is the serum alkaline phosphatase level. Bone marrow biopsy may show abnormal cells. CT scans of the chest, abdomen, and pelvis help in the staging process. Liver and kidney function tests are performed. Lymphangiograms of the lower extremities may be done.

TREATMENT

As mentioned in the discussion of lymphomas, treatment depends on the stage of the disease and ranges from combination chemotherapy with or without irradiation to massive combination chemotherapy and full-body irradiation. The earlier that the disease is discovered and treatment begins, the better the prognosis is. Hodgkin's disease may be cured.

Non-Hodgkin's Lymphoma

SYMPTOMS AND SIGNS

Non-Hodgkin's lymphomas or lymphosarcomas are a group of closely related malignant neoplasms of the lymphatic system. As with Hodgkin's disease, primary symptoms include painless enlargement of lymph nodes and fatigue. Other lymphatic tissue, such as tonsils and adenoids, also may be enlarged, and the patient additionally experiences fever, night sweats, weight loss, and malaise along with coughing and dyspnea.

ETIOLOGY

The etiology is uncertain; however, infectious (including Epstein–Barr virus), environmental, immunologic, and genetic factors have been postu-

lated. In one system, there are five recognized categories of non-Hodgkin's lymphoma:

1. Low-grade B cell lymphoma (mucosa-associated lymphoid tissue [MALT])
2. Centrocytic lymphoma
3. Malignant histiocytic (peripheral T cell) lymphoma
4. Sclerosing large-cell mediastinal lymphoma
5. Large-cell anaplastic lymphoma

There are many other systems for categorizing lymphomas.

DIAGNOSIS

Lymph node and bone marrow biopsies are performed to rule out Hodgkin's disease. As with Hodgkin's disease, blood studies are conducted, and staging of the disease is performed.

TREATMENT

As mentioned in the discussion of lymphomas, treatment depends on the stage of the disease and ranges from combination chemotherapy with or without irradiation to massive combination chemotherapy and full-body irradiation. The earlier that the disease is discovered and treatment begins, the better the prognosis is.

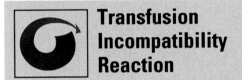

Transfusion Incompatibility Reaction

SYMPTOMS AND SIGNS

Transfusion incompatibility results when the blood or blood product transfused has antibodies to the recipient's RBCs or the recipient has antibodies to the donor's RBCs. This hypersensitivity reaction can range from mild to fatal. Most severe transfusion reactions are incompatibility related and are characterized by hemolysis or **agglutination.** Other forms include bacterial, allergic, and circulatory overload transfusion reactions. The severity of the reaction depends on the amount of incompatible blood that is transfused and prior transfusion reactions of the patient.

The patient with incompatibility reaction who is receiving the blood transfusion experiences chills, fever, and tachycardia. The patient with a more severe reaction has severe back pain, vomiting, diarrhea, hives or rash, a substernal tightness, and dyspnea. The patient becomes hypotensive and progresses to a state of circulatory collapse. As the condition worsens, there is bleeding from the puncture site, blood in the urine, and eventually renal failure.

The most frequent transfusion reaction is associated with WBCs or WBC remnants in donor blood. It is febrile and short lived, ceasing when the transfusion is halted, and there is no hemolysis or allergic response.

The patient experiencing an allergic reaction exhibits hives and itching and possibly bronchial spasms and **anaphylaxis.**

ETIOLOGY

ABO- and Rh-incompatible blood causes an antigen–antibody reaction that produces hemolysis (destruction of RBCs) or agglutination (clumping of RBCs that obstructs the flow of blood through capillaries). Histamine and serotonin are released from mast cells and platelets. Disseminated intravascular coagulation (DIC) usually is triggered (see Disseminated Intravascular Coagulation), with resulting coagulation problems.

DIAGNOSIS

Any sign of chills, fever, hives, back pain, or dyspnea during the transfusion alerts the health-care professional attending the patient to a possible reaction. Blood and urine specimens are examined, along with the used blood, to confirm an incompatibility and the presence of hemolysis or activated coagulation.

TREATMENT

Transfusion protocol mandates that a set of baseline patient vital signs be taken before the start of a transfusion. During the first 15 minutes, the patient is observed closely, and assessment of vital signs is repeated. The monitoring of vital signs and observation of the patient continue at designated intervals until the procedure is completed. At the first indication of any symptoms or signs of reaction, the blood transfusion is stopped immediately. Blood and urine samples are obtained from the patient and sent to the laboratory, along with the remaining untransfused blood. Mild reactions are treated with antihistamines, and anaphylaxis is treated aggressively according to institutional protocol.

Prevention is the best form of treatment. Careful typing and crossmatching of the blood product is mandatory. Two attendants must check the patient information with that on the blood bag and orders before starting the transfusion.

Clotting Disorders

CLASSIC HEMOPHILIA

SYMPTOMS AND SIGNS

Classic hemophilia is a hereditary bleeding disorder resulting from deficiency of clotting factors. The condition can be mild, moderate, or severe. Any unusually prolonged bleeding episode, easy bruising, hematomas, or excessive nosebleeds in a male child suggest hemophilia. The first sign of hemophilia may be ecchymosis at birth or bleeding from a circumcision. Joint swelling and pain are indicative of bleeding in the joints.

ETIOLOGY

An X-linked genetic disorder in males, hemophilia is transmitted by the asymptomatic carrier mother to her son. Factor VIII, a clotting factor in the intrinsic clotting cascade, is functionally inactive. Any minor trauma can initiate the bleeding episode.

DIAGNOSIS

Diagnosis is made by the clinical picture and a thorough history. Clotting studies indicate normal platelet count, bleeding time, and prothrombin time (PT); prolonged partial thromboplastin time (PTT); and a factor VIII assay of 0 to 30%.

TREATMENT

Hemophilia cannot be cured; however, treatment prevents crippling deformities. Concentrated factor VIII (antihemophilic factor [AHF]) is administered to stop the bleeding. Transfusions of whole blood may be necessary. The patients are encouraged to avoid situations that initiate bleeding episodes. There are documented cases of human immunodeficiency virus (HIV) infection resulting from transfusion with contaminated or infected blood products.

DISSEMINATED INTRAVASCULAR COAGULATION

SYMPTOMS AND SIGNS

Disseminated intravascular coagulation is a condition of simultaneous hemorrhage and thrombosis. It is a syndrome that occurs secondary to other diseases. Oozing of blood from needle puncture sites, mucous membranes, or incisions may be noted, as may bleeding in the form of **purpura,** wound hematomas, or **petechiae. Hematemesis, hematuria,** and bloody stools may be present. The patient is weak, reports headaches, and experiences air hunger and tachycardia. Disseminated intravascular coagulation follows a major event, such as obstetric complications, septicemia, trauma, burns, hypothermia, and extensive tissue destruction.

ETIOLOGY

Thrombin activates the production of fibrin, causing clots to form where they are not needed (i.e., in the microcirculation). The thrombin also causes platelet **aggregation,** forming more clots. Additionally, the fibrinolytic system is activated by the presence of thrombin in the plasma; thrombin causes excessive fibrinolysis and additional bleeding. Predisposing factors include hypotension, hypoxemia, acidosis, and stasis of capillary blood. Any of these factors may be the result of the aforementioned major precipitating events.

DIAGNOSIS

Diagnosis is made from the clinical picture; a thorough history, including a probable precipitating event; and laboratory studies. Platelet count and fibrinogen levels are decreased, whereas PT is prolonged.

TREATMENT

Administration of intravenous heparin inhibits the formation of additional microthrombi and prevents the aggregation of platelets. Platelet replacement and plasma-clotting factors are administered when serious hemorrhage is present. The condition is life threatening and often fatal.

Summary

Disease of the heart, a common cause of illness and death, may affect the heart muscle itself, the great vessels leading to and from the heart, the cardiac valves, the coronary vessels, or the conduction system of the heart. The consequences of heart disease are circulatory disturbances that together cause heart failure. Many diagnostic tests are available for evaluation of patients with cardiac disease, allowing for more accurate diagnosis and a specific program of treatment.

• Coronary artery disease caused by atherosclerosis or arteriosclerosis may lead to symptoms of cardiac ischemia, called angina pectoris. Severe cardiac ischemia causes death of cardiac tissue, called myocardial infarction.
• Hypertensive heart disease, the most prevalent cardiovascular disorder in the United States, can be managed by drug therapy, diet, and lifestyle management.
• Congestive heart failure results when the pumping action of the heart is not able to meet the body's demand for blood. Right-sided failure leads to cyanosis and peripheral edema; left-sided failure causes pulmonary congestion and edema of the extremities.
• Enlargement of the myocardium and ventricular dysfunction (cardiomyopathy) may cause symptoms of congestive heart failure. Treatment depends on the type of cardiomyopathy: dilated, hypertrophic, or restrictive.
• Pericarditis, myocarditis, and endocarditis are infections of the heart, most of which originate from pathogens carried by the blood.
• Rheumatic fever, a systemic disease, can lead to cardiac involvement and valvular damage such as mitral stenosis. A complete course of antibiotic therapy is necessary to help prevent complications.
• A 12-lead electrocardiogram (ECG) is used to diagnose types of cardiac arrhythmias.
• Shock is a life-threatening condition with many possible causes that deprives vital organs of oxygen and nutrients.

- Emboli can cause pulmonary obstruction, cerebral vascular accidents (stroke), myocardial infarction, or lodge in vessels of an extremity.
- Atherosclerosis is responsible for most myocardial and cerebral infarctions.
- Aortic aneurysms may require surgical repair before leakage or rupture.
- Immediate intervention is necessary for thrombophlebitis to prevent thrombus from becoming an embolus.
- Stress and smoking can aggravate Raynaud's disease.
- Anemia can result from reduction in the quantity of red blood cells or of hemoglobin; cells are deprived of oxygen.
- Agranulocytosis (neutropenia) must be treated aggressively to restore the body's ability to control infection; the underlying cause also must be addressed.
- In leukemia, malignancy of the blood-forming organs, the abnormal proliferation of red or white blood cells leads to infiltration of other organs.
- Acute myelocytic leukemia is the most common adult leukemia; with treatment, it can be kept in remission for a long time and even cured.
- Acute lymphocytic leukemia, more common in children, requires aggressive treatment for survival.
- Lymphangitis may be manifested by a red streak at the point of infection; without treatment, it can lead to cellulitis and generalized infection.
- Hodgkin's disease can be differentiated from non-Hodgkin's lymphoma by the presence of Reed-Sternberg cells in lymphatic tissue.
- Transfusion incompatibility is a hypersensitivity reaction that can range from mild to anaphylactic.
- Classic hemophilia is a hereditary deficiency of clotting factors passed on by the asymptomatic carrier mother to her son.

Review Challenge

REVIEW QUESTIONS

1. What are common symptoms of cardiovascular disease?
2. How would you describe the pathology in coronary artery disease?
3. How is the patient likely to describe the pain in angina pectoris?
4. How do the symptoms of myocardial infarction differ from those of angina pectoris?
5. Why is angioplasty used for myocardial infarction?
6. What conditions can cause cardiac arrest? What is the time frame for cardiopulmonary resuscitation (CPR)?
7. What is the diagnostic criteria for essential hypertension?
8. What happens when the pumping action of the heart is inadequate? How can congestive heart failure be treated?
9. Which conditions may lead to cor pulmonale?
10. How is pulmonary edema treated?
11. To what does cardiomyopathy refer and how is it treated?
12. How does endocarditis affect the cardiac valves?
13. Why is rheumatic fever described as a systemic disease? Which infection often precedes it?
14. What is the relationship between rheumatic fever and valvular heart disease?
15. What are the sources of cardiac arrhythmias? How are they diagnosed?
16. Why is shock considered a life-threatening emergency? What are the signs and symptoms?
17. What is cardiac tamponade?
18. What is the relationship between venous thrombosis and pulmonary emboli?
19. What is the difference between arteriosclerosis and atherosclerosis? Why are both conditions a threat to health?
20. How might an aneurysm be detected? When are they a serious threat?
21. What is the relationship of phlebitis to thrombophlebitis? Why should the clinician avoid massage of the affected area?

22. What medical intervention is available for severe varicose veins?
23. Which conditions may precipitate an episode of Raynaud's disease?
24. What are the presenting symptoms of anemia?
25. What are some possible causes of anemia?
26. How are the following anemias distinguished: aplastic, sickle cell, hemolytic, iron deficiency, hemorrhagic, and pernicious?
27. What are some usual causes of agranulocytosis?

28. What are typical symptoms in all types of leukemia?
29. Which leukemia is considered more a disease of later life?
30. How does lymphedema differ from lymphangitis?
31. Which lymphoma is characterized by the presence of Reed-Sternberg cells in lymphatic tissue?
32. What symptoms does a patient experience with a transfusion incompatibility reaction?
33. How is classic hemophilia treated?

REAL-LIFE CHALLENGE

Essential Hypertension

A 46-year-old man reports intermittent headaches and lightheadedness for about 3 months. In the past 2 weeks, he has had several episodes of epistaxis. Vital signs are T—98.6°, P—106, R—20, BP—168/98. His weight is 265 lbs, and his height is 5 feet, 11 inches.

History reveals that the patient has high stress level employment requiring extensive travel with overnight stays. He regards himself as a high achiever. Family history discloses that his father died at 53 years of age of a CVA and that his mother at 69 years of age has CHF and hypertension. His brother has a history of hypertension, and his two sisters are alive and well. The patient smokes one pack of cigarettes a day and has for 30 years.

The patient is advised to stop smoking or at least cut down on the number smoked a day. Additionally, he is advised to begin a weight reduction and exercise program and to reduce sodium intake. If possible, he also should reduce stressful situations. Medications ordered are a beta blocker, atenolol and an ACE inhibitor, ramipril. The patient is instructed to return in 1 week for re-evaluation. Essential hypertension is a suspected diagnosis.

Questions

1. What factors contribute to this patient's experiencing the symptoms and signs of essential hypertension?
2. Why would his onset of symptoms be considered insidious?
3. Why couldn't the diagnosis of essential hypertension be confirmed on the initial encounter?
4. Why might a diuretic be ordered?
5. What is the significance of the family history?
6. What is the action of calcium channel blockers in the treatment of essential hypertension?
7. If not controlled, what complications may evolve from the essential hypertension?
8. How important in the diagnosis was the symptom of epistaxis?

Anemia

A 32-year-old woman reports being tired all the time, her heart beating too fast, having difficulty catching her breath, and experiencing some lightheadedness. She appears quite pale. Vital signs are T—98.4°, P—118, R—26, BP—100/68.

The patient is married, has three children ages 7 years, 4 years, and 6 months, and is employed outside of the home. She says she can scarcely make it out of bed in the morning and can just barely make it through the day. She has had four episodes of syncope in the past week. Menstrual periods have been regular but heavy. She denies any observable blood in urine or stools. A CBC with differential is ordered. The RBC count is below normal and normocytic, hemoglobin is 9, hematocrit is 27, and WBC and platelet counts are normal. The patient is diagnosed with iron deficiency anemia and encouraged to rest and increase dietary intake of red meat, liver, and egg yolks. Supplementary iron is prescribed in the form of ferrous sulfate tablets, and the patient is instructed to return to the office in 1 week for follow-up.

Questions

1. What might have been the cause of the iron deficiency anemia in this patient?
2. What causes the RBC count to be microcytic? Macrocytic?
3. What is the importance of the absence of blood in the stool or urine?
4. What might be the connection with the previous pregnancy?
5. Which type of food, in addition to the red meat, liver, and egg yolks, would be helpful in increasing the hemoglobin?
6. What might blood tests show if this were sickle cell anemia?
7. Compare hemolytic anemia with iron deficiency anemia.
8. As the hemoglobin improves, what changes might be expected in vital signs?

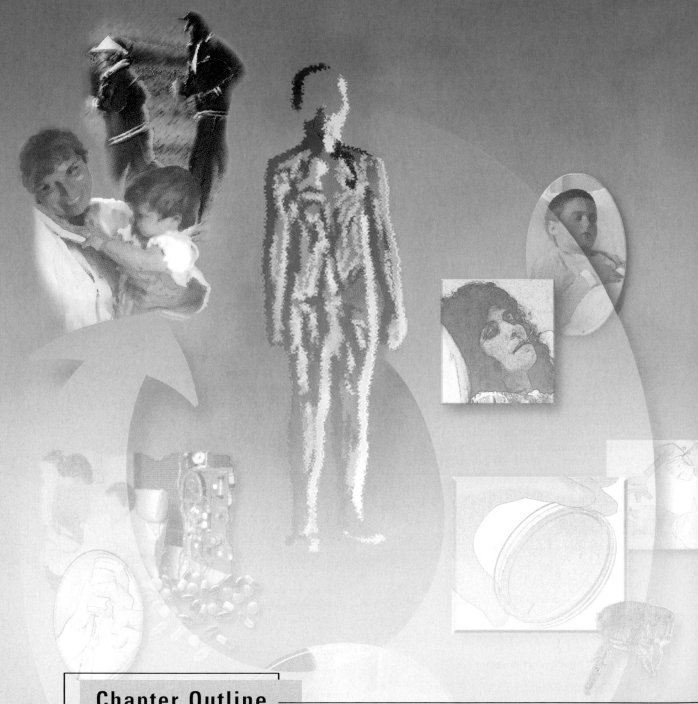

Chapter Outline

Diseases and Conditions of the Urinary System

Learning Objectives

After studying Chapter 11, you should be able to:

1. Explain how pathologic conditions of the urinary system threaten homeostasis and result in illness.
2. Explain the diagnostic value of urinalysis.
3. Relate the symptoms and signs of acute glomerulonephritis.
4. Describe how immune mechanisms are suspected to be a causative factor of acute and chronic glomerulonephritis.
5. Distinguish between hemodialysis and peritoneal dialysis.
6. Identify the hallmark sign of nephrosis.
7. List some nephrotoxic agents.
8. Explain why acute renal failure is considered a clinical emergency.
9. Discuss treatment measures available to prolong life for the patient with chronic renal failure.
10. Identify the etiology and diagnosis of pyelonephritis.
11. Describe hydronephrosis.
12. Describe the common symptoms of renal calculi, and list possible complications.
13. List causes of infectious cystitis and urethritis.
14. Describe diabetic nephropathy.
15. Contrast neurogenic bladder with stress incontinence.
16. Describe the polycystic kidney, and discuss the treatment options.
17. Identify those most at risk for renal cell carcinoma and bladder tumors.

Key Terms

azotemia	(**ah**–zoh–**TEE**–me–ah)	fulguration	(full–gue–**RAY**–shun)
catheterization	(**kath**–eh–ter–eye–**ZAY**–shun)	glomeruli	(gloh–**MER**–you–lye)
		glomerulonephritis	(gloh–**mer**–you–low–neh–**FRY**–tis)
creatinine	(kree–**AT**–in–in)		
cystoscopy	(sis–**TOSS**–ko–pee)	glomerulosclerosis	(gloh–**mer**–you–low–sklee–**ROW**–sis)
dialysate	(dye–**AHL**–ih–sate)		

hemodialysis	(**he**–meh–dye–**AHL**–ih–sis)	nephrotoxic	(**neff**–row–**TOCKS**–ick)
hydronephrosis	(**high**–droh–neff–**ROW**–sis)	oliguria	(ohl–ih–**GOO**–rhee–ah)
immunosuppressive	(**im**–you–noh–sue–**PRESS**–ihv)	peritoneal dialysis	(**per**–ih–toe–**NEE**–al dye–**AHL**–ih–sis)
lithotripsy	(**LITH**–oh–**trip**–see)	pyelonephritis	(**pye**–eh–low–neh–**FRY**–tis)
nephrectomy	(neh–**FRECK**–toh–me)		
nephropathy	(neh–**FROP**–ah–thee)		

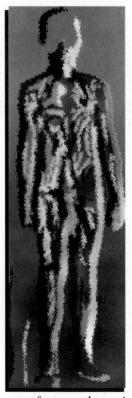

Orderly Function of the Urinary System

The urinary system is responsible for producing, storing, and excreting urine; this prevents the body from becoming **toxic. Homeostasis** is ensured by cleansing the blood of the waste products of metabolism and regulating the normal balance of water, salts, and acids in the body fluids. The urinary system includes the kidneys, which manufacture the urine and play a role in the regulation of systemic blood pressure, and the accessory structures, which transport and store urine in the bladder until it is excreted voluntarily through the urethra. The organs of the urinary system consist of two kidneys, two ureters, the urinary bladder, and the urethra (Fig. 11–1).

Each kidney is composed of about 1 million microstructures called **nephrons** (Fig. 11–2). The nephrons, the units of function in the kidney, are responsible for filtration, reabsorption, and secretion of urine. The urine is transported from the nephron to the renal pelvis and then to the ureters. The kidney has many other functions, including the secretion of *renin,* a hormone that raises blood pressure, and *erythropoietin,* which acts as a stimulus to red blood cell (RBC) production. It also has a role in the activation of vitamin D.

Infection, scarring, toxic **necrosis,** or trauma of the urinary tract can result in disturbances of renal function that allow urea (the nitrogenous waste of metabolism in urine) or extracellular fluid and electrolytes to accumulate in the blood. Congenital or acquired structural defects and tumors cause obstructive diseases of the urinary system. Other important diseases of the urinary tract are immunologic disorders, circulatory disturbances, cystic disease, and metabolic disorders (e.g., diabetes mellitus).

The function of the urinary system frequently is evaluated by urinalysis (Table 11–1) and blood tests (Table 11–2). Normal results demonstrate proper filtration, absorption, and elimination of metabolic waste and precise fluid and electrolyte balance. Other tests for urinary tract disorders include culture and sensitivity tests to determine appropriate antibiotic therapy, radiologic tests that visualize structural abnormalities, cystoscopy (see Fig. 11–4), and biopsy of lesions.

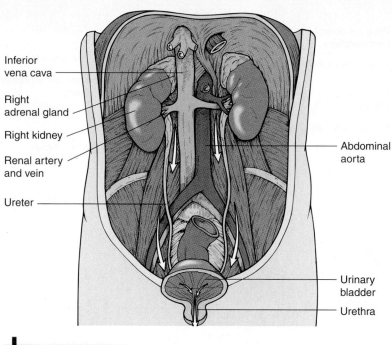

Inferior vena cava

Right adrenal gland

Right kidney

Renal artery and vein

Ureter

Abdominal aorta

Urinary bladder

Urethra

Figure 11–1

Normal urinary system.

Usually symptoms of urinary diseases reflect an accumulation of waste products in the blood and electrolyte imbalances in the body. Common symptoms include:

Nausea
Loss of appetite
Fever
Headache and body aches
Flank or low back pain
Bloody urine
Edema
Decreased urinary output
Hypertension
Pruritus

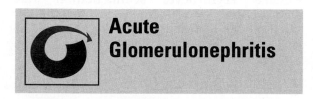

Acute Glomerulonephritis

SYMPTOMS AND SIGNS

Acute glomerulonephritis is an inflammation and swelling of the **glomeruli** (see Fig. 11–2) of both kidneys. It can be a primary disease of the kidney or may develop secondary to a systemic disease. It is marked by proteinuria (protein in the urine), edema, and decreased urine volume. **Hematuria** can range from insignificant to a sudden onset of urine that is grossly bloody (gross hematuria). The urine may appear dark or may be described as coffee colored. Occurring most frequently in children and adolescents, this disease process usually follows a streptococcal infection by 1 to 2 weeks (poststreptococcal glomerulonephritis). Hypertension related to altered renal function and fluid retention is possible, accompanied by headaches, and visual disturbances, **malaise, anorexia,** and a low-grade fever. Flank or back pain develops as a result of swelling of the kidney tissue.

ETIOLOGY

This condition usually follows an infection caused by group A beta-hemolytic streptococcus. It also can be **idiopathic** or may result from an immune reaction that causes circulating **antigen–antibody** complexes to become trapped within the network of capillaries of a glomerulus. In some cases, the antigen is endogenous (arising

NEPHRON

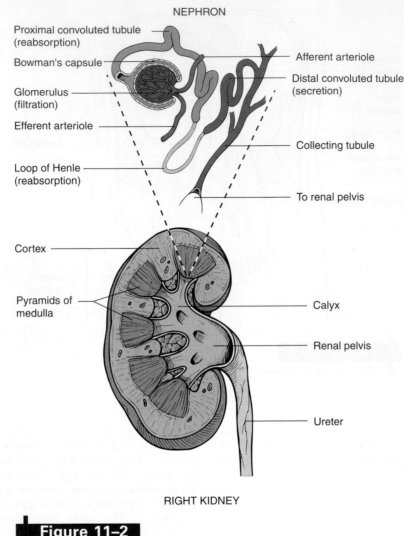

Proximal convoluted tubule
(reabsorption)

Bowman's capsule

Glomerulus
(filtration)

Efferent arteriole

Loop of Henle
(reabsorption)

Afferent arteriole

Distal convoluted tubule
(secretion)

Collecting tubule

To renal pelvis

Cortex

Pyramids of
medulla

Calyx

Renal pelvis

Ureter

RIGHT KIDNEY

Figure 11–2
Kidney and its functioning structures.

from within) as an accompaniment of tumors. The injury to the glomeruli results in a decrease in the rate of filtration of the blood, with retention of water and salts in the body.

DIAGNOSIS

The diagnosis is made by the clinical picture, clinical history, and urinalysis. The urine shows gross blood and the presence of RBCs, **white blood cells** (WBCs), renal tubular cells, and **casts.** Proteinuria may be present because of increased permeability of the glomerular membrane. Blood tests show elevated **blood urea nitrogen (BUN), hypoalbuminemia,** and an elevated **erythrocyte sedimentation rate (ESR).** Kidney-ureter-bladder (KUB) radiographic films and ultrasonography may reveal bilateral enlargement of the kidneys. Renal **biopsy** may confirm the diagnosis.

TREATMENT

No specific therapy is available for the post-streptococcal type of glomerulonephritis other than antibiotic therapy, if infection is still

TABLE 11-1 ➤ Routine Urinalysis*

	NORMAL	ABNORMAL	PATHOLOGY
Characteristics			
Color and clarity	Pale to darker yellow, and clear	Very pale	Excessive water
		Cloudy, milky, white blood cells	Pus, urinary tract infection
		Hematuria, red blood cells, reddish to reddish brown	Bleeding in infection, calculi, or cancer
Odor	Aromatic	Fishy	Cystitis
		Fruity	Diabetes mellitus
		Foul	Urinary tract infection
Chemical nature	pH is generally slightly acidic, 6.5	Alkaline	Infections cause ammonia to form
Specific gravity	1.003–1.030—reflects amount of waste, minerals, and solids in urine	Higher—causes precipitation of solutes	Kidney stones, diabetes mellitus
		Lower—polyuria	Diabetes insipidus
Constituent Compounds			
Protein	None, or small amount	Albuminuria	Nephritis, renal failure, infection
Glucose	None	Glycosuria	Faulty carbohydrate metabolism, as in diabetes mellitus
Ketone bodies	None	Ketonuria	Diabetic acidosis
Bile and bilirubin	None	Bilirubinuria	Hepatic or gallbladder disease
Casts	None—or small number of hyaline casts	Urinary casts composed of red or white blood cells, fat, or pus	Nephritis, renal diseases, inflammation, metal poisoning
Nitrogenous wastes	Ammonia, creatinine, urea, and uric acid	Azoturia, creatinine, and urea clearance tests disproportionate to normal BUN/creatinine ratio	Hepatic disease, renal disease
Crystals	None to trace	Acidic urine, alkaline urine, hypercalcemia, metabolism error	Not significant unless the crystals are large (stones); certain types interpreted by physician
Fat droplets	None	Lipoiduria	Nephrosis

BUN, blood urea nitrogen.
* *Routine urinalysis is a physical, chemical, and microscopic examination of urine for abnormal elements that may help to estimate renal function and furnish clues of systemic disease. This table includes some important characteristics and elements screened for in basic urinalysis. Other normal constituents of urine that are studied routinely for diagnosis include calcium, potassium, sodium, phosphorus, creatinine, and volume in a 24-hour period.*

present, and rest. **Diuretics** help to control edema and hypertension. Sodium intake is restricted to prevent circulatory overload and convulsions. Occasionally, corticosteroids are used if an immune reaction is the suspected cause. Most cases resolve, and the patient recovers spontaneously.

TABLE 11-2 ➤ Some Renal Diagnostic Tests

TEST	DESIGNED TO EVALUATE
Clearance test	Rate of glomerular filtration
Concentration and dilution tests	Functional capacity of renal tubular cells to adaptively retain and/or eliminate water
Serum creatinine and BUN	Capacity to eliminate end products of protein metabolism
Protein in urine	Permeability of glomerular membrane

BUN, blood urea nitrogen. *From Miller M: Pathophysiology: Principles of Disease. Philadelphia: WB Saunders, 1983.*

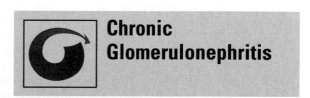

Chronic Glomerulonephritis

SYMPTOMS AND SIGNS

Chronic glomerulonephritis is a slowly progressive, noninfectious disease that can lead to irreversible renal damage and renal failure. At first, it is **asymptomatic;** then subclinical progression of the disease leads to hypertension, he-

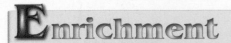

DIALYSIS AND KIDNEY TRANSPLANTATION

In the United States, end-stage renal disease (ESRD) develops in an average of 1.3 in 10,000 people each year. In renal failure, the kidneys no longer can process blood and form urine. Therapy should begin before the development of ultimately fatal uremic symptoms. Dialysis or kidney transplantation, if successful, offers rehabilitation and extended life to patients with ESRD.

Dialysis

Dialysis filters out unwanted elements from the blood by diffusion across a semipermeable membrane; these wastes usually are removed by the healthy kidneys. Thus, the proper fluid, electrolyte, and acid–base balances are maintained in the body. Two methods used to dialyze the blood are hemodialysis and peritoneal dialysis (see Fig. 11–3). Even though these procedures do not cure renal failure, many patients are stabilized after 10 to 15 years of treatment.

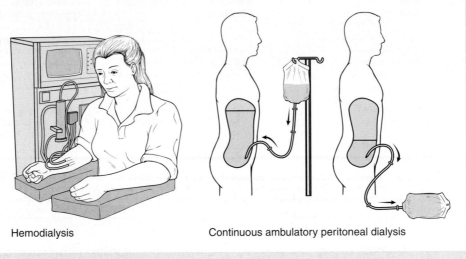

Hemodialysis

Continuous ambulatory peritoneal dialysis

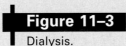

Figure 11–3

Dialysis.

Hemodialysis. Hemodialysis can take place in the home or at a hospital. It removes impurities or wastes from the patient's blood by using an artificial kidney (hemodialyzer). Access to the blood stream is created surgically in the arm or leg with an internal fistula, which allows the blood to pass from the patient's body to the semipermeable membrane in the machine. The cleaned blood then returns to the patient in a procedure that takes 8 to 12 hours, divided into several sessions a week.

Peritoneal Dialysis. Peritoneal dialysis is carried out in the patient's own body by using a **dialysate** solution and the peritoneal membrane to filter out the harmful toxins and excessive fluid. The clean dialyzing fluid passes into the peritoneal cavity through a permanent indwelling peritoneal catheter, and wastes diffuse across the peritoneal membrane into the fluid. The contaminated fluid then is drained and replaced with fresh fluid.

⊃ Continuous ambulatory peritoneal dialysis (CAPD) takes place without a machine by allowing the solution to drain by gravity into a dialysis bag worn around the waist.

> This procedure takes about 15 minutes and is repeated 3 to 4 times a day and once at night.
> ⊃ Continuous cycling peritoneal dialysis (CCPD) takes place while the patient sleeps, using a cycling machine.
> ⊃ Intermittent peritoneal dialysis (IPD) takes several hours, 3 to 5 times a week, and usually is done in a clinic.
>
> ## Kidney Transplantation
>
> Kidney transplantation is a surgical placement of a donor kidney into a patient with irreversible renal failure. Used synergistically with clinical dialysis, kidney transplantation is one of medicine's success stories. Kidney transplantation leads the field of organ replacement, with many patients on waiting lists. **Immunosuppressive** agents are used to prevent or treat rejection syndrome. Sophisticated evaluation of the donor and the recipient to find a good human leukocyte antigen (HLA) match offers the best chance for a good prognosis.
>
> Seventy-five percent of the 10,000 kidney transplants done annually in the United States are performed on patients with diabetes with renal failure, hypertensive renal disease, and glomerulonephritis.

maturia, proteinuria, **oliguria,** and edema. In the later stages with increasing renal failure, the hypertension becomes severe with **azotemia.** When the kidneys fail to remove urea from the blood, the body compensates by attempting to excrete urea through the sweat glands. Tiny crystals of urea appear on the skin, and this condition is termed *uremic frost.* The patient experiences fatigue, malaise, nausea, vomiting, **pruritus,** and **dyspnea.**

ETIOLOGY

Immune mechanisms are suspected as a major cause of chronic glomerulonephritis; antigen–antibody complexes lodge in the glomerular capsular membrane, triggering an inflammatory response and glomerular injury. Primary renal disorders and multisystem diseases such as systemic lupus erythematosus are other causes.

DIAGNOSIS

The diagnostic studies are the same as those used for acute glomerulonephritis: urinalysis, blood tests, radiographic studies, ultrasonography, and renal biopsy. The findings include signs of advanced renal insufficiency, rising BUN and serum **creatinine** levels, and grossly abnormal findings on urinalysis. Renal biopsy and the use of sophisticated tools such as electron microscopy and immunofluorescence are valuable in determining treatment and prognosis.

TREATMENT

The goals of treatment are to control edema, to treat the hypertension, and to prevent congestive heart failure and **uremia.** The patient is given supportive measures for comfort. Medical treatment includes the administration of antihypertensives, diuretics, and antibiotics if urinary tract infection (UTI) develops. Protein, salt, and fluid intake may be limited in the diet. The patient may require **dialysis** (see Fig. 11–3 in Enrichment on dialysis and kidney transplantation) or may be a candidate for kidney transplantation.

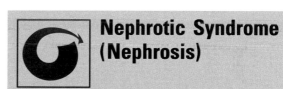

Nephrotic Syndrome (Nephrosis)

SYMPTOMS AND SIGNS

Nephrotic syndrome, a disease of the basement membrane of the glomerulus, is secondary to a number of renal diseases and a variety of systemic disorders. Nephrotic syndrome encompasses a group of symptoms sometimes referred to as the protein-losing kidney. The patient loses excessive amounts of protein, mainly albumin, in the urine (proteinuria). The excessive loss of protein in the urine results in depressed plasma protein levels (hypoalbuminemia). There is diminished glomerular filtration, with retention of water and sodium, resulting in edema and hypertension. The syndrome includes microscopic or gross hematuria. Plasma lipid levels are elevated, but the reason for this is not understood. Sloughed-off fat bodies can be found in the urine. The patients are especially susceptible to infections.

TABLE 11–3 ➤	Nephrotoxic Agents
Solvents	Nonsteroidal anti-inflammatory
Carbon tetrachloride	drugs
Methanol	Iodinated radiographic contrast
Ethylene glycol	media
Heavy metals	Antineoplastic agents
Lead	Miscellaneous compounds
Arsenic	Acetaminophen
Mercury	Amphetamines
Pesticides	Heroin
Antibiotics	Silicon
Kanamycin	Cyclosporine
Gentamicin	Poisonous mushrooms
Polymyxin B	
Amphotericin B	
Colistin	
Neomycin	
Phenazopyridine	

Adapted from: Phipps WJ, Long BC, Woods NF (eds): Medical-Surgical Nursing, Concepts and Clinical Practice, 5th ed. St Louis: Mosby-Year Book, 1995.

The syndrome causes the patient to feel lethargic and depressed, with loss of appetite. He or she appears pale and puffy around the eyes, has swollen ankles (pitting edema), and gains weight. Skin irritation related to edema may be present.

ETIOLOGY

Nephrotic syndrome is caused by increased permeability of the glomerulus, indicating renal damage. This condition may follow an attack of glomerulonephritis or it may be the result of exposure to certain toxins or drugs (Table 11-3), pregnancy, or kidney transplants. Metabolic diseases such as diabetes mellitus, certain infections, and allergic reactions are conditions that may lead to nephrotic syndrome.

DIAGNOSIS

The diagnosis is made from the clinical picture and from the presence of gross proteinuria and lipiduria (the presence of fatty casts) in a 24-hour urine specimen. Abnormal serum values, including hypoalbuminemia and **hyperlipidemia,** support the diagnosis. If renal tumor is suspected, a renal biopsy with histologic study is indicated.

TREATMENT

Effective treatment begins by addressing the underlying cause. Dietary intake of protein is adjusted to the glomerular filtration rate (GFR), and sodium intake is lowered to control edema. A course of corticosteroids, such as prednisone, may have the positive effect of controlling the proteinuria for some patients. Urine output must be monitored. If the condition does not improve with treatment, the syndrome can progress to end stage renal disease.

Acute Renal Failure

SYMPTOMS AND SIGNS

Acute renal failure (ARF), a sudden and severe reduction in renal function, is a common clinical emergency because nitrogenous waste products begin to accumulate in the blood, quickly causing an acute uremic episode. Initially, symptoms include oliguria, gastrointestinal disturbances, headache, drowsiness, and other alterations in the level of consciousness. A host of other symptoms can occur, depending on the underlying cause, the degree of impairment, and the BUN.

ETIOLOGY

The causes of acute renal failure are classified as those that result in diminished blood flow to the kidney (e.g, circulatory shock or heart failure), those that involve intrarenal damage or disease (e.g., glomerulonephritis), and those that result from mechanical obstruction of urine flow. Of special concern is intrarenal damage, which can be prevented by control of exposure to substances known to be nephrotoxic, including drugs, insecticides, organic solvents, and cleaning agents (see Table 11-3). Whatever the cause, sudden renal dysfunction disrupts other body systems and, if left untreated, can lead to death.

DIAGNOSIS

Blood tests and urinalysis reveal many abnormal findings associated with oliguria and the retention of nitrogenous wastes. The BUN, serum creatinine, and potassium levels are elevated in the blood. Other diagnostic studies include kidney scans, ultrasonograms, radiographic films, and **intravenous pyelograms.**

TREATMENT

Determining the cause of acute renal failure, if possible, is crucial in medical management to reduce the risk of permanent kidney damage. However, the goal is to reverse the decreased renal perfusion. All body systems are monitored and supported as needed through the uremic crisis. The patient may be evaluated for dialysis. Fluid intake and output are balanced to avoid overload. Careful nutritional support is important to replace protein in the right proportions to avoid **metabolic acidosis.** Sodium and potassium intake is controlled as well. Drug therapy may include antihypertensives, diuretics, and anti-infective agents because infection is a common complication in acute renal failure.

In many cases, with prompt treatment, ARF is reversible and recovery is rapid and complete.

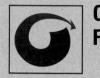

Chronic Renal Failure

SYMPTOMS AND SIGNS

Chronic renal failure (CRF) results from the gradual and progressive loss of nephrons (see Fig. 11–2), with irreversible loss of renal function and gradual onset of uremia. The systemic effects eventually can be manifested in any and all body systems. The patient feels weak, tired, and lethargic. Hypertension and edema result from the retention of fluids in the body as the condition progresses. As the uremic syndrome worsens, many other symptoms and signs are generated: **arrhythmias,** muscle weakness, dyspnea, metabolic acidosis, nausea, vomiting, **ulceration** of the gastrointestinal mucosa, and hair and skin changes.

ETIOLOGY

There are numerous causes of CRF, including primary diseases or infections of the kidney such as glomerulonephritis, **pyelonephritis,** and polycsytic kidneys. Often, it is the end stage of chronic renal diseases or of chronic obstruction of the outflow of urine.

DIAGNOSIS

Blood studies show elevated BUN, serum creatinine, and potassium levels, along with decreased hemoglobin level and **hematocrit.** Urinalysis is grossly abnormal, with excessive protein, glucose, leukocytes, and casts; the 24-hour urine volume is greatly decreased. Diagnostic studies include radiographic KUB films, renal

ultrasonograms, kidney scans, intravenous pyelograms, and renal arteriograms.

TREATMENT

The underlying cause, if known, must be treated. The patient is evaluated for dialysis or kidney transplantation to prolong life. Diet and nutritional modifications control protein and sodium intake to reduce the work of the diseased kidney. Fluid intake and output are monitored and regulated. Drug therapy includes the administration of diuretics, antihypertensives, anti-infective agents, and **antiemetics.** The patient is given supportive care and kept as comfortable as possible. There are many possible complications, so the prognosis is uncertain.

Pyelonephritis

SYMPTOMS AND SIGNS

Pyelonephritis, the most common type of renal disease, is an inflammation of the renal pelvis and connective tissues of one or both kidneys. It usually is caused by infection, pregnancy, or **calculi.** Pus collects in the renal pelvis, with the formation of **abscesses.** The patient experiences rapid onset of fever, chills, nausea and vomiting, and flank (lumbar) pain. This usually is preceded by a UTI with urinary frequency and urgency. The patient may report a foul odor to the urine with hematuria and **pyuria.** There is tenderness in the suprapubic region, the abdomen becomes rigid, and a tender enlarged kidney may be palpated. Urinalysis results show abnormal constituents, including urinary casts.

ETIOLOGY

Pyelonephritis usually is caused by bacteria that ascend from the lower urinary tract to the kidneys; it is less commonly caused by hematogenous or lymphatic spread of bacteria. Obstruction and stasis of urine by **renal calculi** (kidney stones), tumors, and benign prostatic **hypertrophy** predispose the kidneys to infection. Stasis of urine allows invading bacteria, usually *Escherichia coli,* to cause the infectious process. Women are more at risk because sexual activity or poor perineal hygiene can introduce bacterial contamination into the urinary tract. Catheterization or diagnostic procedures such as **endoscopic** examination can directly introduce organisms into the urinary bladder. The infection then moves upward in the urinary tract (ascending infection) to one or both kidneys.

DIAGNOSIS

The diagnosis is made by the clinical picture and urinalysis of a **clean-catch urine specimen** that shows increased WBCs and RBCs with the presence of bacteria, pus, protein, and casts. Blood cultures and urine cultures can identify the causative organism. Radiographic studies reveal kidneys that appear swollen or enlarged.

TREATMENT

The treatment of choice consists of intravenous or oral antibiotics, usually penicillin or cephalosporin, given for a full 7 to 10 days. Increased fluid intake to dilute the urine and bed rest are urged. Unless patients are at high risk for UTI, they respond well to treatment without recurrences. In more complicated cases, surgery may be indicated to relieve obstruction or to correct an anomaly.

Hydronephrosis

SYMPTOMS AND SIGNS

Hydronephrosis is an abnormal dilation of the renal pelvis caused by pressure from urine that cannot flow past an obstruction in the urinary tract (Fig. 11–4*A*). If the obstruction is severe and prolonged, there are **fibrotic** changes and loss of function of the involved nephrons. Hydronephrosis is usually a chronic condition, with destruction of the kidneys that transpires without pain or symptoms. Its detection often is accidental during radiographic examination or ultrasonography of the abdomen. A vague backache and diminished urine output may be the only symptoms that the patient can identify. If an infection accompanies the condition, the patient may experience fever, chills, hematuria, and pyuria, and the kidney may be palpable.

ETIOLOGY

Dilation of the renal pelvis is caused by buildup of pressure in the kidney because of an

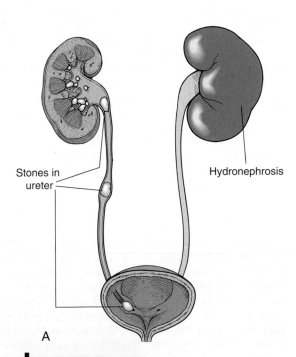

Stones in
ureter

Hydronephrosis

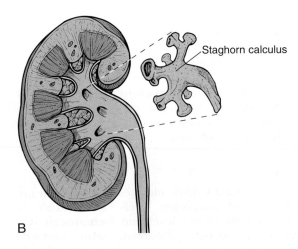

Staghorn calculus

A

B

Figure 11–4
Renal calculi.

obstruction. Usually, the right kidney is affected, but both can be involved. The cause of the obstruction could be renal calculi, tumors, inflammation caused by infections, prostatic hyperplasia (enlargement), or congenital abnormalities. During pregnancy, the enlarged uterus can cause hydronephrosis.

DIAGNOSIS

The first indication of hydronephrosis is usually the result of investigation of other abdominal structures. Follow-up contrast studies of the ureter and the kidney need to be done. A retrograde pyelogram is necessary. Cystoscopy (see Fig. 11–5 in the Enrichment on cystoscopy) to rule out an obstruction by a tumor of the bladder or prostate is helpful.

TREATMENT

The treatment of hydronephrosis depends on the underlying cause of the obstruction and the duration of the condition. When obstruction is discovered early, the source can be identified and removed by surgical intervention. Usually after 2 months, the kidney is no longer functional; therefore, surgical intervention is not indicated. Concurrent infection necessitates antibiotic therapy.

Renal Calculi

SYMPTOMS AND SIGNS

Renal calculi are stones in the kidney or elsewhere in the urinary tract, formed by the concentration of various mineral salts (see Fig. 11–4A). They can be solitary or multiple and vary in size; a larger stone formed in the shape of the renal pelvis is known as a staghorn calculus (Fig. 11–4B). Small stones can be passed spontaneously, unnoticed. The patient's symptoms vary with the degree of obstruction. If there is infection or blockage from the calculi, the patient experiences sudden severe pain in the flank area, known as renal colic, with urinary urgency and other urinary abnormalities. Other symptoms include nausea and vomiting, hematuria, fever, chills, and abdominal distention. Blood in the urine can be the result of trauma caused by the presence of small stones, which may be gravel-like or sand-like in consistency, or larger stones, such as staghorn calculi. Hydronephrosis can de-

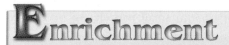

Enrichment

CYSTOSCOPY

Cytoscopy allows direct examination and treatment of the urinary tract. A cystoscope is inserted through the urethra (Fig. 11–5); this instrument has its own lighting system, a viewing scope, and a passage for catheters and surgical devices. Cystoscopy is used to obtain biopsy specimens for diagnosis and to remove stones or tumors.

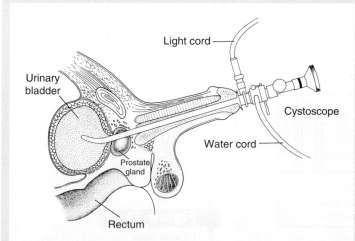

Figure 11–5

Cystoscopy. (From Chabner D: The Language of Medicine, 5th ed. Philadelphia: WB Saunders, 1996, p 208. Used with permission.)

velop if urine is prevented from flowing past the calculi.

ETIOLOGY

Often, the cause is unknown, although there seems to be a hereditary tendency for certain types of stones. Kidney stones are formed when there is an excessive amount of calcium or uric acid in the blood. Males are more prone to kidney stones than females, and the occurrences increase from the age of 30 years up to and including the 50s. Calculi form when there are sources of crystals in the urine, along with the absence of crystalline inhibitors, and the urine is supersaturated with poorly soluble substances.

Risk factors include prolonged dehydration, prolonged immobilization, infection, urinary stasis from obstruction, long-term ingestion of certain medications, and metabolic factors such as **hyperparathyroidism** and gout.

DIAGNOSIS

The diagnosis is made by the family history, clinical picture, urinalysis, radiographic KUB studies, **intravenous urogram,** renal ultrasonogram, and computed tomography (CT) scans. The patient is encouraged to strain the urine to capture any stones that are passed during urination so that they can be analyzed in the labora-

tory. The existence of metabolic disorders can be investigated with blood tests.

TREATMENT

The goals of medical care are to remove the calculi, treat pain and infection, and resolve causative factors. These measures should prevent permanent kidney damage and recurrence of calculi.

The treatment begins with pain relief during the evaluation. Location and size of the calculi indicate the course of treatment. Small calculi (<3 mm) may be treated by observation with fluid hydration in hopes that the stone will pass naturally. Large calculi can be removed by any of several surgical procedures. Attempts are made to crush stones that are too large to pass down the ureter, those in the pelvis of the kidney that will not move, and stones that are trapped in the proximal portion of the ureter. Extracorporeal shock wave lithotripsy (ESWL) (see Fig. 11–6) is the procedure that attempts to crush the stones and then allow the small particles to flush out naturally.

A surgical procedure using a ureteroscope to capture the stone in a basket and remove it is attempted for stones trapped in the distal aspect of a ureter. If the procedure of capturing the stone is unsuccessful, electrohydraulic lithotripsy (EHL) or laser lithotripsy is attempted to break the stone apart into small particles to be flushed

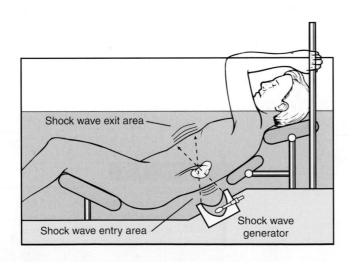

Shock wave exit area

Shock wave entry area

Shock wave generator

Figure 11–6
Lithotripsy.

out of the system. This procedure usually is done under general anesthesia and with the aid of fluoroscopy. After removal of the calculus, the ureter is visualized via the ureteroscope, and often the pelvis of the kidney also is inspected for any scarring, damage, or pathology. A stent is placed in the pelvis of the kidney extending into the urinary bladder as a means of preventing edema and spasms of the ureter and subsequent occlusion of the ureter. The stent is removed in 2 to 5 days.

Stones in the urinary bladder often pass spontaneously. When this does not happen, an attempt to remove bladder stones is done during cystoscopy. When previously mentioned procedures are unsuccessful in removing the calculi, surgical intervention in the form of percutaneous nephrolithotomy may be indicated to remove the stones before permanent damage is caused. A small incision is made into the kidney, and the stone is shattered by ultrasound or EHL. Rarely, when the preceding procedures are unsuccessful, surgical incision of the kidney is done to remove the stone.

Depending on the chemical composition, some kidney stones can be dissolved or prevented from forming with medication. Often the patient may pass small or microscopic stones naturally and without pain. The patient is encouraged to drink 8 to 12 glasses of water a day and may be given diuretics to prevent urinary stasis. Patients are encouraged to strain their urine to catch any stones or particles of stones that may be passed spontaneously.

Urine and blood chemistry measurements and stone analysis lend clues toward which preventative measures are likely to help. Prevention includes modification of diet, exercise, and adequate fluid intake to minimize the chance of stone formation.

Infectious Cystitis and Urethritis

SYMPTOMS AND SIGNS

Cystitis, inflammation of the urinary bladder, and urethritis, inflammation of the urethra, are two common forms of lower UTI. The inflammation and infection cause the patient to experience urinary urgency, frequency, and even incontinence. Additionally, the patient may have pain in the pelvic region and low back, spasm of the bladder, fever and chills, and a burning sensation with urination. The color of the urine may be dark yellow, or pink or red if blood is present.

ETIOLOGY

The usual cause of cystitis and urethritis is an ascending bacterial invasion of the urinary tract. The most frequent causative microorganism is *E. coli,* followed by *Klebsiella, Enterobacter, Proteus,* and *Pseudomonas.* Sexually transmitted diseases can cause cystitis and urethritis. Other sources are viruses, fungi, parasites, and inflammation due to chemotherapy or radiation. Lesions can develop in the bladder secondary to inflammation, intensifying the symptoms.

DIAGNOSIS

The diagnosis is from the clinical picture, urinalysis of a clean-catch urine specimen, urine culture, and cystoscopy. Urinalysis shows dark yellow, pink, or red urine with abnormal urinary sediment and possibly blood and pus. Microscopic examination of the urine shows RBCs (occult blood), increased numbers of epithelial cells or leukocytes, and bacteria. The urine may have a foul odor. The urine culture grows the causative agent for identification. Cystoscopy shows a reddened inflamed bladder wall. Tenderness in the suprapubic region and pain in the lower back may be elicited on palpation.

TREATMENT

Treatment consists of organism-specific antibiotic or urinary antiseptic therapy such as amoxicillin (Amoxil), and trimethoprim-sulfamethoxazole (Bactrim DS, Septra DS). Increased fluid intake is encouraged, as is regular, complete evacuation of the bladder.

Diabetic Nephropathy

SYMPTOMS AND SIGNS

Diabetic nephropathy refers to the renal changes resulting from diabetes mellitus, a systemic endocrine disease caused by failure of the pancreas to release enough insulin into the body (see Diabetes Mellitus in Chapter 4). These changes, called **glomerulosclerosis,** can be expected eventually in all insulin-dependent diabetics, increasing their morbidity and mortality. Clinical manifestations, once they begin, include urinary retention, hypertension, nausea, and protein in the urine. UTI and pyelonephritis are common complications.

ETIOLOGY

Diabetic glomerulosclerosis is a complication of diabetes mellitus; lesions of the glomeruli eventually cause the filtration rate to decrease. Insufficient control of blood glucose levels and blood pressure in the diabetic patient may hasten the deterioration of renal function.

DIAGNOSIS

Blood tests reveal an elevated BUN level and an increase in cholesterol level. Urinalysis shows protein and pus in the urine. The diagnosis is confirmed by radiographic studies of the kidneys and renal biopsy.

TREATMENT

Diabetic persons vary in their susceptibility to renal failure, so the treatment plan is individualized. Medical control of the diabetes and blood pressure is important, as is prompt treatment of infection. Fluid intake and output should balance, with the use of diuretics if needed. A diet for patients with diabetes, with low-protein and low-fat modifications, may be recommended. Dialysis or evaluation for kidney transplantation may be part of the long-term management of ESRD.

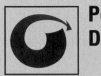

Polycystic Kidney Disease

SYMPTOMS AND SIGNS

Polycystic kidney disease is a slowly progressive and irreversible disorder in which normal renal tissue is replaced with multiple grape-like cysts (Fig. 11-7). The condition is bilateral, with

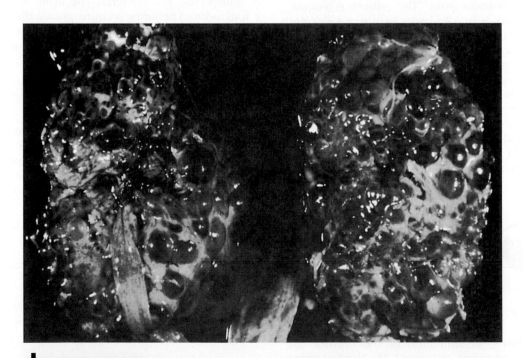

Figure 11-7

Polycystic kidney disease. (From Robbins S, Kumar V: Basic Pathology, 4th ed. Philadelphia: WB Saunders, 1987, p 485. Used with permission.)

cysts that form from dilated nephrons and collecting ducts. Eventually, the kidneys become grossly enlarged, with compression of surrounding tissue leading to impaired renal function and renal failure. As the kidneys become dilated, they are palpable on physical examination. The patient experiences lumbar pain, hematuria, and systemic hypertension and is more prone to renal infections and renal calculi.

ETIOLOGY

Polycystic kidney disease is inherited, but may not be manifested until adolescence or adulthood. It is not clearly understood why the cysts form.

DIAGNOSIS

The diagnosis is made by the clinical picture and renal function tests such as urinalysis, which shows gross blood, proteinuria, and pus. Radiographic films and intravenous pyelogram show enlarged kidneys with irregular outlines and a spidery appearance throughout.

TREATMENT

Because polycystic disease cannot be cured, treatment of this ESRD consists of dialysis and kidney transplantation. Management of UTIs is necessary, as is management of hypertension.

 Neurogenic Bladder

SYMPTOMS AND SIGNS

Neurogenic bladder is a dysfunction of urinary bladder control consisting of difficulty in emptying the bladder or urinary incontinence. Causative factors may alter the symptoms and signs of this condition. Some patients with sensory-related problems experience hesitancy and decreased volume of the urinary stream. Others may experience urinary retention resulting from decreased or absent stimuli to void. If the condition is the result of motor paralysis, the patient has the sensation of a full bladder but is unable to initiate the stream to empty. The patient with uninhibited neurogenic bladder is not able to control the voiding pattern and is persistently incontinent of small amounts of urine. In reflex neurogenic

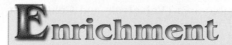

URINARY INCONTINENCE

Normally, as the bladder distends with urine, a reflex is stimulated to initiate voluntary urination (micturition); the sphincters of the bladder and the pelvic diaphragm relax, the bladder muscles contract, and the bladder empties. Urinary incontinence is partial or total loss of voluntary control of the bladder with inability to retain urine. The causes vary from muscle or sphincter impairment to nerve damage or structural abnormalities.

This condition is very prevalent in the elderly, commonly because of overactivity of the bladder musculature, resulting in urgency and incontinence with an inappropriately small volume of urine. Incontinence sometimes is experienced temporarily after the stretching of muscles during childbirth. Children may experience a form termed *enuresis,* or bedwetting. Older women may experience "stress incontinence" resulting from postmenopausal changes in the pelvic musculature that allow intra-abdominal pressure to surpass intraurethral pressure. Other types of overactive bladder—or frequency and urge incontinence—are the subject of much-noted current research. Neurologic damage such as brain damage or spinal cord injury may result in permanent incontinence.

Incontinence is treated or managed according to the degree, the type, and the cause. Antispasmodic agents, adult diapers, "bladder training," estrogen therapy for women, and pelvic muscle exercises are some of the therapeutic measures that may be tried. Chronic indwelling catheters are avoided in the management of incontinence because of the prevalence of infection.

bladder, normal sensation is absent, with uncontrolled bladder contractions occurring, resulting in spontaneous voiding of spurts of urine. With autonomous neurogenic bladder, all sensations and contraction capabilities are absent, resulting in inability to void without applying pressure to the suprapubic area (**Valsalva's** and Credé's maneuvers).

ETIOLOGY

An insult to the brain, spinal cord, or the nerves supplying the lower urinary tract, whether by trauma or disease process, may result in the inability to empty the bladder of urine or to maintain continence. Damage may be caused by cerebrovascular accident, spinal cord trauma, tumors, neuropathies, herniated lumbar disks, poliomyelitis, spinal cord lesions, or myelomeningocele.

DIAGNOSIS

The diagnosis is based on a history of trauma or a disease process, the clinical picture, and urodynamic studies that assess bladder function. Urine flow rate may be evaluated by a uroflow-meter, a device for continuous recording of urine flow in milliliters per second.

TREATMENT

The treatment is directed toward prevention of UTIs and attempts to restore some normalcy in function. Providing means of storage of urine and bladder emptying are of primary importance. Usually, there is no cure for the neurologic deficit that caused the bladder dysfunction. Catheterization (see Fig. 11–8 in Enrichment on catheterization), whether intermittent or indwelling, is necessary to help the patient to maintain a decent quality of life. Drug therapy with parasympathomimetic agents may be indicated in some cases. Surgery and the use of external collection devices are other alternatives. Possible complications include hydronephrosis and renal failure.

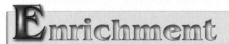

Enrichment

URINARY CATHETERIZATION

Urinary catheterization involves the insertion of a catheter into the urinary bladder through the urethra for the withdrawal of urine (Fig. 11–8) or for irrigation of the bladder with a therapeutic solution. Strict sterile technique is necessary to prevent cystitis. Urinary catheterization is indicated to empty the bladder before surgery, to obtain a sterile urine specimen, to relieve urinary retention, and to treat incontinence (an indwelling catheter is attached to a drainage bag when the patient is incontinent).

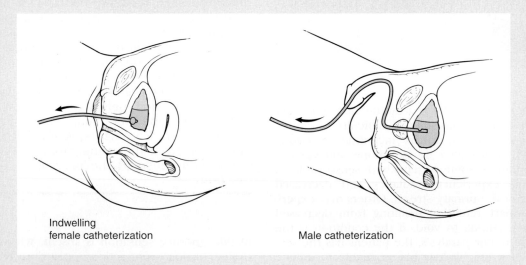

Indwelling female catheterization

Male catheterization

Figure 11–8

Urinary catheterization.

Stress Incontinence

SYMPTOMS AND SIGNS

Stress incontinence is a symptom, a sign, and a diagnosis. It occurs when increased abdominal pressure forces urine through the bladder sphincter. The patient (usually female) experiences leakage of urine on coughing, sneezing, laughing, lifting, or running, without prior urgency. The patient is unable to control the leakage during physical exertion.

ETIOLOGY

This embarrassing disorder is caused by weakening of the pelvic floor muscles and the urethral structure. Trauma to the area from childbirth is the most common cause. Pressure from pregnancy also may be the cause. The hormonal changes of aging and menopause make the condition more common in older women. Certain medications and obesity can precipitate the disorder.

DIAGNOSIS

The symptoms clearly point to the diagnosis. Endoscopy and cystogram voiding reveal abnormal bladder position, with leakage provoked by coughing or straining.

TREATMENT

The treatment consists of exercises (Kegel's exercises, or pelvic floor muscle tightening), estrogen replacement, drug therapy, surgical repair, or collagen injections.

Renal Cell Carcinoma

SYMPTOMS AND SIGNS

Renal cell carcinoma, or malignancy of the kidney, can begin anywhere in the kidney or may be secondary to another primary carcinoma elsewhere in the body. The tumor tends to grow slowly but can invade surrounding tissue or **metastasize** at any time. The most frequent present-ing symptoms are hematuria, weight loss, and nagging pain or a dull ache in the flank area. A firm mass in the abdomen can be palpated on physical examination. The patient is likely to be a man in his sixth or seventh decade; the male : female ratio is 2 : 1.

ETIOLOGY

The cause of renal cell cancer is unknown; heavy cigarette smoking has been implicated as a predisposing factor.

DIAGNOSIS

Laboratoy tests include a CBC; ESR, which may be elevated; urinalysis; and renal biopsy studies. Radiographic studies (KUB), ultrasonography, **magnetic resonance imaging (MRI),** and CT help to stage the tumor.

TREATMENT

Early treatment with radical nephrectomy is the best approach for a cure. The cancer resists radiation and chemotherapy, so the prognosis is poor in advanced cases. The medical management includes psychological support and the administration of pain medication.

Bladder Tumors

SYMPTOMS AND SIGNS

Tumors of the bladder are uncommon, but when they occur they are almost always malignant. They appear as multiple lesions that originate in the lining of the bladder. Bladder cancer can occur at any age; however, the patient is more likely to be older than 50 years of age, white, and male. Symptoms frequently include intermittent gross hematuria, dysuria, and nocturia. Other symptoms relate to the type and size of the tumor. Unfortunately, the disease may be asymptomatic until it has invaded underlying tissue and metastasized.

ETIOLOGY

Although the cause of bladder tumors is not known, risk factors include certain environmental and industrial **carcinogens,** cigarette smoking, coffee drinking, and the use of artificial sweeteners.

DIAGNOSIS

Diagnostic studies include urinalysis for hematuria and cytologic studies for malignant cells. Endoscopy with biopsy confirms the diagnosis. Once identified, the bladder tumor is classified by staging and grading to evaluate its malignant potential and to determine the best treatment plan.

TREATMENT

The goal of treatment is to arrest tumor growth and to eradicate the malignancy. Treatment options are determined by the pathologic grading and staging of the malignancy. Surgical procedures include resection of the tumors or laser **fulguration,** followed by chemotherapy or radiation. The patient is taught to watch for signs of hematuria and the importance of follow-up endoscopy. There is a variable prognosis, and recurrence is possible.

Summary

The healthy urinary system is constantly filtering blood to remove the waste products of protein metabolism and to regulate water, electrolytes, and acid–base balance in the body. Among other important functions are the regulation of blood pressure (secretes renin), the control of red blood cell production (secretes the hormone erythropoietin), and the activation of vitamin D. The urinary tract is susceptible to bacterial infection, toxins, antibody-mediated disease, obstructive disorders, genetic diseases, malignancy, circulatory disturbances, and metabolic disorders.

- Urinalysis examines urine for abnormal elements that may help estimate renal function and furnish clues to systemic disease.
- Acute inflammation and swelling of the glomeruli (acute glomerulonephritis) can be primary or secondary to systemic infection, as in post-streptococcal glomerulonephritis.
- Chronic glomerulonephritis, a chronic noninfectious disease, can result in renal damage and renal failure.
- Dialysis provides an artificial kidney to filter out unwanted elements from the blood in renal failure. Many candidates for kidney transplantation are diabetics with renal failure.
- The patient with nephrotic syndrome (increased permeability of the glomerulus) loses excessive amounts of protein (proteinuria), leading to depressed protein plasma levels (hypoalbuminemia).

- Diminished blood flow to the kidneys, intrarenal disease, or obstruction of urine flow to the kidneys can result in acute renal failure.
- Chronic renal failure may require dialysis or kidney transplantation, or both, to prolong life.
- Pyelonephritis and hydronephrosis are conditions that can result from obstructive conditions of the urinary tract.
- Where a kidney stone lodges and its size, shape, and composition determine symptoms and the approach to treatment.
- Ascending bacterial invasion of the urinary tract can result in pyelonephritis, infectious cystitis, or urethritis.
- Eventually, those afflicted with insulin-dependent diabetes mellitus may suffer diabetic nephropathy.
- Polycystic kidney disease, an inherited condition, causes irreversible impaired renal function.
- Neurogenic bladder, the inability to properly empty the bladder or to maintain urinary continence, is the result of an insult to the brain or the nerves that control the bladder. Leakage of urine (stress incontinence) is frequently the result of weakening of the pelvic floor muscles or the urethral structure.
- Tumors of the urinary tract tend to be malignant and to affect older people.

Review Challenge

REVIEW QUESTIONS

1. Specifically, how does the urinary system work to maintain homeostasis?
2. What are some of the common symptoms of urinary system diseases?
3. What are the etiologic factors of acute glomerulonephritis? Chronic glomerulonephritis?
4. What are some examples of abnormal findings in a urinalysis?
5. Which individuals may require dialysis? Kidney transplant?
6. What are the classic clinical symptoms and signs of nephrosis? What causes nephrosis?
7. Why is acute renal failure considered a clinical emergency?
8. When is renal failure irreversible?
9. How would a patient with pyelonephritis describe his or her symptoms?
10. How might organisms be introduced into the urinary tract and cause pyelonephritis?
11. Which condition is a complication of urinary tract obstruction? What are some causes of urinary tract obstruction?
12. What are the risk factors for renal calculi?
13. What are the etiologic sources of infectious cystitis and urethritis?
14. How does diabetes mellitus contribute to diabetic nephropathy?
15. How would you describe the polycystic kidney?
16. How would you compare the pathology of neurogenic bladder to that of stress incontinence?
17. When may catheterization be indicated?
18. What is the treatment and prognosis for renal cell carcinoma? For bladder tumors?

REAL-LIFE CHALLENGE

Cystitis

A 35-year-old woman reports pain in pelvic region and lower back, frequency and urgency of urination, and burning on urination. The onset of symptoms was approximately 4 hours before the office visit.

Vital signs are T—100.5°, P—96, R—18, BP—130/88. A clean catch urine specimen is obtained, and it is pink in color and has a foul odor. The urine specimen is sent to the laboratory for a urinalysis and culture and sensitivity.

The examination reveals tenderness over the bladder. Microscopic examination of the specimen reveals blood, pus, leukocytes, and bacteria.

A diagnosis of cystitis was made, and trimethoprim-sulfamethoxazole (Bactrim DS) was prescribed. The patient was encouraged to force fluids and was instructed to call the office the next day to report her progress.

Questions

1. What is another term for cystitis?
2. What additional symptoms might a patient with cystitis exhibit?
3. What is the usual cause of cystitis?
4. Why is a urinalysis important in diagnosing cystitis?
5. Why would the urine have a foul odor?
6. Why would a culture and sensitivity be important in the treatment of cystitis?
7. What alternative drug therapy is available to treat cystitis?
8. Why would the patient be encouraged to force fluids?

REAL-LIFE CHALLENGE

Renal Calculus

The wife of a 42-year-old man called the office stating that within the past hour her husband had a sudden onset of severe pain in his left side and back. He also has experienced nausea and vomiting. Questioning revealed the pain to be in the left flank area and quite severe. She also noted that the pain radiated down toward the scrotum and that he was experiencing pressure in the perineal area and the frequent urge to urinate. A renal calculus was suspected, and the patient's wife was advised to transport him to an emergency facility.

Vital signs were T—99.6°, P—96, R—20, BP—124/88. A urine specimen was obtained, and the dipstick indicated blood in the urine.

The abdomen was slightly distended, the left flank area exhibited tenderness on palpation, and tenderness was noted over the bladder. A renal calculus was suspected, and a KUB, intravenous pyelogram, and ultrasound of the kidneys was ordered. An intravenous (IV) line was started, and the patient was given 2 mg of morphine sulfate IV push.

The KUB revealed a suspicious area 8 cm distal to the origin of the left ureter. The IVP confirmed the presence of a 3.5-mm calculus distal to the ureteral origin. The renal ultrasound indicated hydronephrosis of the left kidney. The patient was admitted for observation and for pain management.

Questions

1. What causes renal calculi to form?
2. Why would patients' symptoms vary?
3. What would be the significant symptom or symptoms leading to suspicion of renal calculi?
4. What is renal colic?
5. What would cause blood in the urine?
6. What is the cause of hydronephrosis?
7. Why would the patient be instructed to strain all urine?
8. What are the treatment options for the patient with renal calculi?
9. Why would IV morphine be given?

RESOURCES

National Kidney and Urologic Diseases Information Clearinghouse
3 Information Way
Bethesda, MD 20892-3580
301-468-6345

American Association of Kidney Patients
100 South Ashley Drive, Suite 280
Tampa, FL 33102
800-749-2257
(http://www.aakp.org)

American Kidney Fund
6110 Executive Blvd, Ste 1010
Bethesda, MD 20852
800-638-8299
(http://www.arbon.com/kidney)

American Foundation for Urologic Disorders
1126 N Charles Street
Baltimore, MD 21201
800-242-2387
(http://www.afun.org)

American Urological Association
1120 N. Charles Street
Baltimore, MD 21201
(http://www.auanet.org)

Help for Incontinent People (HIP)
PO Box 8310
Spartanburg, SC 29305-8310
800-BLADDER

Interstitial Cystitis Association of America
51 Monroe St, Ste 1402
Washington, DC 20850
800-435-7422
(ICAmail@ichelp.org)

National Kidney Foundation
30 East 33rd St, Ste 1100
New York, NY 10016
800-622-9010

Polycystic Kidney Research Foundation
 4901 Main St, Ste 200
 Kansas City, MO 64112-2634
 800-PKD-CURE
 (pkdcure@pkrfoundation.org)

National Organ Procurement and Transplantation Network
 1100 Boulders Pkwy, Ste 500
 PO Box 13770
 Richmond, VA 23225
 804-330-8500

Incontinence Organizations
 PO Box 8547
 Silver Spring, MD 20907
 800-358-9295

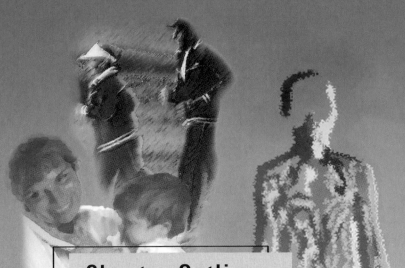

Chapter Outline

Diseases and Conditions of the Reproductive System

After studying Chapter 12, you should be able to:

1. Identify risk factors for sexually transmitted diseases (STDs).
2. Explain what is meant by a silent STD, and state an example.
3. Name the complications of untreated gonorrhea.
4. Recall how trichomoniasis is diagnosed.
5. Explain how genital herpes is transmitted.
6. Explain why women with genital herpes are advised to have regular Pap (Papanicolaou) smears.
7. Describe the stages of untreated syphilis.
8. Explain why hepatitis B is classified as sexually transmitted.
9. List the possible causes of dyspareunia in men and women.
10. Name drugs that can contribute to impotence.
11. Name a common causative factor in male and female infertility.
12. Explain the value of prostate-specific antigen (PSA) as a screening test.
13. Discuss the medical interventions for prostatic cancer.
14. Explain how varicocele may contribute to male infertility.
15. Relate the reason that physicians encourage monthly testicular self-examinations for younger men.
16. Explain what causes the dysmenorrhea associated with endometriosis.
17. Discuss the importance of early diagnosis and prompt treatment of pelvic inflammatory disease.
18. Discuss the advantages and possible risks of hormone replacement therapy for the postmenopausal woman.
19. Explain how uterine prolapse, cystocele, and rectocele may be corrected surgically.
20. List the risk factors for cervical cancer.
21. Name the leading cause of deaths attributed to female reproductive system disorders.
22. List some possible causes of ectopic pregnancy.
23. Explain how a pregnant woman is monitored for toxemia.
24. Describe abruptio placentae.
25. List factors that place women at higher risk for cancer of the breast.

Key Terms

amenorrhea	(ah–**men**–o–**REE**–ah)	multiparous	(mul–**TIP**–ar–us)
autoinoculation	(**aw**–toh–in–**ock**–u–**LAY**–shun)	orchitis	(or–**KYE**–tis)
		pessary	(**PESS**–ah–ree)
chancre	(**SHANG**–ker)	primipara	(pry–**MIP**–ah–rah)
colporrhaphy	(kol–**POUR**–ah–fee)	prolapse	(pro–**LAPS**)
curettage	(**ku**–reh–**TAHZH**)	prostatectomy	(**pros**–tah–**TECK**–toh–me)
dysmenorrhea	(**dis**–men–oh–**REE**–ah)		
		psychosexual	(**sigh**–ko–**SEKS**–you–al)
dyspareunia	(**dis**–pah–**RUE**–nee–ah)		
		salpingo-oophorec-tomy	(sal–**ping**–go–oh–ouf–oh–**RECK**–toh–me)
dysuria	(dis–**YOU**–ree–ah)		
genitourinary	(**jen**–ih–toe–**YU**–rih–nar–ee)		
		septicemia	(sep–tih–**SEE**–me–ah)
hysterosalpingogra-phy	(**hiss**–ter–oh–**sal**–pin–**GOG**–rah–fee)	spermicidal	(**spur**–mih–**SIGH**–dal)
		ultrasonography	(uhl–tra–son–**OGG**–rah–fee)
laparoscopy	(lap–ar–**OS**–ko–pee)		
leiomyoma	(**lye**–o–my–**OH**–ma)	urethritis	(**you**–ree–**THRYE**–tis)
menorrhagia	(**men**–oh–**RAY**–jee–ah)	vaginismus	(vaj–in–**IZ**–mus)
		varicocele	(**VAR**–ih–ko–seel)
metrorrhagia	(**met**–roh–**RAY**–jee–ah)		

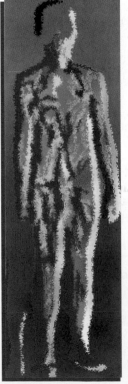

The Normal Functioning Reproductive Systems

The reproductive process in humans is sexual and involves the union of two sex cells, one male and one female. Sex organs are not differentiated in early embryonic development, and therefore gender is difficult to identify. As the fetus develops, male or female definition becomes evident. The organs of the reproductive system usually are classified in two groups: the gonads (testes and ova-ries), which produce germ cells and hormones, and the series of ducts necessary for the transportation of the germ cells.

The male reproductive system functions in the mechanism for the transfer of the sperm cells to the female for fertilization of the ovum. The testes produce the sperm and the hormones necessary for the development and maintenance of the secondary sex characteristics. The sperm is transported through the series of ducts beginning with the epididymis, the ductus deferens, and the ejaculatory ducts. The seminal vesicles, the prostate gland, the bulbourethral glands, and the penis are accessory organs that help to propel the sperm on its journey to meet the egg (Fig. 12-1).

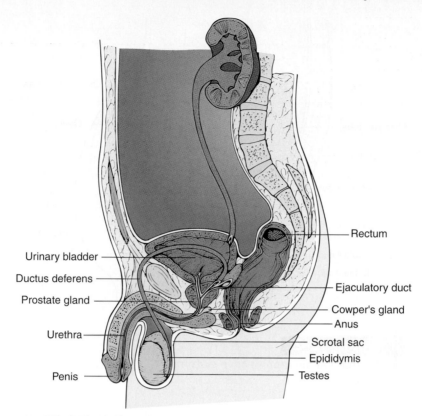

Urinary bladder
Ductus deferens
Prostate gland
Urethra
Penis

Rectum
Ejaculatory duct
Cowper's gland
Anus
Scrotal sac
Epididymis
Testes

Figure 12–1

Normal male reproductive system.

The female reproductive system provides nourishment for and enables the development of the fertilized ovum. The ovaries produce and release the egg and the hormones necessary for the development of secondary sex characteristics and for maintenance of a pregnancy. The ductal system for transport, nourishment, and growth of the fertilized ovum includes the fallopian tubes, the uterus, the cervix, the vagina, and the external genitalia (Fig. 12–2).

The breasts are accessory organs of reproduction and are two milk-producing glands (Fig. 12–3). When a woman is pregnant, the breast tissue is stimulated by both ovarian and placental hormones to prepare for lactation. It is stimulated further after delivery by lactating hormones to produce and release milk for nourishment of the infant.

The process of reproduction requires that the egg be fertilized by the sperm. After release from the ovary, the egg progresses down the fallopian tube. If pregnancy is to ensue, the egg is met, about a third of the way down the fallopian tube, by the sperm cell. After fertilization takes place, the **zygote** continues to travel down the fallopian tube to the uterus, where it eventually attaches to the uterine lining (**endometrium**) to be nourished and to grow. The placenta forms within the uterine wall and provides a mechanism for the exchange of nourishment and waste products between the mother and the developing fetus. A normal gestational period is 38 weeks after conception, at which time the birth process begins with labor and subsequently, the infant is delivered.

The menstrual cycle is regulated by gonadotropic hormones produced by the anterior pituitary gland, which causes the ovaries to produce estrogen and progesterone. During menstruation, the endometrium (the disintegrated endometrial cells along with secretions and blood cells) is shed via the vagina. This is followed by the ovarian production of estrogen, causing the ovum to mature and to be released from the ovary. The development of the corpus luteum follows, and progesterone and additional estrogen are secreted into

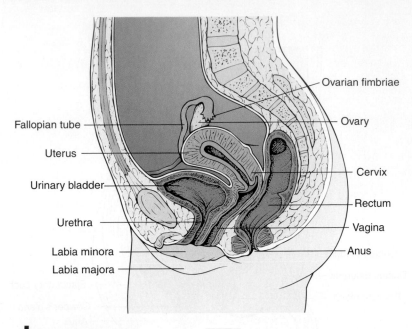

Figure 12–2

Normal female reproductive system.

the bloodstream to stimulate the growth of the endometrium in preparation for implantation of the fertilized ovum. If pregnancy does not ensue, the endometrium again is shed through menses in anticipation of the next cycle and a possible pregnancy.

Both the male and female reproductive systems are vulnerable to many disease entities, whether STDs, malignancy, benign growths, or chemical imbalances. Abnormal reproductive system function sometimes is the result of functional, structural, or emotional causes. Often,

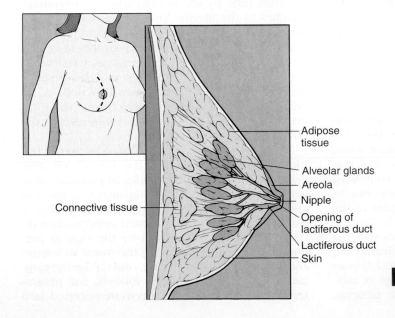

Figure 12–3

Normal female breast.

complications develop during pregnancy, some severe and some merely aggravating. This chapter attempts to explore the most common disease entities, conditions, and complications of both reproductive systems.

Sexually Transmitted Diseases

There are more than 20 infectious diseases spread by sexual contact, all of which can damage health or even threaten life. STDs, sometimes called venereal diseases, are among the most common contagious diseases in the United States. No one is immune, and it is possible to have more than one of the STDs simultaneously. The infections are transmitted from one person to another through bodily fluids such as blood, se-

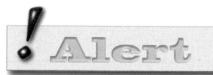

RISK FACTORS FOR SEXUALLY TRANSMITTED DISEASES

- ⟳ Sex with someone whose past sexual history one does not know
- ⟳ Drug use with sharing of needles
- ⟳ Sex with many people
- ⟳ Sexual intimacy with someone who has been diagnosed with an STD or one who is being treated for an STD
- ⟳ Exposure with skin-to-skin contact in the presence of any open lesion, such as a chancre or a wart
- ⟳ Use of alcohol or other drugs that may cloud one's judgment about a sexual encounter
- ⟳ Hemophilia
- ⟳ Transfusion of blood or blood products
- ⟳ Babies being carried by an HIV-positive mother
- ⟳ Breast-fed infants of an HIV-positive mother
- ⟳ Lack of education or concern about risky sexual behavior

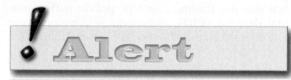

INFECTION CONTROL AND UNIVERSAL PRECAUTIONS

Guidelines. Treat body fluids as if infected and remember to use the following precautions:

1. Practice frequent and thorough hand washing.
2. Report any accidental needle sticks.
3. Wear personal protective equipment, including mask, gown, gloves, and goggles.
4. Use caution with laboratory specimens.
5. Dispose of contaminated sharps in designated biohazard containers. *Caution:* Do not recap or break needles.
6. Use proper linen disposal containers.
7. Use clean mouthpieces and resuscitation bags.
8. Obtain hepatitis B vaccination for occupational exposure to blood.
9. Use proper decontamination techniques.

men, and vaginal secretions during vaginal, anal, or oral sex; some are spread by direct contact with infected skin.

STD rates in the United States are among the highest in the world and are growing. Attempts to control this rampant public health problem are focusing on research studies, education, and prevention campaigns. Prevention messages point out high-risk sexual behavior patterns and lifestyles, and warn of possible predisposing health problems.

CHLAMYDIA

SYMPTOMS AND SIGNS

Chlamydia, the most common bacterial infection, sometimes is called the silent STD because symptoms are often absent and thus sexual transmission occurs unknowingly. A high percentage of women have no symptoms before dangerous complications start. More common than gonorrhea and the leading cause of **pelvic inflammatory disease (PID)**, chlamydia is a major cause of female sterility. Conversely, 75% of men have symptoms 1 to 3 weeks after exposure.

Early female symptoms include a thick vaginal discharge with a burning sensation and itching, abdominal pain, and **dyspareunia.** Infected men experience discharge from the penis, with a burning sensation and itching, and a burning sensation when urinating, the latter caused by urethritis. The scrotum may be swollen. Frequently, the inguinal lymph nodes are enlarged in either sex. A small transient lesion and skin irritation may be noticed. Newborns can acquire chlamydia during birth from the infected mother, resulting in conjunctivitis, blindness, arthritis, or overwhelming infection.

ETIOLOGY

Chlamydia trachomatis, an intracellular bacterium, is the cause of chlamydia and usually is transmitted by sexual contact. The site of primary infection is usually around the genitals but can be oral or anal, depending on sexual practice.

DIAGNOSIS

In the laboratory, swab cultures specifically reveal the parasite *C. trachomatis* in the infected person's body fluids. A **Giemsa stain** of cell scrapings to test for the presence of **antibodies** and **antigen**-specific **serologic** studies are done.

TREATMENT

Antibiotic therapy is given to both partners, beginning with a single injection, and followed with a course of oral antibiotics, such as doxycycline and erythromycin. Prompt treatment can cure the infection and avoid complications such as PID and problem pregnancy.

GONORRHEA

SYMPTOMS AND SIGNS

Gonorrhea, also a common infection of the genitourinary tract, causes symptoms and complications similar to those of chlamydia in male and female patients. A **purulent** discharge from the male or female genitourinary tract and dysuria are often present, but can vary in severity. Up to 50% of men are **asymptomatic,** so they may unknowingly continue to spread the infection, making transmission difficult to control. The disease also can infect eyes and throat or become systemic.

ETIOLOGY

Infection with the common bacterium *Neisseria gonorrhoeae* usually results from sexual transmission. Because transmission is also possible during birth, it is necessary to protect newborns from eye infections that can lead to blindness. Therefore, prophylactic erythromycin salve is administered routinely at birth.

DIAGNOSIS

Laboratory cultures of infectious body secretions and microscopic examination of exudate with a **Gram stain** are done to identify the *N. gonorrhoeae* organism.

TREATMENT

Ceftriaxone, penicillin, or tetracycline administration is started as soon as the diagnosis is made. After the antibiotic therapy, follow-up culture studies are ordered to ensure a complete cure because some strains are antibiotic resistant. Neglecting treatment of a gonococcal infection can lead to complications, including PID, septicemia, and septic arthritis. With early treatment, the prognosis is good.

TRICHOMONIASIS

SYMPTOMS AND SIGNS

Approximately 15% of people who are sexually active have a protozoal infection of the lower genitourinary tract called trichomoniasis. However, most infected men and women are asymptomatic. This contributes to spreading the unrecognized infection as well as delaying treatment.

The initial symptoms for male and female patients include urethritis with dysuria and itching. In addition, women may notice a profuse greenish yellow discharge from the vagina that may subside without treatment; still, the presence of infection remains, and it can become chronic.

ETIOLOGY

Trichomoniasis is a protozoal infection caused by *Trichomonas vaginalis* and usually is transmitted through sexual contact.

DIAGNOSIS

A wet preparation of vaginal secretions or discharge from the male urethra is studied for the microorganism *T. vaginalis.* Urinalysis also may reveal the organism. The cervix is examined for the presence of small hemorrhages with a strawberry-like appearance.

TREATMENT

If the laboratory culture is positive, anti-infective drugs are given vaginally or orally.

The prognosis is good if both partners receive medical treatment, including a follow-up examination that ensures that the infection is cured completely. Failure to treat both partners causes reinfection, called a ping-pong vaginitis.

GENITAL HERPES

SYMPTOMS AND SIGNS

Genital herpes is caused by herpes simplex virus type 2 (HSV-2). It is an infection of the skin of the genital area, with **ulcerations** spread by direct skin-to-skin contact, causing painful genital sores similar to cold sores (Fig. 12–4).

The initial episode may go unnoticed. More commonly, one or more blister-like lesions are noted somewhere on the genitals or around the anus. Systemic influenza symptoms, swollen glands, fever, headache, and painful urination also may be present. The condition is infectious when sores are present, but some people, called "shedders," can transmit the virus without symptoms. Subsequent outbreaks can occur for months or years because the virus hides in the nervous system and lies dormant between flare-ups.

ETIOLOGY

One in six adults carries the highly contagious HSV-2; it usually is transmitted sexually with skin-to-skin contact.

Because of the presence of open lesions, there is an increased risk of contracting acquired immunodeficiency syndrome (AIDS) during sexual acts between persons infected with HSV-2 and those who are positive for human immunodeficiency virus (HIV).

DIAGNOSIS

The presence of the characteristic lesions on the male or female genitalia is noted during physical examination. Tissue culture laboratory techniques are used to identify the HSV-2 virus and to confirm the diagnosis.

TREATMENT

There is no cure, but prescription drugs currently are available to reduce the duration and frequency of outbreaks. These drugs include acyclovir (Zovirax), famciclovir (Famvir), and valacyclovir (Valtrex). In some cases, the body's own immunity makes the episodes less severe. The

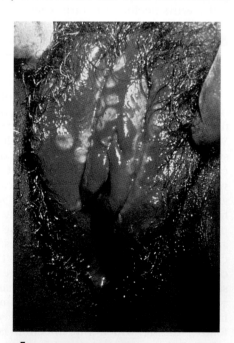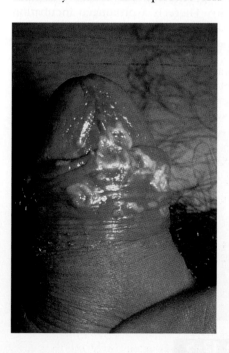

Figure 12–4

Genital herpes in the female *(left)* and the male *(right)*. (From Behrman RE, Kliegman RM, Arvin AM: Slide Set, Nelson Textbook of Pediatrics, 15/E. Philadelphia, WB Saunders, 1996.)

presence of sores in the genital area and the fear of transmitting or acquiring herpes contributes to emotional stress and social embarrassment. Also, women with genital herpes need to be watched more carefully for cervical cancer. A Pap (Papanicolaou) smear every 6 months is recommended. Finally, a cesarean section may be indicated because the virus is dangerous to the newborn.

GENITAL WARTS (CONDYLOMATA ACUMINATA)

SYMPTOMS AND SIGNS

Condyloma acuminatum is a genital infection that causes raised cauliflower-like growths in or near the vagina or rectum or along the penis (Fig. 12–5). These genital warts are usually painless, but they may itch or burn. These contagious lesions appear several weeks to several months after direct skin-to-skin contact during sexual intercourse with an infected person. The discomfort experienced varies with the size, number, and location of the warts.

ETIOLOGY

A virus called the human papillomavirus (HPV) is the cause of genital warts and usually is transmitted sexually. There is a prolonged incubation period of 1 to 6 months.

DIAGNOSIS

Genital warts can be identified by their appearance, but sometimes a biopsy is suggested to rule out carcinoma. The wart must be differentiated from a syphilitic lesion.

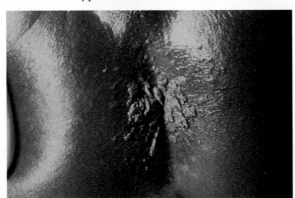

Figure 12–5

Genital warts. (From Behrman RE, Kliegman RM, Arvin AM: Slide Set, Nelson Textbook of Pediatrics, 15/E. Philadelphia, WB Saunders, 1996.)

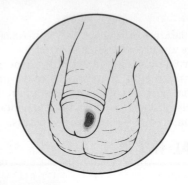

Figure 12–6

Chancre of primary syphilis.

TREATMENT

The treatment is chemical or surgical removal of the warts; however, recurrence is common. Topical drug therapy to remove the warts includes a keratolytic agent such as podofilox and trichloroacetic acid. Some genital warts go away without treatment.

Studies show that women with genital HPV infection are at greater risk for cervical cancer. Because the warts spread more rapidly during pregnancy, a cesarean section may be necessary if the warts occlude the birth canal.

SYPHILIS

SYMPTOMS AND SIGNS

Syphilis begins with the presence of a painless but highly contagious local lesion on the male or female genitalia, called a chancre (Fig. 12–6). Without early treatment during the primary stage, it becomes a systemic, chronic disease that can involve any organ or tissue. In 1 to 2 months when the primary lesion heals, the causative organism (the *Treponema pallidum* spirochete) has disseminated throughout the body and multiplied, producing lesions wherever the organisms are most prevalent: skin, lymph nodes, cardiovascular system, brain, and spinal cord. The disease continues to be contagious during the secondary stage, when there is systemic manifestation, which can present numerous symptoms. Then a latent period, lasting from 1 to 40 years, may follow, during which the infection is generally subclinical or asymptomatic. In the tertiary, or late, stage, the lesions, called gummas, have invaded body organs and systems, causing widespread damage to the point of being disabling and life threatening.

ETIOLOGY

Syphilis is caused by infection with the *T. pallidum* spirochete through sexual contact or other direct contact with infected lesions or infected body fluids. Congenital transmission can occur during pregnancy.

DIAGNOSIS

A smear taken from the primary lesion is examined microscopically for the spiral bacteria *T. pallidum*. Antibodies can be detected in the patient's serum, and this is the most common means of recognition.

TREATMENT

Syphilis can be cured with a course of antibiotic therapy using penicillin G. If the patient is allergic to penicillin, other antibiotics are used. It is best to treat the disease in the early stage, before irreversible damage occurs in the body.

CHANCROID

SYMPTOMS AND SIGNS

Chancroid, also called soft chancre, is a bacterial infection of the genitalia that causes a necrotizing ulceration and lymphadenopathy. The shallow and painless lesion appears on the skin or mucous membrane, at the site of entry, 7 to 10 days after sexual contact with an infected person. Usually, the ulcer deepens and becomes purulent and can be spread to other areas of the body by autoinoculation.

ETIOLOGY

The causative agent of chancroid is the bacterium *Haemophilus ducreyi*.

DIAGNOSIS

In the laboratory, Gram stain smears of the **exudate** are done to confirm cause of the infection.

TREATMENT

The patient usually responds well to antibiotic therapy. Sometimes, the lesions need to be drained surgically. Good personal hygiene is advised. The patient is told to keep the infected areas clean and dry and to refrain from sexual contact during the entire time of treatment.

HEPATITIS B

SYMPTOMS AND SIGNS

Hepatitis B, or serum hepatitis, is an inflammation of the liver that causes liver cell destruction and necrosis. The systemic symptoms of viral hepatitis B result from the inflammation, progressive destruction, and swelling of the liver. The patient feels ill initially and eventually may have a variety of symptoms, including digestive disturbances, fever, weight loss, **jaundice,** fatigue, and abdominal pain.

ETIOLOGY

Hepatitis B is considered sexually transmitted because the mode of transmission includes contact with blood, semen, vaginal secretions, and saliva. Most infections result from sexual contact or blood exchange from sharing contaminated needles. Health-care providers are at risk for infection from accidental inoculation from a contaminated needle puncture or scratch; therefore, all patients must be considered potential sources of the disease, and universal precautions must be practiced.

DIAGNOSIS

First, the patient's history may point to how the disease was transmitted and the source of the infection. Then laboratory testing for liver function and increased levels of enzymes (transaminase and alkaline phosphatase) that indicate hepatic damage is ordered. When the patient is jaundiced, there are high levels of bilirubin in the blood and urine. There is an increase in the **prothrombin time (PT),** indicating a decrease in the ability of the blood to clot. The detection of gamma globulin, specifically hepatitis B antibodies, in the blood confirms the diagnosis.

TREATMENT

There is no cure, so the patient is given medication to control nausea, is encouraged to rest, and is made as comfortable as possible. In most cases, the liver heals and regenerates, but this takes time, perhaps several months.

In 1982, an effective vaccine (Heptavax B) was developed and currently is available to those at high risk. This includes health-care workers and all persons who handle bodily fluids; among the general population, intravenous drug users, homosexual men, and inner-city heterosexuals are at greatest risk.

Sexual Dysfunction

The most common male and female sexual dysfunctions are discussed briefly. Sexual health and proper sexual functioning are important to human beings for the pleasure they provide and the closeness they nurture in a relationship and for reproduction. To fulfill these purposes, individuals need to be free from organic disease and psychosexual disorders.

Ideally, the human sexual response cycle progresses from a state of desire or arousal, through orgasm, to resolution or a feeling of well-being and relaxation. This cycle depends on a balance and interplay among the mind, the nervous system, and biogenic physical factors.

DYSPAREUNIA

SYMPTOMS AND SIGNS

Either men or women can experience dyspareunia, recurrent painful or difficult sexual intercourse, but it is more common in women. The nature of the pain (superficial or deep) and the amount of pain, as well as the conditions under which it occurs, are significant because the possible causes are diverse for men and women.

ETIOLOGY

In a woman, organic causes such as an intact **hymen,** insufficient lubrication, the presence of an STD, or the use of a spermicide may cause superficial pain during sexual intercourse. Other conditions that cause deeper pelvic pain during intercourse include **endometriosis,** PID, and the presence of cysts or tumors in the genitourinary tract or pelvis.

The condition can have a psychological basis from past trauma, sexual abuse, or fears, including a fear of pregnancy. Anxiety alone can be sufficient to cause **vaginismus.** Allergic reactions to spermicidal creams and jellies or even to semen can cause irritation, itching, and burning.

In a man, causes of dyspareunia might include anatomic abnormalities, such as a "bowed" erection, a tight foreskin, and prostatitis. Lesions on the penis and urethritis secondary to an STD are other causes. Frequently, anxiety or guilt points to psychosexual dysfunction as the root of the problem.

DIAGNOSIS

A careful history of the type and nature of the pain experienced during intercourse is significant. A physical examination, with laboratory tests depending on the possible causes, helps to determine the basis of the dyspareunia.

TREATMENT

Treatment of male or female dyspareunia is based on the cause. The use of lubricants during intercourse or a gentle stretching of the vaginal opening is helpful in some cases. Underlying conditions such as infection are treated. In more complex situations, corrective surgery may be required. The patient may be advised to address any psychosexual dysfunctions through counseling.

ERECTILE DYSFUNCTION/ IMPOTENCE

SYMPTOMS AND SIGNS

Erectile dysfunction (ED)/impotence is the inability of a man to perform sexual intercourse, usually because he is unable to attain or maintain an erection of the penis sufficient for satisfactory sexual activity. It is a common disorder, affecting most men at some time during their lives. The condition can be temporary or may become chronic.

ETIOLOGY

Sexual arousal causes the arteries in the penis to relax and dilate, thus allowing an increased blood flow to the penis. The expansion and hardening of the penis cause a compression of the veins carrying blood away from the penis, resulting in an erection. Anything that impedes the nerve response or that alters the necessary blood flow pattern results in failure of an erection.

Often, ED/impotence has a psychological basis in depression, unconscious guilt, or some kind of anxiety about sex. Sexual trauma, repressed inhibitions, depression, stress, and discordant relationships are other possible contributing factors. Chronic fatigue and stress also can impair sexual function.

There are numerous physical or medical conditions that play a significant role in ED. Medical conditions affecting the blood vessels and restricting blood flow to the penis include diabetes mellitus, hypertension, heart disease, and hypercholesterolemia. Neurologic elements, such as nerve insult resulting from prostate surgery and spinal cord or pelvic or perineal trauma, may interrupt the impulse transmission between the central nervous system and the penis. Medications prescribed to treat hypertension and depression can have a side effect of ED. Other common offenders are alcohol, recreational drugs, antihistamines, and diuretics.

DIAGNOSIS

A medical history and physical examination to reveal any underlying medical causative factors are necessary. The history should include information regarding disease history of the patient and his family members, such as diabetes mellitus, hypertension, heart disease, cerebral vascular accidents, spinal cord injuries, and vascular or renal disease; any surgery or trauma to the pelvic area; medications that the patient currently is or previously has taken; lifestyle, including smoking habits and alcohol consumption; stress levels; and relationship with sexual partner. Laboratory tests to rule out organic disease aid the physician in making the diagnosis.

TREATMENT

Sometimes, the treatment is as simple as making changes in medications being taken or discontinuing them. Other courses of remedies are more complex and take time, such as programs for substance abuse or psychological counseling. Interventions such as psychoanalysis, discussion, behavioral modification, and sensate exercises are aimed at restoring the patient's ability to complete the entire sexual response cycle. Other approaches include penile implants, external vacuum devices, and penile injection therapy.

A more recent approach is oral drug therapy with sildenafil citrate (Viagra). During sexual stimulation, nitric oxide is released in the corpus cavernosum, initiating an enzymatic cascade, ultimately resulting in relaxation of the smooth muscle of corpus cavernosum and an inflow of blood. Sildenafil citrate enhances the effect of nitrous oxide, consequently assisting the male to have an erection satisfactory for desired sexual activity. Sexual stimulation is necessary for sildenafil citrate to assist with the erection, and at recommended dosage, it has no effect in the absence of sexual stimulation.

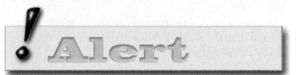

PRECAUTIONS CONCERNING SILDENAFIL CITRATE (VIAGRA)

Men in whom underlying cardiovascular disease has made sexual activity inadvisable should not take sildenafil citrate. An additional warning is advised for men who have had a heart attack, stroke, or life-threatening arrhythmia in the past 6 months. Other factors that preclude the use of Viagra include a history of hypotension, hypertension, unstable angina, retinitis pigmentosa, and any anatomic deformity of the penis.

Side effects may include headache, flushing, stomach pain, or mild temporary vision changes, including changes in color perception and blurred vision. It is advisable to take the smallest possible dose to achieve an erection. Additionally, experiencing a prolonged erection (more than 4 hours) is an indication to notify a physician.

Any male experiencing chest pain after taking sildenafil citrate should seek immediate emergency medical assistance and should advise emergency personnel of the use of sildenafil citrate. Furthermore, concurrent use of any form of nitrate drug therapy or short-acting nitrate drug may initiate life-threatening hypotension.

FRIGIDITY

SYMPTOMS AND SIGNS

Frigidity is the lack of sexual desire or response in a woman.

ETIOLOGY

Rarely, underlying medical problems can cause nerve damage that results in frigidity. More common contributing factors include specific medications being taken, chronic fatigue, stress, and depression. More complicated psychological causes such as rape and past sexual abuse may exist.

DIAGNOSIS

A physical examination with a medical and sexual history should help to identify any physical or psychological causes.

TREATMENT

When the dysfunction is primary, proper stimulation or the use of sensate focus exercises may be all that is required to solve the problem. Inhibited female orgasm can stem from a psychological obstacle; a troubled relationship between the partners is an example. In this case, a behaviorist approach of counseling both partners may bring positive results and fulfillment. Once any causes have been addressed and treated, good results are expected.

PREMATURE EJACULATION

SIGNS AND SYMPTOMS

When a man regularly ejaculates during foreplay, or too early after a minimum amount of stimulation, he may not be able to satisfy his partner or impregnate a woman. The problem is fairly common in young men and is not serious.

ETIOLOGY

Often, premature ejaculation has a psychological basis that may stem from guilt or anxiety. A troubled or negative relationship with the sex partner could contribute. Certain diseases such as infections and degenerative neurologic conditions are possible causes.

DIAGNOSIS

The diagnosis is based on patient history and a medical evaluation with a physical examination and laboratory tests to rule out pathologic conditions. Taken into consideration are all factors that affect stimulation during foreplay and ejaculation.

TREATMENT

Any underlying physical causes are treated, and psychological factors are addressed.

Certain techniques that help delay ejaculation or control male stimulation during lovemaking are suggested to the female partner. This allows more time for the woman to reach orgasm and enables ejaculation to occur after penetration of the vagina.

MALE AND FEMALE INFERTILITY

SIGNS AND SYMPTOMS

With regular, unprotected intercourse, approximately 90% of couples conceive within 1 year. The inability of a couple to conceive can originate from female or male factors, or both.

ETIOLOGY

In a man, insufficient number or mobility of sperm can cause infertility. The presence of an STD or any infection or blockage in the genitourinary tract is another familiar cause. Less commonly, structural anomalies, genetic diseases, or endocrine disorders result in sterility. The presence of a **varicocele** can lower the sperm count. Finally, other causes include injuries that affect the blood or nerve supply, radiation exposure, exposure to pollutants, chronic stress, and hormonal imbalances.

In a woman, the causes include

- STDs or other infections of the reproductive organs
- Ovulatory dysfunction or failure to ovulate
- Blocked fallopian tubes
- Congenital structural or chromosomal disorders
- Scar tissue from infection, ectopic pregnancy, or surgery
- Tumors
- Endometriosis
- Antisperm antibodies in the female vaginal secretions
- Medications that compromise fertility

DIAGNOSIS

After a physical examination and an interview of both partners, specific testing procedures are determined. Sometimes, the cause of infertility is diagnosed quickly and easily. If not, the clinical observation and therapeutic approaches can become time consuming and expensive.

In men, a complete history, with special attention to childhood diseases, is followed by a thorough physical examination for any structural abnormalities. Semen analysis is essential. Genetic and endocrine disorders are ruled out.

In women, ovulatory function is established by charting the menstrual cycle. Hormone levels are studied by blood tests. The fallopian tubes and uterine cavity are visualized by hysterosalpingography to determine tubal patency. In some cases, **laparoscopy** may be necessary to rule out endometriosis or chronic infection. The patient is evaluated for the aforementioned cause.

TREATMENT

Each treatment plan is individual, depending on the problems that surface in the medical and psychological evaluation. Unless the condition is untreatable, the course of action to achieve pregnancy may include treatment of infection, surgery to remove blockage, and the use of fertility drugs or artificial insemination.

When possible, the prevention of causative factors that lead to sterility is preferable because only about one half of the couples treated for infertility achieve pregnancy.

Male Reproductive Diseases

The most common diseases of the male reproductive system are those affecting the prostate gland. The gland can become inflamed or enlarged as a result of bacteria and cause urinary problems. Common symptoms are

- Any urinary symptoms, such as frequency, urgency, incontinence, and dysuria
- Pain, swelling, or enlargement of any of the reproductive organs
- Any sexual dysfunction, such as ED/impotence

EPIDIDYMITIS

SYMPTOMS AND SIGNS

Symptoms of inflammation of the epididymis can include fever, **malaise,** and pain. The epididymis may become enlarged, tender, and hard. There may be groin and scrotal tenderness with severe pain in the testes. Walking may be difficult for the patient, as he tries to protect a painful scrotum.

ETIOLOGY

N. gonorrhoeae and *C. trachomatis* are the most common causes of epididymitis. *Escherichia coli, Staphylococcus,* and *Streptococcus* are other bacterial causes of this condition. Epididymitis also can result from a urinary tract infection, prostatitis, and STDs such as gonorrhea and syphilis. Tuberculosis, mumps, removal of the prostate gland (prostatectomy), trauma, and the prolonged use of an indwelling catheter also may predispose the patient to epididymitis.

DIAGNOSIS

Physical examination, urinalysis, and urine cultures are used to make the diagnosis of epididymitis. The patient also may have an elevated **white blood cell (WBC) count.**

TREATMENT

Antibiotic treatment combined with the administration of **analgesics,** rest, and the avoidance of alcohol and spicy foods are beneficial. Use of a scrotal support also may be helpful. Epididymitis usually responds well to treatment. Scarring may occur, which can lead to sterility, if treatment is delayed. This is especially true if the disease is bilateral.

The best prevention for epididymitis is the early treatment of urinary tract infections. Condom use during sexual intercourse also is recommended.

ORCHITIS

SYMPTOMS AND SIGNS

Inflammation of the testes is caused by viral or bacterial infection or injury. It may affect one or both testes, causing swelling, tenderness, and acute pain. The patient also may experience chills, fever, nausea, vomiting, and general malaise.

ETIOLOGY

Orchitis is typically a consequence of infection from the mumps virus. Other viruses and bacteria also can cause this condition, and it may follow epididymitis. About one half of severe cases result in atrophy of the affected testicle. If both sides are affected, sterility results.

DIAGNOSIS

Urinalysis, **serologic** study, or throat cultures may be used to isolate or identify causative agents, such as the mumps virus. The patient's clinical history to determine exposure to mumps or other related disease may be beneficial.

TREATMENT

If the orchitis is bacterial, appropriate antibiotic treatment should be started immediately. There is no specific treatment of the mumps virus–induced orchitis. Bed rest usually is prescribed, along with certain adrenal steroid drugs to reduce fever and swelling in severe cases. The use of a scrotal support also may be helpful.

To prevent orchitis related to mumps virus, all

adult men who have not had a clinical case of mumps should be vaccinated.

TORSION OF THE TESTICLE

SYMPTOMS AND SIGNS

Torsion of the testicle is a condition in which one testicle is twisted out of its normal position. The major symptom that the man experiences is a sudden, severe pain in one testicle. The pain can be so severe that it causes nausea and even vomiting. When the torsion occurs, the scrotum becomes swollen, red, and tender. Torsion can cause the blood vessels supplying the testicle to become kinked, which in turn prevents blood flow to and from the affected testicle.

ETIOLOGY

The cause of this condition is a sudden, extreme twist or torsion. It can happen while sleeping.

DIAGNOSIS

Diagnosis is made by the patient history and a gentle physical examination by the physician. Gentle manipulation may be tried to untwist the testicle.

TREATMENT

No treatment is needed if the testicle can somehow untwist itself. Immediate relief from the pain and swelling follows. If this does not occur, surgery is necessary. Delaying surgery can result in permanent damage to the testicle.

Prognosis is good if treatment is received promptly when the torsion does not correct itself. Even if the condition corrects itself, and pain is relieved, the torsion may recur. With surgery, the testicle is untwisted and stitched into position so that the problem cannot recur.

VARICOCELE

SYMPTOMS AND SIGNS

In varicocele, the veins of one of the testicles become abnormally distended, and then swelling around the testicle occurs. This is a rather mild disorder that is more uncomfortable than painful. A varicocele may be especially uncomfortable in hot weather or after exercise and may be relieved temporarily by lying down. Because the increased presence of venous blood raises the temperature within the scrotum, varicocele may contribute to a lower sperm count.

ETIOLOGY

There is no apparent cause of or prevention for varicocele; however, it may be congenital and usually occurs in the 15- to 25-year-old age group.

DIAGNOSIS

The patient history, physical symptoms, and an examination by the physician confirm the diagnosis.

TREATMENT

Treatment consists of relieving the symptoms. This can be accomplished by wearing tight-fitting underwear or by using an athletic supporter. If the varicocele affects fertility, surgery can remove the distended veins. However, the results may not justify the risks of the surgery. Results vary and depend on the severity of the distention.

PROSTATITIS

SYMPTOMS AND SIGNS

Inflammation of the prostate gland is more common in men older than 50 years of age. The prostate may be enlarged and tender, and in some instances, pus may be seen at the tip of the penis. The patient may be asymptomatic or may experience acute symptoms in mild or sporadic forms. He has pain and a burning sensation during urination. Other common symptoms include low back pain, fever, muscular pain or tenderness, and urinary frequency.

ETIOLOGY

The cause of inflammation of the prostate is not always known. It may be either bacterial or nonbacterial. Bacterial causes may include gonococci from a patient with gonorrhea, *E. coli* that has caused a urinary tract infection, *Staphylococcus, Streptococcus,* or *Pseudomonas.*

DIAGNOSIS

Urinalysis, urine culture, and a rectal examination are used to diagnose prostatitis.

TREATMENT

The usual treatment consists of **antimicrobial** ampicillin therapy. Sitz baths, rest, an increase in fluid intake, and the administration of analgesics also may be ordered by the physician.

The prognosis for acute prostatitis is good because it responds well to treatment. The outlook for chronic prostatitis is not as favorable. Complications such as epididymitis, cystitis, and urethritis can occur. Chronic prostatitis has the potential to develop from recurrent urinary tract infection, urethral obstruction, and acute urinary retention. The best prevention for prostatitis is the early treatment of urinary tract infections with the prescribed antibiotics.

BENIGN PROSTATIC HYPERPLASIA

SYMPTOMS AND SIGNS

Enlargement of the prostate gland is a common condition in men older than 50 years, and the frequency increases with age. The usual signs and symptoms may include difficulty in starting urination, a weak stream of urine, or inability to empty the bladder completely. Urinary frequency, including nocturia, or fecal incontinence, and in severe cases, inflammation and symptoms of renal disease, have been seen.

ETIOLOGY

The cause of benign prostatic hyperplasia (BPH) is not completely understood but seems to be associated with the aging process and hormonal and metabolic changes. As the prostate gland enlarges, it compresses either the neck of the bladder or the urethra, causing obstruction of the urinary flow.

DIAGNOSIS

The usual diagnosis is made by the patient history and a rectal examination by a physician. To confirm the diagnosis, the physician may order a urinalysis, urine culture, **intravenous pyelogram** (IVP), or a cystoscopy.

TREATMENT

Treatment of BPH may be symptomatic and include sitz baths, catheterization, and massage of the prostate gland. Drug therapy with alpha-adrenergic blockers, including tamsulosin hydrochloride (Flomax), doxazosin mesylate (Cardura), and terazosin hydrochloride (Hytrin), may be prescribed to relax the tightened muscles inside the prostate and relieve symptoms; finasteride (Proscar), which claims to shrink the enlarged prostate gland, may be prescribed in some cases. Surgical treatment, transurethral resection, may be performed to remove any urinary tract obstruction. The prognosis for BPH is good with intervention; however, if left untreated, infection may reach the kidneys. Complications of this condi-

tion may include cystitis, dilation of the ureters, **pyelonephritis, hydronephrosis,** and uremia.

Prevention of benign prostatic hyperplasia is unknown. Physicians highly recommend that older men have regular prostate examination to detect any enlargement.

PROSTATIC CANCER

SYMPTOMS AND SIGNS

Cancer of the prostate gland is the second leading cause of cancer death in men, after lung cancer. Prostatic cancer tends to spread or **metastasize,** often to the pelvis or spine, before it is discovered. The usual symptoms, when present, are those associated with urinary obstruction. These include weak or interrupted urine flow, urinary frequency, difficulty starting or stopping urine flow, urinary retention, hematuria, and pain or burning on urination. Additionally, there may be continuing pain in the lower back, pelvis, or upper thighs. These symptoms often are also common to BPH or an infection or inflammation of the prostate gland.

ETIOLOGY

The cause of cancer of the prostate is unknown, and there are no specific risk factors, except that it becomes increasingly common with age. Recent studies suggest that dietary fat may be a contributing factor and that in a small percentage of cases, an inherited predisposition may be responsible.

DIAGNOSIS

Blood testing for the **prostate-specific antigen (PSA)** is valuable in detecting this disease when the levels of prostatic antigens are elevated. Refer to Table 12–1 for PSA values. A digital rectal examination is helpful to the physician in diagnosing prostatic cancer to identify any irregular or abnormally firm area typical of cancer. Transrectal ultrasound helps to differentiate normal prostate tissue and prostate tumors. A **biopsy** is necessary to confirm the diagnosis.

TREATMENT

Treatment of prostatic cancer depends on the stage of the disease, the age and physical condition of the patient, and risks and benefits of each treatment option. Surgical interventions include radical prostatectomy and transurethral resection of the prostate. Radical prostatectomy has the potential for the complications of ED/impotence and urinary incontinence. Hormonal therapy af-

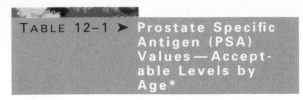

AGE (YR)	ACCEPTABLE LEVELS
Up to 40	0–2 ng/ml
40–50	0–4 ng/ml
50–60	0–5 ng/ml
60–70	0–6 ng/ml

TABLE 12–1 ➤ Prostate Specific Antigen (PSA) Values—Acceptable Levels by Age*

* PSA blood tests are reported as ng/ml.
PSA is considered a marker in the screening for prostatic cancer. Zero to 4 ng/ml usually are considered to be in the normal range; 4–10 ng/ml are considered borderline; values >10 ng/ml are considered as high. However, increasing age makes slightly higher values acceptable.
Any increase of 20% or more in the PSA value in 1 year's time is suspicious and requires further investigation.
The PSA screening is to be completed before the digital rectal examination. A constant increase in the PSA leads to suspicion of prostate cancer. PSA levels that fluctuate up and down usually are not indicative of cancer but of an inflammatory process in the prostate or of benign prostatic hypertrophy. PSA is a screening tool and must be combined with a digital rectal examination for a more accurate screen. Men older than 50 years of age are encouraged to have prostate screening on an annual basis.

fects hormone levels in an attempt to inhibit cancer cell growth. Orchiectomy (surgical removal of a testicle) may be considered as an additional method to reduce hormone levels. Radiation therapy may be tried to kill cancer cells and shrink tumors. Chemotherapy may be useful in treating advanced stages or recurrence of the cancer after other treatments. Watchful waiting and careful observation without aggressive intervention is sometimes considered for men older than 70 years of age, those with significant coexisting illnesses, and those who are apprehensive of the side effects of the more aggressive approaches. If the patient is older than 60 years of age when the cancer is discovered, he probably will outlive it and die of some unrelated cause. However, if the cancer has metastasized, the prognosis is generally poor.

TESTICULAR CANCER

SYMPTOMS AND SIGNS

Tumor of the testis is rare and usually occurs in men younger than 40 years of age. It is the most common type of cancer in men between the ages of 20 and 35 years. The first sign is often a painless lump discovered in the testicle.

ETIOLOGY

The cause of cancer of the testes is essentially unknown. If not treated in the early stages, the cancer can spread through the lymphatic system to the lymph nodes in the abdomen, chest, and neck, and eventually to the lungs. Other predisposing factors include undescended testicle (cryptorchidism), an inguinal hernia during childhood, and a history of mumps.

DIAGNOSIS

Palpation of the testes by the physician is generally how the diagnosis is made. It is confirmed by a biopsy.

TREATMENT

Surgical removal of the diseased testicle, followed by radiation therapy and chemotherapy, is the usual treatment. The surgery usually leaves one testicle intact, so it is unlikely to have an effect on either potency or fertility.

The prognosis varies according to the cancer's cell type and the stage of the disease. Because there is no direct lymphatic connection between the two testicles, the disease is unlikely to spread from one testicle to the other. With early detection and treatment, the chances for complete recovery are excellent. Physicians recommend and encourage all men to perform monthly testicular self-examinations.

Female Reproductive Diseases

The female reproductive organs are affected by disease in several ways. First, microorganisms can invade the organs, allowing infections to occur. Second, tumors, both benign and malignant, and cysts can develop in the reproductive organs. Common symptoms are

- Any abnormal vaginal discharge or itching
- Lower pelvic or abdominal pain
- Menstrual symptoms, such as pain (dysmenorrhea), absence of menstruation (amenorrhea), scanty menstruation (oligomenorrhea), irregular menstruation (metrorrhagia), and heavy menstrual flow (menorrhagia)
- Fever
- Pain during sexual intercourse (dyspareunia) or any sexual dysfunction

PREMENSTRUAL SYNDROME

SYMPTOMS AND SIGNS

Premenstrual syndrome (PMS) is a syndrome of physical and emotional symptoms that appear during the days immediately preceding the occurrence of menstrual flow and subside with its onset.

The female patient may notice changes related to the hormone levels that fluctuate monthly to prepare her for ovulation and pregnancy. Some changes, such as increased energy and sexual desire, are positive. Other symptoms, which can range from mild to severe, may be troublesome. The most common include tension and irritability, headache, fatigue, restlessness, feelings of sadness, breast tenderness, and joint pain. Some women experience edema, a bloated feeling, and abdominal pain as well.

ETIOLOGY

The cause is not certain, but the higher estrogen level before menstruation contributes to the symptoms related to retention of fluids. PMS occurs only in ovulating females.

DIAGNOSIS

The patient may be asked to observe and record her menstrual symptoms monthly. There are no specific medical tests to diagnose PMS; however, blood testing may be done to rule out general medical problems. Symptoms subside within 2 to 3 hours after the onset of menses. PMS can be confused with depression.

TREATMENT

The treatment of PMS is directed toward the relief of symptoms. Reduced dietary intake of sodium, moderate exercise, the administration of mild analgesics and **diuretics,** and emotional support are helpful. In addition, some women notice less breast tenderness when they eliminate caffeine from their diet. In severe cases, antidepressant medication or hormone therapy may be indicated.

AMENORRHEA

SYMPTOMS AND SIGNS

The absence of menstrual periods, whether temporary or permanent, is known as amenorrhea. This condition is classified as either primary, if menstruation has not occurred by the age of 18 years, or secondary, if a woman who has been having regular menses has a delay or absence of menstruation for a period of 6 months.

ETIOLOGY

In primary amenorrhea, the cause is generally the result of a late onset of puberty. However, it can be caused by an abnormality in the reproductive system or hormonal imbalances. These conditions usually are not suspected unless the girl has reached 18 years of age and still is not having periods. The causes of secondary amenorrhea are mainly hormone related. Pregnancy is one cause, but emotional factors, illness, malnutrition, sudden weight loss or gain, athletic training, and ovarian or pituitary tumors also may cause amenorrhea. Neither primary nor secondary amenorrhea presents any health risks when the underlying cause can be determined and corrected.

DIAGNOSIS

The diagnosis of amenorrhea is made by the physician after a thorough pelvic examination and diagnostic procedures. The pelvic examination rules out any physical abnormalities or pregnancy. Blood and urine samples detect any hormonal problems, and radiographic studies, laparoscopy, and biopsy detect tumors.

TREATMENT

For primary amenorrhea, no treatment may be necessary if all test results indicate that no physical abnormalities are present. If periods do not begin on their own, hormone therapy usually can start the menstrual cycle. Secondary amenorrhea may necessitate long-term hormone therapy, when pregnancy has been ruled out. Certain preventive measures can reduce the chance of amenorrhea developing. These measures include the reduction of emotional problems, control of weight, and a balanced exercise program.

DYSMENORRHEA

SYMPTOMS AND SIGNS

Painful periods are one of the most frequent gynecologic problems. If the pain begins within 3 years of the onset of menstruation, it is called primary dysmenorrhea; it is not associated with a pathologic disorder. In secondary dysmenorrhea, the woman has been having periods for longer than 3 years before she begins having pain. Symptoms range from a dull pain in the abdomen or back to sharp abdominal cramping. Pain also may radiate to the thighs and genitalia. The symptoms are generally worse at the beginning of a period.

ETIOLOGY

In primary dysmenorrhea, the cause is thought to be the result of normal hormonal changes associated with menstruation. Secondary dysmenorrhea is more likely to be caused by an underlying disorder or disease condition, including pelvic infections, fibroids, endometriosis, and cervical **stenosis.**

The prognosis for dysmenorrhea is good when the underlying causes are corrected. Primary dysmenorrhea often abates after a woman gives birth.

DIAGNOSIS

The diagnosis is made after a complete patient history and pelvic examination by the physician. A laparoscopy and a dilation and curettage (D & C) also may be used to confirm the diagnosis.

TREATMENT

Nonsteroidal anti-inflammatory drugs (NSAIDs), whether prescription or over the counter, are generally all that is necessary for pain relief. The use of a heating pad on the abdomen also may be helpful. Fibroids and cervical stenosis may necessitate surgery. In the absence of specific

pathologic conditions, the best remedy for dysmenorrhea is the use of oral contraceptives, which usually produce lighter and more regular periods.

OVARIAN CYSTS

SYMPTOMS AND SIGNS

Ovarian cysts are fluid-filled sacs that form on or near the ovaries. These cysts can become large before any symptoms appear. The patient may notice a painless swelling in the lower abdomen that feels firm to the touch or may experience pain during sexual intercourse. Urinary retention can result when a large cyst presses on the area near the bladder. Vaginal bleeding or an increase in hair growth on the body may occur if a cyst affects hormone production. A cyst also can cause an ovary to twist on its blood supply, which causes severe abdominal pain, nausea, and even a fever. The risk from a torsion of an ovary is that it may rupture and cause **peritonitis.**

ETIOLOGY

There are two basic types of ovarian cysts: physiologic cysts (those caused by normal functioning of the ovary) and neoplastic cysts. Neoplastic cysts are either benign or malignant and are not directly related to structures normally present in the ovary. Most ovarian cysts are physiologic, resulting from ovarian follicle growth or a corpus luteum that persists too long.

DIAGNOSIS

An ultrasonogram is done to view the ovaries indirectly. Laparoscopy with direct vision of the ovaries or even surgical removal may be appropriate if cysts are not physiologic because cancer must be ruled out.

TREATMENT

Benign physiologic cysts are common, and small cysts seldom necessitate any treatment. Large cysts sometimes can be drained during laparoscopy or can even be removed. This often can be done without affecting the ovary. Cysts that are drained are more likely to recur than those that are removed. Small physiologic cysts usually disappear spontaneously. Several months of oral contraceptive therapy (birth control pills) often resolve larger physiologic cysts without surgery.

Enrichment

MITTELSCHMERZ

Mittelschmerz is the term applied to unilateral pain in the region of an ovary occurring mid-cycle at ovulation. This dull pain has a duration of a few minutes to a few hours and can indicate the time of ovulation for couples attempting to conceive.

Although the etiology is unknown, a leakage of follicular fluid into the abdomen during ovulation may be the cause. Occasionally, the pain is severe enough for the woman to seek medical care. A history of occurrence at the menstrual cycle midpoint and the elimination of other pelvic or abdominal causes lead to the diagnosis of mittelschmerz. Mild analgesics provide pain relief.

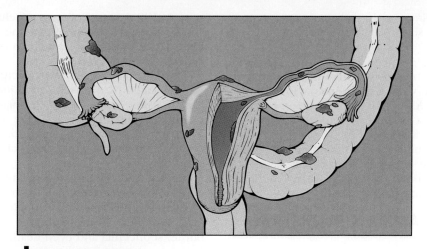

Figure 12-7
Usual sites of endometriosis.

ENDOMETRIOSIS

SYMPTOMS AND SIGNS

Endometriosis occurs when endometrial tissue implants outside the uterus in the pelvic cavity or in the abdominal wall (Fig. 12-7). Although it is considered a benign condition, the severe symptoms of endometriosis are troublesome. Acquired dysmenorrhea, beginning before and extending several days after menstruation, is a classic symptom. There is constant pain and cramping in the lower abdomen, the vagina, and the back. The woman, usually of childbearing age, also may experience heavy menses, pelvic pain during intercourse, and even painful defecation. Complications include infertility, **ectopic** pregnancy, and spontaneous abortion.

ETIOLOGY

When functioning endometrial tissue grows outside the uterine cavity, it responds to the ovarian hormones as the endometrium (lining of the uterus) does during the normal menstrual cycle. These misplaced islands of endometrial tissue usually implant on other pelvic organs, where they imitate the menstrual cycle, irritating the surrounding tissues. The thickening and sloughing (bleeding) in unnatural areas and the ensuing cysts, scar tissue, and adhesions are the basis of much pain and discomfort. It is not known what causes the lining tissue of the uterus to break away and travel to other parts of the body. The use of tampons may foster displacement of endometrial tissue up through the fallopian tubes during menstruation; therefore, their use is discouraged.

DIAGNOSIS

During the pelvic examination, the physician may be able to detect multiple tender nodules, as well as the presence of ovarian cysts. Laparoscopy may confirm the diagnosis and help to stage the extent of endometrial implant or adhesions according to size, character, and location (Fig. 12-8). The treatment then can be deter-

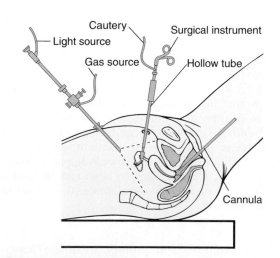

Figure 12-8
Laparoscopy.

mined, depending on the woman's age, general health, and the severity of her symptoms.

TREATMENT

Conservative treatment with various hormones is indicated for younger patients who desire to have children. Although there is no cure, pregnancy, nursing a baby, or menopause brings remission of symptoms because the aberrant tissue tends to shrink under these conditions. In severe cases or in the presence of ovarian masses, a total hysterectomy with bilateral salpingo-oophorectomy may be indicated.

PELVIC INFLAMMATORY DISEASE

SYMPTOMS AND SIGNS

PID is a mild to serious infection that involves some or all of the female reproductive organs. The infection can occur after miscarriage, childbirth, or abortion; however, it is most common in young **nulliparous** females and is not necessarily involved with a pregnancy. The symptoms are those of an active infection: fever, chills, malaise, a foul-smelling vaginal discharge, backache, and a painful, tender abdomen. The white blood cell (WBC) count is elevated.

ETIOLOGY

The causative organism, one that is sexually transmitted or a common vaginal bacterium, can enter the body through the vagina and travel up through the cervix into the pelvic cavity. Young sexually active women and those who use intrauterine devices (IUDs) for contraception are at higher risk.

DIAGNOSIS

The vaginal examination is painful because of the swelling and inflammation. A specimen is taken for Gram stain and sensitivity studies. This allows the physician to prescribe an antibiotic that is specific in action against the bacteria that are found. A laparoscopy can be done to look for an **abscess** or hepatic involvement, or even to confirm the diagnosis if cervicovaginal cultures are negative. Ultrasonography also can be useful by showing a mass (possible abscess) or fluid in the **cul-de-sac.**

TREATMENT

Early diagnosis and prompt treatment lessen the degree of damage to the reproductive system. The treatment plan begins with aggressive antibiotic therapy, the administration of analge-

sics, and bed rest. Follow-up includes education about measures to minimize the risks and the importance of early treatment to prevent complications.

The inflammation of the structures of the pelvis can cause scar tissue (adhesions) to form. If the adhesion forms in the fallopian tubes, it can cause infertility or increase the risk of ectopic pregnancy. In addition, adhesions can develop rapidly between any of the pelvic organs and structures.

Serious and life-threatening complications can develop without effective treatment. Peritonitis can spread the infection throughout the abdominal cavity, or, if the infection becomes blood borne, septicemia and even death may result.

LEIOMYOMAS AND FIBROIDS

SYMPTOMS AND SIGNS

Leiomyomas are noncancerous (benign) tumors of the smooth muscle within the uterus. Fibroids are also benign tumors but are composed of fibrous tissue. They may vary in number, size, and location within the uterus. Leiomyomas and fibroids are the most common tumors of the female reproductive system, and they tend to calcify after menopause. These tumors may not cause any symptoms at all. If symptoms do occur, they may include pelvic pain and pressure, constipation, urinary frequency, abnormal bleeding, and heavy or prolonged periods. The latter symptom is the most common.

ETIOLOGY

The cause of leiomyomas and fibroids is unknown. Their development is stimulated by estrogen, and they occur only in the premenopausal woman.

DIAGNOSIS

Diagnosis is made by pelvic examination and the patient history. Definitive diagnosis can be by ultrasonography; occasionally, small fibroids are discovered incidentally at laparoscopy. In the case of abnormal bleeding, a D & C procedure or endometrial biopsy usually is done to rule out **adenocarcinoma** of the uterus.

TREATMENT

Treatment generally depends on the severity of the symptoms, the patient's age, and the woman's desire for childbearing. In women of childbearing age, surgery can be done to remove the tumors, or if bleeding continues, removal of the uterus (hysterectomy) is recommended. Only rarely do leiomyomas become malignant, and there is no known method for the prevention of either leiomyomas or fibroids.

VAGINITIS

SYMPTOMS AND SIGNS

Inflammation of the vagina is common and is not dangerous, although it can be irritating and painful. A foul-smelling or greenish yellow vaginal discharge is the principal symptom. The discharge causes itching, burning, and soreness of the vulva.

ETIOLOGY

Vaginitis can be caused by a variety of organisms; however, it frequently is caused by an organism called *Trichomonas,* which usually is transmitted through sexual intercourse. It is likely that the sex partner also will have the infection. The infection does not cause any symptoms in the man, but if he is carrying the organism, he can reinfect the woman. Vaginitis also can occur after menopause. With the loss of estrogen, the vaginal lining changes and becomes more susceptible to infections.

DIAGNOSIS

The physician does a pelvic examination and swabs the vagina. Specimens from the vagina and cervix are analyzed for the presence of the *Trichomonas* organism.

TREATMENT

Depending on what the cultures and wet preparation examination show, treatment can consist of hormonal therapy, the administration of antibiotics, or the use of steroid creams. If the vaginitis has been transmitted sexually, both partners need to be treated. With proper treatment, the inflammation usually clears up in about a week.

TOXIC SHOCK SYNDROME

SYMPTOMS AND SIGNS

Toxic shock syndrome (TSS) is a systemic disease of menstruating females who use tampons, specifically the superabsorbent type. Superabsorbent tampon use may predispose the woman to a *Staphylococcus aureus* infection. The most common symptoms include a high fever, rash, skin peeling, and decreased blood pressure (hy-

potension). Other symptoms and signs that might be experienced are gastrointestinal symptoms, neuromuscular disturbances, and an elevation of the liver enzyme levels.

ETIOLOGY

The cause of TSS is thought to be an increase in staphylococcal toxin production in the presence of the synthetic fibers found in the superabsorbent tampons. These fibers are responsible for removing magnesium from the vagina. This then creates an ideal environment for the bacteria to produce the toxins. The synthetic fibers also have been found in surgical dressings. This may explain why some cases of TSS in non–tampon users have been reported. These synthetic fibers are no longer in use, but physicians advise women who use tampons to avoid the superabsorbent type, to use them only during the daytime, and to change them frequently. This prevents the possibility of TSS.

DIAGNOSIS

A diagnosis of TSS is based on the patient's history of tampon use, the physical symptoms, and elevated liver enzyme levels.

TREATMENT

Therapy for TSS includes the replacement of fluids to counteract shock and the use of prescribed antibiotics to treat the infection. If treatment is delayed, death can result because of the overwhelming shock.

MENOPAUSE

SYMPTOMS AND SIGNS

Menopause (change of life or climacteric) is the cessation of menstrual periods. Fluctuation in the menstrual cycle and flow are noted, with periods becoming lighter and less frequent. Hot flashes and night sweats commonly are reported as a mild to intolerable nuisance; vaginal dryness and skin changes appear. Many women experience transient to troublesome psychological symptoms, including depression, poor memory, anxiety, sleep disorders, and loss of interest in sex.

ETIOLOGY

Between 45 and 55 years of age, a woman's ovaries gradually produce less estrogen, resulting in the cessation of ovulation and menstruation. This and other changes in the pituitary hormone levels result in physical and psychological changes. This natural process can be induced artificially by a bilateral oophorectomy, or removal of both ovaries.

DIAGNOSIS

A patient history suggests menopause. The blood serum levels of follicle-stimulating hormone are elevated, and the estrogen levels are low.

TREATMENT

Hormonal changes can be noted in blood serum levels, and these chemical changes increase the incidence of cardiac disease and osteoporosis in the postmenopausal female. To help to protect against these diseases and to relieve the other aforementioned symptoms, some physicians are in favor of hormone replacement therapy (HRT). Each woman needs to be evaluated to weigh the side effects and risks against the benefits of HRT.

Menopause cannot be prevented, and the prognosis is generally good.

UTERINE PROLAPSE

SYMPTOMS AND SIGNS

Prolapse of the uterus is a downward displacement of the uterus. It occurs when the pelvic floor muscles and ligaments become extremely overstretched or weakened. Feelings of heaviness, discomfort, and backache are common symptoms. In some women, **stress incontinence** develops; in other women, prolapse has the opposite effect, and urination becomes more difficult. Bowel movements also may become more difficult.

ETIOLOGY

Uterine prolapse results when the pelvic floor muscles weaken from childbirth or old age. As the muscles and ligaments become overstretched, they no longer can hold the uterus in place, so it falls or sags downward. This causes a lump or bulge to occur on the vaginal wall. Occasionally, the prolapse is so severe that it bulges

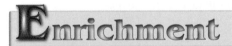

Hormone Replacement Therapy

HRT has assumed an important role in the health care of postmenopausal women. The treatment regimen is highly individualized after results of a complete history, physical examination, and pretreatment screening tests. Such therapy concurrently entails the use of estrogen and progesterone in women with a uterus and estrogen only in women without a uterus. The April 1999 issue of *Pharmacy Times* listed Premarin as the most frequently filled prescription (new and refills) in the United States in 1998; Estrace ranked 123rd and estradiol, its generic form, ranked 150th. Prempro, a combination of estrogen and progestin, ranked 16th; Provera, a form of progestin, was listed as number 149. HRT not only helps to lessen the effects of menopause, such as hot flashes and skin, hair, cardiovascular, urinary, and emotional changes, but also helps to decrease the risks of cardiovascular disease and osteoporosis. A possibility for increased risk of breast cancer must be considered by the woman as she weighs the pros and cons of replacement therapy.

Estrogen alone is prescribed for the woman whose uterus has been surgically removed, whereas HRT includes both estrogen and progestin and is indicated for the menopausal and postmenopausal woman who still has her uterus. These two drugs may be administered concurrently on a continuous basis, or there may be a recommendation for a cyclic administration to women with a uterus to prevent an increased risk of endometrial hyperplasia and carcinoma. Women who take the progestin in a cyclic manner may experience withdrawal bleeding during each cycle.

HRT is contraindicated in postmenopausal women with estrogen-dependent tumors of the breast or uterus, liver disease, cardiovascular disease, any history of blood clots, and certain other medical conditions. Each woman is unique, and side effects are common; thus, modification of therapy may be required.

out of the vagina. This is called a complete prolapse. This condition can be uncomfortable and inconvenient, but there is no risk to general health, unless the prolapsing organ ulcerates or bleeds or the urethra becomes completely obstructed.

DIAGNOSIS

The prolapse is visible on inspection if it is protruding from the vagina. A speculum examination can reveal the descent of the rectum or bladder.

TREATMENT

Treatment consists of strengthening the muscles of the pelvic floor, losing weight if the woman is overweight, and eating a high-fiber diet to prevent bowel straining. If there is no improvement, the woman may be fitted with a **pessary.** This device is inserted into the vagina to support the uterus. Most commonly, surgery is necessary to correct serious prolapse.

CYSTOCELE

SYMPTOMS AND SIGNS

Cystocele is a downward displacement of the urinary bladder into the vagina (Fig. 12-9). This disorder causes the female patient to experience pelvic pressure, frequency, urgency, and incontinence of urine, including stress incontinence.

ETIOLOGY

This condition results from trauma to the fascia, muscle, and pelvic ligaments during pregnancy and delivery or from atrophy of the pelvic floor muscles with age.

DIAGNOSIS

Diagnosis is made by the clinical picture and physical examination findings.

TREATMENT

Treatment consists of exercises to strengthen the pelvic floor muscles (Kegel exercises), which involve voluntary isometric tightening of the pelvic floor muscles, including stopping the flow of urine midstream. Muscle tone may be improved with estrogen therapy. Surgical repair is anterior vaginal **colporrhaphy.**

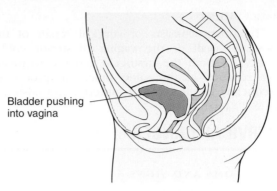
Bladder pushing into vagina

Cystocele

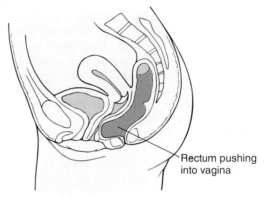
Rectum pushing into vagina

Rectocele

Figure 12–9
Cystocele and rectocele.

RECTOCELE

SYMPTOMS AND SIGNS

A rectocele is the protrusion of the rectum into the posterior aspect of the vagina, causing the female patient to experience a bearing-down feeling and constipation (see Fig. 12-9). She also may have incontinence of gas and feces or may experience difficulty in fecal evacuation.

ETIOLOGY

Similar to a cystocele, a rectocele occurs when the posterior wall of the vagina is weakened, allowing a protrusion of the rectum into the vagina. This also is a result of trauma to the area during childbirth, although the patient may not exhibit symptoms until years after the pregnancy.

DIAGNOSIS

Diagnosis is by the clinical picture and physical examination findings.

373

TREATMENT

Treatment consists of surgical repair of the posterior wall of the vagina (posterior colpoplasty). If both the cystocele and the rectocele are repaired at the same time, the procedure frequently is referred to as anterior and posterior (A & P) repair.

CERVICAL CANCER

SYMPTOMS AND SIGNS

The two main symptoms of cervical cancer are a watery, bloody vaginal discharge, which may be heavy and foul smelling, and bleeding between menstrual periods, after intercourse, or after menopause; however, the most common sign is the abnormal Pap smear test result. Later, there may be a dull backache, and the patient experiences general ill health. Carcinoma of the cervix is one of the most easily diagnosed forms if found in the early stages.

ETIOLOGY

Development of the earliest stage of cervical cancer (carcinoma in situ) into an advanced malignancy can be slow. Ulceration of the cervix occurs, causing vaginal discharge and bleeding. If left untreated, the tumor becomes inoperable. Risk factors include being sexually active at an early age and having multiple sexual partners or partners who have a history of multiple sexual partners. Exposure to sexually transmitted infections with certain types of HPV expands risk factors. Additionally, it is postulated that cigarette smoking and low socioeconomic status contributes to increased risk factors.

DIAGNOSIS

The Pap smear test was developed specifically to detect this form of cancer. By obtaining scrapings from the cervix and cervical os and examining them microscopically, cellular abnormalities can be detected.

TREATMENT

Surgery, followed by radiation therapy, is the usual treatment of choice. The surgery may involve removing the cervix and the rest of the uterus (hysterectomy), the ovaries (bilateral oophorectomy), and the fallopian tubes (bilateral salpingectomy). The prognosis is excellent if the disease is detected in the earliest stage, when cancer has not spread beyond the uterus. There is no known method for prevention of cervical cancer, but practicing good feminine hygiene and limiting the number of sexual partners may be beneficial.

When the cancer is in the in situ stage, less drastic treatment options include cryotherapy, electrocoagulation, laser ablation, or local surgery on the involved cervical tissue.

VAGINAL CANCER

SYMPTOMS AND SIGNS

The two major symptoms of cancer of the vagina, a rare form of cancer, are **leukorrhea** and a bloody vaginal discharge.

ETIOLOGY

Cancer of the vagina is usually a **squamous cell** type. Another, less common type is adenocarcinoma, which has been linked to the synthetic hormone diethylstilbestrol (DES). DES has been used to prevent spontaneous abortions. The cancer tends to develop in the daughters of mothers who received DES during their pregnancies.

DIAGNOSIS

A diagnosis of vaginal cancer can be made after a complete pelvic examination is performed and a Pap smear and biopsy are examined by a **pathologist.** The patient's family history is also valuable in the diagnosis.

TREATMENT

Treatment of vaginal cancer can consist of surgical excision of the tumor, if small, and radiation or chemotherapy. The prognosis depends on the stage of tumor development when discovered. There is no known method to prevent cancer of the vagina.

LABIAL OR VULVAR CANCER

SYMPTOMS AND SIGNS

Cancer of the vulva begins as a small hard lump, which tends to grow slowly and develops into an ulcer. The ulcer becomes thickened in time and may weep or even bleed. If the ulcer is not treated, it spreads (metastasizes). Squamous cell carcinoma of the vulva is the most common form and is a disease mainly of postmenopausal women.

ETIOLOGY

The cause of this condition is not known. It was once thought to be linked to vulvar dysplasia. Now, as with cervical cancer, vulvar cancer is associated more clearly with pelvic infection and with venereal warts. As with any cancer, the complete etiology is not understood.

DIAGNOSIS

If the physician suspects cancer, she or he performs a biopsy of the ulcer and possibly a dilation and curettage to check for **metastases.**

TREATMENT

The usual treatment of vulvar carcinoma is either surgical removal of the growth and surrounding skin or removal of all or part of the vulva itself. The latter procedure is known as a vulvectomy. Depending on the size of the tumor, lymph glands in the groin also may be removed. Radiation therapy also is used sometimes in combination with the surgery. The prognosis is only fair, with an overall 5-year survival rate of 60%.

OVARIAN CANCER

SYMPTOMS AND SIGNS

The ovaries are a common site for cancer to develop, and ovarian cancer is the leading cause of deaths attributed to the female reproductive system. Early detection is difficult because of placement of the ovaries deep within the pelvis. Symptoms of this often "silent" cancer do not appear until the disease is well advanced and pressure develops on adjacent structures, such as the bladder. There also may be lower abdominal pain, weight loss, and general poor health. Sometimes, the whole abdomen enlarges as it fills with fluid (ascites) from the tumor. Vague persistent digestive disturbances, such as stomach discomfort, flatus, and distention, indicate the need for further investigation.

ETIOLOGY

Cancer of the ovaries occurs when there is abnormal tissue development. The cause of this development is unknown. Pregnancy and oral contraceptive drugs may reduce the risk. A history of breast cancer or familial history of ovarian or breast cancer increases the risk.

DIAGNOSIS

If any of the symptoms are noticed, a physician should be seen immediately. The probable recommendation is a visual examination of the ovaries with a laparoscope (laparoscopy) and a biopsy. Routine screening includes periodic thorough pelvic examinations. Diagnosis may be assisted by transvaginal ultrasound and a blood test that identifies tumor marker CA125.

TREATMENT

Treatment options include surgery, radiation therapy, and chemotherapy. Surgery is performed to remove not only the affected ovary, but also the other ovary and the fallopian tubes (bilateral salpingo-oophorectomy). The uterus also may be removed (hysterectomy), as well as nearby lymph glands, to ensure that all the tumor has been removed. When the tumor is detected in the very early stages and the woman wishes to have children, only the affected ovary is removed. Radiation therapy or anticancer (cytotoxic) drugs, or both, then usually are administered to prevent the cancer from recurring or, if it has already metastasized, to slow down the progression. If fluid has accumulated in the abdomen (ascites), it can be removed with a syringe and needle. This procedure is called a *paracentesis.* The prognosis varies according to whether the tumor has metastasized. If the tumor is not discovered early and treated promptly, the cancer can be fatal within a few years.

ENDOMETRIAL CANCER

SYMPTOMS AND SIGNS

The disease usually begins with the development of endometrial thickening (hyperplasia), abnormal tissue development (dysplasia), and carcinoma in situ. Ulcerations of the endometrium develop, and as blood vessels erode, vaginal spotting or bleeding occurs. This bleeding is irregular and may be accompanied by a white or yellow mucous discharge (leukorrhea). Late manifestations of this cancer include pain and systemic symptoms.

ETIOLOGY

Endometrial carcinoma most often occurs in postmenopausal women who have never had children. It also is associated with prolonged estrogen stimulation. Early menarche, late menopause, use of tamoxifen, estrogen replacement therapy, never being pregnant, and a history of failing to ovulate may contribute to increased risk. Including progesterone with estrogen replacement therapy appears to offset the increased risk of HRT for women who still have their uterus. Other conditions associated with this disease include hypertension, diabetes mellitus, obesity, gallbladder disease, and infertility.

DIAGNOSIS

Diagnosis is made after visual examination of the endometrium and microscopic examination of biopsied tissue samples.

TREATMENT

Surgical removal of the ovaries and uterus, combined with radiation therapy, is the usual treatment. With surgical and radiation therapy, the overall survival rate can be 75 to 80%. This high rate occurs because most of these cancers develop after menopause; thus, any abnormal bleeding is easily recognized.

Conditions and Complications of Pregnancy

Most pregnancies progress to term uneventfully (Fig. 12–10). Occasionally, complications ranging from worrisome or annoying conditions to life-threatening complications affecting the mother or the fetus occur. Complications can develop at any point in the gestational period, emphasizing the importance of early and continual prenatal care and opportunities for patient education.

MORNING SICKNESS

SYMPTOMS AND SIGNS

The patient with morning sickness experiences transient nausea or vomiting, usually on arising. This generally occurs between the 6th and 12th week in the pregnancy, often as the first sign of pregnancy.

ETIOLOGY

It is believed that elevated estrogen, progesterone, and **human chorionic gonadotropin (hCG)** levels are responsible for the nausea and vomiting. In some cases, emotions may trigger the episodes.

DIAGNOSIS

Diagnosis is made by symptoms and a positive pregnancy test result.

TREATMENT

The nausea and vomiting usually subside by the end of the first trimester. The patient is encouraged to eat small amounts of food at frequent intervals. She also is advised that eating soda crackers before getting up may help. *No medication has been approved by the U.S. Food and Drug Administration (FDA) for this condi-*

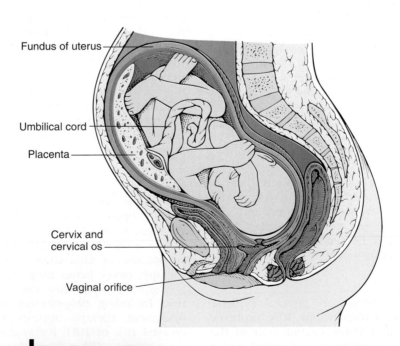

Figure 12–10

Normal uterine pregnancy.

tion; however, several medications are used universally. If the condition becomes severe, it is termed hyperemesis gravidarum.

HYPEREMESIS GRAVIDARUM

SYMPTOMS AND SIGNS

Hyperemesis gravidarum, excessive vomiting of pregnancy, occurs when the pregnant patient experiences frequent, severe episodes of nausea and vomiting, weight loss, and dehydration, being unable to keep either food or liquid in the stomach. If it is untreated, fluid and electrolyte imbalances can cause acid–base disturbances in the baby as well as in the mother.

ETIOLOGY

As with morning sickness, it is thought that elevated estrogen and progesterone levels are responsible for this condition. Again, emotions may play a big part in the onset and severity of the vomiting. The patient is unable to ingest any food or liquid without vomiting.

DIAGNOSIS

Diagnosis is made by the symptoms, weight loss, and signs of dehydration, which disturb the serum electrolyte balance. Serum electrolyte levels are monitored to detect any potassium depletion or **acidosis.**

TREATMENT

In severe cases, the patient usually is treated with intravenous fluid and electrolyte replacement, and all food and fluids are withheld. The acidosis must be corrected by the intravenous fluid and electrolyte replacement. Sedatives or **antiemetics** are administered to control nausea and vomiting. Hyperemesis gravidarum can be treated in the hospital but more often is dealt with through home nursing services. It usually subsides as the pregnancy progresses into the second trimester.

SPONTANEOUS ABORTION (MISCARRIAGE)

SYMPTOMS AND SIGNS

The naturally occurring termination of a pregnancy before the fetus is viable is a spontaneous abortion, or miscarriage. The pregnant patient presents with vaginal bleeding and cramping pelvic pain. When pulse rate is increased and blood pressure is lowered, the vital signs are indicative of shock. Usually, the patient has missed at least one menstrual period and has positive results of hCG testing. Vaginal examination reveals bleeding from the mouth of the cervix, an enlarged uterus, and dilation of the cervix (Fig. 12–11). These symptoms occur at any time during the first trimester of pregnancy. If miscarriage occurs early in the second trimester, there can be a leakage of **amniotic fluid** from the vagina. The term abortion indicates that the fetus is less than 20 weeks' gestation and weighs less than 500 g.

ETIOLOGY

The etiology is unknown; however, approximately 10 to 15% of all pregnancies terminate in spontaneous abortion. It is believed that many spontaneous abortions are the result of a maldeveloped or genetically abnormal fetus. Occasionally, the cervix is incompetent and begins to dilate. Other causes may be infection, drug ingestion, and blood group incompatibility.

DIAGNOSIS

Diagnosis is made from the clinical picture and pelvic ultrasonography (see Fig. 12–12 in the Enrichment on ultrasonography).

TREATMENT

If bleeding is not severe, the mother is treated conservatively with bed rest. Although not rou-

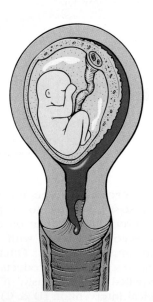

Figure 12–11

Miscarriage.

377

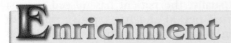

ULTRASONOGRAPHY

Ultrasonography is a technique in which high-frequency intermittent sound waves are reflected off tissue. The various densities of the tissue then are displayed on a screen, and still pictures can be taken to record the image.

Pelvic ultrasonography is specific for the lower abdominal tissue, including the uterus, adnexa, and fetus. This noninvasive, nonradiating, painless technique is helpful in diagnosing fetal anomalies, fetal age and size (Fig. 12–12), fetal position, the condition and placement of the placenta, and many other conditions of the female reproductive system.

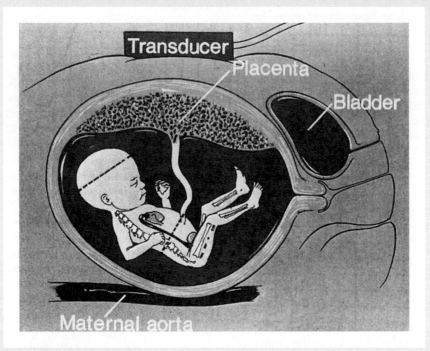

Figure 12–12

Ultrasonography. (From Hadlock FP: The role of fetal biometry in obstetric sonography. In: Putman CE, Ravin CE: Diagnostic Imaging. Philadelphia: WB Saunders, 1988, p 1969. Used with permission.)

tine, cervical **cerclage** may be attempted in the form of a purse-string suture to keep the cervix closed. This procedure is done on only the patient in the second trimester with a history of habitually incompetent cervix. Often, the pregnancy terminates, and the products of conception are expelled spontaneously. If bleeding is severe, surgical intervention (D & C) is indicated after negative results of hCG testing. Blood replacement may be indicated in these cases.

ECTOPIC PREGNANCY

SYMPTOMS AND SIGNS

An ectopic pregnancy occurs when the fertilized ovum implants and grows in a structure outside the uterus, most commonly the fallopian tube (Fig. 12–13). Sometimes, the first sign of this type of problem pregnancy occurs when the patient experiences a sudden onset of severe

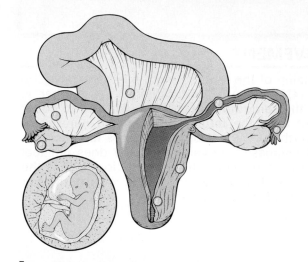

Figure 12–13

Sites of ectopic (tubal) pregnancy.

lower abdominal pain, which may be accompanied by vaginal bleeding. If blood vessels are ruptured, vital signs may become indicative of shock. Testing for hCG, the hormone of pregnancy, is positive. hCG levels begin to fall with fetal **demise.**

ETIOLOGY

Ectopic pregnancies have been known to develop on an ovary, the intestine, or the outer wall of the uterus and even in the vaginal canal. Often, the fertilized ovum cannot follow the normal progression to the uterus because of blockage of the fallopian tube resulting from adhesions, PID, recurrent infections, or congenital conditions.

DIAGNOSIS

Diagnosis is made by evaluating the clinical picture. Pelvic examination may reveal a tender pelvic mass, which then is scrutinized further by endovaginal ultrasonography. The uterus may be enlarged but smaller than expected for the date of the last menstrual period.

TREATMENT

The usual treatment is surgery to terminate the pregnancy. Prompt diagnosis and intervention are essential to save the patient's life. Replacement of lost blood is necessary. Attempts are made to preserve the ovary and tube; however, this is not always successful, and the patient may not be able to conceive at a later date.

PREMATURE LABOR

SYMPTOMS AND SIGNS

Premature labor occurs when the pregnant woman in the late second or early third trimester begins experiencing contractions, spotting, or leakage of amniotic fluid. A vaginal examination may reveal cervical dilation or **effacement;** pelvic ultrasonography also may demonstrate dilation or effacement.

ETIOLOGY

The etiology is unknown.

DIAGNOSIS

Uterine contractions, cervical effacement and dilation, and/or rupture of the amniotic membranes (bag of waters [BOW]) before the expected date of confinement (EDC) signal the onset of premature labor.

TREATMENT

The treatment consists of monitoring the patient, fetal heart tones (FHTs), and fetal movement (see Fig. 12–14 in the Enrichment on fetal movement). Drug therapy includes the administration of terbutaline sulfate (Brethine) or magnesium sulfate. It is hoped that labor can be postponed until the fetus can develop to maturity.

TOXEMIA, PREECLAMPSIA, AND ECLAMPSIA

SYMPTOMS AND SIGNS

Hypertension that is pregnancy induced can be associated with the potentially life-threatening disorder toxemia. The pregnant patient, usually in the third trimester, experiences sudden weight gain with edema, primarily in the face, hands, and feet. Headaches, dizziness, spots before the eyes, and nausea and vomiting may occur. The blood pressure is elevated, and protein is found in the urine. Both mother and fetus can be in danger.

ETIOLOGY

The etiology of this condition, which is unique to pregnant females, is unknown; however, poor nutrition and above-normal sodium intake are possible contributing factors. It occurs most frequently in **primiparas** who are 12 to 18 years old or older than 35 years.

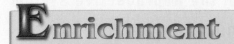

FETAL MOVEMENT

Fetal movement is an indicator of the well-being of the fetus. Some physicians have the expectant mother use a kick chart (Fig. 12–14) to record fetal activity. The mother is instructed to relax each day at approximately the same time for 30 minutes and to count the number of times that she feels movement from the fetus. The expected number of movements varies from patient to patient; nevertheless, the mother becomes familiar with the pattern of her baby and can be aware of decreased movement. If she does not feel movement in the 30-minute period, she is instructed to repeat the observation later in the day. If fetal movement remains absent or decreased from the norm, she is to notify her physician, who can investigate and evaluate the fetal status further.

KICK COUNT SHEET

1. Lie down for 30 minutes after breakfast, lunch, and dinner.
2. Count the number of times that you can feel the baby move. Record on the chart.
3. If the baby moves fewer than 6 times after you eat for 2 times in a row (e.g., breakfast and lunch call the office. If the total number of times in 1 day is 50% less than for the previous day call the office. (e.g., Tuesday total = 40 and Wednesday total = 16.)

Date	Breakfast	Lunch	Dinner	Total

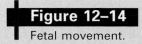

Figure 12–14

Fetal movement.

The toxemic patient is preeclamptic before any convulsions occur. If the toxemia is allowed to progress to eclampsia, the patient experiences convulsions, which may result in **abruptio placentae** (separation of the placenta from the uterine wall) and fetal or maternal demise.

DIAGNOSIS

Diagnosis is made by the clinical picture, the serum electrolyte levels, elevated blood albumin level, and exaggerated reflexes.

TREATMENT

Monitoring the patient's blood pressure, weight, and urine protein level is customary in prenatal care. As the pregnancy progresses, the monitoring becomes more frequent. At the first indication of signs and symptoms of toxemia, the patient is encouraged to use no added salt in the diet. If the toxemia becomes more severe (e.g., spots before the eyes, headache, and higher blood pressure), the patient may be hospitalized and monitored. The room is kept dark and quiet to decrease any stimuli, in an effort to prevent convulsions. FHTs and fetal movement are monitored closely. Medications are given to decrease blood pressure.

Termination of the pregnancy resolves the condition. Usually within 24 to 48 hours, the patient's blood pressure returns to normal levels, edema subsides, and protein is no longer present in the urine.

Good prenatal care and diet help substantially in decreasing the frequency and severity of toxemia. Other possibilities being explored are calcium supplementation and low-dose aspirin therapy.

ABRUPTIO PLACENTAE

SYMPTOMS AND SIGNS

When the placenta separates from the uterine wall too early during pregnancy and causes the mother to hemorrhage, generally in the third trimester, the pregnant patient experiences sudden, severe abdominal pain with board-like rigidity and a large amount of bright vaginal bleeding. Vital signs are indicative of shock, with an increased pulse rate that is weak and thready, falling blood pressure, and cool, clammy, moist, pale skin. The patient is apprehensive. FHTs decrease and have no variability, indicating impending fetal demise. Fetal activity or movement is decreased.

ETIOLOGY

Abruptio placentae is a separation of the placenta from the uterine wall, either complete or partial (Fig. 12–15). Marginal or complete cases have massive bright bleeding, whereas concealed cases have no visible bleeding but have extreme abdominal pain with board-like rigidity.

Trauma or seizures can cause the separation; however, in many cases, the cause is unknown.

DIAGNOSIS

Diagnosis, if time permits, is made by pelvic ultrasonography along with the clinical picture. Often, the abruptio placentae is so severe and sudden that the clinical picture is the only basis for treatment.

TREATMENT

When indicated, decreasing fetal heart rate and maternal shock demand immediate surgical intervention. Maternal or fetal mortality rate depends on the severity of the abruptio placentae and prompt intervention. Blood replacement may be indicated.

PLACENTA PREVIA

SYMPTOMS AND SIGNS

Placenta previa occurs when the placenta that is implanted in the lower uterine segment en-

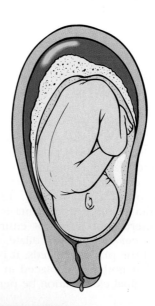

Figure 12–15
Abruptio placentae.

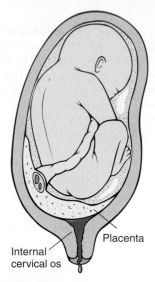

Figure 12–16
Placenta previa.

croaches on the internal cervical os, causing bleeding. The patient experiences painless, bright vaginal bleeding, usually in the last trimester of pregnancy. Occasionally, the patient has experienced painless vaginal bleeding earlier in the pregnancy. The abdomen is soft and nontender. Vital signs may be indicative of shock, with the pulse being rapid and thready and the blood pressure falling. Fetal heart rate may indicate that the blood supply to the fetus is compromised.

ETIOLOGY

The etiology is unknown, although there appears to be an increased incidence in breech presentation.

DIAGNOSIS

Diagnosis is made by a pelvic ultrasonogram that shows the placenta implanted over the cervical os. In a complete placenta previa, the placenta totally overlies the os (Fig. 12–16). In a partial placenta previa, the placenta is implanted low in the uterus but does not entirely overlie the os. As the cervix begins to dilate, the vessels tear loose and the placenta bleeds. It is of utmost importance that nothing be placed in the vagina and that no vaginal examination be performed.

TREATMENT

To control the mother's hemorrhaging and to save the baby, treatment of complete placenta previa is immediate surgical termination of the pregnancy with delivery of the infant by cesarean section. Partial placenta previa of nonterm pregnancies may be treated conservatively by observing the mother in a hospital. Surgical intervention is employed when the fetus is nearer to term or if the bleeding becomes profuse.

HYDATIDIFORM MOLE

SYMPTOMS AND SIGNS

The patient with a hydatidiform mole, a developmental anomaly of conception, experiences symptoms that mimic those of pregnancy. Toward the end of the third month of gestation, she begins to experience bright red or brownish vaginal bleeding. The bleeding may be spotting in nature or may be continuous. The uterus increases in size, out of proportion to the gestational age. The patient also may experience nausea and vomiting. The hCG levels are elevated, but no FHTs are present. The signs and symptoms of toxemia may be present as early as 20 weeks of gestation.

ETIOLOGY

This developmental anomaly of conception occurs when the chorionic villi develop into a mass of clear grape-like vesicles (Fig. 12–17). Usually, no fetus is present. There may be a paternal genetic link.

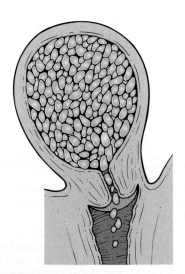

Figure 12–17
Hydatidiform mole.

DIAGNOSIS

Diagnosis is made by the clinical picture, the absence of FHTs, abnormally elevated hCG levels, and ultrasonogram.

TREATMENT

The mole normally is not expelled spontaneously, so surgical intervention is indicated, with the usual treatment being evacuation of the

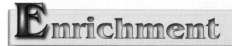

USUAL AND UNUSUAL PRESENTATIONS

Most fetuses present in the **cephalic,** or **vertex** (head first), presentation; however, some present in other manners, such as footling **breech** (feet first), frank breech (buttocks), or transverse lie (across the uterus) (Fig. 12–18). Even some of the cephalic presentations (brow or chin) cause complications that may prevent a normal vaginal delivery. In the abnormal presentations, delivery is accomplished by cesarean section.

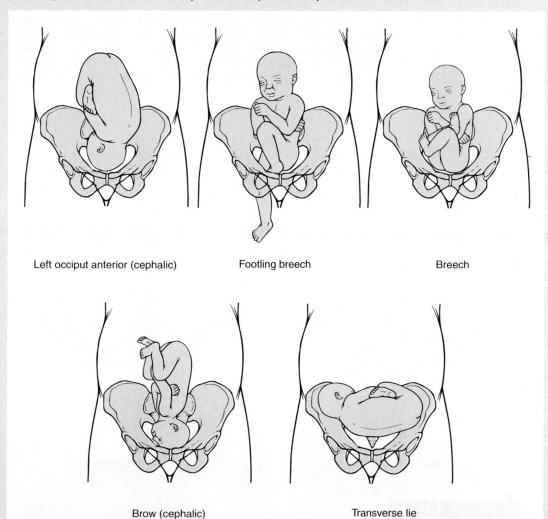

Left occiput anterior (cephalic)   Footling breech   Breech

Brow (cephalic)   Transverse lie

Figure 12–18

Fetal presentations.

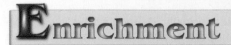

MULTIPLE PREGNANCIES

Multiple pregnancies are occurring more frequently (Fig. 12–19). Treatment of infertility contributes to this increase, because drugs such as clomiphene citrate (Clomid) are given to stimulate ovulation. These drugs frequently cause numerous ova to be released at ovulation, thus providing the sperm with multiple opportunities for fertilization. During the in vitro fertilization process, several fertilized ova are implanted in the hope that at least one successful pregnancy will ensue. Sometimes, the ovaries release more than one ovum in a natural course of events. Identical twins result when the fertilized zygote divides.

Problems associated with multiple pregnancies are numerous. The mother is at greater risk for toxemia. She experiences dyspnea, frequency of urination, constipation, edema of the feet and legs, and heartburn at an earlier time in the pregnancy than does the mother with a single fetus. Often, the expectant mother of triplets, quadruplets, quintuplets, or sextuplets is hospitalized by the beginning of the third trimester and restricted to bed rest. The fetuses are monitored frequently and usually must be delivered by cesarean section. The size of the multiple pregnancies generally makes it impossible for the pregnancy to continue to term. This may result in very small immature infants who need intensive nursing care and monitoring.

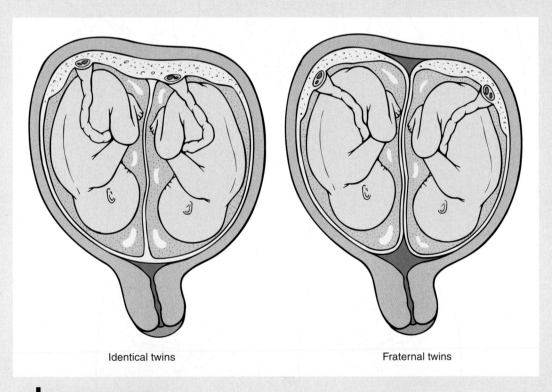

Identical twins   Fraternal twins

Figure 12–19
Multiple pregnancies.

uterus by D & C. Observation for hemorrhage is important. This condition can be a precursor to choriocarcinoma, and the patient must be instructed to have frequent follow-up examinations. Some patients receive chemotherapy in the form of antimetabolite drugs.

Diseases of the Breast

Ranging from mild to fatal, diseases of the breast necessitate frequent screening, including monthly self-examinations and routine mammograms as prescribed by the physician. Although diseases of the breast are most common in women, men do experience diseases of the breast. Any deviations of the breast tissue such as lumps, indentations, nipple crusting, or leaking should be cause for concern and investigation.

MAMMARY DYSPLASIA OR CYSTIC DISEASE OF THE BREAST

SYMPTOMS AND SIGNS

The female patient with mammary fibroplasia experiences an uncomfortable feeling in the breasts. Lumps and cysts, single or multiple, smooth and rounded, can be palpated in one or both breasts. The breasts are tender on palpation, and the patient may experience shooting pains in the breast tissue.

ETIOLOGY

The etiology is unknown. There is an increase in the formation of fibrous tissue and a hyperplasia of the epithelial cells of the ducts and glands, resulting in a dilation of the ducts. Cystic disease is the most common disease of the female breast, usually occurs between the ages of 35 and 50 years, and could be endocrine related.

DIAGNOSIS

Prompt diagnosis is made by palpation and by mammogram to differentiate cystic disease from malignant **neoplasm.**

TREATMENT

There is no specific treatment of this condition. Some physicians aspirate the cysts with a needle. The patient should wear a firm support-

ing bra, and caffeine intake should be avoided. The patient needs to be made aware of the importance of breast self-examination and of annual mammograms. The lumps and cysts of the disease can mask malignant lumps.

MASTITIS

SYMPTOMS AND SIGNS

Acute puerperal mastitis is the inflammation of breast tissue during lactation. The nursing mother experiences pain, redness, and heat in the breasts at either the beginning or end of the lactation period. The breasts are hot and feel doughy and tough. There is a discharge from the nipple.

ETIOLOGY

Bacteria invade the milk ducts and cause inflammation and occlusion. Milk stagnates in the lobules, producing a dull pain. The baby, nursing staff, or even the mother's own body may be the source of the infection.

DIAGNOSIS

Diagnosis is made by the clinical picture.

TREATMENT

Treatment includes having the mother stop breast-feeding immediately. A firm, good-supporting bra should be worn, heat may be applied to the area, progesterone may be prescribed, and chemotherapy in the form of antibiotics is implemented. The mother needs to be instructed in good personal hygiene, especially in hand-washing techniques.

FIBROADENOMA

SYMPTOMS AND SIGNS

The female patient in her late teens or early 20s feels a firm, round, movable mass in the breast. She experiences no pain or tenderness.

ETIOLOGY

The etiology is unknown.

DIAGNOSIS

Diagnosis is made by palpation, the clinical picture, and mammogram.

TREATMENT

Treatment of this benign tumor of the breast is surgical removal.

CANCER OF THE BREAST

SYMPTOMS AND SIGNS

The patient (usually female) discovers a small nontender lump in the breast tissue. Generally, this isolated lump is in the upper outer quadrant of the breast. The painless lesion may cause a retraction of the skin over the breast or may have a dimpling effect. There may be an orange-peel appearance to the skin **(peau d'orange).** Visual examination may reveal that the breasts are asymmetric, and there may be nipple retraction. In advanced stages of untreated lesions, the nodule becomes fixed to the chest wall and axillary masses develop, as does ulceration. Breast pain is not a common factor in early breast cancer.

ETIOLOGY

The etiology is unknown, although there are factors that appear to put the patient in a higher risk group. The risk is increased in women who have a family history of breast cancer or a history of exposure to radiation or carcinogens, women older than 40 years of age, women who have never been pregnant, women whose first pregnancy occurred after the age of 35 years, women who experience early menarche, and women whose menopause occurred after the age of 50 years.

DIAGNOSIS

Diagnosis includes palpation of the lesion, mammography, and biopsy, either aspiration or surgical. The final confirmation is made by biopsy.

Early detection by mammography is possible before any palpable lesions are detected. Early detection increases survival and treatment options.

TREATMENT

Treatment is usually surgical and may incorporate radiation therapy and/or chemotherapy. Surgical treatment may be a **lumpectomy,** partial **mastectomy,** modified radical mastectomy, total mastectomy, or a full radical mastectomy. Radiation may be done before surgery to shrink the mass or may be done postoperatively in an attempt to destroy any remaining malignant cells. Some oncologists elect to administer chemotherapy to the patient as an adjunct to radiation or as an independent treatment. Chemotherapeutic agents include antimetabolites, alkylating agents, mitotic inhibitors, hormones, antibiotics, and immunotherapeutic drugs. Combinations of the drugs are individualized for each patient. Bone marrow transplant and stem cell rescue are alternative treatments that are being studied.

Early detection and treatment is of primary importance in breast cancer, as it is for any cancer. Monthly breast self-examinations, annual examinations by the physician, and mammograms as recommended by the physician are screening tools that can detect malignancy before metastasis occurs and enable early treatment that can reduce the number of deaths due to breast cancer.

PAGET'S DISEASE OF THE BREAST

SYMPTOMS AND SIGNS

Paget's disease of the breast is carcinoma of the mammary ducts. The female patient, usually older than 45 years, experiences a mild crusting, scaling type of change in the tissue of one nipple. It may itch or burn and eventually spreads to the areola. If it is left untreated, ulceration of the tissue results. The nipple may retract.

ETIOLOGY

The etiology of this form of carcinoma is unknown.

DIAGNOSIS

Diagnosis is made by the clinical picture and biopsy of the lesion.

TREATMENT

Treatment is surgical removal of the breast.

Summary

Both the male and female reproductive systems are vulnerable to many disease entities. Some directly hinder reproductive capacities because of functional, structural, or emotional causes. Other disease conditions interfere with the process of elimination of wastes, and certain conditions potentially lead to systemic involvement. Currently, STDs are a burgeoning threat to general well-being and a specific peril to healthy reproduction. Cancers afflicting male and female organs of the reproductive system, some associated with natural or therapeutic hormone activity, endanger health and longevity.

- Public education focuses on the known risk factors for the more than 20 STDs.
- Chlamydia, gonorrhea, trichomoniasis, chancroid, and syphilis are STDs that all respond well to a prompt and complete course of antibiotic therapy. Preventive vaccine is available for those at risk for hepatitis B.
- STDs and other infections of the reproductive tract cause scarring that may contribute to female infertility. Some of the other causes are congenital disorders, tumors, endometriosis, and ovulatory dysfunction.
- Male infertility may result from various conditions causing insufficient number or mobility of sperm, including structural anomalies, genetic diseases, endocrine disorders, varicocele, and injuries.
- Careful investigation of the cause (anatomic, chemical, or psychological) precedes appropriate treatment of sexual dysfunction.
- Benign prostatic hyperplasia is a common disorder in older men that may respond to symptomatic treatment or require surgical resection (transurethral resection).
- Bacterial infections of the prostate gland, the epididymis, or the testes require symptomatic measures and antimicrobial therapy.
- Regular physical examination, monitoring of PSA levels, and biopsy are beneficial for early detection of prostatic cancer; time is of the essence in preventing metastasis to other pelvic organs.
- Secondary dysmenorrhea may be caused by pelvic infections, fibroids, endometriosis, or cervical stenosis.
- Ovarian cysts can be physiologic or neoplastic, small or very large, benign or malignant; precise diagnosis requires ultrasonogram or laparoscopy to determine treatment.
- Endometriosis, or endometrial tissue growing outside the uterine cavity, causes abnormal menstrual pain and bleeding; complications of pregnancy may occur.
- Early diagnosis and treatment of pelvic inflammatory disease (PID) lessens damage to the reproductive system.
- The pros and cons of hormone replacement therapy (HRT) must be weighed for each postmenopausal woman.
- Uterine prolapse, cystocele, and rectocele all share birth trauma as an etiologic factor.
- Early detection of cervical cancer is possible by regular screening with a Papanicolaou (Pap) smear. Conversely, early detection of ovarian cancer is difficult.
- Toxemia, abruptio placentae, and placenta previa are conditions of pregnancy that threaten the well-being of the baby and pregnant woman.
- Cystic disease of the breast and fibroadenoma are both benign conditions; cancer of the breast and Paget's disease are malignant conditions requiring surgical and medical intervention.

387

Review Challenge

REVIEW QUESTIONS

1. What are the risk factors for sexually transmitted diseases (STDs)?
2. Why is chlamydia referred to as the silent STD?
3. What are the possible complications of untreated gonorrhea?
4. What is meant by the term "ping-pong" vaginitis?
5. What is the pathologic course of genital herpes? How is it treated? Can it be cured?
6. How is genital herpes contracted?
7. Why is early diagnosis and treatment of syphilis important?
8. What is the primary mode of transmission of hepatitis B? Who is at risk?
9. Which prevention measures are recommended for those at high risk for hepatitis B?
10. What are some of the diverse causes of dyspareunia in men and women?
11. Which drugs may contribute to male impotence?

12. What are the possible causes of male and female infertility? Are any preventable?
13. How is benign prostatic hyperplasia treated? What are the possible complications?
14. What are the possible causes of epididymitis? Of orchitis?
15. What are the symptoms and signs of torsion of the testicle?
16. What is a varicocele? How may it be a factor in male infertility?
17. Why is PSA screening valuable? Why is early detection of prostatic cancer vital?
18. What is often the first sign of testicular cancer?
19. What are some of the common symptoms of female reproductive diseases?
20. What are some possible causes of primary and secondary dysmenorrhea?
21. How is mittelschmerz related to ovulation?
22. What is the pathology associated with endometriosis?
23. Why is pelvic inflammatory disease (PID) a serious condition? What is the etiology?

24. What are the most common tumors of the female reproductive system?
25. What organism is commonly the cause of vaginitis?
26. What is toxic shock syndrome (TSS)?
27. What are the advantages and possible side effects of hormone replacement therapy (HRT)?
28. Which etiologic factor do uterine prolapse, cystocele and rectocele have in common?
29. What are the risk factors for cervical cancer? How is cervical cancer detected by the Papanicolaou (Pap) smear?
30. What is the leading cause of death attributed to female reproductive system disorders? Why is it referred to as a "silent" cancer?
31. What are the possible causes of ectopic pregnancy?
32. What are the clinical indications of toxemia?
33. What is the life-threatening complication that may occur in abruptio placentae? In placenta previa?
34. What are the factors that place women at a higher risk for cancer of the breast?

REAL-LIFE CHALLENGE

Endometriosis

A 35-year-old woman presents with dysmenorrhea, often having onset of pain the day before onset of menses. The pain occasionally continues a few days after menses have ceased. She describes the pain as constant cramping-type pain in the lower abdomen, vagina, and back. The patient describes her menstrual flow to be unusually heavy and also states that she has pain with defecation.

The patient is a gravida iii para ii with a history of a miscarriage 5 years ago. Her living children are 7 and 11 years of age. The patient

also states that she has been unable to conceive after 3 years of unprotected intercourse. She also reveals a history of use of tampons during the past 10 years.

The pelvic examination reveals generalized tenderness throughout the pelvis. Vital signs are: T — 98.8°, P — 88, R — 16, BP — 106/74. Endometriosis is suspected, and the patient is given the choice of conservative treatment with hormones or a laparoscopy to visualize the condition of the reproductive organs. The Pap smear result is negative.

Questions

1. What is the cause of endometriosis?
2. What is the significance of the obstetric history?
3. Why would the patient experience pain before menses?
4. What other pelvic organs might be involved?
5. Why would hormone therapy be prescribed?
6. What other types of treatment may be used?
7. What is the significance of the patient being unable to conceive?

REAL-LIFE CHALLENGE

Benign Prostatic Hyperplasia

A 60-year-old man reports urinary frequency and nocturia 3 to 4 times a night. On questioning, he reveals having difficulty starting urination and a weak stream of urine. He also states that he thinks he is not completely emptying his bladder. The symptoms have had an insidious onset.

The examination reveals a well-nourished 60-year-old man with vital signs as follows: T—98.6°, P—72, R—14, BP—116/78. His skin is warm, dry, and pink. A PSA test is ordered, and results return at 5 ng/ml. The subsequent digital rectal exam (DRE) reveals an enlarged prostate gland with no nodules or depressions. The urinalysis results are normal, and the urine cultures are negative.

Drug therapy with tamsulosin hydrochloride (Flomax) is ordered. The patient is instructed to have a repeat PSA test in 6 weeks and to return for follow-up DRE. The diagnosis is possible BPH.

Questions

1. What is the underlying reason for the urinary symptoms?
2. What are "normals" for PSA?
3. What causes the prostate to enlarge?
4. Why is the PSA drawn before the DRE?
5. What are treatment options other than drug therapy?
6. What might be the side effects of drug therapy?
7. What might be the side effects of surgical treatment of BPH?
8. What symptoms of BPH are similar to symptoms of cancer of the prostate?

RESOURCES

Women's National Health Resource Center
120 Albany Street, Suite 820
New Brunswick, NJ 08901
877-986-9472

National AIDS Hotline
U.S. Public Health Service
800-342-AIDS (2437)
800-344-7432 (Spanish)

Impotence Information Center
PO Box 9
Minneapolis, MN 55440
800-843-4315

American Society of Plastic and Reconstructive Surgeons (ASPRS)
444 East Algonquin Road
Arlington Heights, IL 60005-4664
704-228-9900
(http://www.plasticsurg.com)

CDC National STD Hotline
Centers for Disease Control and Prevention
800-227-8922

American College of Obstetricians and Gynecologists (ACOG)
409 12th St SW, PO Box 96920
Washington, DC 20090-6920
800-673-8444

American Cancer Society
1599 Clifton Rd
Atlanta, GA 30329
800-ACS-2345

Planned Parenthood Federation of America, Inc.
810 Seventh Ave

New York, NY 10019
212-541-7870

American Society for Reproductive Medicine
1209 Montgomery Highway
Birmingham, AL 35216-2809
205-978-5000
asrm@asrm.org

American Venereal Disease Foundation
Box 385
University of Virginia
Charlottesville, VA 22908

Endometriosis Association
8585 North 76th Place
Milwaukee, WI 53223
800-992-3636

National Alliance of Breast Cancer Organizations
9 E 37th St, 10th Floor
New York, NY 10016
800-719-9154

North American Menopause Society
PO Box 94527
Cleveland, OH 44101
216-844-8748
info@menopause.org

Sex Information and Education Council of the US
130 West 42nd St, Ste 2500
New York, NY 10036
212-819-9770

National Cervical Cancer Coalition (NCCC)
16501 Sherman Way, Ste 110
Van Nuys, CA 91406
800-685-5531

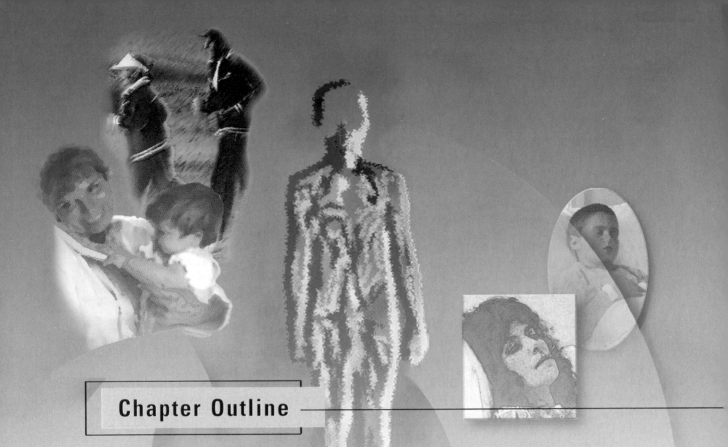

Chapter Outline

Neurologic Diseases and Conditions

After studying Chapter 13, you should be able to:

1. Name the main components of the nervous system.
2. List some of the problems to which the nervous system is susceptible.
3. Describe how data are collected during a neurologic assessment.
4. Name the common symptoms and signs of a cerebrovascular accident (CVA).
5. Name the three vascular disorders that may cause a CVA.
6. Define a transient ischemic attack (TIA).
7. Distinguish between (a) epidural and subdural hematomas and (b) cerebral concussion and cerebral contusion.
8. Describe three mechanisms of spinal injuries.
9. Name the goals of treatment of spinal cord injuries.
10. Explain the neurologic consequences of the deterioration or rupture of an intervertebral disk.
11. Describe the symptoms of migraine.
12. Explain why cephalalgia sometimes is considered a symptom of underlying disease.
13. Describe first aid for seizures.
14. Explain how the symptoms of Parkinson's disease are controlled.
15. Describe the progression of amyotrophic lateral sclerosis (ALS).
16. Distinguish between trigeminal neuralgia and Bell's palsy.
17. List the diagnostic tests used for meningitis and explain how the causative organism is identified.
18. Name the common causes of encephalitis.
19. Explain the pathologic course of Guillain-Barré syndrome.
20. Explain what is meant by postpolio syndrome.

Key Terms

aphasia	(ah–**FAY**–zee–ah)	cephalalgia	(sef–ah–**LAL**–jee–ah)
aura	(**AW**–rah)	chorea	(ko–**REE**–ah)
autonomic	(aw–toe–**NOM**–ic)	concussion	(kon–**KUSH**–un)

contusion	(kon–**TOO**–zhun)	hemiparesis	(**hem**–ee–**PAR**–ee–sis)
craniotomy	(**kray**–nee–**OTT**–toe–me)	hemiplegia	(**hem**–ee–**PLEE**–jee–ah)
demyelination	(dee–**my**–eh–lih–**NAY**–shun)	neurotransmitter	(**new**–roh–**TRANS**–mit–er)
diplopia	(dip–**LOW**–pee–ah)	paraplegia	(par–ah–**PLEE**–jee–ah)
epidural	(ep–ih–**DUR**–al)		
fasciculation	(fa–**sik**–you–**LAY**–shun)	parasympathetic	(**par**–ah–**sim**–pa–**THET**–ik)
hematogenous	(**he**–mah–**TOJ**–eh–nus)	paresis	(pah–**REE**–sis)
		quadriplegia	(**kwod**–rih–**PLEE**–jee–ah)
hematoma	(hem–ah–**TOE**–mah)		

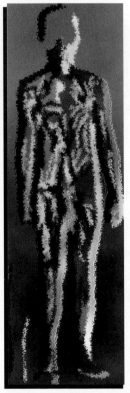

Orderly Function of the Nervous System

The nervous system is a complex, sophisticated, and elaborate network of many interlaced nerve cells (neurons) that make up the brain (Fig. 13-1 *A*), the spinal cord (Fig 13-1 *B*), and the nerves. Electrical impulses are carried throughout the body by the neurons (Fig. 13-1 *C*). This entire system regulates and coordinates the body's activities and produces reponses to stimuli, which help the body to adjust to changes in its environment, both internal and external.

The nervous system is composed of two divisions, the central nervous system (CNS) and the peripheral nervous system (PNS). The CNS includes the brain and spinal cord. Its job is to process and store sensory and motor information and to govern consciousness. For example, the structures of the brain that control the intellectual functions of thinking, willing, remembering, and deciding, as well as those that control personality, are located in the frontal lobe of the cerebrum. Coordination, equilibrium, and posture are coordinated in the cerebellum area of the brain. The hypothalamus regulates the secretion of hormones from the pituitary gland and regulates many visceral activities. Five pairs of the 12 cranial nerves originate in the medulla oblongata, an extension of the spinal cord; the medulla also contains vital centers that help regulate heart rate, blood pressure, and respiration. All the sensory and motor nerve fibers pass through the medulla oblongata, connecting the brain and the spinal cord. The spinal cord, a continuation of the medulla oblongata, extends to the first lumbar vertebra. It is divided into 31 segments, each giving rise to a pair of spinal nerves that act like a telephone switchboard, or reflex center, carrying impulses to and from the brain (Fig. 13-1 *D*).

The vast network of nerves throughout the rest of the body is part of the PNS (Fig. 13-2 *A*). Peripheral nerves connect with the spinal cord at many levels, and the information (impulses) they carry travels to and from the brain and spinal cord. Sensory (afferent) nerves transmit impulses from parts of the body (e.g., skin, eye, ear, and nose) to the spinal cord and brain. Motor (effer-

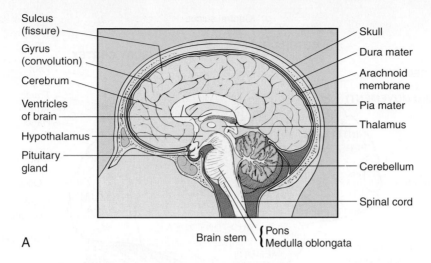

A

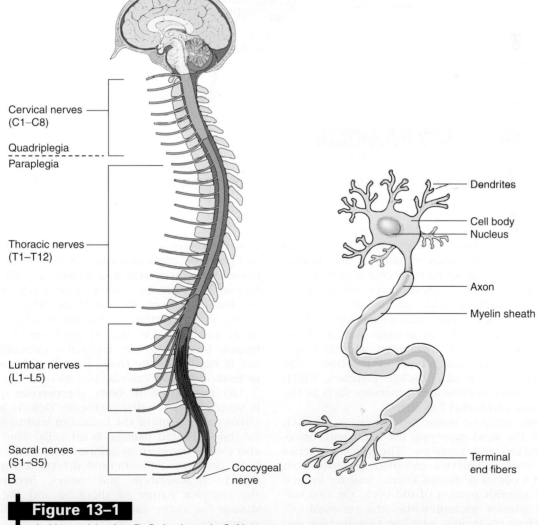

B

C

Figure 13–1

A, Normal brain. *B,* Spinal cord. *C,* Neuron.

Illustration continued on following page

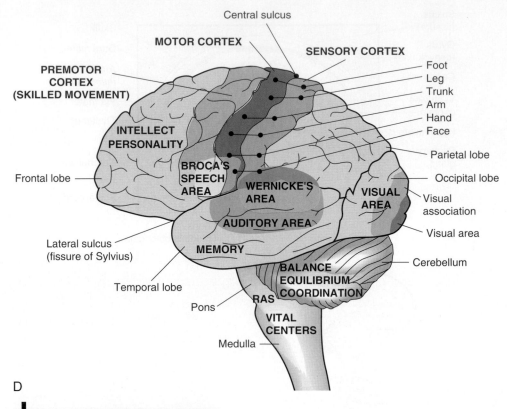

D

Figure 13–1 *Continued*

D, Functional areas of the brain. (From Gould BE: Pathophysiology for the Health-Related Professions. Philadelphia: WB Saunders, 1997, p 323. Used with permission.)

ent) nerves transmit impulses away from the CNS and produce responses in muscles and glands. The PNS contains 12 pairs of cranial nerves (Fig. 13-2 *B*), 31 pairs of spinal nerves (Fig. 13-2 *C*), and the sympathetic and parasympathetic nerves. The sympathetic and parasympathetic nerves make up the autonomic nervous system (ANS), which regulates the involuntary muscle movements and glandular actions of the body. The PNS also controls all conscious activities, which greatly affect unconscious processes such as the heart rate and bowel functions.

There are four major blood vessels on each side of the head supplying the brain with essential oxygen and nutrients. The carotid arteries (two internal and two external) originate from the two common carotid arteries and are located in the anterior portion of the neck; the two vertebral arteries, located within the vertebral column (Fig. 13-3), join with the two anterior and posterior cerebral arteries and the two arterior and posterior communicating arteries to form the brain's vascular system in a roughly circular configuration of arteries known as the circle of Willis. Branches from the circle of Willis supply blood to all portions of the brain (Fig. 13-4). Areas of the brain that depend on a single branch for survival are especially vulnerable to any disruption in the blood flow (e.g., thrombus or **embolus**) (see Vascular Disorders).

Like the rest of the body, the nervous system is susceptible to varied problems. Defects in the circulatory system of the brain can lead to vascular disorders and damage brain cells. The brain also can be damaged by injuries, infections, metabolic derangement, inherited defects, congenital defects, degeneration, and tumors. Because of the complex nature of the CNS and the PNS damage to them can cause extremely diverse symptoms.

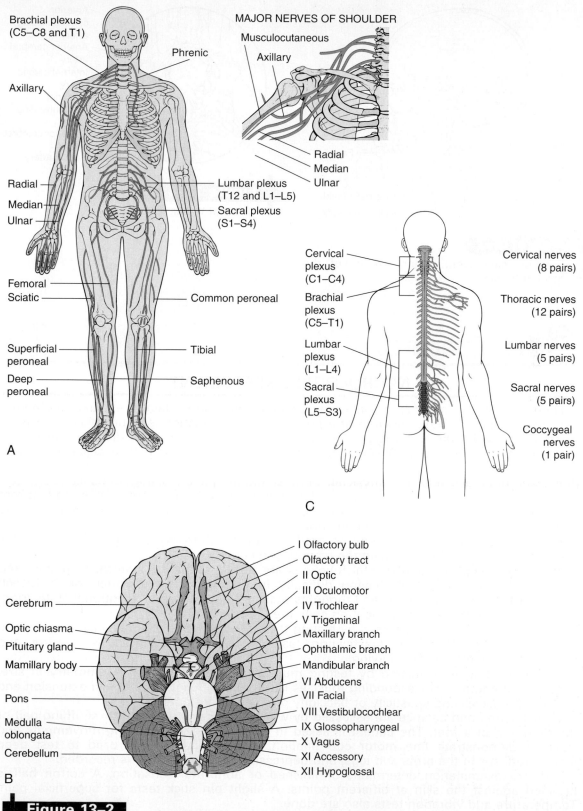

Brachial plexus
(C5–C8 and T1)

Phrenic

Axillary

MAJOR NERVES OF SHOULDER

Musculocutaneous

Axillary

Radial

Median

Radial

Ulnar

Median

Lumbar plexus
(T12 and L1–L5)

Ulnar

Sacral plexus
(S1–S4)

Femoral

Sciatic

Common peroneal

Superficial
peroneal

Tibial

Deep
peroneal

Saphenous

A

Cervical
plexus
(C1–C4)

Cervical nerves
(8 pairs)

Brachial
plexus
(C5–T1)

Thoracic nerves
(12 pairs)

Lumbar
plexus
(L1–L4)

Lumbar nerves
(5 pairs)

Sacral
plexus
(L5–S3)

Sacral nerves
(5 pairs)

Coccygeal
nerves
(1 pair)

C

Cerebrum

Optic chiasma

Pituitary gland

Mamillary body

Pons

Medulla
oblongata

Cerebellum

B

I Olfactory bulb
Olfactory tract
II Optic
III Oculomotor
IV Trochlear
V Trigeminal
Maxillary branch
Ophthalmic branch
Mandibular branch
VI Abducens
VII Facial
VIII Vestibulocochlear
IX Glossopharyngeal
X Vagus
XI Accessory
XII Hypoglossal

Figure 13–2

A, Peripheral nervous system. *B,* Cranial nerves. *C,* Spinal nerves.

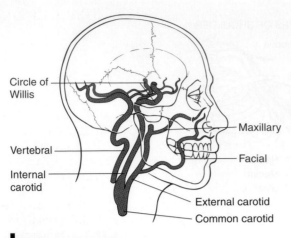

Figure 13-3

Cerebral circulation: major arteries of the head and neck.

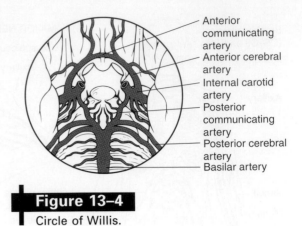

Figure 13-4

Circle of Willis.

Enrichment

NEUROLOGIC ASSESSMENT

Neurologic assessment relies on a step-by-step collection of data to evaluate the neurologic status and cognitive function of a person. The examination is appropriate after head trauma occurs or cranial surgery is performed or when a neurologic disorder, such as a brain tumor, is suspected. Observations and findings are graded on a scale and documented. The assessment is done within the constraints of circumstances (e.g., the location [the scene of an accident or a physician's office] and the patient's state of consciousness).

Neurologic assessment begins with a thorough medical history, noting past and current problems, and a record of medications being taken. The patient's comprehension and judgment are noted during the examination.

The patient's mental status may be graded with the Glasgow Coma Scale, which is a standardized system for assessing the response to stimuli.

Next, more sophisticated mental functions are tested, including speech, language, and written skills. Is the patient having difficulty in putting words together, or is speech slurred? Do the patient's ideas and thoughts make sense? Behavior, emotional state, long-term and recent memory and attention span are observed.

The cranial nerves are assessed by testing the patient's sense of smell, visual acuity and eye movements, muscles of mastication, taste perception, facial muscles, hearing, and tongue movements and swallowing.

Motor function is evaluated by testing muscle tone and strength. Asymmetry in size, shape, or strength of corresponding muscles may be significant. Changes in extension and flexion of muscles and spasticity or flaccidity of muscles are noted.

Coordination and balance are assessed by watching for unsteadiness or shuffling gait or the dragging of a foot. The patient is asked to perform rapid alternating movements and tasks to demonstrate fine motor coordination. A reflex hammer is used to test deep tendon reflexes in the arms and legs; and depression or hyperactivity is recorded.

Sensory examination determines diminished or abnormal sensation. A cotton ball is brushed against the skin at different points. A slight pin stick tests for superficial pain. Temperature and vibration tests also are done.

Findings lead the clinician to begin focusing on any problem area. The need for further testing also is indicated as abnormal assessment findings emerge.

Common problems within the nervous system that necessitate attention from health-care providers include:

- Headaches
- Dizziness
- Muscle weakness
- Tremors
- Motor disturbances, other disturbances of movement, or paralysis
- Radiating pain
- Memory impairment
- Altered levels of consciousness
- Drowsiness
- Sensory disturbances or numbness
- Speech disturbances
- Visual disturbances

Vascular Disorders

CEREBROVASCULAR ACCIDENT (STROKE)

SYMPTOMS AND SIGNS

A cerebrovascular accident (CVA), or stroke, occurs when the brain is damaged by a sudden disruption in the flow of blood to a part of the brain or by bleeding inside the head. It is the number one cause of adult disability. Because there is inadequate blood supply, the physical and mental functions controlled by the affected area fail to operate properly. The brain tissue in this area becomes bloodless (Fig. 13-5 *A*).

The symptoms and signs of a stroke reflect the portion of the brain affected (Fig. 13-5 *B*). Common stroke symptoms include

- Sudden severe headache
- Sudden **dysphasia,** or difficulty understanding language
- Sudden weakness, numbness, or paralysis of the face, or **hemiparesis**
- Sudden confusion or impaired consciousness
- Sudden loss of vision, blurred vision, or **diplopia**
- Sudden **dysphagia**
- Sudden onset of dizziness, loss of balance, or loss of coordination

A severe stroke can result in coma and death. Early recognition of symptoms and prompt medi-

cal intervention can help reduce the chances of disability and death.

ETIOLOGY

A CVA is usually the result of one of three types of vascular disorders: cerebral thrombosis (clot), cerebral hemorrhage, and cerebral embolism (moving clot). These vascular disorders most often are caused by atherosclerosis (see Atherosclerosis in Chapter 10) and hypertension (high blood pressure). Strokes also can result from blood disorders, **arrhythmias,** systemic diseases (e.g., diabetes mellitus and syphilis), **hyperlipidemia,** rheumatic heart disease, or head trauma. A high-fat diet, lack of exercise, cigarette smoking, obesity, and a family history of atherosclerotic disease are contributing factors.

CVAs caused by an embolus or hemorrhage often have a sudden onset, whereas strokes caused by a thrombus usually appear more gradually. A cerebral thrombosis occurs if one of the cerebral arteries becomes narrowed because of **plaque** buildup from atherosclerotic disease. This thrombus, or clot, can enlarge until it partially or completely blocks blood flow to the artery, starving the tissue it feeds of oxygen.

A cerebral embolism is also a blockage, but it is caused by a foreign object, or embolus. This embolus can be a piece of arterial wall, a small blood clot from a diseased heart, or a bacterial clot; usually, platelet **fibrin** from an ulcerated arterial wall of the heart or valve of the heart is the causative factor. It is carried in the bloodstream until it becomes wedged in a blood vessel and obstructs the flow of blood to an area of the brain.

With a cerebral hemorrhage, the cerebral artery is not blocked, but ruptures, filling the surrounding brain tissue with blood. The initial effects of a hemorrhage may be more severe than those of a thrombosis or embolism, and the long-term effects are much more serious.

DIAGNOSIS

Physical examination of the patient leads the physician to suspect a CVA and to gauge impairments on a functional scale. It can be confirmed by **magnetic resonance imaging (MRI), computed tomography (CT),** cerebral angiography, or electroencephalography (EEG). Blood tests for bleeding and clotting disorders may be done.

TREATMENT

Immediate appropriate medical intervention (within 3 hours) on onset of stroke symptoms may limit brain damage and thereby improve the

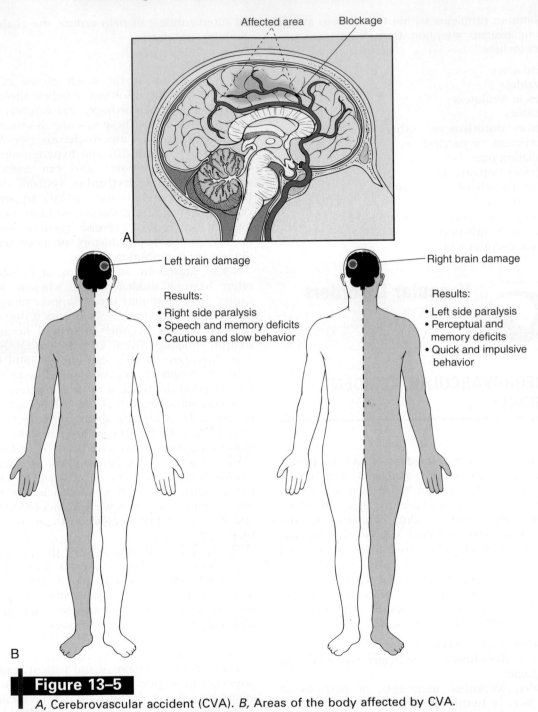

Affected area   Blockage

A

Left brain damage   Right brain damage

Results:
• Right side paralysis
• Speech and memory deficits
• Cautious and slow behavior

Results:
• Left side paralysis
• Perceptual and memory deficits
• Quick and impulsive behavior

B

Figure 13–5

A, Cerebrovascular accident (CVA). *B,* Areas of the body affected by CVA.

prognosis. **Anticoagulants** (warfarin sodium [Coumadin]), thrombolytic agents, and antiplatelet medications (aspirin) may be given. Surgery to improve circulation within the cerebral arteries or to remove clots is considered. Other therapeutic measures include surgery to repair broken or bleeding blood vessels and drugs to prevent or reverse brain swelling. Long-term treatment for CVA depends on the size and location of the stroke and the presence and severity of impairments. Brain cells destroyed do not recover and are not replaced; patients can learn new ways of functioning and use other undamaged brain cells. The goal of medical treatment is to restore lost functions and treat underlying disorders. A team approach to rehabilitation includes family members and a medical team of speech, physical, and occupational therapists; nurses; and doctors. Recovery varies in rate of improvement and degree of rehabilitation; some permanent disability may remain. Prevention of stroke includes positive lifestyle changes to reduce controllable risk factors such as smoking, excesses in diet and alcohol consumption, untreated high blood pressure, and uncontrolled diabetes. Other risk factors include family history of stroke and age.

TRANSIENT ISCHEMIC ATTACK

SYMPTOMS AND SIGNS

Transient ischemic attacks (TIAs) are temporary episodes of impaired neurologic functioning caused by an inadequate flow of blood to a portion of the brain. TIAs often are referred to as little strokes because they resemble a stroke caused by an embolism. The individual may report sudden weakness and numbness down one side of the body, dizziness, dysphagia, dysphasia, or confusion. Usually, TIAs do not cause unconsciousness. These little strokes are often recurring episodes, lasting from just seconds to hours, with symptoms gradually subsiding. The symptoms of a true stroke last for longer than 24 hours, but TIAs are often important signals of an impending stroke (CVA). The symptoms, like those of a stroke, depend on which part of the brain is affected.

ETIOLOGY

The most common cause of TIA is a piece of plaque, formed by atherosclerosis, that breaks away from the wall of an artery or heart valve and travels to the brain (Fig. 13-6). This is known as an embolus or moving clot. Platelet fibrin emboli from an arterial **ulcer** are frequently causative. Arterial vascular spasms and minute blood clots also may be etiologic factors.

DIAGNOSIS

A physical examination and history are the first steps in diagnosing the problem. Next is determining the source of a possible embolus. A likely source of emboli is the carotid arteries. Cranial MRI scan, CT scan, and an EEG are all helpful in confirming the diagnosis; however, all can appear normal.

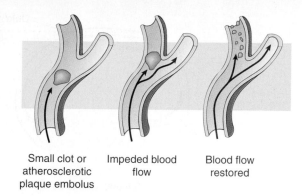

Small clot or atherosclerotic plaque embolus | Impeded blood flow | Blood flow restored

Figure 13-6
Embolus causing transient ischemic attack.

TREATMENT

Treatment depends on the location of the TIA and the underlying cause. Anticoagulants commonly are used during an episode to lessen the frequency or chance of recurrences. In certain cases, surgery may be attempted to increase the blood flow to the affected area.

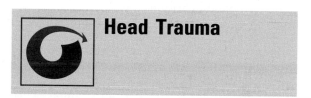

Head Trauma

EPIDURAL AND SUBDURAL HEMATOMAS

SYMPTOMS AND SIGNS

An epidural hematoma is a collection or mass of blood that forms between the skull and the dura mater, the outermost of the three meningeal layers covering the brain (Fig. 13-7). With a subdural hematoma, the blood collects or pools between the dura mater and the arachnoid membrane, the second meningeal membrane (see Fig. 13-7). The resulting pressure on the brain from either of these hematomas can result in impaired functioning of the brain, or possible death.

Symptoms of an epidural hematoma typically appear within a few hours of injury. They include sudden headache, dilated pupils, nausea and often vomiting, increased drowsiness, and perhaps hemiparesis. Eventually, if the hematoma is not treated promptly, unconsciousness, coma, and death occur. Deterioration of the patient's

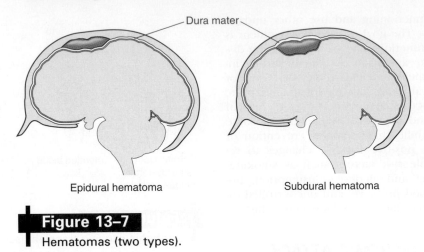

Epidural hematoma

Subdural hematoma

Figure 13-7

Hematomas (two types).

condition can be rapid. This is a neurologic emergency.

Subdural hematomas often exhibit symptoms similar to those of an epidural hematoma, except that the onset is delayed because of a slower accumulation of blood. This delayed onset may mimic the symptoms of a TIA, stroke, or dementia. Diplopia is a frequent occurrence in patients with a subdural hematoma.

ETIOLOGY

Both types of hematomas result when blood from ruptured vessels seeps into and around the meningeal layers. Head trauma is the usual cause; a blow to the head can cause an epidural hematoma, or the head's striking an immovable object can cause a subdural hematoma. Subdural hematomas frequently occur among the elderly as a result of falls. Cerebral hematomas usually follow skull fractures.

DIAGNOSIS

The clinical picture of the patient, along with a history of recent head trauma, suggests to the physician the possibility of either an epidural or a subdural hematoma. Cranial radiographic films, CT scans, and cerebral arteriograms locate the hematoma and rule out other causes of the symptoms. Suspicion of the condition is vital.

TREATMENT

If the person loses consciousness because of head trauma, rapid medical attention is needed. A **craniotomy**, cranial trephination (bur hole, a hole made in the skull with a drill to relieve pressure by draining off the blood that has accumulated), may be necessary. This procedure is performed to remove the accumulated blood and

to **cauterize** the bleeding vessels if increasing intracranial pressure indicates a life-threatening situation. When this procedure is performed promptly, a complete recovery is possible. A patient not losing consciousness but displaying symptoms, either immediate or delayed, should be seen by a physician as soon as possible for evaluation.

CEREBRAL CONCUSSION

SYMPTOMS AND SIGNS

With a cerebral concussion, there is an immediate loss of consciousness. It often is referred to as being "knocked out." This may last from a few seconds to several minutes, and may be followed by a varying period of **amnesia,** lasting from 12 to 24 hours. Respirations become shallow, pulse rate is depressed, and there is flaccid muscle tone. Symptoms appearing after the person has regained consciousness may include headache, nausea, vomiting, diplopia or blurred vision, and photophobia (sensitivity to light). These persons may exhibit an irritability, decreased levels of concentration, and amnesia.

ETIOLOGY

A concussion is an injury resulting from impact with a blunt object, either by a blow or from a fall. A concussion causes a disruption of the normal electrical activity in the brain, but the brain itself usually is not injured (Fig. 13-8).

DIAGNOSIS

A complete neurologic examination, along with a history of the injury, is needed. CT scan indicates no evidence of damage to the brain

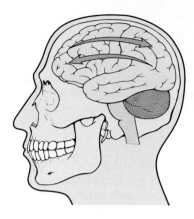

Concussion

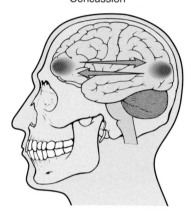

Contusion

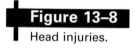

Figure 13–8

Head injuries.

tissues. History from others (e.g., relative, friend, observer, and ambulance staff) is vital.

TREATMENT

The usual treatment of a concussion is quiet bed rest with observation of the patient for signs of behavioral changes. The patient should be awakened every 4 hours. Any changes noted, including changes in the level of consciousness, could indicate a progressive brain injury.

CEREBRAL CONTUSION

SYMPTOMS AND SIGNS

A cerebral contusion is more serious than a concussion. This injury to the brain involves bruising of tissues along or just beneath its surface. The symptoms and signs of a contusion vary, according to the site and extent of the injury, and persist for longer than 24 hours. They may range from temporary loss of consciousness to coma. When conscious, the person may report a severe headache and hemiparesis. The person may appear drowsy and lethargic or hostile and combative.

Permanent damage to the brain may result from a contusion due to subdural and epidural hematomas (see Epidural and Subdural Hematomas), causing impaired intellect, dysphasia, paralysis, epilepsy, impaired gait, and continuing stupor.

ETIOLOGY

A contusion of the brain is caused by a blow to the head or an impact against a hard surface, as in an automobile accident. The twisting or shearing force against the two hemispheres of the brain when colliding with the cranial bones may damage structures deep within the brain (see Fig. 13-8). A contusion often is associated with a skull fracture.

DIAGNOSIS

A thorough neurologic examination is necessary, as well as a medical history of the injury. CT scans reveal the location and extent of brain damage. Cranial radiographic films rule out a possible skull fracture.

TREATMENT

Patients with a cerebral contusion need to be hospitalized to monitor their vital signs and to enable rapid medical intervention if required. Specific treatment is provided according to the site and severity of the contusion.

DEPRESSED SKULL FRACTURE

SYMPTOMS AND SIGNS

When a portion of the skull is broken and is pushed in on the brain, causing injury, it is said to be a depressed skull fracture (Fig. 13-9). The symptoms depend on the site of the fracture. For example, a bone fragment pressing on the motor area of the brain may cause hemiplegia (Fig. 13-10). Characteristically, symptoms from a depressed fracture are not progressive. They tend to remain static until the depressed bone is elevated, and the pressure is relieved. Epilepsy is a common complication of depressed skull fractures.

See Figure 13-9 for additional types of skull fractures.

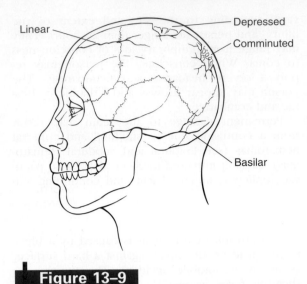

Figure 13–9

Skull fractures.

ETIOLOGY

Direct impact on the skull with a blunt object is the most frequent cause of depressed fractures. Industrial injuries and automobile accidents are two of the many possible causes. The fractured bone from a depressed fracture may cut an artery or vein, causing hemorrhage in the brain.

DIAGNOSIS

Physical examination of the patient most likely reveals a defect in the skull. Cranial radiographic films indicate if and where the brain is being crushed. CT scans show the presence of life-threatening cerebral edema.

TREATMENT

The treatment is aimed at relieving the intracranial pressure. A craniotomy is performed, and

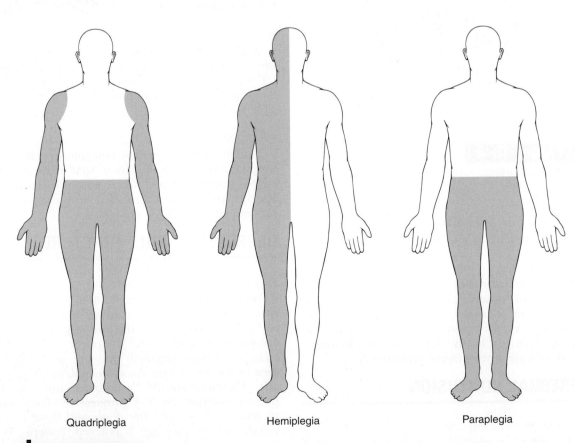

Quadriplegia   Hemiplegia   Paraplegia

Figure 13–10

Types of paralysis.

the depressed bone is elevated back into place. Head protection is worn until the fracture has at least partially healed.

Spinal Cord Injuries

PARAPLEGIA AND QUADRIPLEGIA

SYMPTOMS AND SIGNS

If the spinal cord is injured, a part or parts of the body inferior to the point of injury may be affected. The damage to the cord may be only temporary, but it usually leads to some degree of permanent disability because nerve pathways control many bodily functions and actions. Paraplegia results in the loss of motor and sensory control of the trunk of the body and lower extremities. Loss of bowel, bladder, and sexual function is also common. Quadriplegia results in paralysis of the lower extremities and usually the trunk, with either partial or total paralysis in the upper limbs. There also may be hypotension, hypothermia, bradycardia, and respiratory problems. In some patients, respiration is maintained or assisted by mechanical ventilation.

ETIOLOGY

Generally, spinal cord injuries causing paraplegia and quadriplegia are the result of vertebral fractures or vertebral dislocation. The site of the injury, the type of trauma to the cord, and the severity of the trauma determine whether the person is paraplegic or quadriplegic (see Fig. 13-10).

Trauma to the thoracic and lumbar regions of the spine (T1 and below) usually results in paraplegia (see Fig. 13-1 B). Vertical compression and hyperflexion of the spine usually produce this injury. Trauma to the cervical vertebrae (C5 or above) may result in quadriplegia. Injuries between C5 and C7 in the cervical vertebrae may produce varying degrees of **paresis** to the shoulders and arms. Damage occurring above C3 is usually fatal. The usual cause of this fatal injury is hyperextension or flexion of that portion of the

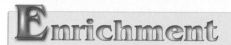

BASILAR SKULL FRACTURE

A basilar skull fracture is a fracture of the bones of the floor of the cranial vault (see Fig. 13–9). This injury usually results from a massive insult to the cranium during a motor vehicle accident or other violent trauma in which the head is struck anteriorly or laterally in the mid-portion. As with other head injuries, symptoms, signs, and treatment depend on the area involved and the extent of the fracture. **Raccoon eyes** and **Battle's sign** are manifestations of basilar skull fracture, and these signs alert the physician to order imaging of the cranial vault for further investigation. Cerebrospinal fluid (CSF) flowing from the ears or nares may be associated with a skull fracture. The level of consciousness is assessed, as are other neurologic signs. Treatment is similar to that of head injuries, with surgical intervention to relieve intracranial pressure. Occasionally, the severity of the fracture causes severing of the pituitary stalk, resulting in **panhypopituitarism**.

spine. Mechanisms of spinal cord injury are presented in Fig. 13-11.

DIAGNOSIS

A complete assessment of neurologic functioning is needed. Spinal radiographic films, MRI scans, and CT scans are ordered to determine the type and extent of injury.

TREATMENT

The goals of treatment of all spinal cord injuries include restoration of the normal alignment and stability of the spine; decompression of the spinal cord, nerves, and vertebrae; and early rehabilitation of the patient. These goals may involve surgery or using specialized medications and procedures. The prognosis for a person with a spinal cord injury always is guarded. However, the earlier treatment is begun, the better the prognosis.

403

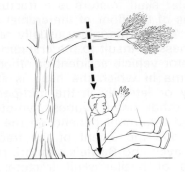

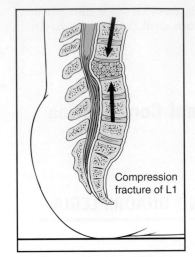

Compression of vertebrae

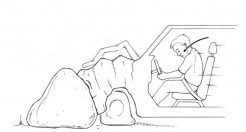

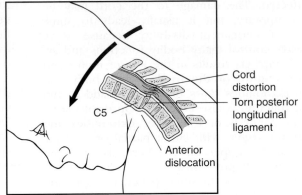

Hyperflexion of neck

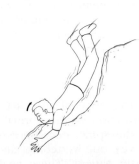

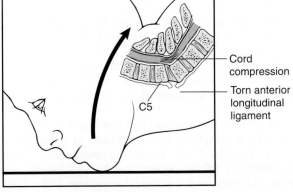

Hyperextension of spine

Figure 13–11

Spinal injuries.

Intervertebral Disk Disorders

DEGENERATIVE DISK DISEASE

SYMPTOMS AND SIGNS

The degeneration or deterioration of the intervertebral disk results in pain in the areas served by the spinal nerves of the involved disk space. The pain radiates down the nerve path, is burning and constant, and can become **intractable.** The constant back pain and severe pain that radiates down one or both legs may be accompanied by loss of some motor functions in the legs.

ETIOLOGY

The degeneration usually is mechanical and is the result of constant wearing on the disk. A misalignment of the vertebrae causes a continual rubbing on the disk involved, resulting in inflammation and gradual destruction of the disk. The inflammation eventually involves the spinal nerve roots and causes scarring. A sequela is spinal **stenosis,** in which the nerve roots become trapped in the **foramen** as they leave the spinal canal.

DIAGNOSIS

The clinical picture and a history of previous back involvement leads to investigation with various types of imaging, including radiographic films, CT scan, MRI scan, and myelogram with contrast to show the disk status. The narrowing of the intervertebral spaces is consistent with the condition. **Electromyogram** (EMG) and neurologic testing demonstrate the involvement of dependent nerves and also measure the nerve conduction. The observation of neurologic deficits, including footdrop and the dragging of a leg when walking, adds to suspicion of the degeneration.

TREATMENT

Conservative treatment involves resting the back and lower extremities. Bracing the back is helpful. Analgesics and nonsteroidal anti-inflammatory drugs (NSAIDs) are prescribed for pain relief. Surgical intervention includes spinal fusion and freeing of the spinal nerve roots from entrapment. In severe cases, nerve blocks, the use of **transcutaneous electrical nerve stimulation (TENS)** units, or a continuous infusion of morphine, by pump, into the epidural space may be employed to treat intractable pain.

HERNIATED AND BULGING DISK

SYMPTOMS AND SIGNS

Intervertebral disks are soft pads of cartilage located between each of the vertebrae that make up the spine. Each disk acts as a shock-absorbing cushion for the vertebrae and gives the back its flexibility for movement. Within each of these disks is a gelatinous center called the nucleus pulposus, which is surrounded by a circular wall-like structure, an annulus. A herniated disk, also known as a ruptured or slipped disk, is the rupture of the nucleus pulposus through the annular wall of the disk and into the spinal canal (Fig. 13-12 *A* and *C*). The nucleus pulposus is contained within the annular wall in a bulging disk (Fig. 13-12 *B*), thus the protrusion into the spinal canal is not as severe. The rupture can cause severe back pain and even disability if it presses against or pinches the spinal nerves. Sudden, sharp pain that worsens with movement results. It may radiate from the back to the buttocks, thigh, and leg following the distribution of the impinged nerve and causing paresthesia and muscle weakness in the leg. When this pain results from pinching of the sciatic nerve, it is known as sciatica (Fig. 13-13). Most herniated disks occur in the lower back, between the fourth and fifth lumbar vertebrae or the fifth lumbar and first sacral vertebrae (lumbosacral area). Ruptured disks in the cervical region of the spine often produce pain and weakness in the arms and neck. Pain from injury to a disk can be either unilateral or bilateral. A herniated disk is a serious condition and necessitates immediate medical attention. It occurs more often in men than in women.

ETIOLOGY

Herniated and bulging intervertebral disks usually result from accumulated trauma (e.g., improper body mechanics when lifting) or sudden impact. Poor posture and the aging process can cause the disks to degenerate. The rupture may occur at the time of the trauma or shortly thereafter.

DIAGNOSIS

A thorough history of the back pain is important. Physical examination of the back is performed to rule out other causes of the patient's symptoms. The diagnosis of lumbar disk hernia-

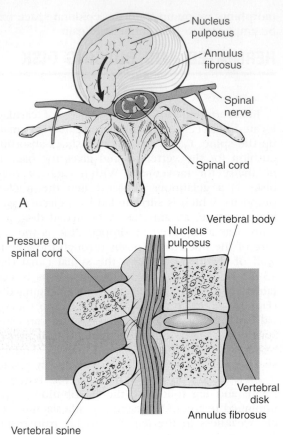

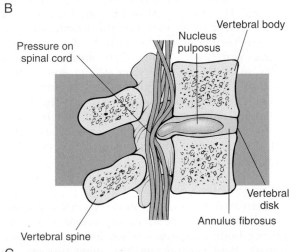

A, Herniated disk. Nucleus pulposus protrudes through annulus fibrosus, putting pressure on spinal cord and spinal nerve. B, Bulging disk (lateral view). Nucleus pulposus contained in annulus fibrosus. C, Herniated disk (lateral view). Nucleus pulposus through annular wall (annulus fibrosus) and pressure on the spinal cord.

406

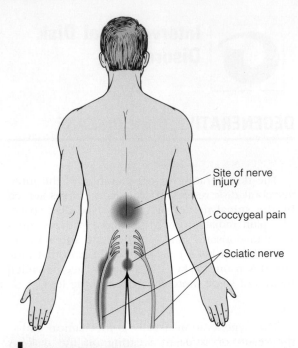

Figure 13–13

Radiation of sciatic nerve pain.

tion can be considered if the patient has sciatic pain when the physician performs a straight leg raising test. The physician may order a CT scan, an MRI study, or a myelogram to help to confirm the diagnosis.

In a bulging or contained disk herniation, the disk material is herniated through the inner annulus but not the outer annulus, so the contained material can still distort the path of the nerve with resulting pain. In more severe herniation, which is considered noncontained, the nucleus pulposus penetrates both the inner and outer layers of the annulus.

TREATMENT

Conservative treatment consists of bed rest for 24 to 48 hours, traction, the use of hot or cold packs, and the administration of muscle relaxants and analgesics, such as aspirin and ibuprofen. A back brace for a herniated lumbosacral disk or a cervical collar for a herniated cervical disk may prove beneficial in relieving some of the discomfort.

When conservative treatment is not successful, surgical excision of the herniated disk may be needed. Procedures include percutaneous diskectomy, in which a needle is introduced into the intravertebral space and the encroaching portion of the nucleus pulposus is aspirated (for uncomplicated disk herniation); microdiskectomy, involving a small surgical incision, allowing the offending material to be aspirated; diskectomy as a surgical procedure combined with laser ablation and evaporation of the disk; or removal of the disk along with a laminectomy with fusion of the vertebrae.

Some patients may be treated with an enzyme called chymopapain. It is injected directly into the disk with the hope that it will dissolve the nucleus pulposus. This process is called chemonucleolysis and is considered controversial because of potentially serious complications, namely paralysis of a leg or an arm or death from anaphylactic shock.

Often pain from bulging disks resolves with rest and drug therapy.

SCIATIC NERVE INJURY—SPINAL STENOSIS

SYMPTOMS AND SIGNS

Sciatic nerve injury is a pathologic condition. It is brought about by trauma, degeneration, or rupture of the nucleus pulposus within intervertebral disks L4 through S1. The degeneration or rupture of the nucleus pulposus exerts pressure directly on the sciatic nerve, or on other closely positioned spinal nerves, sending impulses down the sciatic nerve. Rupture of one or more disks or their nuclei produces severe, sharp pain radiating from the sciatic nerve down the leg and to the foot (see Fig. 13-13). The pain may be continuous or intermittent, and areas of the skin supplied by the affected nerves may feel numb. A rupture of the nucleus pulposus posteriorly, toward the neural canal, results in pressure on the sciatic nerve and causes low back pain. Anterior or lateral ruptures may or may not produce symptoms. Resulting symptoms depend on the extent of the rupture, the proximity of the nerves to the site, and the strength of the muscles and ligaments surrounding the spine. Nerve injury can produce severe disability, which may be temporary or permanent. Persons with sciatic nerve involvement may be so uncomfortable that they are unable to sit or stand.

Spinal stenosis, a narrowing of the spinal canal, often is termed sciatica because of the compression on the spinal cord and spinal nerve roots. Patients with spinal stenosis also report back pain and pain radiating down the legs and in the buttocks, thighs, or calves, which increases with walking or exercise. Additionally, they may experience numbness in the same areas that is worse when standing, walking, or exercising. A weakness in the legs may be noted. Reflexes in the lower extremities often are asymmetric, and there may be decreased sensation.

ETIOLOGY

Trauma to the sciatic nerve may result from a fall, poor body mechanics, or gunshot or stab wounds. The aging process can lead to the degeneration of the disk or the nucleus pulposus. An inflammatory autoimmune response may prompt more rapid degeneration within a disk. The aging process, along with arthritic changes, may cause a narrowing of the spinal canal and the foramen where the spinal nerves exit the vertebrae. Formation of osteophytes on the foramen where the spinal nerves exit also can cause pain that radiates down the leg. A congenital narrowing of the spinal canal also may be involved.

DIAGNOSIS

After a medical history is obtained and physical examination is performed, the physician may order several diagnostic tests. These tests include spinal radiographic films, MRI scan, CT scan, myelogram or diskogram, and blood serum studies. Vascular integrity is assessed and insufficiency ruled out. Often a radiograph of the spine shows degenerative changes along with a narrowed spinal canal. EMG studies may show neurologic changes.

TREATMENT

Conservative treatment may include bed rest on a firm mattress for 24 to 48 hours, the use of a back brace, ultrasound diathermy with massage, and iontophoresis. After the acute pain and inflammation have subsided, an exercise program to strengthen the back and abdominal muscles may be ordered. Drug therapy consists of analgesics (e.g., aspirin [acetylsalicylic acid, ASA] and acetaminophen [Tylenol]), muscle relaxants (e.g., diazepam [Valium] and methocarbamol [Robaxin]), and anti-inflammatory medications (e.g., piroxicam [Feldene], ibuprofen [Motrin, Advil, and Nuprin], and naproxen [Naprosyn]). For severe pain not controlled by the aforementioned medications, narcotic drugs (e.g., meperidine [Demerol], codeine, morphine, and oxycodone-aspirin [Percodan]) may be necessary.

Physical therapy, including applications of heat and cold or gentle massage (myofascial release), may help with acute pain. Corticosteroid

407

injections may relieve pain; however, they will not cure the spinal stenosis or sciatica. Often, leaning forward while sitting relieves the pain in the back.

Disabling pain or increasing weakness may necessitate surgical intervention. If a disk is causing the pain, then removal of part or all of the disk or nucleus pulposus (diskectomy or microdiskectomy), spinal fusion, or chemical dissolving, by an enzyme, of the nucleus pulposus (chemonucleolysis) may be helpful. Surgery may not relieve low back pain caused by underlying conditions such as osteoarthritis.

Functional Disorders

HEADACHE

SYMPTOMS AND SIGNS

A headache (**cephalalgia**) is pain in the head that is not confined to any one nerve distribution area. It may be acute or chronic and located in the frontal, temporal, or occipital regions of the head. Cephalalgia also may be confined to only one side of the head or over one or both eyes. The type of pain may vary from dull and aching to almost unbearable. It can be an intense intermittent pain, throbbing pain, pressure pain, or penetrating pain driving through the head. Brain tissues themselves never ache because they do not contain sensory nerves; however, meninges do have pain receptors. Sensitivity in this area exists in only the meninges, the skin and muscles covering the skull, and many nerves that travel from the brain to the head and face.

Headaches are commonly experienced and usually are self-limiting. Cephalalgia is sometimes a symptom of an underlying disorder or disease (e.g., hypertension, stroke, brain tumor, and **encephalitis**). In most cases, however, headaches are caused by nothing more serious than fatigue or tension.

Some types of headaches are not symptoms of underlying disorders but are considered a specific disease. One of these is the cluster headache in which the pain is generally severe, developing around or behind one eye. The affected eye may tear. Cluster headaches usually occur at night and continue occurring for several weeks

or months, then disappear for some time, even years. Another example of a severe type of headache is the migraine (see Migraine).

ETIOLOGY

Many factors can irritate the pain-sensitive tissues or structures in the head, either alone or in combination, and produce headaches. Examples are stress, too little or too much sleep, overeating or drinking, a stuffy or noisy environment, and heavy physical labor, either indoors or outdoors. From a physiologic standpoint, however, there are actually only two causes of headaches. The first cause is strain on facial, neck, and scalp muscles resulting from tension. This is called a tension headache. The second cause is edema within the blood vessels of the head, which results in change in arterial size. This is called a vascular headache.

DIAGNOSIS

The medical history is vitally important in identifying a pattern to the headaches and is helpful in detecting any underlying causes. Physical examination and neurologic testing are necessary if a recurring pattern of headaches is revealed. Cranial and spinal radiographic films, an EEG, and a cranial CT scan may be ordered to rule out organic causes.

TREATMENT

The cause of the headache determines the type of treatment chosen. If the physician does not find an underlying cause of the headache, the use of **analgesics** (e.g., aspirin, acetaminophen, and NSAIDs), muscle relaxants, minor tranquilizers, and muscle massages, and relaxation with a warm bath are effective in providing temporary relief from a headache.

MIGRAINE

SYMPTOMS AND SIGNS

Periodic severe headaches that may be completely incapacitating and almost always are accompanied by other symptoms, such as nausea and vomiting, **anorexia,** intense hemicranial or bilateral throbbing pain, and visual signs and symptoms, are known as migraine headaches. Before the onset of the headache, many persons who experience migraine headaches have visual **auras:** flashing lights, zigzagging lines, or areas of total darkness. Photophobia is another warning sign. The nature of each attack varies from person to person, but there is usually a warning period during which the person feels abnormally fatigued and irritable. Other less common symptoms that occur occasionally are numbness or tingling in one arm or one side of the body, dizziness, and temporary mental confusion.

These headaches may begin in adolescence or early adulthood, become less frequent and intense with age, and affect women nearly twice as frequently as men.

ETIOLOGY

Despite much medical research, it is not known why some people are subject to migraines or what triggers them. Certain factors do appear to be involved in many cases. Susceptibility to migraines, for instance, tends to appear in families, leading to a strong suspicion of inherited or genetic aspects of the disorder. In some cases, certain foods (e.g., aged cheese, chocolate, and red wine) have been found to provoke an attack.

The biologic cause of migraines may be changes in the cerebral blood flow. This is presumably attributable to vasoconstriction followed by vasodilation of the cerebral and cranial arteries.

DIAGNOSIS

A medical history of recurring, severe headaches, preceded by any combination of the aforementioned symptoms or signs, suggests the diagnosis. An EEG, a CT scan, and possibly an MRI scan may be ordered to rule out any organic conditions.

TREATMENT

In some cases, the treatment is simply bed rest in a quiet, darkened room and the administration of analgesics at the first sign of attack. For other patients, drug therapy in the form of vasoconstrictors, to constrict dilated blood vessels, and **antiemetics,** to control vomiting, may be needed. The use of **ergot** preparations has been effective for some patients in forestalling an impending attack or lessening the symptoms of an ongoing attack. Beta-blocking drugs and tricyclic antidepressant drugs can be prescribed. Sumatriptan succinate (Imitrex) is used for pain relief. Relaxation therapy or biofeedback has been used successfully to lessen the number of migraines for some people.

EPILEPSY

SYMPTOMS AND SIGNS

Epilepsy is a chronic brain disorder, characterized by sudden episodes of abnormal intense electrical activity in the brain, which result in seizure activity. The recurring seizures may entail involuntary contractions of muscles (convulsions) with disturbances of consciousness and sensory phenomena. Epilepsy takes many forms, with a variety of manifestations; there are more than 30 types of seizures, and it is possible to have more than one type. Epileptic seizures are classified as partial or generalized. Status epilepticus is a complication of prolonged seizure activity.

Partial seizures do not involve the entire brain but arise from a localized area in the brain. The effects may involve the hand or face, with motor signs such as a rhythmic twitching of a group of muscles or compulsive lip smacking or picking at clothing. Behavioral, psychic, and sensory manifestations (auras) can occur. There is usually amnesia of the attack. However, there is not loss of consciousness.

Generalized seizures cause a diffuse electrical abnormality within the brain and include absence (petit mal) and tonic–clonic (grand mal) attacks. Absence seizures, also called petit mal epilepsy, consist of a brief change in the level of consciousness indicated by staring, blinking, or blankly staring, with loss of awareness of surroundings. The episodes last only a few seconds and can occur many times a day, if not treated. Absence seizures occur most often in children and young adults.

Tonic–clonic seizures (grand mal epilepsy) may begin with a loud cry, followed by falling to the ground and loss of consciousness. During the tonic phase, the body stiffens and the tongue may be bitten. Prolonged contraction of the respiratory muscles causes the patient to become **cyanotic.** Then there are generalized rhythmic muscle spasms followed by relaxation, the clonic phase. The patient may be incontinent of urine and feces. The seizure subsides in 1 to 2 minutes, but consciousness may be regained slowly. The person may be drowsy, confused, and weak; report headache; and have no memory of the event.

Status epilepticus occurs when one seizure follows another with no recovery of consciousness between attacks. This is considered a medical emergency that requires immediate anticonvulsant therapy to prevent cerebral anoxia, hyperpyrexia, vascular collapse, and even death.

ETIOLOGY

In idiopathic epilepsy, there is no apparent cause for the abnormal electrical discharge, although there may be a greater frequency in some families.

In symptomatic epilepsy, a known abnormality in the brain resulting from a pathologic process, genetic or acquired, seems to trigger seizures. Pathologic conditions associated with seizure disorder include scar tissue on the cerebral cortex from infection or trauma, cortical **neoplasms,** cerebral edema, and CVAs (strokes). Others are birth trauma (cerebral palsy), drug toxicity (e.g., alcohol), and other conditions that deprive the brain of oxygen.

DIAGNOSIS

Not all seizures imply epilepsy; thus a medical history is essential. An EEG shows semispecific brain activity, suggesting epilepsy; MRI also may be helpful. Classification of epilepsy is based on the location of the abnormal activity and its dura-

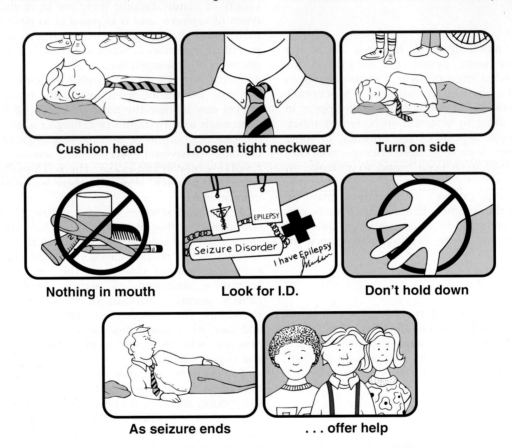

Cushion head   **Loosen tight neckwear**   **Turn on side**

Nothing in mouth   **Look for I.D.**   **Don't hold down**

As seizure ends   **. . . offer help**

Most seizures in people with epilepsy are not medical emergencies. They end after a minute or two without harm and usually do not require a trip to the emergency room.

But sometimes there are good reasons to call for emergency help. A seizure in someone who does not have epilepsy could be a sign of serious illness.

Other reasons to call an ambulance include:

- A seizure that lasts more than 5 minutes
- No "epilepsy" or "seizure disorder" I.D.
- Slow recovery, a second seizure, or difficult breathing afterward
- Pregnancy or other medical I.D.
- Any signs of injury or sickness

Figure 13–14

First aid for seizures. (From Epilepsy Foundation of America, Landover, MD, 1990.)

tion. CT scan shows structural changes in the brain, such as tumors, scars, and malformations. Cerebral angiography may identify vascular changes in the brain. A skull radiographic film may reveal evidence of fracture, separation of cranial sutures, or movement of the pineal gland. Blood serum chemistry changes may indicate metabolic disease, drug toxicity, or hypoglycemia.

TREATMENT

Anticonvulsant medications are the treatment of choice for epilepsy; more commonly used drugs include phenytoin (Dilantin), carbamazepine (Tegretol), primidone (Mysoline), and valproate. Close monitoring and adjustments of dosage for good therapeutic control are essential. In rare cases, surgical intervention may be necessary to excise an identifiable lesion in the brain. Certain restrictions may be necessary. For instance, depending on state regulations, a license to drive a motor vehicle may not be issued unless the person has been seizure free, with treatment, for a specific period. Emotional support for the patient and the family is made available. Because this disease often is feared and misunderstood, education is necessary to dispel myths. First aid instructions are available for grand mal seizures (Fig. 13–14).

PARKINSON'S DISEASE

SYMPTOMS AND SIGNS

Parkinson's disease is a common, slowly progressive neurologic disorder characterized by the onset of recognizable disturbances: a "pill-rolling" tremor of the thumb and forefinger, muscular rigidity, slowness of movement, and postural instability. Usually **insidious** in onset, the symptoms, which vary from person to person, may be associated with aging until the recognizable paradigm of Parkinson's disease emerges. The posture is stooped, and the patient moves with a peculiar shuffling gait: the head is bowed, the body is flexed forward, the knees are slightly bent, and there is a tendency to fall (Fig. 13–15). The face takes on a mask-like or expressionless appearance, speech is muffled, and swallowing is difficult. Gradual changes in behavior and mental activity are noted in some patients as the disease progresses. The mean age of onset is 60 years, but there are many cases in younger persons. Parkinson's disease afflicts more men than women, and the usual life span after diagnosis is 10 years.

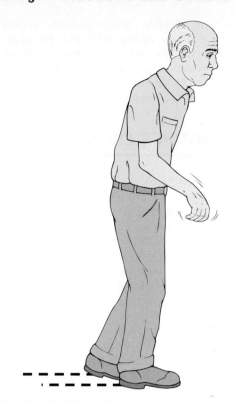

Figure 13–15
Typical shuffling gait and posture of Parkinson's disease.

ETIOLOGY

It is not known what causes degeneration of nerves in the motor system of the brain stem. A deficiency of dopamine, a **neurotransmitter** manufactured in the midbrain, has been clinically demonstrated in patients with Parkinson's disease. Parkinsonism (as a syndrome) also occurs in poisoning, after encephalitis, and in patients given certain major tranquilizers and certain antihypertensive drugs.

DIAGNOSIS

The diagnosis is made from the characteristic history and careful neurologic examination. Decreased dopamine levels may be noted in the urine.

TREATMENT

Parkinson's disease cannot be cured; therefore, medical management consists of supportive measures and control of symptoms with the administration of drugs such as levodopa, carbidopa, antidepressants, and anticholinergics for tremor and rigidity. Many patients report improvement when taking deprenyl. Physical therapy helps the patient to maximize his or her mobility within the limitations of the disease. The patient is given every possible supportive measure to encourage independence and self-care.

HUNTINGTON'S CHOREA

SYMPTOMS AND SIGNS

Huntington's chorea (Huntington's disease) is a hereditary degenerative disease of the cerebral cortex and basal ganglia; progressive atrophy of the brain occurs. The chronic, progressive chorea (ceaseless, uncontrolled, involuntary movements) has an insidious onset, with the loss of musculoskeletal control exhibited by subtle, semipurposeful movements. Typically, the arms and face are the first areas to be involved, with movements ranging from mild fidgets to tongue smacking. Speech difficulties are experienced and the emotional state deteriorates, followed by dementia. There is a disruption in the personality displayed by the untidy and careless appearance of the individual. Personality changes are noted by apathetic, moody behavior, a loss of memory, and onset of paranoia. The onset of symptoms typically is in early middle age.

ETIOLOGY

Although the exact etiology of this condition is uncertain, it is transmitted by an **autosomal**-dominant trait that can be inherited by either sex.

DIAGNOSIS

There is no definitive way to diagnose this condition, except through careful neurologic appraisal and by detection of the defective gene through DNA analysis. A history of progressive chorea and dementia, along with a familial trait, leads to further investigation. A cerebral CT scan shows brain atrophy.

TREATMENT

There is no cure for this progressively deteriorating condition; therefore, treatment is supportive, symptomatic, and protective. Haloperidol lactate (Haldol) and fluphenazine hydrochloride (Prolixin) are prescribed in an attempt to control choreic movements and to reduce agitation. Eventually, institutionalization may be necessary to provide the necessary care for the deteriorating condition of the patient.

AMYOTROPHIC LATERAL SCLEROSIS

SYMPTOMS AND SIGNS

Amyotrophic lateral sclerosis (ALS), also known as Lou Gehrig's disease, is a progressive, destructive motor neuron disease with resulting muscular atrophy. Fasciculations (small local involuntary muscular contractions) and accompanying atrophy and weakness are noted in the forearms and hands. These patients progress to difficulties in speech, chewing, swallowing, and breathing; eventually, a ventilator is required. There is no sensory neuron involvement, and the mind is not affected. ALS characteristically affects men slightly more often than women, with onset after the age of 50 to 60 years.

ETIOLOGY

Although the etiology of ALS is uncertain, some cases may be caused by autosomal inherited traits.

DIAGNOSIS

The clinical picture of upper and lower motor neuron involvement without any sensory neuron involvement leads to further investigation. EMG and muscle **biopsy** are employed to confirm nerve, not muscle, involvement. Over a period of several months, the diagnosis is confirmed by the typical progression of the disease.

TREATMENT

With no known cure for the condition, a team approach to treatment consists of supportive measures and control of symptoms. Death usually occurs within 6 to 10 years after onset. Pulmonary management is vital.

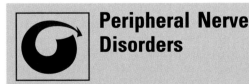

Peripheral Nerve Disorders

PERIPHERAL NEURITIS

SYMPTOMS AND SIGNS

Peripheral neuritis, the degeneration of peripheral nerves, affects the distal muscles of the extremities. Unless the precipitating factors are severe infection or chronic alcohol intoxication, the onset is insidious. Clumsiness and loss of sensation in the hands and feet are followed by a flaccid paralysis and a wasting of muscles in these areas. Deep tendon reflexes become diminished, and there is a tenderness in the atrophied muscles. The skin may take on a glossy, red appearance, and sweating is decreased. With leg and foot involvement, footdrop may be experienced. Some patients have pain in the affected regions.

ETIOLOGY

Chronic alcohol intoxication; toxicity from arsenic, lead, carbon disulfide, benzene, or phosphorus; infectious diseases, including mumps, pneumonia, and diphtheria; metabolic or inflammatory disorders, including diabetes, rheumatoid arthritis, gout, and systemic lupus erythematosus; and certain nutritional deficiency diseases are all causative factors. The nerve degeneration leads to muscle weakness and sensory loss.

DIAGNOSIS

The history, combined with the clinical picture of characteristic motor and sensory involvement, leads to additional investigation. Motor and sensory nerve impairment usually is detected by EMG.

TREATMENT

The first step in effective treatment is to ascertain the cause and, if possible, to correct or eliminate the condition. **Toxic** substances need to be removed, if possible, and vitamin and nutritional deficits corrected. Underlying disease processes are treated or controlled. When chronic alcoholism is the cause, the patient must avoid all alcohol in any form. Supportive measures, such as the administration of anticonvulsants and tricyclic antidepressants, rest, and physical therapy, are employed to relieve pain.

TRIGEMINAL NEURALGIA (TIC DOULOUREUX)

SYMPTOMS AND SIGNS

Trigeminal neuralgia, or tic douloureux, is pain of the area innervated by the fifth cranial nerve, the trigeminal nerve. The transient, excruciating pain radiates along the fifth cranial nerve distribution and can affect any of the three branches (Fig. 13-16). When the ophthalmic branch is affected, pain is experienced in the eye and forehead. The maxillary branch involves the

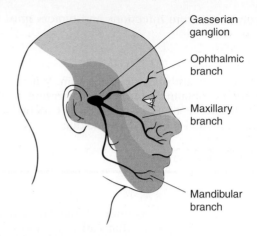

Figure 13–16
Trigeminal nerve (fifth cranial nerve) and branches.

nose, upper lip, and cheek. The mandibular branch involves the lower lip, the outer portion of the tongue, and the area of the cheek close to the ear. Additionally, there may be involvement of several branches. The pain is always unilateral and does not cross midline because only one side of the face is involved. The abrupt and sudden onset of pain is triggered by mechanical or thermal stimulation. These persons sleep poorly and may be undernourished and dehydrated because chewing, swallowing, or any touching of the area may set off the pain.

ETIOLOGY

The cause is uncertain, although some cases have been found to be related to compression of a nerve root by a tumor or vascular lesion. Occasionally, trigeminal neuralgia is a sequela to multiple sclerosis or herpes zoster. Most cases have no identified cause.

DIAGNOSIS

The reports of an excruciating pain that has an abrupt onset and a duration of seconds to minutes on one side of the face suggest trigeminal neuralgia. Observation of the patient, both during an attack and at normal times, demonstrates the presence of pain. The patient avoids touching the face to prevent triggering an attack. Because a draft or breeze may set off the pain, the face is protected and temperature extremes are avoided. No impairment of sensory or motor function is noted. The episodes may last from months to years and then subside. Sinus or tooth

413

involvement from infections and tumors must be ruled out.

TREATMENT

Analgesics are prescribed for pain. When relief cannot be obtained, surgical intervention to dissect the nerve roots is performed. Patients who smoke are advised to avoid smoking.

BELL'S PALSY

SYMPTOMS AND SIGNS

Bell's palsy is a disorder of the facial nerve (seventh cranial nerve) that causes a sudden onset of weakness or paralysis of facial muscles. The severity of paralysis varies widely. The patient may be aware of pain or a drawing sensation behind the ear, followed by an inability to open or close the eye and drooping of the mouth with drooling of saliva. Frequently, the disorder is first noticed in the morning, having developed overnight. Initially, the patient is unable to smile, whistle, or grimace, and the facial expression is distorted (Fig. 13–17). Taste perception may be diminished, contributing to loss of appetite. The condition is usually unilateral. It may be transient or permanent and usually occurs between 20 and 60 years of age, in men and women alike.

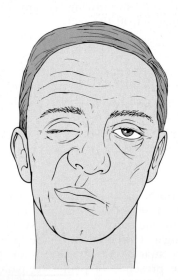

Figure 13–17

Bell's palsy. Note on the affected side that the forehead is not wrinkled, the eye does not close completely, and the mouth is drooping.

ETIOLOGY

The cause of Bell's palsy is not always certain. The symptoms result from blockage of impulses from the facial nerve (cranial nerve VII) caused by compression of the nerve in the bony canal. Bilateral facial paralysis has been noted in a small percentage of people with Lyme disease.

DIAGNOSIS

Bell's palsy is diagnosed from symptoms and signs and the characteristic history. The differential diagnosis includes CVA (stroke) and autoimmune disease.

TREATMENT

Early treatment is critical. The application of warm moist heat, gentle massage, and facial exercises to stimulate muscle tone are recommended. Prednisone may be prescribed to reduce edema of the facial nerve. Analgesics also may be required. Inability to close the eye may result in dry, sore eyes; artificial tears and an eye patch for protection from outside elements may be needed unless the case is mild. Electrotherapy stimulates the nerve and prevents atrophy of muscles. Complete recovery is possible if the disease is treated early, and recovery frequently occurs spontaneously, especially in younger individuals. Patients who smoke are advised to avoid smoking.

 Infectious Disorders

MENINGITIS

SYMPTOMS AND SIGNS

Meningitis is an inflammation of the meninges, the membranous coverings of the brain and spinal cord. Early symptoms include vomiting and a headache that increases in intensity with movement or shaking of the head. Attempts of the examiner to move the head reveal **nuchal rigidity,** a stiffness of the neck that resists any sideward or flexion-extension movements of the head; this is a classic sign. Positive Kernig's sign (resistance to leg extension after flexing the thigh on the body) and Brudzinski's sign (neck flexion causes flexion of the hips from a supine position) indicate meningeal irritation. Deep tendon reflexes increase, and the patient exhibits irritability, photophobia, and a hypersensitivity of the skin. Seizures caused by cortical irritation can be late manifestations of the process. Drowsiness may progress to stupor and coma.

ETIOLOGY

The infection can originate directly from the brain, spinal cord, or sinuses. Open head injuries are additional portals of entry for the offending bacteria. *Haemophilus influenzae, Neisseria meningitidis,* and *Streptococcus pneumoniae* are the bacteria responsible for most meningeal infections; however, the causative microorganism can be either bacterial or viral.

DIAGNOSIS

The clinical picture alerts the physician to the possibility of meningitis. A diagnostic **lumbar puncture** reveals increased cerebrospinal fluid (CSF) pressure and the presence of **white blood cells** (WBCs), protein, and glucose in the CSF. Culture of the CSF with resulting growth of microbes confirms the diagnosis. The CSF may appear cloudy because of the presence of the WBCs.

TREATMENT

Meningitis is treated aggressively with intravenous antibiotic therapy. Anticonvulsive drugs are administered to control seizure activity. Aspirin or acetaminophen are given for the headache. Stimuli are kept at a minimum; the room is kept dark and quiet.

ENCEPHALITIS

SYMPTOMS AND SIGNS

Encephalitis, an inflammation of the brain tissue, may have an insidious or sudden onset. Primary symptoms include a headache and elevated temperature. The patient experiences a stiffness in the neck and back, muscular weakness, restlessness, visual disturbances, and lethargy. Mental confusion progresses to disorientation and even coma.

ETIOLOGY

The inflammation leads to cerebral edema and subsequent cell destruction. It is caused by viruses or the toxins from chickenpox, measles, or mumps. Most cases are the result of a bite from an infected mosquito. Eastern equine, western equine, and Venezuelan equine encephalomyelitis and St. Louis encephalitis are forms of encephalitis encountered in the United States.

DIAGNOSIS

The clinical picture leads the physician to further investigation, including a lumbar puncture; the CSF pressure is elevated. Blood and CSF studies reveal the virus. The EEG is abnormal.

TREATMENT

Antiviral agents are effective against only the herpes simplex encephalitis. Otherwise, treatment is symptomatic, with mild analgesics for pain, **antipyretic** drugs for elevated temperature, anticonvulsants for seizure activity, and antibiotics for any intercurrent infection.

GUILLAIN-BARRÉ SYNDROME

SYMPTOMS AND SIGNS

Guillain-Barré syndrome is an acute, rapidly progressive disease of the spinal nerves. A numbness and tingling of the feet and hands are experienced at the onset, followed by increasing muscle pain and tenderness. Progressive muscle weakness and paralysis usually start in the lower extremities and move up the body in 24 to 72 hours. Although most patients experience an ascending paralysis occasionally, some patients have a descending weakness and paralysis. There is a potential for respiratory insufficiency as well as difficulty swallowing.

ETIOLOGY

Knowledge of the etiology is limited, but the syndrome is thought to have an autoimmune basis. The condition has been known to follow a respiratory infection or gastroenteritis in 10 to 21 days. **Demyelination** of the nerves occurs with the syndrome.

DIAGNOSIS

Confirmation is made by elevated protein level in the CSF, which peaks in 4 to 6 weeks. Leukocyte count is normal, as is CSF pressure.

TREATMENT

Hospitalization usually is required for observation. Treatment is supportive. **Plasmapheresis** washes the plasma to remove antibodies, thereby shortening the time of recovery. Intravenous human immunoglobulin may be beneficial. Prognosis varies, but recovery is usually complete.

BRAIN ABSCESS

SYMPTOMS AND SIGNS

A brain abscess, a collection of pus, can occur anywhere in the brain tissue (Fig. 13–18). The primary symptom is a headache. Other symptoms and signs depend on the location and extent of the abscess. Generally, the patient exhibits symptoms and signs of increased intracranial pressure, including nausea and vomiting, visual disturbances, unequal pupil size, and seizures. Many times, the eyes look toward the insult, moving to the side of the head where the abscess is located. Nuchal rigidity may be noted.

ETIOLOGY

CNS abscesses may be the result of a local infection or may be secondary to infections elsewhere in the body. Common causative organisms are staphylococci, streptococci, or pneumococci. Any occurrence that breaches the integrity of the CNS, including head trauma and a craniotomy wound, may be the portal of entry for the microorganisms. The abscess may be secondary to another infectious process, including sinusitis, otitis, dental abscess, subdural empyema, and bacterial endocarditis (Fig. 13–19).

DIAGNOSIS

A history of infection, especially of the sinuses or ear, or an insult to the CNS coupled with the characteristic clinical features of increased intracranial pressure suggests an abscess. An EEG and CT scans are used to verify the diagnosis. Lumbar puncture is contraindicated because the in-

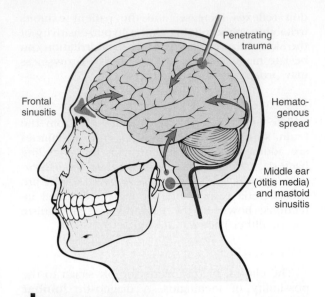

Figure 13–19

Bacterial infections of the central nervous system. Infectious organisms may reach the brain through several routes: hematogenously; by direct entry because of penetrating trauma; or by direct spread from adjacent structures, such as the inner ear or the nasal sinuses. (From Damjanov I: Pathology for the Health-Related Professions. Philadelphia: WB Saunders, 1996, p 507. Used with permission.)

creased intracranial pressure may cause the brain stem to herniate, with death resulting.

TREATMENT

Intravenous antibiotics are administered to resolve the infection. Mannitol or steroids are prescribed to reduce cerebral edema. Surgical drainage of the abscess may be necessary to relieve intracranial pressure and to culture the offending organism. Additional treatment is supportive.

POLIOMYELITIS AND POSTPOLIO SYNDROME

SYMPTOMS AND SIGNS

Poliomyelitis is a viral infection of the anterior horn cells of the gray matter of the spinal cord and a selective destruction of the motor neurons. This highly contagious disease is no longer the threat to humankind that it was before the 1960s. The Salk and Sabin vaccines have virtually eliminated poliomyelitis in the western world.

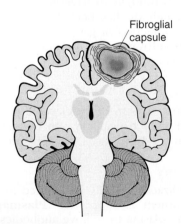

Figure 13–18

Brain abscess.

The patient with poliomyelitis has a low-grade fever, a profuse discharge from the nose, and **malaise.** These symptoms are followed by a progressive muscle weakness, stiff neck, nausea and vomiting, and a flaccid paralysis of the muscles involved. Atrophy of the muscles follows, with decreased tendon reflexes, then muscle and joint deterioration.

Poliomyelitis that involves the muscles supplied by spinal nerves is termed spinal, whereas involvement of the muscles supplied by cranial nerves (gray matter of the medulla) is termed bulbar.

ETIOLOGY

The poliovirus enters the body through the nose and throat and crosses into the gastrointestinal tract. Traveling by way of the bloodstream, the virus progresses to the CNS. The incubation period is 7 to 21 days. Poliovirus is transmitted from person to person by infected oropharyngeal secretions or feces that contain the virus.

DIAGNOSIS

The clinical symptoms along with possible exposure to an infected person are the primary tools of diagnosis. Isolation of the poliovirus from throat washings or from feces confirms the diagnosis. When the CNS is involved, cultures of CSF are positive for poliovirus.

TREATMENT

Treatment is supportive. Analgesics are administered for pain relief, along with moist heat applications. Bed rest is indicated until the acute stage is resolved. Physical therapy, including the use of braces, may be necessary. When there is respiratory involvement, respiratory support with mechanical ventilation may be necessary. Prevention by means of Sabin and Salk vaccines has rendered poliomyelitis almost nonexistent in the world.

Three distinct serotypes of poliovirus exist: types 1, 2, and 3. All three types can be found worldwide, and immunization with the Sabin trivalent oral vaccine affords immunity to all three forms. There also is a monovalent Sabin vaccine, which grants immunity to only one form, as does the Salk vaccine. Persons with **immunosuppressive** conditions should not be given the trivalent vaccine because they are at risk for contracting poliomyelitis. Additionally, any immunosuppressed person should not come in contact with feces or nasal secretions of a recently vaccinated person. Two poliovirus vaccines currently are licensed in the United States: inactivated poliovirus vaccine (IPV) and oral poliovirus vaccine (OPV).

Postpolio syndrome occurs later in life in persons who have previously experienced the disease. Functional deterioration of muscles is accompanied by loss of strength. The progressive weakness begins 30 years or more after the initial attack and involves already affected muscles. Fasciculations and muscular atrophy may accompany the weakness. Treatment is supportive, and generally the prognosis is good.

Intracranial Tumors (Brain Tumors)

Intracranial tumors are benign or malignant neoplasms, classified as primary or secondary, occurring in any structural area of the brain (Fig. 13-20). The signs and symptoms are specific to the tumor's location.

Primary tumors, benign or malignant, arise from neuroglial (connective tissue) cells that are part of intracranial brain structures. Secondary tumors, which are more common, are malignant neoplasms that **metastasize** from a primary site elsewhere in the body (e.g., lungs, breast, ovaries, colon, and pancreas). Brain tumors are named according to the tissues from which they originate.

SYMPTOMS AND SIGNS

Regardless of the type, symptoms and signs result from displacement and compression of normal brain tissue by the tumor, causing progressive neurologic deficits, expansion of the brain (cerebral edema), and increased intracranial pressure. Headaches, vomiting, dizziness, double

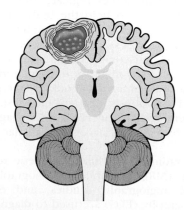

Figure 13-20
Brain tumor.

vision, and disturbances of muscle strength and coordination are likely initial symptoms and necessitate medical evaluation. Neurologic assessment findings are associated with particular regions affected by destruction of neural tissue. Changes in personality and mental function, seizures, paralysis, **aphasia,** and sensory disturbances are possible clinical manifestations. Edema of the optic nerve (papilledema) can be seen with an **ophthalmoscope.** Hydrocephalus and herniation of the brain are potential complications. Other studies may identify the primary site of a metastatic brain tumor.

ETIOLOGY

The cause of brain tumors is unknown, except as described previously.

DIAGNOSIS

Tumor localization may be determined by brain scan, cerebral angiogram, CT scan, skull radiographic films, and EEG. Lumbar puncture may reveal increased pressure in the CSF and the presence of tumor cells. A biopsy of the tumor provides important diagnostic information about the type of tumor.

TREATMENT

If operable, the brain tumor is excised. Surgery, radiation, and chemotherapy may be used in combination. Drug therapy is used to control seizures and pain. Fear, anxiety, and depression can be addressed in individual counseling or group therapy. Physical therapy and other appropriate rehabilitation is made available.

Summary

The nervous system is responsible for consciousness, memory, and intelligence; it also receives and transmits all sensory stimuli and interprets all stimuli. Other functions include controlling or influencing all muscular activities in the body and affecting glandular function. Diseases of the nervous system discussed in this chapter are related to vascular disorders, head or spinal cord trauma, infections, tumors, peripheral nerve disorders, and functional disorders.

- Neurons that make up the brain, spinal cord, and peripheral nerves regulate and coordinate body activities and help the body to adjust to the internal and external environment.
- A neurologic assessment evaluates the neurologic status and cognitive function of a person and may lead the clinician to focus further testing on a problem area as findings emerge.
- Cerebral thrombosis, cerebral embolism, or cerebral hemorrhage can result in damage to the brain referred to as a cerebrovascular accident (CVA).
- Cranial radiographic films, magnetic resonance imaging (MRI), computed tomography (CT), cerebral angiography studies, and electroencephalography (EEG) are used to diagnose cerebral vascular disorders and head trauma.
- Subdural hematomas may exhibit delayed symptoms because of a slower accumulation of blood.

- Cerebral concussion causes a temporary disruption of the normal electrical activity in the brain; a cerebral contusion or a depressed skull fracture involves brain injury.
- The site of vertebral fracture or vertebral dislocation determines the type of paralysis (quadriplegia or paraplegia).
- Degeneration of an intervertebral disk causes radiating pain down a nerve path and may be accompanied by loss of motor function.
- Injury to the sciatic nerve caused by trauma, degenerative changes, or spinal stenosis can result in severe pain and produce temporary or permanent disability.
- Cephalalgia can be (a) a benign self-limiting condition, (b) a symptom of underlying disease, or (c) considered a specific disease as in cluster headache or migraine.
- Epilepsy, a chronic brain disorder, can be idiopathic or secondary to certain pathologic conditions.
- First aid for seizures includes recognizing when it is necessary to call for emergency help.
- Parkinson's disease, a slowly progressive neurologic disorder, has recognizable disturbances; as a syndrome, parkinsonism can be triggered by certain drugs.
- Huntington's chorea refers to the onset of ceaseless, uncontrolled, involuntary movements

and loss of musculoskeletal control, followed by progressive speech difficulties and dementia.

- The clinical picture of amyotrophic lateral sclerosis (ALS), also known as Lou Gehrig's disease, reflects progressive destruction of motor neurons resulting in muscular atrophy.
- Peripheral nerve disorders include peripheral neuritis (affecting distal muscles of extremities), trigeminal neuralgia (involving severe pain along the fifth cranial nerve) and Bell's palsy (a disorder of the facial nerve causing weakness or paralysis of facial muscles).

- The causative organism of meningitis is frequently bacterial but also may be viral. Encephalitis is often viral and can be the result of a bite from an infected mosquito.
- Guillain-Barré syndrome has been known to follow a respiratory infection or gastroenteritis.
- The occurrence of brain abscess may be a local infection or secondary to infection elsewhere in the body.
- The signs and symptoms of intracranial tumors are the result of displacement and compression of normal brain tissue.

Review Challenge

REVIEW QUESTIONS

1. What does the central nervous system comprise? The peripheral nervous system?
2. What are some possible causes of disease of the nervous system?
3. How is the nervous system evaluated during a diagnostic examination?
4. What are the three vascular disorders that may result in a cerebrovascular accident (CVA)?
5. How does a transient ischemic attack (TIA) differ from a CVA?
6. What are some of the likely causes of epidural and subdural hematomas? Which condition is more likely to have a delayed onset of symptoms?
7. Which condition is more serious, a cerebral concussion or cerebral contusion? Why?
8. What is the relationship between the location of a spinal cord injury and the signs and symptoms?
9. Which diagnostic findings may indicate a degeneration or rupture of an intervertebral disk?
10. How does spinal stenosis contribute to sciatic pain?
11. Are headaches always a symptom of an underlying disease? What are some causative factors of cephalalgia?

12. What are the classic signs and symptoms of migraine?
13. What are the different types of epileptic seizures? What are the first aid guidelines?
14. What are the characteristic signs and symptoms of (a) Parkinson's disease, (b) Huntington's chorea, and (c) amyotrophic lateral sclerosis (ALS)?
15. What are some causative factors of peripheral neuritis?
16. How does a patient with trigeminal neuralgia typically describe the pain?
17. What is the clinical appearance of a person with Bell's palsy?
18. What is the diagnostic significance of nuchal rigidity in the presence of headache and photophobia?
19. What are the possible etiologic agents of encephalitis?
20. What is the pathologic progression of Guillain-Barré syndrome?
21. How do infectious organisms reach the brain? How is a brain abscess treated?
22. What is postpolio syndrome?
23. How are intracranial tumors classified, and what determines the symptomatology?

REAL-LIFE CHALLENGE

Epilepsy

A 26-year-old man was previously (2 weeks prior) in a motor vehicle accident (MVA) with closed head injury. Recovery was uneventful, and the patient was dismissed from the hospital. The patient returned to work 2 days ago. The patient's wife called the office to state that she awakened this morning to find her husband having seizure-type activity. The patient was responsive but appeared confused.

The patient was transported to a hospital.

Vital signs were T—98.4°, P—72, R—18, and BP—116/78. The patient was responsive but not oriented to time, place, or person, appearing postictal. An EEG was ordered, as was a cerebral CT scan. The patient was diagnosed with seizure activity (epilepsy) secondary to the cerebral trauma received in the previous MVA. The patient was placed on antiseizure medication and admitted for observation.

Questions

1. What patient or family teaching regarding patient activity is indicated?
2. What is the significance of the cerebral trauma to the onset of seizure activity?
3. As what type of epilepsy is this seizure activity classified?
4. Compare the three types of epilepsy as per seizure activity, treatment, and predisposing factors.
5. Which other diagnostic tests might be ordered?
6. Describe appropriate first aid intervention for a grand mal seizure patient.
7. Explain status epilepticus.

REAL-LIFE CHALLENGE

Transient Ischemic Attack (TIA)

The wife of a 67-year-old man called the office and reported that her husband awoke this morning with weakness and numbness of the right side. He had difficulty getting out of bed and complained of intermittent episodes of dizziness. He also was experiencing difficulty speaking. The patient has a history of hypertension and is taking enalapril maleate (Vasotec) and propranolol hydrochloride (Inderal). The wife was advised that her husband should be seen in an emergency care facility, and an ambulance was called for transport.

On examination in the emergency facility, the patient was found to have diminished strength in the right hand and foot, diminished movement in the right arm and leg and had slurred speech. Vitals signs were T—98.6°, P—106 and irregular, R—22, and BP—172/96. Oxygen therapy was started. Reflexes were diminished, as was pain response on the right side, including the extremities.

A cerebral MRI scan, CT scans, an EEG, skull radiographs, and an ECG were ordered. The ECG showed atrial fibrillation. Approximately 6 hours postonset, the symptoms began to resolve, with improvement in feeling and movement of the right extremities. Speech slowly became less slurred. The patient was diagnosed as having a TIA and was scheduled for follow-up evaluation. He was started on anticoagulant therapy.

Questions

1. What is the importance of the right-side involvement and slurring of speech?
2. Why would ambulance transportation to an emergency facility be recommended?
3. What is the significance of the elevated blood pressure?
4. Explain the difference between a TIA and a CVA.
5. In which area of the brain would the diminished circulation and subsequent reduced oxygenation be anticipated?
6. Why would anticoagulant therapy be prescribed?
7. Research the importance of the ECG result indicating atrial fibrillation.

RESOURCES

Epilepsy Foundation of America
4351 Garden City Dr
Landover, MD 20785
800-EFA-1000
(http://www.efa.org)

National Headache Foundation
428 W St James Place
Chicago, IL 60616
800-843-2256
800-523-8858 in Illinois
(http://www.headaches.org)

Huntington's Disease Society of America
158 West 29th St
New York, NY 10001-5300
800-345-4372
212-242-1968 in New York
(curehd@idt.net)

American Paralysis/Spinal Cord Hotline
2200 Kernan Dr
Baltimore, MD 21207
800-526-3456

American Paralysis Association
500 Morris Ave
Springfield, NJ 07081
800-225-0292
(http://www.paralysis.org)

National Spinal Cord Injury Association
545 Concord Ave, No 29
Cambridge, MA 02138-1122
800-962-9629

National Spinal Cord Injury Hotline
545 Concord Ave, No 29
Cambridge, MA 02138-1122
800-526-3456
800-638-1733 in Maryland

National Stroke Association
96 Inverness Dr East, Ste 1
Englewood, CA 80112-5112
800-STROKES

National Parkinson Foundation
1501 NW Ninth Ave
Miami, FL 33136
800-327-4545
800-433-7022 in Florida

Parkinson's Disease Foundation
Columbia University Medical Center
710 W 168th St
New York, NY 10032
800-457-6676

American Parkinson Disease Association
1250 Hylan Blvd, Ste 4-B
Staten Island, NY 10305
800-223-2132

American Brain Tumor Association
2720 River Rd, Ste 146
Des Plains, IL 60018

Guillain-Barré Syndrome Foundation International
PO Box 262
Wynnewood, PA 19096
215-667-0131
(http://www.webmast.com/gbs)

Brain Injury Association
1776 Massachusetts Ave, NW, Ste 1000
Washington, DC 20036
800-444-6443
(http://www.biausa.org)

Independent Living for the Handicapped
1301 Belmont St, NW
Washington, DC 20009
202-797-9803

The ALS Association National Office
27001 Agoura Road, Suite 150
Calabasas Hills, CA 91301-5104
818-880-9007
(http://www.alsa.org)

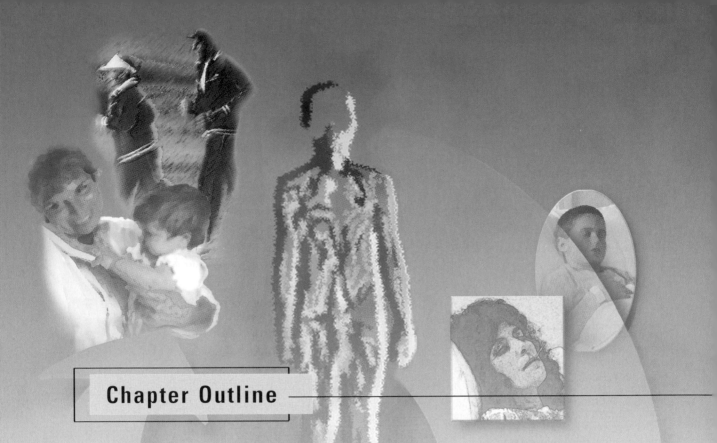

Chapter Outline

Mental Disorders

Learning Objectives

After studying Chapter 14, you should be able to:

1. Name some contributing factors to mental disorders.
2. List some of the many causes of mental retardation.
3. Describe the characteristic manifestations of autism.
4. List some examples of tic disorders.
5. Describe the progressive degenerative changes in an individual with Alzheimer's disease.
6. Explain important factors in the treatment of Alzheimer's disease.
7. Explain the cause of vascular dementia.
8. Relate treatment options for alcohol abuse.
9. Name the classic signs and symptoms of schizophrenia. Explain what is included in the multidimensional treatment plan.
10. Explain why bipolar disorder is considered a major affective disorder. Describe the treatment approach.
11. Explain the difference between reactive depression and a major depressive disorder.
12. Name the distinguishing characteristics of personality disorders.
13. Discuss how each type of anxiety disorder prevents a person from leading a normal life.
14. Explain how post-traumatic stress disorder differs from other anxiety disorders.
15. Explain how a somatization disorder is diagnosed.
16. Discuss the relationship between anxiety and conversion disorder.
17. Describe Munchausen syndrome.
18. Contrast insomnia to narcolepsy.

Key Terms

affect	(**AF**–feckt)	endarterectomy	(**end**–ar–ter–**EK**–toh–me)
amyloid	(**AM**–ih–loyd)		
autism	(**AW**–tism)	hallucination	(ha–loo–sih–**NAY**–shun)
catatonic	(kat–ah–**TOH**–nic)		
circadian	(sir–**KAY**–dee–an)	hypoxia	(**hi**–**POX**–ee–ah)
cognitive	(**KOG**–nih–tive)	ischemia	(is–**KEY**–me–ah)
deficit	(**DEAF**–ih–sit)	malinger	(ma–**LING**–er)
delusion	(dee–**LOO**–zhun)	mutism	(**MYOO**–tizm)

narcissistic	(nar–sis–**SIST**–ik)	psychotic	(sigh–**KOT**–ik)
neurosis	(noo–**ROH**–sis)	schizoid	(**SKIZ**–oyd)
paranoid	(**PAR**–ah–noid)		

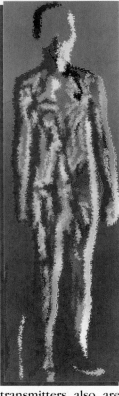

Mental Wellness and Mental Illness

At some time in life, almost every person is affected by mental disorders, either personally or by the involvement of a family member or friend. Stress is considered a contributing factor of mental disorders. Other factors are hereditary or congenital, accidental, traumatic, or drug toxicity related. Chemical imbalances in the brain and its neurotransmitters also are postulated to be causative factors. The specific causes of mental illness remain unclear in many cases.

Mental illness has been linked to stress imposed by modern society. Pressures imposed by life circumstances can be a source of personal pain and distress. Mental wellness or being in a good state of mental health is variable and a relative state of mind. When healthy individuals have the capacity to cope and adjust in a reasonable manner to the ongoing stresses of everyday life, they are considered to be in a state of mental wellness.

Psychological pain is real and intense. Subsequently, impaired or pathologic coping skills emerge in people's behavior. Some coping behaviors are conscious, and some are not easily controlled because they are unconscious. Certain disorders in thinking, perceiving, and behavior can be organized into clusters of signs and symptoms. These clusters become diagnostic criteria and a part of a total physical and psychological evaluation. The American Psychiatric Association's *Diagnostic and Statistical Manual of Mental Disorders,* fourth edition (DSM-IV), is the accepted reference that offers guidelines for criteria used in the clinical setting when diagnosing a mental disorder. In addition to diagnostic criteria, the DSM-IV provides the practitioner a standardized diagnosis code, similar to the ICD-9 (International Classification of Diseases, 9th rev) coding system.

Mental disorders include those of congenital and hereditary origins. Other categories such as maladaptive disorders, phobias, anxiety, depression, addiction, and psychotic disorders have uncertain or unknown causes and possibly more than one contributing factor. Mental disorders cause mild to severe disruption in a person's ability to function in interpersonal relationships, self-care, and occupational settings. In some disorders, the person may experience psychotic symptoms that are incapacitating.

Some mental disorders, in which oxygen and nutrient deprivation with necrosis result in the death of brain cells, are permanent and cannot be reversed. Supportive therapy or custodial care often are the only interventions available.

Modern therapeutic approaches include control of symptoms with psychotropic drugs, including antipsychotic drugs, antidepressants, anxiolytics (antianxiety agents), central nervous system (CNS) stimulants, and antimanic agents; hospitalization during acute episodes; psychotherapy; and group therapy. Outpatient treatment is available and preferred in many cases.

 Mental Retardation

Mental retardation, or developmental disability, is not a disease but a wide range of conditions with many causes. There is an interference with the developmental processes, resulting in alterations in the acquisition of intellectual skills and adaptive functioning in a variety of areas, including social and interpersonal skills, self-care, communication, self-direction, health, and safety. Additionally, there is a reduced level of behavioral performance. General intellectual functioning is subaverage, and there are noticeable deficits in adaptive behavior. This condition is manifested during the developmental period and before the age of 18 years.

SYMPTOMS AND SIGNS

During early childhood, persons with mild intellectual impairment often appear normal because there are no obvious physical defects. The first indication may be observed at school, when there appears to be a failure to progress intellectually and socially at a normal rate. Persons who have an underlying condition that is responsible for the impairment usually exhibit early symptoms of the underlying condition (e.g., Down syndrome). Occasionally, delayed development of communication and motor skills is suspected; however, confirmation of the disability is not obtained until the child enters school. Delayed adaptive behavior, coupled with difficulties with schoolwork, leads to further evaluation and the diagnosis of mental retardation.

ETIOLOGY

Mental retardation has numerous causes, many of which are unidentifiable. The predisposing factors include heredity (inborn errors of metabolism, genetic disorders, or chromosomal abnormalities); early alterations of embryonic development (Down syndrome or damage from **toxins**); prenatal, perinatal, or postnatal conditions (prematurity, **hypoxia,** viral infections, or trauma); general medical conditions (infections, trauma, or poisoning); and environmental influences. Any condition that compromises the

blood supply to the developing brain, depriving it of oxygen and nutrients, can result in neurologic damage and mental retardation. Some examples are placental insufficiency, cord or head compression during the perinatal period, failure to breathe at birth, prematurity, and viral infections of the mother in the prenatal period or of the infant or child after birth. Trauma of any type that causes hypoxia or anoxia also may contribute to the deficit.

DIAGNOSIS

Diagnosis involves observation and confirmation of the intellectual capabilities and adaptive behavior of the child. A lack of control of emotions and reduced socialization skills are noted. Intellectual testing using standardized tests, such as Wechsler Intelligence Scales for Children—Revised, Stanford-Binet, and Kaufman Assessment Battery for Children, to score an intelligence quotient (IQ) also is considered. Acceptable terminology for intelligence testing based on the IQ determined by the Binet test is:

110 to 90—average
70 to 50—mild retardation
50 to 35—moderate retardation
35 to 20—severe retardation
Below 20—profound retardation

The IQ measurement is only one factor considered, and slight error can occur in testing; therefore, allowances should be made for borderline scores, and possible testing with other instruments should be considered before a diagnosis is made.

Criteria for the diagnosis of mental retardation include subaverage general intellectual functioning accompanied by significant limitations in adaptive functioning. There must be limitations in at least two of the following areas: communication, home living, self-care, social or interpersonal skills, self-direction, and health and safety. Onset must be before 18 years of age.

TREATMENT

Once the deficit occurs, the brain cells die and cannot be restored. However, the child can be trained and, in some cases, even educated to perform various level tasks. Underlying causes should be treated, and intervention may prevent or delay progression of the condition.

Many mildly to moderately retarded persons are able to function in society. Patients whose retardation is severe or profound may be institutionalized for needed daily care.

Learning Disorders

SYMPTOMS AND SIGNS

The person with learning disorders exhibits difficulty in acquiring a skill in a specific area of learning, such as reading, writing, and mathematics. This lower level of achievement occurs despite the child's normal (sometimes above-normal) intelligence or adequate schooling. Many of these individuals become school dropouts, have low self-esteem, and feel demoralized. They also may exhibit deficits in social skills.

ETIOLOGY

The etiology of this condition is uncertain, although there may be underlying abnormalities in **cognitive** processing. Deficits in visual perception, language processes, attention, or memory may contribute to the problem.

DIAGNOSIS

In addition to normal variations in academic attainment being ruled out, so should inadequate schooling, language barriers, lack of opportunity, and poor teaching.

TREATMENT

Some children who are learning disabled also may be diagnosed with hyperactivity and therefore may respond to drug therapy. Other children may respond favorably to special instructional techniques. It is hoped that continuing research will help in developing additional treatments for children who have learning disabilities.

Communication Disorders

Often, children exhibit difficulties in communication. These disorders may be psychologically based and are listed in the DSM-IV.

STUTTERING

SYMPTOMS AND SIGNS

Stuttering is defined as frequent repetitions or prolongations of sounds or syllables. These constitute a disturbance of the time patterning and normal fluency of speech that is inappropriate for the child's age. There also may be broken words, filled or unfilled pauses in speech, word substitutions, or word repetitions. Onset usually occurs between 2 and 7 years of age.

ETIOLOGY

Although the etiology is uncertain, there may be genetic factors involved. There appears to be a familial tendency toward stuttering, with the condition occurring more frequently in males. Parents also may unwittingly cause anxiety in their child by overreacting to mild speech limitation. Anxiety appears to be a major factor that creates and maintains stuttering.

DIAGNOSIS

Observation of the speech pattern is usually all that is needed for the diagnosis. However, hearing should be assessed, and any hearing difficulty should be ruled out.

TREATMENT

Speech therapy is helpful in the treatment. The condition may resolve spontaneously.

Pervasive Development Disorders

Characteristic of pervasive development disorders is severe impairment in several areas of development, including communication and social interaction skills. Particular behaviors involving failure to develop peer relationships and interactions with others, including lack of nonverbal communication and reciprocation of emotions, can be present. This impairment is related directly to the person's developmental level or mental age. Autism is a pervasive development disorder.

AUTISTIC DISORDER

SYMPTOMS AND SIGNS

Autistic disorder (autism) is a syndrome of extreme withdrawal and obsessive behavior. It has its onset in infancy, and manifestations are apparent by the second or third year of age. Socialization and communication, activities, and interests are markedly impaired. The impairment is noted in nonverbal behaviors, such as eye-to-eye gaze, facial expressions, and other forms of nonverbal communication. Seizures may be present. Additionally, there is a failure to establish normal peer relationships and to seek shared enjoyment. Communication impairments include delayed or absent verbal communication, inability to initiate a conversation, and repetitive use of inappropriate language. The child does not initiate age-appropriate play activities. Repetitive motions, often self-destructive, may be noted, along with an inflexibility for change and a compulsion for sameness. These youngsters display a persistent preoccupation with objects and may have a memory for certain lists or facts.

Four symptoms that are nearly always present are social isolation, cognitive impairment, language deficits, and repetitive naturalistic motions. The autistic child exhibits resistance to any change.

ETIOLOGY

The etiology is uncertain; however, evidence indicates that there may be an organic factor. The occurrence is more frequent in males.

DIAGNOSIS

Usually, observation of the behavior is all that is needed for the diagnosis. The child exhibits impairment in social interaction and communication, restricted repetitive patterns of behavior, and delayed or abnormal patterns of symbolic or imaginative play.

TREATMENT

Behavioral therapy and self-instructed training have been helpful for some autistic children. It is most beneficial when parents also are trained in behavioral techniques, with the goal of helping these children to learn some adaptive responses, enabling them to function outside of custodial care.

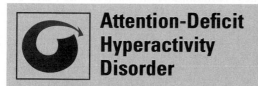

Attention-Deficit Hyperactivity Disorder

SYMPTOMS AND SIGNS

Attention-deficit hyperactivity disorder (ADHD) is a condition of persistent inattention leading to hyperactivity and impulsivity. Typical behavior can be observed at any age; however, symptoms are usually present before the age of 7 years. Failure to give close attention to details; careless mistakes; messy work, which is performed carelessly; and difficulty in sustaining attention and completing tasks are manifestations of the condition. There is an avoidance of activities that require a sustained attention, effort, concentration, and organization. An inability to sit quietly without fidgeting or squirming or even to remain seated denotes hyperactivity. Inappropriate running and climbing, difficulty in playing, and excessive talking are other signs of the condition.

A display of impatience, difficulty in waiting for one's turn, frequent interruptions, and failure to listen to directions are manifestations of impulsivity. The inability to organize and define goals makes it difficult to perform simple tasks, such as picking up toys.

Any aspect of this behavior may be displayed at home, school, work, or social occasions. There seems to be an exaggeration of the behavior in group situations.

ETIOLOGY

The cause is uncertain; however, there appears to be a familial pattern.

DIAGNOSIS

Diagnosis involves the observation of behavior and an evaluation that the inattention is not age appropriate. The inattention must last for longer than 6 months and involve at least two of the following settings: home, school, work, and social activities. Persistent hyperactivity and impulsivity also must meet the aforementioned criteria. Some of the symptoms are present before the age of 7 years. There is an impairment in functioning as a result of the behavior.

TREATMENT

An effective treatment for some children is the use of amphetamines, such as dextroamphetamine sulfate (Dexedrine), methylphenidate hydrochloride (Ritalin), and mixed salts of a single-entity amphetamine product (Adderall). Other successful treatments have been in the use of behavioral therapy — rewarding appropriate behavior to extinguish inappropriate behavior.

Tic Disorders

Tic disorders involve sudden, rapid, recurrent motor movement or vocalization that is non-rhythmic. The tics are irresistible; however, they may be suppressed for varying lengths of time and diminish during sleep. Eye blinking, facial grimacing, coughing, and neck jerking are examples of simple motor tics. Making facial gestures, jumping, touching, and stamping are examples of complex motor tics. Simple vocal tics include throat clearing, sniffing, snorting, and grunting. The repetition of words out of context, the use of socially unacceptable words, and the repetition of one's own words or of the last sound heard are examples of complex vocal tics.

TOURETTE'S DISORDER

SYMPTOMS AND SIGNS

Tourette's disorder, also known as Gilles de la Tourette's syndrome, is a syndrome of multiple motor tics coupled with one or more vocal tics, which may appear simultaneously or at different periods. The location, nature, and number of tics tend to change over time. Typically, the head is involved. Other body parts such as the torso or upper and lower limbs may be involved. Clicks, grunts, yelps, barks, and snorts are examples of vocal tics. Additionally, the uttering of obscenities may be present.

ETIOLOGY

The etiology is uncertain. Incidence is more common in males.

DIAGNOSIS

The observation of symptoms is usually enough for diagnosis. Onset may be as early as 2 years of age but is before the age of 18 years. Remissions may occur; however, the syndrome is of lifelong duration. Usually, the severity of the symptoms diminishes, and the symptoms may even disappear by early adulthood.

To meet diagnostic criteria, the tics must be both motor and vocal, although not necessarily displayed at the same time. They occur several times a day over a period of a year without a tic-free period of longer than 3 months. There is significant impairment in functioning at work or in socialization, and the condition is not the result of substance use or a general medical condition.

TREATMENT

Some patients with Tourette's disorder have improved with the administration of haloperidol lactate (Haldol).

Dementia

Dementia involves a progressive, general deterioration of mental faculties, including deterioration of perceiving, thinking, and remembering. There is an abnormal decline in cognitive functioning. The irreversible brain damage may be the result of compromised blood flow to the brain from atherosclerosis, thrombi, or trauma. Additionally, toxins, metabolic conditions, organic disorders, infections, tumors, or Alzheimer's disease may be responsible for the deterioration. The onset may be slow and insidious or may be sudden, depending on the cause.

ALZHEIMER'S DISEASE

SYMPTOMS AND SIGNS

Alzheimer's disease is a progressive degenerative disease of the brain in which there is a typical profile in the loss of mental and physical functioning. It is the most frequent cause of deterioration of intellectual capacity, or dementia. It is most common in people older than 65 years of age, and its frequency increases in people older than 80 years of age. Onset is gradual and insidious, with early signs including loss of short-term memory, inability to concentrate, incapacity for learning new things, impairment of reasoning, and subtle changes in personality. As its course continues, communication skills decline, and the patient struggles to find the right words, uses meaningless words, or interjects nonsensical phrases. Over a span of 5 to 10 years, there is profound deterioration of intellectual ability and physical capability. The patient becomes increasingly dependent on a caretaker. There is diminished response to stimulation by the outside world, and the person seems emotionally detached. The patient may exhibit restlessness, sleep disturbances, disorientation, hostility, or combativeness. Eventually, the patient is bedridden and ultimately dies of intercurrent infection or other complications.

ETIOLOGY

The cause of Alzheimer's disease is not known, but the disease is age related and may have a genetic basis in some families. Research has focused on an abnormality found on chromosome 21 as a genetic link. Persons with Down syndrome (a syndrome also linked to an abnormality on chromosome 21) show the same brain changes as patients with Alzheimer's disease. In later life, people with Down syndrome have the clinical symptoms of Alzheimer's disease. Other causal theories regarding Alzheimer's disease include biochemical changes in brain growth, an autoimmune reaction, infection with a slow virus, toxic chemical excess, chemical deficiency, blood vessel defects, and a deficiency of neurochemical factors in the brain. Research shows a higher rate of occurrence in people with history of head trauma.

DIAGNOSIS

It is difficult to obtain direct evidence of Alzheimer's disease. Once other causes of organic brain disease have been ruled out, diagnostic criteria for Alzheimer's disease include evidence of memory and cognitive disturbances. As the disease progresses, neurologic examination reveals sensory and motor deficits. In later stages, diagnostic studies include brain scans, which may detect brain atrophy, widened sulci, and enlarged cerebral ventricles. Positive diagnosis is possible after death, when evidence of brain atrophy and characteristic lesions in the cerebral cortex can be found on pathologic examination of the brain. The brain shows loss of neurons and the presence of **senile plaques,** which include microscopic deposits of **amyloid** material. Neurofibrillary tangles are also evident (Fig. 14–1). However, some of the same postmortem anomalies may be found in persons who never were diagnosed with or exhibited symptoms of Alzheimer's disease. Alzheimer's disease is one of the most overdiagnosed or misdiagnosed mental functioning disorders of older adults because it is not easily distinguished from other dementias that result from excessive use of medication, depression, brain tumors, subdural hematomas, and certain other metabolic diseases.

TREATMENT

There is no known cure for Alzheimer's disease; therefore, the treatment is supportive and is geared to helping alleviate symptoms. Drug therapy to help alleviate cognitive symptoms includes tacrine hydrochloride (Cognex) or donepezil hydrochloride (Aricept). Antipsychotic or neuroleptic agents including haloperidol, antianxiety agents including alprazolam (Xanax) and buspirone hydrochloride (BuSpar), and selective serotonin reuptake inhibitor (SSRI) antidepressants including paroxetine hydrochloride (Paxil) are used to manage behavioral symptoms. In addition to reducing symptoms and decreasing suffering, treatment aims to increase the ability of the patient to cope and to decrease the frustration level. As the patient's ability for self-care declines, general management of fluid intake, adequate nutrition, and personal hygiene is necessary. Treatment provides the patient with opportunities to be mobile and to maintain remaining mental abilities for as long as possible. Provisions to protect the patient from injury are employed.

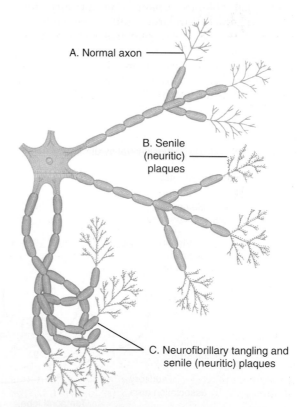

A. Normal axon

B. Senile (neuritic) plaques

C. Neurofibrillary tangling and senile (neuritic) plaques

Figure 14–1

Neurofibrillary tangles and senile plaques found in patient with Alzheimer's disease. (From Black JM, Matassarin-Jacobs E: Medical-Surgical Nursing, 5th ed. Philadelphia: WB Saunders, 1997, p 864. Used with permission.)

Finally, emotional support for the patient and the family or caregiver is vital because the disease forces enormous adjustments on them.

Research continues to delve into the etiology of Alzheimer's disease. It is hoped that determining the cause may lead to prevention because currently there is no way to reverse the neurologic damage created by the disease. Early diagnosis and drug therapy may help to slow the course of the disease.

VASCULAR DEMENTIA

SYMPTOMS AND SIGNS

Decreased blood flow to the brain can result from narrowed and stenosed arteries. Functional areas of the cerebrum are pictured in Figure 14–2. The resulting hypoxia and diminished nourishment to the brain cells causes a general loss in intellectual abilities. Changes in memory, judgment, abstract thinking, and personality are noted. A disregard for personal hygiene is observed, along with apathy, disorientation, and inappropriate responses. Depression, anxiety, and irritability often are involved. Restlessness, sleeplessness, **hallucinations,** and psychotic tend-

encies appear as the condition advances. Stupor and coma are final stages.

ETIOLOGY

As atherosclerotic plaque progresses in the carotid and cerebral arteries, blood flow is diminished to brain tissue. Prolonged hypoxia with resulting **ischemia** leads to irreversible **necrosis** and death of the brain cells. When the blockage is caused by an embolism, the hypoxia is sudden and complete. Small aneurysms may be responsible for minute cerebral bleeds. When the cerebral cortex is involved, cognitive capabilities are compromised. (See Cerebrovascular Accident [Stroke] in Chapter 13.)

DIAGNOSIS

Because symptoms of atherosclerotic involvement have an insidious onset, the family often does not notice the subtle changes taking place. When the person's personal hygiene deteriorates, along with memory and judgment, family members may become aware of a problem. A thorough history with physical and neurologic examination is necessary to rule out other causes of the altered behavior. Vascular assessment of the carotid and cerebral arteries may yield informa-

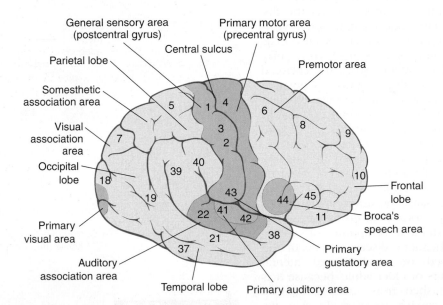

Figure 14–2

Map of the lateral surface of the cerebral cortex showing some of the functional areas. Areas 4, 6, and 8 are motor areas; areas 1, 2, 3, 41, 42, and 43 are primary sensory areas; and areas 9, 10, 11, 18, 19, 22, 38, 39, and 40 are association areas. (From Solomon EP: Introduction to Human Anatomy and Physiology. Philadelphia: WB Saunders, 1992. Used with permission.)

tion about compromised blood flow. Cerebral arteriograms or magnetic resonance imaging (MRI) arteriograms confirm the presence of the condition.

TREATMENT

Treatment is aimed at increasing the blood supply to the brain. Drug therapy may be helpful in increasing the blood flow. When the carotid arteries are compromised, surgical intervention in the form of carotid **endarterectomy** may lessen extension of the condition. Brain cell death is irreversible. As the condition progresses, institutionalization may be necessary for the patient's safety and care.

DEMENTIA DUE TO HEAD TRAUMA

SYMPTOMS AND SIGNS

Reduced intellectual capabilities and cognitive functioning may result from trauma to the head. After a head injury, the person exhibits reduced mental status and is unable to perform many of the cognitive tasks that were possible before the injury. Intelligence testing shows decreased capabilities.

ETIOLOGY

Trauma to the head causes an insult to the brain because of edema, increased intracranial pressure, or damage to the vessel walls. The insult results in compromise to the cerebral blood supply. The hypoxia is followed by ischemia and eventually irreversible necrosis of brain cells. (See Head Trauma in Chapter 13.)

DIAGNOSIS

The history of head trauma with decreased level of mental functioning is augmented by a thorough physical and neurologic examination. Imaging studies may include skull radiographic films, computed tomography (CT) scan of the brain, and MRI scan of the brain and cerebral vessels. Subdural or epidural hematomas may be noted, as may any type of skull fracture. **Ventricular shift** is indicative of increasing intracranial pressure. Any neurologic deficit, such as unequal pupils, unequal grips, hemiparesis, and posturing, is indicative of insult to the brain tissue. As the condition progresses, decreased intellectual functioning is noted.

TREATMENT

Treatment involves correcting the insult to the brain to prevent additional damage. After the necrosis has evolved, the damaged tissues cannot be repaired. Therapy and training to maintain what functions remain is attempted. When the damage is severe, the person may have to be institutionalized for care and safety.

Alcohol Abuse

SYMPTOMS AND SIGNS

Alcohol abuse is a disorder of physical and psychological dependence on daily, or regular, excessive intake of alcoholic beverages. The onset can be insidious or can be accelerated by an acute traumatic event. Excessive use of alcohol frequently is associated with anxiety, depression, insomnia, impotence, behavioral disorders, and **amnesia** during intoxication. Repeated heavy drinking of alcohol produces symptoms and signs in nearly every organ system. Common physical findings include frequent infections, hypertension, and gastrointestinal (GI) problems. The patient may report unexplained seizure activity or symptoms of alcohol withdrawal. Prolonged heavy use of alcohol may cause cirrhosis of the liver, pancreatitis, and peripheral neuropathy, resulting in muscle weakness and **paresthesia.** There is also increased risk of cancer of the esophagus, stomach, and other parts of the GI system.

Consequences of chronic alcohol abuse include dysfunction within family and social relationships and disruption in occupational responsibilities. Some people are prone to aggressive or violent behavior, accidents, and threatened or attempted suicide. The person frequently denies inability to control or discontinue alcohol abuse.

ETIOLOGY

There is no single cause of alcohol abuse; nevertheless, a cluster of possible causative factors is considered notable. The origin may include genetic or biologic factors, depression, emotional conflict, social factors, and cultural attitudes. Because the patient history frequently includes a familial pattern of alcohol abuse, genetic factors pose a recognized statistical risk.

TABLE 14-1 ➤ Effects of Rising Blood Alcohol Level (BAL)*

BAL	EFFECTS
0.02	Mild euphoria, decreased inhibitions, slight body warmth, talkativeness
0.05	Noticeable relaxation, decreased alertness, increased self-confidence
0.08	**Legally drunk in some states,** impairment in coordination, judgment, memory, and comprehension
0.10	**Legally drunk in remaining states,** behavior becomes loud or embarrassing; mood swings are noticeable, and reaction time is reduced
0.15	Impaired balance and coordination; appears intoxicated
0.20	Disoriented, mental confusion, dizziness, lethargy, exaggerated emotional states
0.30	Staggering gait, slurred speech, visual disturbances, possible loss of consciousness
0.40	Inability to walk or stand, decreased response to stimuli, vomiting, incontinence, loss of consciousness, possible death ("dead drunk")
0.50	Respiratory effort depressed to point of ceasing, lack of reflexes, body temperature drops, impairment of circulation, possible death; immediate intervention and intense life support measures required to sustain life
0.60	Usually death occurs or has occurred

* Blood alcohol level (BAL) is measured in milligrams of alcohol per 100 ml of blood and reported as milligrams percent. An individual with a BAL of 0.10 has 1/10 of 1% (1/1000) of total blood volume as alcohol. BAL depends on the blood volume (increases with weight) and the amount of alcohol consumed over a given time.

DIAGNOSIS

Screening tests for alcohol abuse include questionnaires that attempt to identify pathologic behavior. Test results may be altered by the person's attempts to deny or hide the addiction. Diagnostic information gathered during physical examination and a medical history may fit the profile of alcohol abuse. Laboratory findings may help to confirm the diagnosis. One sensitive indicator of heavy alcohol intake is a high gamma-glutamyltransferase (GGT) level in the blood. The amount of alcohol consumed may be calculated by using a chart such as is used by law enforcement agencies. Table 14-1 lists the effects of levels of blood alcohol on the brain. Table 14-2 indicates how an individual's weight and the amount of alcohol consumed determines blood alcohol content. Other abnormal laboratory findings emerge with organ system complications resulting from chronic alcohol abuse.

TREATMENT

Rehabilitation consists of a specialized treatment plan that meets the patient's physical and psychological needs and supports abstinence from alcohol. After detoxification (usually not needed), most patients benefit from psychotherapy or group therapy and participation in the 12-step program of Alcoholics Anonymous (AA). Ongoing therapy usually can continue on an outpatient basis. Willing participation in a recovery program on a sustained, as-needed basis usually offers a promising prognosis. Relapses are common and need not represent failure of treatment as long as the patient returns to a program of recovery and abstinence from alcohol. Only a small percentage of patients can ever become "social" or moderate drinkers.

TABLE 14-2 ➤ Blood Alcohol Content*

BODY WEIGHT (LB)	NO. OF DRINKS (1 OZ 86% PROOF LIQUOR, 3 OZ WINE, OR 12 OZ BEER)								
	1	2	3	4	5	6	7	8	9
100	0.032*	0.065†	0.097‡	0.129‡	0.162‡	0.194‡	0.226‡	0.258‡	0.291‡
120	0.027*	0.054†	0.081‡	0.108‡	0.135‡	0.161‡	0.188‡	0.215‡	0.242‡
140	0.023*	0.046*	0.069†	0.092‡	0.115‡	0.138‡	0.161‡	0.184‡	0.207‡
160	0.020*	0.040*	0.060†	0.080‡	0.101‡	0.121‡	0.141‡	0.161‡	0.181‡
180	0.018*	0.036*	0.054†	0.072†	0.090‡	0.108‡	0.126‡	0.144‡	0.162‡
200	0.016*	0.032*	0.048*	0.064†	0.080‡	0.097‡	0.113‡	0.129‡	0.145‡
220	0.015*	0.029*	0.044*	0.058†	0.073†	0.088‡	0.102‡	0.117‡	0.131‡
240	0.014*	0.027*	0.040*	0.053†	0.067†	0.081‡	0.095‡	0.108‡	0.121‡

* Blood alcohol content to 0.05% → Caution.
† Blood alcohol content to 0.05-0.079% → Driving impaired.
‡ Blood alcohol content 0.08% and up → Presumed under the influence.

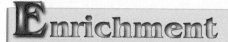

BLOOD ALCOHOL LEVELS

After ingestion, alcohol is absorbed from the GI tract and distributed to all tissues. The rich blood supply to the brain results in a concentration of alcohol in the CNS proportional to blood alcohol concentration. The rate at which alcohol is metabolized in the liver is constant, and only 10 to 15 ml of pure alcohol can be metabolized in 1 hour. Figure 14–3 compares the amount of beer (12 oz), wine (6 oz), or 86% proof liquor (1 oz) that contains 10 to 15 ml of pure alcohol.

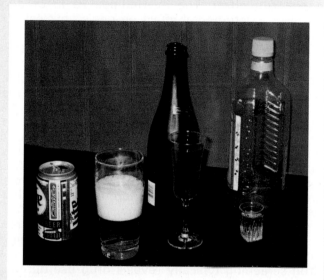

Figure 14–3

Comparison of the amount of beer (12 oz), wine (6 oz), or 86% proof liquor (1 oz) that contains 10–15 ml of pure alcohol. (Courtesy of David L. Frazier, 1999.)

Schizophrenia

SYMPTOMS AND SIGNS

Schizophrenia, a major psychiatric disturbance, is a group of disorders that may result in chronic mental dysfunction, producing varying degrees of impairment. The onset is usually insidious during adolescence or young adulthood. There are **prodromal** signs, such as withdrawal, odd behavior, disheveled appearance, and loss of interest in school or work. The patient may report feeling confused, isolated, anxious, and afraid. In the active phase of schizophrenia, a vast range of severe behavioral and perceptual manifestations is present, with marked social and occupational dysfunction.

One important feature is disorganized thinking, usually reflected by the person's speech and by disturbances in language and communication. For example, the person may switch from one topic to another, speak incoherently, give an unrelated answer to a question, or experience difficulty in speaking at all.

Distortions of perception called hallucinations are a common characteristic of schizophrenia. The patient with auditory hallucinations acknowledges hearing voices that may be threatening, instructive, or conversational. Delusions, which are erroneous beliefs, represent exaggerations or distortions of perceptions or experiences. In persecutory delusion, for instance, people may believe that they are being mistreated, deceived, or stalked. More bizarre delusions may include belief that one's thoughts are controlled by an "alien."

Inappropriate affect (feeling) is another identifying characteristic of schizophrenia. Lack of

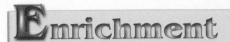

SUBSTANCE ABUSE

Substance abuse is a significant social and medical concern. Altered behavior and medical complications exhibited cross all levels of social, economic, ethnic, racial, educational, and professional backgrounds. Substances abused on a regular episodic basis include but are not limited to alcohol, sedatives, stimulants, opioids, cannabis, hallucinogens, inhalants, caffeine, nicotine, illicit synthetic (designer) drugs, and other chemical substances. These substances, prescribed or illegal, provide the user with a stimulant or depressant effect. The overindulgence in or dependence on chemical substances often leads to a detrimental effect on one's physical and psychological well-being as well as on the welfare of others.

During substance abuse, tolerance to the chemical or drug often develops, necessitating increased amounts of the substance to achieve the desired effect. In addition to tolerance, both physical and psychological dependence can develop. Rapid withdrawal from certain drugs can cause life-threatening and even fatal reactions.

The individual under the influence of drugs often exhibits inappropriate behavior. Judgment often is impaired, and they are at risk for injury to themselves or others when driving or operating machinery when under the influence. They experience multiple social and interpersonal problems. While under the influence of mood-altering drugs, some may appear intoxicated but others may exhibit a fairly normal pattern of behavior. Over an extended period of time, performance and relationships deteriorate. Dependability decreases, legal problems develop, and desperation for more of the desired substance may lead to criminal behavior.

Many prospective and current employers require employees to participate in drug-screening programs. This type of drug screening usually is accomplished in one of two noninvasive methods. A urine sample can be analyzed for drug content. However, urine drug screening typically reveals drug use during the preceding 3 to 4 days. It is possible for an individual to abstain from the drug usage for 4 days and have negative test results. Another method is analysis of a hair sample (Fig. 14–4). Evidence of drug usage stays in

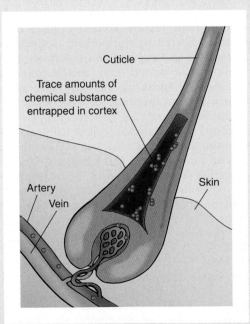

Figure 14–4

The scientific principle behind hair analysis is that as drugs are ingested, they enter our bloodstream, which nourishes our hair follicles. In this way, trace amounts of drugs are deposited in the hair shaft that, when analyzed, can reveal a person's drug history. (With permission from Psychemedics Corporation, Cambridge, MA 1998.)

the hair shaft for approximately 90 days. Drugs are absorbed into the bloodstream and circulated in the blood, which nourishes the hair follicle, leaving trace amounts of residue entrapped in the core of the hair shaft. Washing, bleaching, or dying the hair does not remove the drug residues. Thus, abstinence for a few days does not alter the results of the test. Finally, these tests do not indicate pattern of use or presence of dependence; thus results are to be interpreted and integrated with other clinical data.

Law enforcement officers use a Breathalyzer test for a expeditious evaluation of blood alcohol levels. Blood tests for presence of or specific drug level measurements also are performed. General toxicology drug screening provides only a qualitative detection of drugs. Identified drugs should be confirmed and levels determined by a test specific for that drug. Blood screening for nonspecific drugs usually is accompanied by urine drug screening.

emotional expression (flat affect) or unreasonable outbursts of emotions may be noted.

Behavior may be bizarre or grossly disorganized, unpredictable, agitated, or violent. The patient may assume rigid posturing (**catatonic posturing**), dress in an odd manner, and neglect self-care. Any of these behaviors can stem from the patient's delusional thinking.

As the symptoms and signs persist, the patient's ability to function in interpersonal, social, or occupational relationships deteriorates.

Schizophrenia has subtypes, which are determined by a clustering of characteristics as follows:

Paranoid Type. Paranoid schizophrenia features anger, hostility, violence, grandiose or persecutory delusions, or hallucinations. The patient may be intelligent and well informed.

Disorganized Type. The patient is blatantly incoherent, with delusions that are not systematized into a theme. The patient's feelings are dull, inappropriate, or greatly exaggerated. Behavior may be odd or regressive. There is a history of extreme social impairment and a history of poor functioning and poor adaptation. The condition has a chronic course.

Catatonic Type. Catatonic schizophrenia features either excitement or stupor with mutism, negativism, rigidity, and posturing.

Undifferentiated Type. The behavior is grossly disorganized, and the patient is obviously incoherent, grossly delusional, and hallucinatory. Prominent symptoms of psychosis may fit more than one subtype.

Residual Type. The patient has experienced at least one episode of schizophrenia, but is presently without prominent symptoms. Continuing evidence of illness, such as illogical thinking and odd behavior, may prevent the patient from functioning in the workplace.

ETIOLOGY

The cause of schizophrenia is unknown, although evidence suggests that genetic factors play a substantial role. Close biologic relatives of patients with schizophrenia have a 10-fold increased risk of schizophrenia. Vulnerability to stress and environmental factors are considered contributing catalysts.

DIAGNOSIS

The diagnosis of schizophrenia entails recognition of a group of psychotic signs and symptoms, including dysfunctional thinking, perception, behavior, language and communication, volition, and mental attention. There have been no laboratory findings identified as diagnostic of schizophrenia. Psychological tests that may help in diagnosis include the Rorschach (inkblot) test, the Thematic Apperception Test (TAT), and the Minnesota Multiphasic Personality Inventory (MMPI). Organic causes such as toxic psychosis associated with substance abuse, cerebral arteriosclerosis, and hyperthyroidism should be ruled out.

TREATMENT

During the acute phase of schizophrenia, antipsychotic drugs are used to control symptoms and to allow early release from the hospital. A minimal effective dose for remission of symptoms without troublesome side effects associated with antipsychotic medications is desirable. Subsequent long-term multidimensional treatment combines supportive psychotherapy, drugs, and family involvement. After the patient is stabilized, the goal of treatment is helping the patient to establish a better sense of self with attainment of personal, social, and vocational achievements. Responses to treatment vary, and relapses may occur.

Mood Disorders

In mood disorders, a person experiences a pathologic disturbance in mood that influences all aspects of his or her life. The terms affect and mood are used interchangeably to refer to the outward manifestation of a person's feeling or tone.

BIPOLAR DISORDER

SYMPTOMS AND SIGNS

Bipolar disorder is a major affective disorder with abnormally intense mood swings from a hyperactive, or manic, state to a depressive syndrome. In some cases, symptoms of hyperactivity and depression may coexist. The patient may remain manic for days, weeks, or months before experiencing depression. Assessment findings vary with the type of episode (manic, depressive, or mixed) that the patient is experiencing at the time of medical evaluation.

During a manic episode, the patient is excited, euphoric, and expansive. The person speaks rapidly, with great certitude and conviction. Evidence of thought disorders, such as frequent changes of topics, or flight of ideas may be noted. Patients sleep little and seem to have excessive energy, which leads to overinvolvement in activities. Judgment is impaired, and they may spend money extravagantly. Behavior may appear bizarre, grandiose, or promiscuous. The patient may be delusional or experience auditory hallucinations.

During an episode of depression, the patient's mood becomes lowered, sad, or markedly indifferent (flat affect). Thoughts and speech are slow, and the patient may avoid communication. The patient becomes withdrawn and demonstrates loss of interest in life. Reports of sleep disturbance, loss of appetite, and feelings of guilt are common. There is a marked decrease in physical activity. Suicide may be threatened or attempted.

ETIOLOGY

There is no clear cause of bipolar disorder. Biochemical factors such as alterations of **neurotransmitter** levels in the brain, endocrine disorders, and electrolyte imbalances may play a role. The risk of mood disorders is higher among close relatives of the patient. Emotional or physical trauma may precipitate the onset of bipolar disorder in a predisposed person.

DIAGNOSIS

Bipolar disorder is identified when certain prescribed diagnostic criteria can be documented during physical and psychological evaluation. The mood disturbance must be pervasive and persistent and cause marked impairment over a distinct period of time. Other medical causes, such as organic diseases and psychiatric conditions, must be ruled out.

TREATMENT

After diagnosis, therapeutic treatment is dictated by the specific form of behavior exhibited by the patient. Lithium carbonate is the drug of choice during an acute manic phase of bipolar disease. It may even abate a swing into the depressive phase. During an episode of depression, antidepressants are used with caution because they may trigger a manic episode. Treatment includes a therapeutic milieu, or environment, that meets the patient's physical needs, encourages

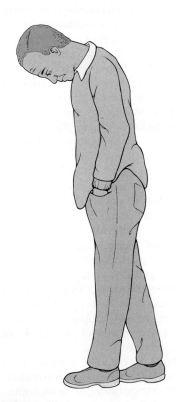

Figure 14–5

Depression.

personal responsibility, and sets reasonable limits and goals for behavior. During this time, the patient may need to be protected from self-injury.

MAJOR DEPRESSIVE DISORDER

SYMPTOMS AND SIGNS

Major depressive disorder is a serious alteration in mood, which may be described as deep and persistent sadness, despair, and hopelessness (Fig. 14-5). Symptoms develop gradually over several days, during which an anxious or brooding appearance may be noted. The person may experience an empty or heavy feeling inside accompanied by a vague sense of loss. An attitude of self-blame, remorse, guilt, or loss of self-esteem may exist. Other symptoms include sleep disturbance (insomnia or hypersomnia), physical sluggishness or fatigue, loss of concentration, and inability to experience pleasure. In addition, a depressed person may have a variety of physical symptoms. Appetite disturbance results in a change in weight. The patient withdraws socially and may admit to having suicidal thoughts; suicidal behavior is common in major depression (Fig. 14-6; Table 14-3).

ETIOLOGY

Major depressive disorder is thought to have a biologic basis and a familial pattern, but the precise cause is not understood. Psychosocial pres-

sures, chronic physical illness, and alcohol dependence are considered predisposing factors. Although many patients blame their environment, it is not considered a cause.

DIAGNOSIS

Major depressive disorder must be differentiated from a reactive type of depression resulting from a difficult or stressful life circumstance; one example is a grief syndrome. Diagnostic criteria used in psychiatric evaluation include a prominent and persistent depressed mood lasting at least 2 weeks, with at least four of any of the aforementioned symptoms documented.

TREATMENT

The most effective treatment is a combination of medication and psychotherapy. Most patients have relief of symptoms and a good prognosis if they respond favorably to antidepressant therapy. Depression may occur as a single episode or may be recurrent. Electroconvulsive therapy (ECT) is helpful when a patient is severely incapacitated, has psychotic features, or does not respond to other therapeutic measures. Family support and education are considered important in the recovery process.

Patients who commit suicide have a high incidence of the hopelessness of acute depression. Often, the suicidal patient wishes to discuss suicidal fears and does not want to die but sees suicide as the only escape from an intolerable

437

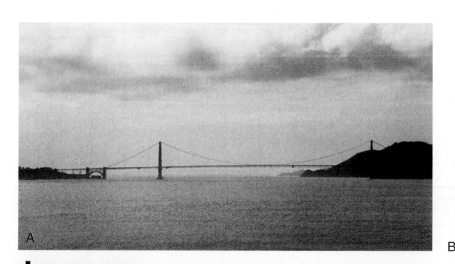

Figure 14–6

A, The Golden Gate Bridge, where many suicide jumps have been made. *B*, Crisis Control Center telephone available for potential jumpers to use to call for help. (Courtesy of David L. Frazier, 1999.)

TABLE 14-3 ➤ Depression on a Continuum

MILD TO MODERATE	SEVERE
Communication	
Slow speech, long pauses before answering; monotone	Slow in extreme; may be mute and not talk at all
Affect	
Crying and weeping, slumping in chair, drooping shoulders, look of gloom and pessimism Anxiety may or may not be manifested **Anhedonia**—inability to experience pleasure	May appear without affect; may be experiencing "nothingness"; can sit for hours staring into space Anhedonia
Thinking	
No impairment in reality testing Thinking is slow, concentration and memory are poor, interest narrows; perspective in situations is lost, e.g., • "Every one always lets me down." • "No one cares." Thoughts reflect doubts and indecisions; thinking is often repetitive in negative cycle: • "Why was I born? What's life all about?" Mild feelings of guilt and worthlessness **May have suicidal ideation**	Grasp of reality may be tenuous Thoughts may indicate delusional thinking, reflecting feelings of • Low self-esteem • Worthlessness • Helplessness • "I'm no good." • "God is punishing me for my terrible sins." • "My insides are rotting." • "My heart has stopped beating." Concentration is extremely poor Preoccupation with bodily symptoms **May have suicidal ideation**
Physical Behavior	
Fatigue and lethargy are hallmark symptoms. They do not prevent the person from working, although the person often works below potential. Initiative and creativity are impaired. Grooming and hygiene usually are neglected.	Severe and extreme chronic fatigue and lethargy markedly interfere with occupational functioning, social activities, or relationships with others Client may show extreme neglect of personal grooming and hygiene
Vegetative Signs	
Sleep—middle or late insomnia, hypersomnia; EEG studies show shortened REM latency Energy is often highest in AM, lowest in PM Eating—may have anorexia or overeat Sexual appetite is diminished Bowels—constipation if psychomotor retardation is present; may have diarrhea if psychomotor agitation is present Psychomotor retardation (slow motor movements)—everything is an effort *or* Psychomotor agitation (agitated depression)—pacing up and down halls, wringing hands	Sleep—usually insomnia; early morning waking at 3:00 or 4:00 AM Energy is often lowest in AM, highest in PM Eating—usually has anorexia; weight loss of more than 5% in 1 month Loss of libido Bowels—usually constipation Psychomotor retardation (most common) *or* Psychomotor agitation

EEG, electroencephalographic; REM, rapid eye movement.
From: Varcarolis EM: Foundations of Psychiatric Mental Health Nursing, 3rd ed. Philadelphia: WB Saunders, 1998, p. 560. Used with permission.

situation. Reluctance to openly discuss suicidal thoughts makes it important to explore understandingly preoccupation with death or comments such as, "People would be better off without me" or "better off dead."

Suicide intervention is an attempt by medical, mental health, and community services to assist the depressed individual through the hopeless situation. Most telephone directories list crisis control centers for crisis intervention. Hospital

Enrichment

GRIEF RESPONSE

The grief response is initiated primarily by the death of a loved one; however, grieving is a normal sequela to any loss, including loss of a function, body part, employment, or other important entity. The patient with a terminal illness is faced with the prospect of total separation and also needs to work through the various stages of grief.

The normal grieving process passes through several phases. The most recognized stages are those identified by Elisabeth Kubler-Ross. The first is denial: "No, I don't believe it." Second is anger: "Why did he or she do this to me?" or "Why is God letting this happen?" The third stage involves bargaining: "If only this task can be accomplished or I can achieve this goal [live long enough], I will do this." Fourth is depression, in which people retreat within themselves and have little or no involvement with their environment. Finally, in the fifth stage, acceptance comes. Not everyone is able to move through these steps, and not everyone moves through them at the same pace or in the same order. Some people cannot express anger at the dead person or at God and do not move on. Many of these people never complete the grieving process, remain in a depressed state, and have reduced coping mechanisms. Medical intervention may be beneficial during depression. However, most people recover with minimal treatment.

Grieving is handled differently in different cultures. Many grieve quietly and privately, whereas others cry, moan, rant, and even throw themselves on the funeral pyre. The important aspect of funerals and viewing the remains is to allow closure of the relationship and to say good-bye (Fig. 14–7 and Table 14–4).

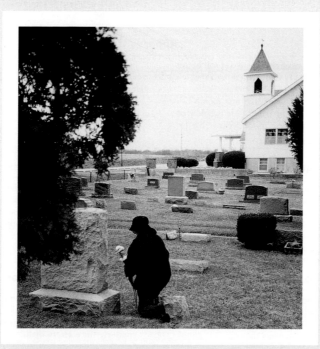

Figure 14–7

Grief response. (Courtesy of David L. Frazier, 1999.)

TABLE 14-4 ➤ Phenomena Experienced During Mourning

SYMPTOMS	EXAMPLES
Sensation of Somatic Distress	
Tightness in throat, shortness of breath, sighing, "mental pain," exhaustion. Food tastes like sand; things feel unreal. Pain or discomfort may be identical to the symptoms experienced by the dead person. Normally symptoms are brief.	A woman whose husband died of a stroke complains of weakness and numbness on her left side.
Preoccupation with the Image of the Deceased	
The bereaved brings up and thinks and talks about numerous memories of the deceased. The memories are positive. This process goes on with great sadness. The idealization of the deceased lets the bereaved relive the gratifications associated with the deceased and helps resolve any guilt the bereaved has toward the deceased. The bereaved also may take on many of the mannerisms of the deceased through identification. Identification serves the purpose of holding onto the deceased. Preoccupation with the dead person takes many months before it lessens.	A man whose wife just died states, "I just can't stop thinking about my wife. Everything I see reminds me of her. We picked up this seashell on our honeymoon. I remember every wonderful moment we had together. The pain is so great, but the memories just keep coming." His friends notice that when he talks, his hand gestures and expressions are very like those of his recently deceased wife.
Guilt	
The bereaved reproaches himself or herself for real or fancied acts of negligence or omissions in the relationship with the deceased.	"I should have made him go to the doctor sooner." "I should have paid more attention to her, been more thoughtful."
Anger	
The anger the bereaved experiences may not be toward the object that gives rise to it. Often, the anger is displaced onto the medical or nursing staff. Often, it is directed toward the deceased. The anger is at its height during the first month but is often intermittent throughout the first year. The overflow of hostility disturbs the bereaved, resulting in the feeling that he or she is going "insane."	"The doctor didn't operate in time. If he had, Mary would be alive today." "How could he leave me like this . . . how could he?"
Change in Behavior (Depression, Disorganization, Restlessness)	
A person may exhibit marked restlessness and an inability to organize his or her behavior. Routine activities take a long time to do. Depressive mood is common as the year passes and as the intensity of the grief declines. Absence of depression is more abnormal than its presence. Loneliness and aimlessness are most pronounced 6 to 9 months after the death.	Six months after her husband died, Mrs. Faye stated, "I just can't seem to function. I have a hard time doing the simplest tasks. I can't be bothered with socializing." "I feel so down . . . so, so empty."
Reorganization of Behavior Directed Toward a New Object or Activity	
Gradually, the person renews his or her interest in people and activities. The grieving thus releases the bereaved from one interpersonal relationship, and new ones are free to take its place.	Twenty months after her husband's death, Mrs. Faye tells a friend, "I'll be away this weekend. I am going fishing with my brother and his friend. This is the first time I've felt like doing anything since Harry died."

From: Varcarolis EM: Foundations of Psychiatric Mental Health Nursing, 3rd ed. Philadelphia: WB Saunders, 1998, p. 548. Used with permission.

440

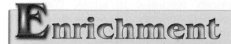

SEASONAL AFFECTIVE DISORDER

Seasonal affective disorder (SAD), also known as seasonal pattern specifier, is a depressive condition that is manifested in a cyclical manner at characteristic times of the year. It has been noted that the depression usually has an onset in the fall of the year, extends through the winter months, and then improves or goes into remission during spring to return in the fall. There may be an occasional summer episode. The episode pattern occurs in successive years. Symptoms include lack of energy, excessive sleeping, overeating, a craving for carbohydrates, and weight gain. The incidence of SAD is greater in women than in men, and younger people appear to be at higher risk than the elderly. The geographic latitude appears to be involved, with the occurrence increasing the higher the latitude and the shorter the daylight hours.

The cause of SAD has been suggested to be an increase in the amount of the hormone melatonin secreted by the pineal gland. Melatonin is produced during dark hours; therefore, it is speculated that an excessive amount affects certain people. The hormone secretion is suppressed by light. Increased amounts of melatonin are associated with lethargy and drowsiness. Drugs have been used to suppress melatonin secretion with some success. Another theory suggests that the body's **circadian rhythm** is delayed in people with SAD, causing the "vegetative" symptoms. This theory supports the use of light therapy, the exposure to bright light for certain periods of time in the morning during the winter months. This treatment also has produced positive results and generated improvement in the depressed state of people with SAD.

emergency departments and law enforcement agencies have resource personnel available for immediate contact to provide support and personal contact. Mental health agencies routinely provide their clients with a 24-hour "hot line" number with which to contact a counselor. Structures that are frequent lethal jumping points, such as bridges, have strategically placed signs with crisis control telephone numbers (see Fig. 14–6A and *B*).

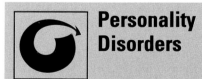

Personality Disorders

SYMPTOMS AND SIGNS

Personality disorders affect the mental aspects of a person and involve chronic, ingrained maladaptive behavior. Disordered patterns of relating, thinking, and perceiving impair social and occupational performance. Although personality disorders typically are recognized during adolescence, they may continue throughout adult life. A history of long-standing problems in interpersonal relationships and occupational difficulties is likely. Personality traits may give the person a reputation for arrogance or painful shyness and rejection of responsibility for behavior. The person tends to project negative feelings and blame others. There are many recognized types of personality disorders, each with unique distinguishing characteristics. Examples of personality disorders include paranoid, schizoid, antisocial, histrionic, and narcissistic disorders.

Paranoid Disorder. The chief traits are suspiciousness and extreme mistrust of others. Patients relentlessly suspect the motives, prejudices, and intent of others as deliberately harmful to themselves. Inappropriately angry and hostile responses are common.

Schizoid Disorder. The person may be described as a loner, aloof and unemotional. He or she avoids close relationships, preferring to remain detached. The opinions of others seem to have little or no effect. The person with schizoid personality disorder has difficulty in expressing ordinary anger or aggression.

Antisocial Disorder. Behavior patterns of the antisocial personality cause frequent conflicts with social values. Troublesome conduct usually emerges by 15 years of age, with truancy, fighting, stealing, history of running away, or cruel behavior. Antisocial persons do not express guilt or learn from their mistakes. Other traits include a propensity for irresponsible and impulsive actions.

Histrionic Disorder. The histrionic person displays overly dramatic and theatrical mannerisms. There is a conscious, or unconscious, pervasive need to be the center of attention. People with this disorder are immature and dependent, constantly seeking approval and reassurance. Behavior or appearance may be inappropriately seductive.

Narcissistic Disorder. The narcissistic personality demonstrates pathologic self-love or grandiose self-admiration. When criticized, the person reacts with rage or humiliation, based on an exaggerated sense of self-importance. There is lack of empathy and a tendency to exploit others. A preoccupation with fantasies of unlimited success is exhibited.

ETIOLOGY

The cause of personality disorders has not been identified. Various theories include possible biologic, social, or psychodynamic origins.

DIAGNOSIS

Diagnosis of personality disorders is based on the documentation of diagnostic criteria defined in the American Psychiatric Association's DSM-IV.

TREATMENT

The treatment of personality disorders depends on the symptoms and involves psychotherapy and, in some cases, drug therapy. Improved coping mechanisms and control of symptoms are the goals of therapy. A trusting relationship between patient and therapist is advantageous because some people with these disorders tend to be noncompliant and resist therapy. Hospitalization may be required during acute episodes that incapacitate the person. Family involvement in group therapy has proved beneficial for some patients.

Anxiety Disorders

SYMPTOMS AND SIGNS

Anxiety is a common form of psychological disorder (Fig. 14-8). For most people, anxiety is just a temporary response to stress. For some people, however, anxiety becomes a chronic problem, and they experience excessive levels of anxiety on a regular basis. They often exhibit anxiety that is inappropriate to the circumstance. Only when anxiety persists and prevents the person from leading a normal life does it become an illness. As a group, anxiety disorders represent the single largest mental health problem in the United States. They can lead to more severe disorders, such as depression and alcoholism.

Anxiety disorders, previously known as neuroses, include three specific disorders or syndromes that are different in behavioral manifestations but share the fact that the person's behavior is dominated by anxiety. The disorders are generalized anxiety disorder and panic disorder, phobic disorder, and obsessive–compulsive disorder.

Generalized Anxiety Disorder and Panic Disorder

Patients with generalized anxiety disorder have a condition known as free-floating anxiety and live in a constant state of apparently causeless anxiety. They constantly worry about previous mistakes and future problems. These individuals dislike having to confront decisions and worry about the ones that they do make. Their constant worrying frequently is accompanied by physiologic symptoms: diarrhea, elevated blood pressure, and sustained muscular tension. Inability to sleep and nightmares are common. Some persons are even prone to panic attacks.

In panic disorder, the anxiety is also unfocused. With a panic attack, the anxiety begins suddenly and unexpectedly, reaching a peak within 10 minutes. This often is accompanied by a sense of impending doom and a feeling that the patients are "going crazy," losing control, or dying. The world may seem unreal (derealization), or the patients may seem unreal to themselves (depersonalization). In addition, these persons may experience palpitations, rapid pulse, pounding heart, sweating, trembling, shortness of breath, chest pain, nausea, paresthesia, dizziness, and chills or hot flashes.

The anxiety characteristic of a panic disorder can be differentiated from generalized anxiety by its sudden, intermittent nature and greater severity. A person is said to have panic disorder if he or she has four panic attacks within a month's time or if one or more attacks have been followed by a persistent fear of having another attack.

```
                    ┌──────────────────────────────┐
                    │ Anxiety Disorders: Stress     │
                    │          Response             │
                    └──────────────────────────────┘
```

Posttraumatic Stress Response

1. The person experienced, witnessed, or was confronted with an event that involved actual, threatened death to self or others, responding in fear, helplessness, or horror

2. The event is persistently reexperienced by
   (a) Distressing dreams or images
   (b) Reliving the event through flashbacks, illusions, hallucinations

3. Persistent avoidance of stimuli associated with trauma:
   (a) Avoidance of thoughts, feelings, conversations
   (b) Avoidance of people, places, activities
   (c) Inability to recall aspects of trauma
   (d) Decreased interest in usual activities
   (e) Feelings of detachment, estrangement from others
   (f) Restriction in feelings (love, enthusiasm, joy)
   (g) Sense of shortened feelings

4. Persistent symptoms of increased arousal (two or more):
   (a) Difficulty falling/staying asleep
   (b) Irritability/outbursts of anger
   (c) Difficulty concentrating

5. Duration more than 1 month:
   • Acute: Duration less than 3 months
   • Chronic: Duration 3 months or more
   • Delayed: If onset of symptoms is at least 6 months after stress

Acute Stress Response

1. The person experienced, witnessed, or was confronted with an event that involved actual, threatened death to self or others, responding in fear, helplessness, or horror.

2. The event is associated with three or more of the following dissociative symptoms:
   (a) Sense of numbing, detachment, or absence of emotional response
   (b) Reduced awareness of surroundings (e.g., "in a daze")
   (c) Derealization
   (d) Depersonalization
   (e) Amnesia for an important aspect of the trauma

3. The event is persistently reexperienced by
   (a) Distressing dreams or images
   (b) Reliving the event through flashbacks, illusions, hallucinations

4. Marked avoidance of stimuli that arouse memory of trauma (thoughts, feelings, people, places, activities, conversations).

5. Marked symptoms of anxiety:
   (a) Difficulty falling/staying asleep
   (b) Irritability/outbursts of anger
   (c) Difficulty concentrating

6. Causes impairment in social, occupational, and other functioning, or impairs ability to complete some memory tasks.

7. Lasts from 2 days to 4 weeks and occurs within 4 weeks of the traumatic event

Figure 14–8

Anxiety disorders.

Phobic Disorder

A phobic disorder is marked by excessive, persistent, and irrational fear and the avoidance of the phobic stimulus. In phobic disorders, the person's excessive anxiety has a specific focus (Fig. 14-9), some object or a situation that presents no realistic danger. Many persons with phobias realize that their fears are irrational but feel powerless to control or prevent them. Phobic persons must design their lives to avoid the things that they fear. When they are confronted by an object or situation that causes them anxiety, they often have a severe attack of anxiety.

Phobias can develop from or against almost anything (Table 14-5).

Obsessive-Compulsive Disorder

Obsessive-compulsive disorder is marked by the presence of obsessions (thoughts) and compulsions (actions). Obsessions are persistent intrusions of unwanted thoughts and compulsions are uncontrollable urges to carry out certain actions. The two features of this disorder usually occur together, but not always. People with obsessions often have thoughts of harm to other individuals, suicide, or sexual acts considered im-

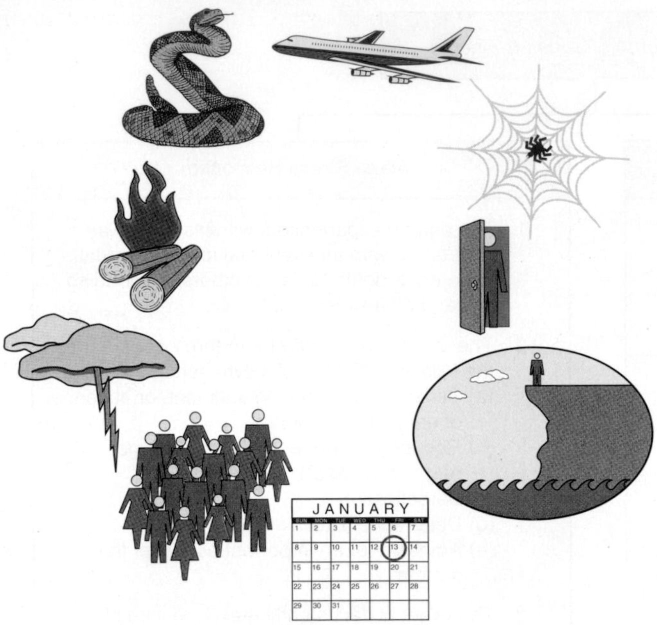

Figure 14–9
Phobias.

444

moral. These people feel as though they have lost control of their minds, which causes them great anxiety. People with compulsions develop senseless actions or rituals that relieve their anxiety temporarily (e.g., excessive hand washing).

ETIOLOGY

There are many theories as to the causes of anxiety disorders. Some anxiety disorders are caused by severe stress. In persons who are anxiety prone, only slight stress, or none at all, can be involved. A physical condition such as hyperthy-roidism (overactive thyroid gland), or a cerebro-vascular disorder, also can produce the symptoms of anxiety. The role of neurotransmitters and genetic factors has been studied. In obsessive–compulsive disorder, there also may be a relation to dysfunctioning in the frontal lobe of the brain.

DIAGNOSIS

The diagnosis of anxiety disorders is made after much investigation into the patient's symptoms and history. In some cases, metabolic testing indicates abnormalities. **Positron-emission**

TABLE 14–5 ➤ Phobias

Acrophobia	Fear of high places	Olfactophobia	Fear of odor
Agoraphobia	Fear of open spaces	Ombrophobia	Fear of rain
Algophobia	Fear of pain	Ophidophobia	Fear of snakes
Androphobia	Fear of men	Pathophobia	Fear of disease
Arachnophobia	Fear of spiders	Pharmacophobia	Fear of drugs
Astrophobia	Fear of storms, thunder, and lightning	Phasmophobia	Fear of ghosts
Avioidphobia	Fear of flying	Phobophobia	Fear of fear
Claustrophobia	Fear of closed or narrow spaces	Ponophobia	Fear of work
Hematophobia	Fear of blood	Pyrophobia	Fear of fire
Hodophobia	Fear of travel	Sitophobia	Fear of food
Hydrophobia	Fear of water	Thanatophobia	Fear of death
Iatrophobia	Fear of physicians	Toxophobia	Fear of being poisoned
Kainophobia	Fear of change	Traumatophobia	Fear of injury
Kakorrhaphiophobia	Fear of failure	Triskaidekaphobia	Fear of the number 13
Lalophobia	Fear of speaking in public	Xenophobia	Fear of strangers
Monophobia	Fear of being alone	Zoophobia	Fear of animals
Ochlophobia	Fear of crowds		

tomography (PET) to detect chemical activity or metabolism of the brain and biochemical studies also have been used.

TREATMENT

If the anxiety prevents the person from living a normal life, a psychiatrist or a practitioner trained in treating psychological problems (e.g., psychologist or psychoanalyst) should be consulted. Many forms of treatment are used by these therapists, depending on their perspective. Hypnosis sometimes is used to help the patient and the therapist to gain access to the unconscious mind. If the anxiety is caused by a specific stress (e.g., job related), steps should be taken to minimize or eliminate the problem. Various methods of relaxation can make the symptoms less severe. Relaxation exercises (e.g., biofeedback) to relax tense muscles or a physical activity such as brisk walking, jogging, or swimming may be beneficial. In addition, or as an alternative, the physician may prescribe an **anxiolytic** drug or recommend psychotherapy. In severe cases of anxiety, a period of hospitalization also may be necessary. If severe anxiety is not treated, psychotic depression may develop.

Post-Traumatic Stress Disorder

SYMPTOMS AND SIGNS

Post-traumatic stress disorders (PTSDs) are different from other anxiety disorders because the cause of the stress is an external event of an overwhelmingly painful nature (Fig. 14-10). The person may experience this disorder for weeks, months, or even years (chronic) after the event through painful recollections or nightmares. People with PTSD go out of their way to avoid being reminded of the painful event. They may be unable to respond to affection and have insomnia and irritability. These individuals also may exhibit strong physiologic responses to any reminder of the event.

Symptoms of PTSD usually appear within a short time after the event. In some cases, however, there is a delayed response (onset). The person may be symptom free for days or months after the event before signs of response to the painful event begin to appear. Usually, however, the symptoms disappear spontaneously in approximately 6 months. Not all people exposed to severe traumatic events have such symptoms. It appears that the likelihood of developing PTSD depends, to some degree, on the person's psychological strength before the event. The likelihood of this disorder also depends on the nature of the event.

ETIOLOGY

Occurrences caused by human actions (e.g., rape, acts of war, and continued abuse) tend to precipitate more severe reactions than those caused by natural disasters (e.g., hurricanes, earthquakes, and floods). In the case of natural disasters, the greater the threat of death and the larger the number of people affected, the greater the likelihood of severe PTSD. The overwhelming experience of a threat to the individual's life is a causative factor.

Children also may be affected by experiencing or observing horror in their lives. Traumatic events include acts of war, in which they have observed family members killed or have been separated from the family unit. Additionally, catastrophic events of nature, in which they have witnessed violent destruction to homes and surroundings, may make them fearful and withdrawn. Abuse also is known to cause PTSD, especially sexual abuse. Recognition of traumatic events in children's lives is essential, as is involving them in therapy.

DIAGNOSIS

Diagnosis is confirmed when the patient experiences intrusive symptoms, both recurrent and distressing recollections of the event, including recurrent dreams and flashbacks of the event. An additional factor in the diagnosis is the individual's persistent avoidance of stimuli associated with the traumatic experience. Hyperarousal in the form of rapid heartbeat, dyspnea, and panic usually are involved.

Children often will re-enact the event, have recurrent dreams or nightmares of the event, or have repetitive patterns of the event in their play.

TREATMENT

The goal of treatment of PTSD is to restore the individual's sense of control. Counseling and drug therapy are used in the treatment. The counseling therapy helps PTSD victims to accept the overwhelming memories without rearranging their lives to avoid the memories. They work to develop a sense of safety and control. Feelings of guilt and self-blame need to be addressed. Cognitive behavior training to increase self-esteem and self-control is employed.

Sleep disturbances must be recognized and treated. Benzodiazepines may be prescribed to assist with regaining normal sleep patterns. Addi-

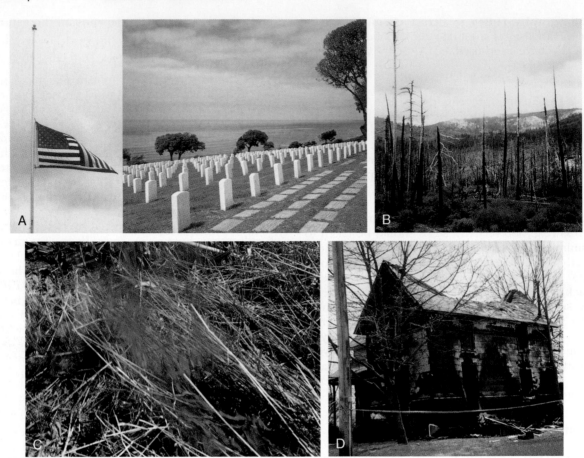

Figure 14–10

Post-traumatic stress disorder sources. *A*, Overwhelming numbers of violent deaths, as in wars; *B*, destruction by fire of one's environment, as in forest fires encroaching on communities; *C*, brush fires suddenly erupting on community property; *D*, fire destroying shelters and property. (Courtesy of David L. Frazier, 1999.)

tionally, antianxiety agents or selective serotonin reuptake inhibitors (SSRIs) may be used as drug therapy. Recovery may be complete in some individuals in a short time, whereas others may never completely recover.

Somatoform Disorders

Somatoform disorders are a group of mental disorders in which the person experiences physical symptoms without the underlying organic cause. These symptoms are not under voluntary control and are real to the affected person. The opposite is true of factitious disorders (Munchausen syndrome) or malingering, in which the patient presents with feigned symptoms for personal or emotional gain. There is no diagnosable general medical condition that is confirmed that accounts for the symptoms.

SOMATIZATION DISORDER

SYMPTOMS AND SIGNS

In somatization disorder, the patient experiences multiple, recurring somatic symptoms that have no underlying clinical pathologic basis. These symptoms have an onset before the age of

30 years and are ongoing for several years. Symptoms include pain related to four or more areas or functions of the body. Additionally, the patient reports GI symptoms (nausea, vomiting, and blood in the stool) other than pain, a symptom related to the reproductive system (e.g., for females, irregular or heavy menses, and for males, erectile or ejaculatory problems), and a neurologic symptom that is without clinical basis.

ETIOLOGY

The etiology is uncertain; however, there appears to be a familial pattern.

DIAGNOSIS

Diagnosis is made after medical conditions are ruled out. Criteria include the presence of four pain symptoms, two GI symptoms, one sexual symptom, and one **pseudoneurologic** symptom. Onset is early in life, before the age of 30 years and the condition is chronic, with never a symptom-free period of longer than 1 year. There is an absence of clinical pathologic change, and no laboratory findings support the symptoms.

TREATMENT

This chronic condition rarely has complete remission. Treatment includes investigating symptoms and ruling out any underlying general medical condition.

CONVERSION DISORDER

SYMPTOMS AND SIGNS

Conversion disorders formerly were termed hysteria. Anxiety is changed (converted) to a physical or somatic symptom. The anxiety is too difficult to face, and as a defense mechanism, the physical symptoms allow the person to escape or avoid a stressful situation. Symptoms include deficits in voluntary motor or sensory functions (paralysis) and are unintentional and preceded by conflicts or other stressors. Clinically significant social and occupational functioning is present.

Sensory symptoms may include **anesthesia, hyperesthesia, analgesia,** and paresthesia. Motor symptoms may include paralysis, tremors, tics, **contractures,** and ambulation disturbances. Speech disturbances may include **aphonia** and **mutism,** whereas visceral symptoms may include headaches, difficulty in swallowing and breathing, choking, coughing, nausea, vomiting, belching, cold and clammy extremities, weight loss, and **pseudopregnancy.** Blindness and seizures also may be noted.

ETIOLOGY

The cause of this psychiatric syndrome is usually a highly stressful situation.

DIAGNOSIS

Diagnosis is made from history of the preceding event and the classic pattern of acute onset of symptoms. A complete physical examination rules out underlying pathologic conditions.

TREATMENT

Treatment is supportive and symptomatic. The course of this disorder is usually short, with many cases resolving in a few weeks. Recurrence is common.

PAIN DISORDER

SYMPTOMS AND SIGNS

Pain disorders include the subtypes that are associated with psychological factors, those associated with both psychological factors and general medical conditions, and those associated with general medical conditions. The pain is severe and lasting and may have a clinical basis. The response to pain depends on the patient's interpretation; however, this type of pain causes an interference with life activities, including occupational, social, and other areas of functioning. The pain may be associated with musculoskeletal disorders (herniated disk, osteoporosis, and arthritis), neuropathies, and malignancies. Chronic pain often causes depression.

ETIOLOGY

The pain may be related to underlying clinical pathologic conditions. Psychological factors may play a role in the onset and severity of the pain. Occasionally, both clinical pathologic and psychological factors contribute to the manifestation of the condition. This condition is not intentionally produced, as is malingering.

DIAGNOSIS

Diagnostic studies may reveal pathologic change. Because pain is subjective and pain disorder may or may not have a clinical basis, it is difficult to determine the extent of the pain and psychological involvement. Long-standing pain may cause depression and even lead to suicide.

TREATMENT

Any underlying identifiable pathologic change is treated. Patients with terminal disease may be

447

given narcotics to relieve intractable pain. Psychotherapy may be of some help.

HYPOCHONDRIASIS

SYMPTOMS AND SIGNS

Hypochondriasis is characterized by patients' reports and symptoms of possible physical illness without any identifiable evidence of the illness. These patients have a preoccupation with illness and have an abnormal fear of disease. The history provided by the patients is generalized, symptoms are vague, and they have difficulty with specifics. There is no conscious faking of symptoms; these patients really do feel the conditions about which they complain.

ETIOLOGY

The etiology of hypochondriasis is uncertain.

DIAGNOSIS

Diagnosis is difficult because these people change physicians and present their symptoms to different health-care providers when they do not receive affirmation of illness. Frequently, laboratory and diagnostic studies reveal no underlying condition. When one does exist, it may be overlooked. Social and occupational relationships suffer from the constant abnormal preoccupation with one's health status.

TREATMENT

Treatment of any underlying conditions is necessary; however, these conditions easily can be missed because of the vagueness of the symptoms reported and the changing of health-care providers. Some patients may benefit from psychotherapy.

MUNCHAUSEN SYNDROME AND MUNCHAUSEN SYNDROME BY PROXY

SYMPTOMS AND SIGNS

Munchausen syndrome, or factitious disorder, occurs when the patient simulates symptoms of illness and presents for no apparent reason other than treatment. The patients feign symptoms and actually can make themselves ill by injecting foreign material to cause a fever. Generally, these patients have extensive knowledge of medical terminology and hospital routines. Munchausen syndrome by proxy occurs when the parent projects the symptoms to the child, usually a preschooler. This parent often stimulates the illness in the child and then presents the child for treatment. The parent denies any knowledge of actual cause and relates the symptoms to be GI, genitourinary, or CNS in nature. As in Munchausen syndrome, the degree of the complaint is limited only by the parent's medical knowledge.

ETIOLOGY

The cause of this behavior is uncertain. There is no external motive other than to assume the sick role.

DIAGNOSIS

These patients present at a hospital or physician's office with reports of fever, anemia, dermatitis, or seizure activity. The symptoms have an atypical clinical course, with laboratory findings that are inconsistent with the symptoms. They have a dramatic flair but give vague answers when questioned closely. When the initial workup indicates no particular disease entity, symptoms change. Multiple invasive procedures are undergone eagerly. There is a history of repeated hospitalizations with no firm evidence of an underlying disease process. Additionally, there is no motive of financial gain, only that of attention.

TREATMENT

Eventually, the behavior is revealed and when confronted with this fact, these patients seek attention at another facility.

Enrichment

MALINGERING

Malingering is the feigning of symptoms for financial or personal gain. The action is deliberate and fraudulent, and the symptoms usually are exaggerated. Various undesirable situations may cause the patient to report symptoms to avoid or delay the situation. Diagnosis is difficult because often the symptoms are subjective and cannot be disproved.

Gender Identity Disorders

SYMPTOMS AND SIGNS

Gender identity is a person's inner sense of maleness or femaleness. The disorder occurs when the person feels as if she or he really should be the opposite sex. Evidence of a strong cross-gender identification is present, and there is a discomfort about the assigned sex. These people also experience a sense of inappropriateness in their gender role.

Boys have a marked preoccupation with feminine activities, including dressing in feminine clothing and playing with traditionally girl toys. Competitive sports and typical boy activity and play are avoided. Some boys remark that they do not want their penis and prefer to have a vagina.

Girls display a dislike for feminine attire and prefer boy-type clothing and short hair. They prefer boys as playmates and engage in typical boy sports and games. Many claim that they will grow a penis and do not want breast growth or menses.

During adulthood, these persons have a strong desire to adopt the role of the opposite sex and to seek out physical change by hormonal or surgical intervention. They are not comfortable as society defines their gender role and prefer to act out as the opposite sex. They take on the characteristics of the other sex and dress accordingly.

Regardless of age, many of these patients experience social isolation and ostracism. They frequently have low self-esteem.

ETIOLOGY

The etiology of the syndrome is uncertain.

DIAGNOSIS

Observation of the behavioral patterns leads to suspicion of gender identity disorder; however, there is no known diagnostic test for this syndrome. Psychological evaluation may reveal the tendency. A strong cross-gender identification persists, along with a discomfort with one's sex or sense of inappropriate gender identification.

TREATMENT

Psychological counseling to recognize and acknowledge the feelings may be of value. Sex alteration with hormone treatment and surgical intervention often helps these patients.

Sleep Disorders

Sleep disorders include insomnia, parasomnias, sleep **apnea,** and narcolepsy. Sleep disorders are assessed by polysomnography, which measures rapid eye movement (REM) and the four non–rapid eye movement (NREM) sleep stages, stages 1, 2, 3, and 4. Stage 1 NREM sleep is considered transitional and occupies 5% of normal sleep time. Stage 2 occupies approximately 50% of normal sleep time and is a deeper sleep. Stages 3 and 4 (slow-wave sleep) are the deepest states and occupy 10 to 20% of sleep time. Stages 3 and 4 lessen in extent with aging and even disappear in some people older than 55 years of age. The average adult requires 6 to 8 hours of continuous sleep, with younger people requiring more and the elderly needing less.

The disorders can be caused by functional or organic disorders, so underlying pathologic conditions must be ruled out or treated.

INSOMNIA

SYMPTOMS AND SIGNS

Insomnia is difficulty in falling asleep or staying asleep. In addition, the person with insomnia arises physically and mentally tired, groggy, tense, irritable, and anxious. Additionally, some people experience extremely early morning awakening and state that their sleep was not restorative.

ETIOLOGY

The cause may be situation related, caused by medical problems, or caused by a change to high altitudes. Additional causes are pain, cardiovascular problems, thyroid conditions, and fever. Stimulants, including caffeine, amphetamines, steroids, alcohol, nicotine, and bronchodilators, cause drug-related insomnia. Psychological causes include anxiety, stress, and even the fear of sleeplessness itself.

DIAGNOSIS

To be diagnosed as insomnia, the sleeplessness must have a duration of longer than 1 month and must interfere with normal functioning in social, occupational, or other areas. A study is conducted of the 24-hour sleep and wakefulness periods, along with an examination of any underlying factors. Polysomnography, a recording of several physiologic variables related to sleep made while the patient is sleeping, indicates poor sleep patterns, including increased stage 1 and decreased stage 3 and 4 periods, along with increased muscle tremors. The person appears fatigued and exhibits no other abnormalities. The occurrence of insomnia increases with age and is more common in females.

TREATMENT

The first step in treatment is to identify and remove the cause; this is followed by an attempt to improve sleep hygiene. Patients are counseled to make changes in lifestyle to relieve tension and reduce stress. They are encouraged to have a regular sleep schedule and to consider the bedroom for sleep and not for worry about stressful situations. Noise and disruptions during the normal sleep time should be eliminated, and daily activities should be increased. There should be a regular bedtime and a regular time for arising. Psychotherapy may be indicated to help to relieve anxiety and stress. As a last resort, hypnotics of the benzodiazepine class may be prescribed.

PARASOMNIAS

SYMPTOMS AND SIGNS

Parasomnias are a group of sleep disorders that include sleepwalking, night terrors, and nightmares. These disorders usually occur in children early in the night. When there is late onset in the elderly, a CNS pathologic process is responsible. People who sleepwalk generally have no memory of the event. They awake confused, with blank expressions on their faces, and are unaware of the environment. Those experiencing nightmares often have vivid recall and remember dreams of fear of attack, falling, and death. These dreams occur late at night.

ETIOLOGY

Several elements, including possible genetic, developmental, psychological, and organic factors, may precipitate the occurrences. Febrile episodes or brain tumors may be causes. Lithium and certain drugs precipitate the condition. There is evidence of increased REM sleep periods and rebound REM sleep because of certain drugs.

DIAGNOSIS

Reports of the episodes lead to further investigation. A thorough history should include any drug consumption. Any underlying cause in the elderly and mature adults should be investigated and diagnosed.

TREATMENT

Protection from injury is primary for the sleepwalking person. The sleepwalking person should not be interrupted or awakened. The occurrence of night terrors is reduced by minimizing the exposure to terror, especially from movies, videotapes, and television programs. Children usually outgrow these conditions. Frequently, adults are treated with diazepam (Valium).

NARCOLEPSY

SYMPTOMS AND SIGNS

Narcolepsy, irresistible daytime sleep episodes, can occur for a few seconds to a half hour in duration. Usually precipitated by sedentary, monotonous activity, narcolepsy attacks occur while driving, sitting in a lecture, or even eating. Normally, the onset is before the age of 25 years. A period of sleep paralysis lasts approximately 1 minute; the person is unable to move, but breathing persists.

ETIOLOGY

There appears to be a familial incidence and possible genetic aberration of REM sleep time.

DIAGNOSIS

The history of repeated episodes suggests narcolepsy. Seizure activity and sleep apnea should be ruled out. Onset is usually during adolescence, producing disturbed night sleep.

TREATMENT

Treatment consists of therapeutic naps and establishing a normal night sleep pattern. Methylphenidate is prescribed. These patients must be warned of the dangers of driving or operating machinery and falling asleep during that time. This chronic disorder is not under voluntary control.

SLEEP APNEA

SYMPTOMS AND SIGNS

Sleep apnea is the intermittent short period of cessation of breathing during sleep. During normal nocturnal sleep, there are periods of breath cessation, which are followed by snorting and gasping. This condition occurs more frequently in men than in women and may be associated with obesity, hypertension, or an airway-obstructive condition. The patient does not feel rested even after several hours of sleep.

ETIOLOGY

There appears to be an inherent predisposition to this condition. Often, a nasal obstruction is the cause. Alcohol ingestion, smoking-related bronchitis, and sleep deprivation are other causes.

DIAGNOSIS

Diagnosis begins with a sleep history. Onset usually occurs in middle age. Daytime sleepiness, sleep attacks, and snoring and snorting episodes also suggest sleep apnea. Sleep laboratory studies confirm the diagnosis when periods of breathing cessation while sleeping are observed.

TREATMENT

Weight loss is encouraged. Protriptyline is prescribed. **Constant positive air pressure** or dental appliances may be tried. Any underlying pathologic condition should be diagnosed and corrected. The patient is advised to avoid the use of any drugs that depress the CNS. **Uvulopalatopharyngoplasty** (UPPP), a surgical procedure to remove portions of the uvula, soft palate, and posterior pharyngeal mucosa, is attempted as a last resort.

Summary

Persistent anxiety, depression, sleep disorder, or somatic preoccupation may be symptoms of an emotional disorder requiring medical intervention. With treatment, most psychiatric conditions are managed to allow recovery and to restore a person's ability to function in interpersonal relationships, self-care, and occupational settings.

- Certain disorders in thinking, perceiving, and behaving can be organized into clusters of signs and symptoms.
- Mental retardation, learning disorders, and communication disorders require diagnostic evaluation of intellectual capabilities and specific recognition of any underlying medical conditions, hereditary causes, and environmental influences.
- Dementia involves a progressive, general deterioration of the mental capacities of perceiving, thinking, and remembering.
- There are many other causes of dementia other than Alzheimer's disease.
- Chronic alcohol abuse produces symptoms and signs in nearly every organ system.
- Schizophrenia, a major psychiatric disturbance, is marked by disorganized thinking, hallucinations, inappropriate affect, and a vast range of behavioral manifestations. Antipsychotic drugs are used to control symptoms.
- Mood disorders represent a pathologic disturbance in mood that interferes with all aspects of an individual's life.
- Major depression can lead to suicidal thoughts and actions that must be taken seriously for effective intervention.
- Bipolar disorder and major depressive disorder manifest a serious alteration in mood, accompanied by various changes in behavior and a variety of physical symptoms. Usually, these conditions respond effectively to a combination of medication and psychotherapy.
- Persons with personality disorders have a history of long-standing maladaptive behavior with unique and distinguishing characteristics.
- Chronic or inappropriate anxiety can become an illness, such as panic disorder, phobic disorder, or obsessive-compulsive disorder.
- Post-traumatic stress disorder is a delayed response to an external traumatic event that produces signs and symptoms of extreme distress.
- Somatoform disorders include a group of mental disorders in which there are physical symptoms without organic cause (as in a conversion disorder) and factitious disorders (as in Munchausen syndrome) or malingering.
- Sleep disorders, including insomnia, parasomnias, sleep apnea, and narcolepsy, can be caused by functional or organic conditions; polysomnography frequently is used as a diagnostic tool.

Review Challenge

REVIEW QUESTIONS

1. What are the contributing factors to mental disorders?
2. What observations may indicate mental retardation?
3. What variants are considered in the diagnosis of a learning disorder?
4. What are the characteristics of a child with autism?
5. What are the diagnostic criteria for a tic disorder?
6. Under which conditions may dementia occur?
7. Why is Alzheimer's disease so difficult to diagnose?
8. How may vascular dementia be related to atherosclerosis?
9. How might head trauma cause dementia?
10. How does repeated heavy alcohol abuse harm the body?
11. What are some effects of a rising blood alcohol level on the brain?
12. Why is schizophrenia termed a major psychiatric disturbance?
13. How does bipolar disorder affect an individual?
14. What is thought to cause a major depressive disorder?
15. What are the phases of the grief process?
16. What are some of the long-standing problems typical of personality disorders?
17. How are the major anxiety disorders classified? How do they differ from each other?
18. Which condition may result as a delayed response to an external painful event?
19. What is a somatization disorder?
20. How is anxiety related to a conversion disorder?
21. Which condition results from preoccupation with illness and abnormal fear of disease?
22. Can severe pain cause illness?
23. How is Munchausen syndrome diagnosed?
24. What is the typical pattern of sleep disorder in (a) insomnia, (b) narcolepsy, and (c) sleep apnea?

REAL-LIFE CHALLENGE

Sleep Apnea

The wife of a 48-year-old man states that she cannot sleep because of the loud snoring of her husband. Questioning reveals that she has noticed that he has periods during which he appears to stop breathing for about 30 seconds when sleeping. The patient has a history of mild alcohol consumption and also of smoking. He is approximately 30 pounds overweight.

Sleep studies are ordered because sleep apnea is suspected. The patient also states that he does not feel rested after sleeping 8 to 9 hours a night.

Questions

1. What is the significance of the loud snoring?
2. Why is a history of social habits (smoking and alcohol consumption) important?
3. What are sleep studies?
4. What may happen if the sleep apnea is not diagnosed?
5. Which treatment may be prescribed?
6. What is the anticipated outcome of the treatment?

REAL-LIFE CHALLENGE

Alzheimer's Disease

A 75-year-old man is diagnosed with Alzheimer's disease. The retired businessman has noticed many memory lapses, primarily in the area of short-term memory and the inability to concentrate. His family noted that his verbalization appears somewhat diminished because he has difficulty expressing his thoughts in an appropriate manner and interjects nonsensical phrases. He becomes agitated quite easily and

has very little interest in grooming and self-appearance. The family has been advised that they may have to have help in the future to care for the patient and that he probably will have to be institutionalized.

Because the patient exhibits both cognitive and behavioral symptoms of Alzheimer's disease, he is treated with donepezil (Aricept) and alprazolam (Xanax).

Questions

1. Who is most likely to exhibit symptoms of Alzheimer's disease?
2. List the typical symptoms.
3. Which interventions may be taken?
4. What are some of the theories that have been advanced regarding the cause of Alzheimer's disease?
5. How is Alzheimer's disease diagnosed?

6. What is the anticipated prognosis for this patient?
7. What differentiates Alzheimer's disease from senile dementia?
8. To what class of drugs does Xanax belong, and what is the expected outcome of its administration?

RESOURCES

Alzheimer's Association
919 N Michigan Ave, Ste 1000
Chicago, IL 60611-1671
800-272-3900
(http://www.alz.org)

National Center for Post-Traumatic Stress Disorder (PTSD)
VA Medical Centers
White River Junction, VT 05009
802-296-5132
ptsd@dartmouth.edu

National Clearinghouse for Alcohol and Drug Information (NCADI)
PO Box 2345
Rockville, MD 20847-2345
800-NCADI64 (622-3464)
(http://www.health.org)

National Institute of Mental Health (NIMH)
Public Inquiries Branch
6001 Executive Blvd, Room 8184 MSC 9663
Bethesda, MD 20892-9663
301-443-4513
nimhinfo@nih.gov

National Council on Aging
409 Third St, SW
Washington, DC 20024
800-424-9046
info@ncoa.org

Al Anon Family Group Headquarters
1600 Corporate Landing Parkway
Virginia Beach, VA 23454-5617
800-356-9996
(http://www.al-anon.alateen.org)

Alateen
888-425-2666

National Autism Hotline
PO Box 507
Huntington, WV 25710-0507
304-525-8014

Autism Society of America
7910 Woodmont Ave, #650
Bethesda, MD 20814-3015
800-3-AUTISM

The International Dyslexia Society
800-ABCD-123

National Foundation for Depressive Illness
PO Box 2257
New York, NY 10116
800-239-1265
(http://www.depression.org)

National Mental Health Association
1021 Prince St
Alexandria, VA 22314-2971
800-969-6642

Tourette Syndrome Association
4240 Bell Blvd, Ste 205
Bayside, NY 11361
800-237-0717

Children with Attention Deficit Disorder
499 NW 70th Ave
Plantation, FL 33317
301-443-1333

Challenge, ADD Association
PO Box 488
West Newbury, MA 01985
508-462-0495

National Alliance for the Mentally Ill
200 No Glebe Rd, #1015
Arlington, VA 22203-3754
800-950-NAMI

Learning Disabilities Association of America
4256 Library Rd
Pittsburgh, PA 15234
412-341-1515

National Chronic Pain Outreach Association (NCPOA)
7979 Old Georgetown Rd, #100
Bethesda, MA 20814
301-652-4948

American Association of Suicidology
4201 Connecticut Ave, Ste 310
Washington, DC 20008
202-237-2280
(http://www.suicidology.org)

Compassionate Friends
PO Box 3696
Oakbrook, IL 60522-3696

Alcoholics Anonymous, General Services
475 Riverside Dr
New York, NY 10018
212-870-3003
(http://www.alcoholics-anonymous.org)

American Psychiatric Association
1400 K St NW
Washington, DC 20005
202-682-6000
apa@psych.org

American Sleep Disorders Association
1610 14th St, NW, Ste 300
Rochester, MN 55901
(http://www.asda.org)

National Alliance for Research on Schizophrenia and Depression
60 Cutter Mill Rd, Ste 404
Great Neck, NY 11021
516-829-0091
(http://www.mhsource.com/narsad.html)

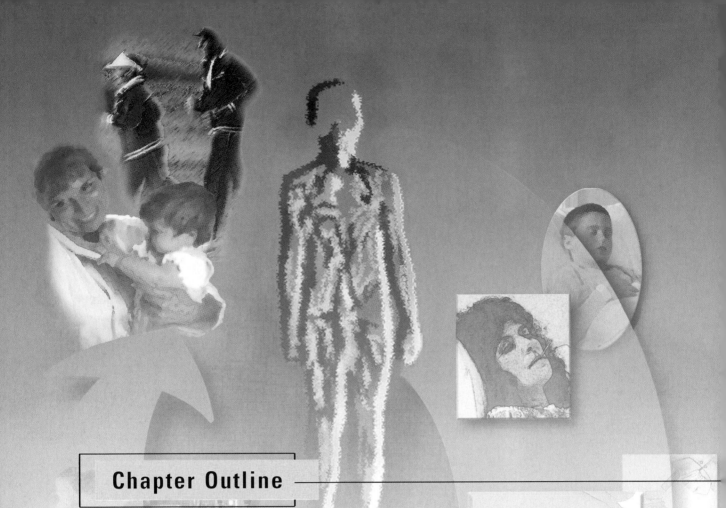

Chapter Outline

Disorders and Conditions Resulting From Trauma

Learning Objectives

After studying Chapter 15, you should be able to:

1. List the major types of trauma.
2. List environmental factors that may result in trauma.
3. Name three factors that generally need to be addressed in open trauma.
4. Distinguish between an abrasion and an avulsion injury.
5. Relate conditions that require prophylaxis with tetanus toxoid.
6. Explain the risk to health-care workers for puncture wounds.
7. Name the conditions classified as thermal insults.
8. Explain the illustration of the rule of nines in adults with burns and how it is used.
9. Describe the possible injuries sustained by (a) electrical shock and (b) lightning.
10. Define hypothermia and name those most at risk.
11. Describe the guidelines for treating (a) frostbite, (b) insect bites, and (c) snake bites.
12. Explain the pathology that results in the pain and numbness of carpal tunnel syndrome.
13. Name the best treatment of child abuse and elder abuse.
14. Explain the importance of immediate intervention in shaken baby syndrome.
15. Discuss special concerns in the diagnosis of (a) battered spouse syndrome, (b) sexual abuse, and (c) rape.

Key Terms

abrasion	(ah–**BRAY**–shun)	cautery	(**KAW**–ter–ee)
analgesic	(**an**–ahl–**GEE**–sik)	débride	(day–**BREED**)
antipyretic	(an–tee–pye–**RET**–tic)	ergonomic	(**er**–go–**NOM**–ic)
antiseptic	(**an**–tih–**SEP**–tic)	hyperabduction	(**high**–per–ab–**DUCK**–
avulsion	(ah–**VUL**–shun)		shun)

hyperthermia	(**high**–per–**THERM**–ee–ah)	laceration	(**lass**–er–**AY**–shun)
hypothermia	(**high**–poh–**THERM**–ee–ah)	prophylaxis	(proh–fih–**LACK**–sis)
		tendinitis	(**ten**–deh–**NYE**–tis)
		vector	(**VECK**–tor)

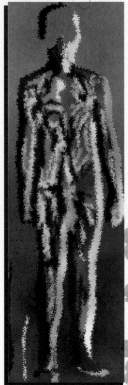

Patient History

Trauma

Although they are not specific disease entities, traumatic occurrences include physical and psychological injury from external force or violence; trauma may be self-inflicted. Regardless of the cause, it can interfere with body functions or the **homeostatic** status of the body, inflict a permanent disability, or may be life threatening. Major types are open trauma, assault trauma, thermal trauma, and psychological trauma. Whether physical or emotional, trauma, including abuse and sexual attack, is prevalent in current society. Physical trauma is the leading cause of death in the United States in young people.

Environmental factors sometimes result in traumatic circumstances. Weather-related conditions often contribute to thermal insults and to motor vehicle or other forms of mechanical or natural accidents. Severe winds and changes in barometric pressure are responsible for trauma to tissue and to the respiratory system. Poisons may result from contaminated ground water, toxins in the air, ingestion of seafood from contaminated sources, or chemical spills. Bites from animals, insects, reptiles, or other sources may occur in special environmental circumstances. High altitudes also can affect body functions. Precaution and prevention are of primary concern in all potentially traumatic circumstances on a continuous basis.

Trauma centers are capable of providing specialized critical care for the seriously injured on a 24-hour basis. Services include a specialized medical team, intensive care measures, and a facility for surgical intervention if needed.

Open Trauma

Open trauma may involve only the skin surface or it may extend to the soft tissue and structures far below the skin. It may be in the form of an abrasion, in which the skin surface is scraped away, or it may be an avulsion, in which the tissue or appendage is torn away. A small area of the skin may be involved, as in a puncture wound, or larger areas may be damaged, as in crushing injuries. All have a commonality, the risk of infection if not appropriately cleaned and dressed. Pain usually is involved in most open trauma.

Bleeding also can be a factor and must be addressed. Some of the injuries need only the basic first aid, whereas others necessitate medical intervention and surgical repair. Regardless of the severity of the injury, appropriate treatment aids healing and lessens scarring. Orthopedic and neurologic traumas are addressed in Chapters 7 and 13, respectively.

ABRASIONS

SYMPTOMS AND SIGNS

Abrasions occur when the outer layers of the skin have been scraped away. The area appears raw, reddened, and painful and has a small amount of bleeding (Fig. 15-1 *A* and *B*). The exposure of sensitive nerve endings causes a burning-type pain in the area. The area may be embedded with small foreign particles.

ETIOLOGY

Abrasions are caused by friction from a rough, hard surface. Frequently called friction burns, floor burns, rug burns, or road rash, the abrasion occurs when the affected body part comes in contact with the rough hard surface in a scraping-type mechanism.

DIAGNOSIS

Diagnosis is made by history and visual inspection.

TREATMENT

Treatment consists of gentle washing or scrubbing of the area with a germicidal soap and water. Any foreign particles, such as gravel and dirt, that have not been removed by cleansing should be removed with forceps. A germicidal ointment or cream then may be applied. A nonadherent dressing may or may not be applied, depending on the size and location of the abrasion. **Prophylaxis** with tetanus toxoid is confirmed or administered if necessary. 7 to 10 years

AVULSION

SYMPTOMS AND SIGNS

In avulsion injuries, a portion of the skin or tissue is torn away, either completely or partially (Fig. 15-2 *A* and *B*). The involved body part may be a limb or appendage, or it may be a soft tissue area anywhere on the surface of the body. The patient usually has severe pain in the area, and bleeding from the wound is common. When the avulsion is partial, the avulsed tissue still is partially attached to the injured part.

ETIOLOGY

The mechanism of this injury is one in which the body part becomes entangled in machinery, clothing, or other means of entrapment, causing the skin, tissue, and bone to be torn and pulled away from the body. If the limb or appendage is severed completely from the body, it is termed an amputation.

DIAGNOSIS

Diagnosis is made by visual inspection of the affected part and by history of the mechanism of injury.

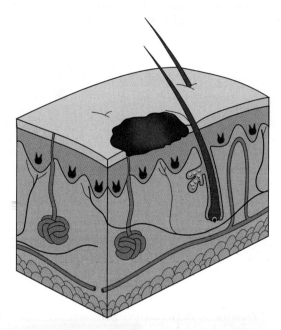

A

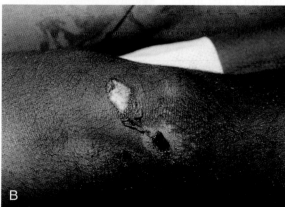

B

Figure 15-1

Abrasion. *A*, Outer layers of the skin are scraped away. *B*, Abrasion wounds of the kneecap caused by a fall to the ground after being struck by an automobile. (*B* from Henry MC, Stapleton ER: EMT Prehospital Care, 2nd ed. Philadelphia: WB Saunders, 1997, p 465. Used with permission.)

459

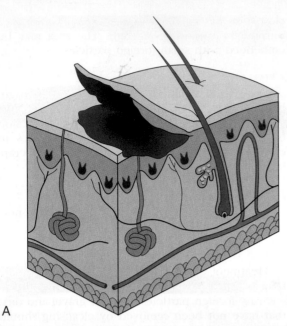

A

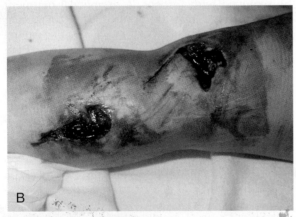

B

460

Figure 15–2

Avulsion. *A*, A flap of skin has been torn away. *B*, Avulsions over the knee and lower leg. (*B* from Henry MC, Stapleton ER: EMT Prehospital Care, 2nd ed. Philadelphia: WB Saunders, 1997, p 467. Used with permission.)

TREATMENT

Treatment consists of controlling the bleeding, cleansing the area, and surgically repairing the tissue. If an amputation has occurred, the stump or remaining area must be cleansed and surgically repaired. The patient probably is treated prophylactically with antibiotics to prevent infection. A sterile dressing is applied to the repaired wound. Tetanus prophylaxis is confirmed or administered if necessary.

See the doctor every week for redness

CRUSHING INJURIES

SYMPTOMS AND SIGNS

A crushing injury may involve any body part, but most frequently, a finger, hand, toe, or foot is involved. The patient experiences pain and may not be able to move the injured part. Soft tissue is compressed, and, depending on the amount of pressure of the crushing mechanism, bone, nerves, and vessels also may be crushed.

ETIOLOGY

The crushing injury occurs when the body part becomes pressed between two hard surfaces. Examples of such injuries are fingers shut in doors, hands or fingers caught in presses, heavy objects being dropped on feet or toes, and compression of any body part in motor vehicle accidents. Falling debris, such as building parts in a storm or earthquake, also can cause crushing injuries.

DIAGNOSIS

Diagnosis is made from history, visual inspection of the body area, and physical examination. Radiographic studies of the injured part also aid in the diagnosis.

TREATMENT

Treatment depends on the severity and location of the injury. When there is an open wound, the area is cleansed and **débrided** if necessary. Immobilization of the affected limb or appendage follows any surgical repair that is indicated. Sterile dressings probably are applied to any open wound or surgical area. If the crushing injury is to the head or trunk of the body, appropriate monitoring of vital signs and surgical intervention is undertaken. Tetanus prophylaxis is confirmed or administered if necessary, and antibiotics may be prescribed as an additional prophylactic measure.

PUNCTURE WOUNDS

SYMPTOMS AND SIGNS

Puncture wounds result when a pointed foreign body penetrates the soft tissue (Fig. 15–3 *A* and *B*). They cause pain and very little bleeding. There may be redness at the site, or there may be no indication of the wound other than the pain. If the foreign body extends out of the wound, it is considered an impaled object (Fig. 15-4).

ETIOLOGY

The puncture wound occurs when a sharp, pointed object penetrates the skin and underlying soft tissue. The offending object may be a needle, a nail, a splinter of glass, wood or metal, a knife, or even a bullet. The object penetrates

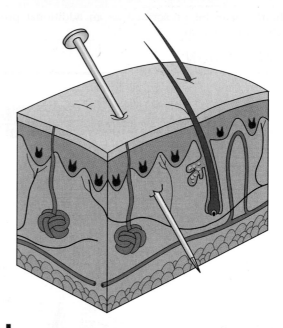

Figure 15–4

Impaled object. A nail is impaled in the skin.

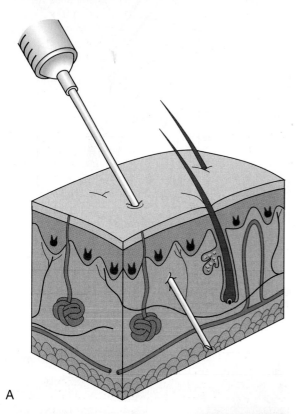

A

the skin, which then closes around the object or point of entry. As a result, bleeding is minimal.

DIAGNOSIS

Diagnosis is made by visual examination, history, and sometimes radiographic studies (if the object can be visualized by imaging).

TREATMENT

Treatment is by removal of the foreign body, along with copious irrigation of the wound. A sterile dressing is applied. Tetanus prophylaxis is confirmed or administered if necessary, and anti-

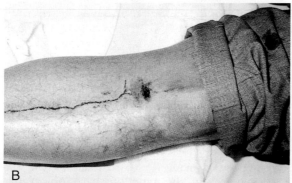

B

Figure 15–3

Puncture wound. *A*, A pointed object has punctured the skin. *B*, Puncture wound of the anterior lower leg. (*B* from Henry MC, Stapleton ER: EMT Prehospital Care, 2nd ed. Philadelphia: WB Saunders, 1997, p 468.) (Courtesy of S.L. Wiener and J. Barrett.)

Enrichment

NEEDLE STICKS

Health-care providers are at risk for puncture wounds from contaminated needle sticks. U.S. Occupational Safety and Health Administration (OSHA) guidelines must be followed to lessen the risk of occurrence and to reduce the likelihood of transmitting acquired immunodeficiency syndrome (AIDS) or hepatitis B.

461

biotics may be prescribed as an additional prophylactic measure.

LACERATIONS ☆ time limit 12 hours

SYMPTOMS AND SIGNS

Lacerations result when the skin and possibly underlying soft tissue are cut by a sharp object.

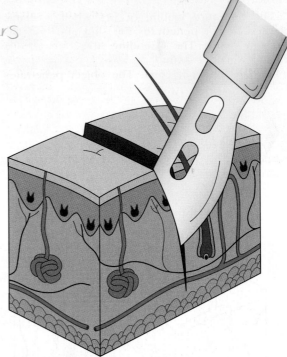

Figure 15–6

Incision. A laceration with smooth edges.

They cause pain and moderate to severe bleeding. The edges of the cut may be smooth, or they may be jagged, depending on the object that did the cutting. The bleeding is generally proportionate to the depth and length of the laceration.

ETIOLOGY

Lacerations occur when a sharp instrument, such as a knife or sharp piece of glass or metal, cuts the skin and underlying soft tissue (Fig. 15–5 A and B).

DIAGNOSIS

Diagnosis is made by visual examination. History may reveal the type of sharp object that caused the injury. A laceration with smooth edges that can be approximated cleanly is termed an incision (Fig. 15–6).

TREATMENT

Lacerations should be cleansed gently with a germicidal soap and water. If the laceration is not too deep and bleeding is controlled, approxi-

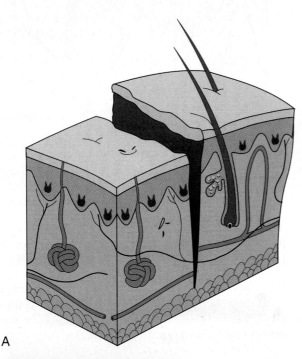

A

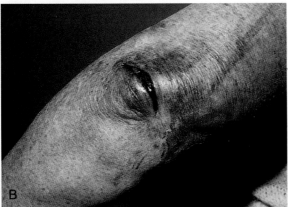

B

Figure 15–5

Laceration. *A*, Skin is cut by a sharp object. *B*, Laceration of the elbow caused by a fall on the street. (*B* from Henry MC, Stapleton ER: EMT Prehospital Care, 2nd ed. Philadelphia: WB Saunders, 1997, p 466.)

462

mating and securing the edges with tape, butterfly dressing, or sterile adhesive strips **(Steri-Strips)** may be the only intervention necessary other than a sterile dressing application. Lacerations that are deep, have jagged edges, or are bleeding need to be débrided and have the edges trimmed for good approximation. Bleeding should be controlled by either **coagulation** or suture. Suturing of the wound is probably necessary. If the laceration is over a movable joint, immobilization of the area is indicated. A sterile dressing should be applied. Tetanus prophylaxis is confirmed and administered if necessary, and

antibiotics may be prescribed as an additional prophylactic measure.

Thermal Insults

Thermal insults can be caused by either heat or cold. These insults can be burns or frostbite. Extremes in temperatures can cause conditions

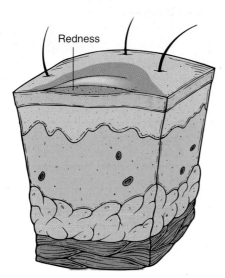

Superficial burn

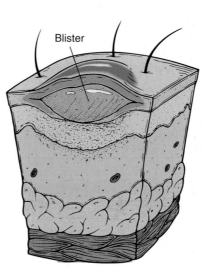

Partial-thickness burn

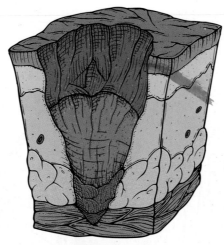

Full-thickness burn

Figure 15–7

Depths of burns. The extent of involvement of layers of the skin.

such as hypothermia, hyperthermia, heat stroke, and heat exhaustion. Regardless of the variance in temperature, most of these conditions, in the severe state, can be life threatening if left untreated. Hypothermia may be a protective factor in cold-water near-drownings.

BURNS

SYMPTOMS AND SIGNS

The patient who has experienced a burn usually has pain. The extent of the burn, along with the surface area involved, usually is related proportionately to the extent of the pain. Depending on the depth and nature of the burn, the skin surface may be reddened, blistered, or charred.

ETIOLOGY

Burns can be caused by flame, heat, scalds, radiation, chemicals, or electricity. The exposure of the skin to any of these causes destruction of the skin. The injury to the underlying soft tissue is proportionate to the duration of the exposure and the intensity of the thermal source.

DIAGNOSIS

Diagnosis is made by visual examination and history. In a flame-type burn, it is necessary to

determine whether the burn occurred inside an enclosure or out in the open. The respiratory state of any patient with a flame-type burn must be assessed. The status of the eyebrows, eyelashes, and nasal hair must be determined. Any singeing of these hairs is indicative that the patient inhaled the flame or superheated air and that the respiratory status may be in grave danger.

Determination of the depth (Fig. 15–7) and extent (Fig. 15–8) of a burn is important. Pain intensity depends on the amount of nerve tissue that is involved or destroyed. Superficial burns involve only the outer layers of the skin and are usually only reddened. These burns are painful. Partial-thickness burns involve all layers of the skin and have blisters and are very painful. Full-thickness burns involve both the skin and the underlying subcutaneous tissue. Prompt assessment of the surface area of the burn is achieved by applying the rule of nines. The rule of nines provides a fast and fairly accurate calculation of the body surface involved. Percentages used to ascertain the burned tissue area in the adult are as follows: head—9%; anterior trunk—18%; posterior trunk—18%; entire right arm—9%; entire left arm—9%; anterior surface right leg—9%; posterior surface right leg—9%; anterior surface left leg—9%; posterior surface left leg—9%; and

464

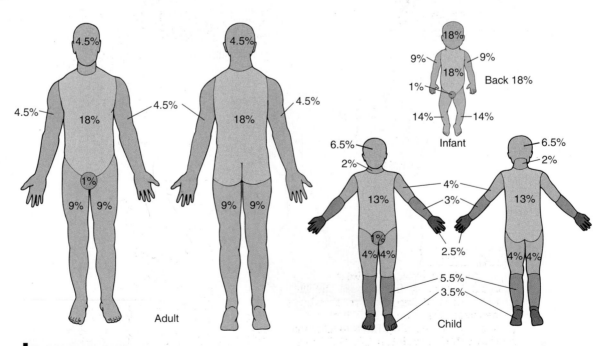

Figure 15–8
Rule of nines.

perineum—1%. Percentages in children and infants are slightly different.

TREATMENT

Treatment depends on the source of the burns. Heat burns (from flame, scalds, or superheated air) should be cooled with cool water and covered with dry sterile dressings until seen by a physician. Sunburns should be cooled with cool water and may be sprayed with antiseptic and analgesic sprays. Chemical burns, other than those caused by lime, should be flushed with cool water for at least 15 minutes, covered with a sterile dressing, and treated by a physician. Electrical burns should be examined for points of entry (rings, belts, necklaces) and exit (knees, toes (Fig. 15-9). These areas should be covered with dry sterile dressings and treated by a physician.

Analgesics are given to treat the pain. Minor burns usually are treated with an antibacterial cream or ointment. Severe burns require specialized treatment, with surgical débridement of the burned tissue and skin grafts if necessary.

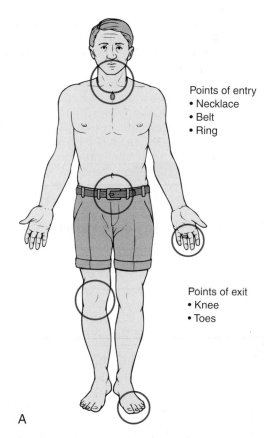

Points of entry
• Necklace
• Belt
• Ring

Points of exit
• Knee
• Toes

A

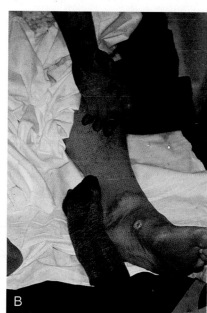

B

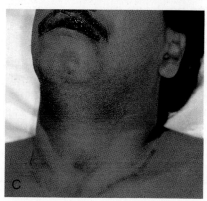

C

Figure 15–9

A, Points of entry and exit for electrical burns. *B,* Exit wound in the foot. *C,* Lightning burst a metal necklace chain on the patient, leaving a burn marking. (*B* and *C* from Henry MC, Stapleton ER: EMT Prehospital Care, 2nd ed. Philadelphia: WB Saunders, 1997, pp 500, 501. Used with permission.)

Patients with severe large-area burns, the elderly and the very young, and those with severe burns to the face, hands, feet, or perineal area usually are admitted to a burn center, where they receive specialized burn care. Respiratory status (if the respiratory tract is involved), fluid and electrolyte balance, and vital signs are monitored. Pain control is accomplished with narcotic analgesics. Tetanus prophylaxis is confirmed or administered if necessary, and antibiotics may be prescribed as an additional prophylactic measure. Skin grafting, including cloned skin and autografts, is used for treatment of extensive destruction of tissue.

ELECTRICAL SHOCK

SYMPTOMS AND SIGNS

Patients who have experienced electrical shock may be in cardiac or respiratory failure. They have a visible burn at the entrance wound and at the exit wound. If conscious, they experience pain at these sites. There also can be a charring of the tissue.

ETIOLOGY

The person with electrical shock experiences tissue damage from the point of entry of the electricity to the point of exit. The current follows the path of least resistance through the body, usually along nerve routes. The current enters the body at the point of contact with the electrical source and exits at the point of grounding (see Fig. 15-9). As the alternating current passes through the body, it may produce muscular contractions, causing the person to be thrown from the source. This can result in lacerations, fractures, or head trauma.

DIAGNOSIS

Diagnosis is made by visual examination and history.

TREATMENT

Treatment consists of maintaining the cardiac and respiratory status. If indicated, cardiopulmonary resuscitation (CPR) must be administered after the patient has been removed from the electrical source. The patient's neurologic and vascular status are assessed for the extent of tissue destruction. Any fractures, lacerations, and head injuries are treated. The burned areas are débrided and dressed with sterile dressings. Pain management is accomplished with narcotic analgesics. Tetanus prophylaxis is confirmed or administered if necessary, and antibiotics may be prescribed as an additional prophylactic measure.

LIGHTNING INJURIES

SYMPTOMS AND SIGNS

Lightning injuries can be classified by the severity of the injury or by the type of strike the person receives. Usually, the severity of the injury is in direct proportion to the intensity of the lightning strike.

The victim of a direct lightning strike is probably in a severely compromised state, unconscious and not breathing. There may be a heartbeat if the **apnea** has not caused cardiac arrest. Clothing may be literally "blown off" the victim, and the victim may have been propelled through the air by the blast. Burns usually are noted in areas of the skin where there is normal moisture, such as the axillae and groin or where metal was touching the body (see Fig. 15-9A). Motor and sensory disturbances are noted, along with possible ruptured **tympanic membranes.** The patient who has experienced moderate contact has less severe symptoms, with altered level of consciousness and skin burns. The person with minor injuries exhibits fairly normal vital signs, some confusion, **amnesia** of preceding events, and some minor muscle or sensory nerve distur-

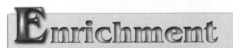

Enrichment

SUNBURN

Exposure to the ultraviolet alpha and beta rays from the sun can cause sunburn, ranging from mild to severe. The person who has experienced at least three severe sunburns with blistering is at risk for the development of skin cancer. Prevention of sunburn includes avoiding exposure from 10 AM to 2 PM, when the sun's rays are the strongest, applying a sunscreen to exposed skin areas, and wearing a hat to protect the scalp and eyes. Those at greatest risk have light or fair skin and freckles and blond or red hair.

bances. All may experience some hearing or visual difficulties.

ETIOLOGY

It is possible for lightning to strike a person in five different ways. When the person is struck directly by the lightning discharge, it is termed a direct strike. When lightning strikes an object that the person is touching, resulting in a transference of the energy, it is termed contact strike. If lightning strikes an object, travels a certain distance, then "jumps" through the air and strikes the person, it is termed side flash. If the current enters the leg of the person, travels through the lower part of the body, and exits out the other leg, it is termed stride potential. Lastly, when the lightning bolt hits the ground and travels to the person by way of the ground, it is termed ground current.

Lightning tends to flow over the surface of the body, often sparing the deeper tissues.

DIAGNOSIS

Diagnosis is made by visual examination and a history of the person's being outdoors with lightning present or inside a structure that is hit by lightning and in contact with a conductive or grounding source. A detailed neurologic assessment should be completed, as should a thorough examination of the surface of the body for burns. A classic fern-like pattern of burn may be noted on the skin. An eye examination should be conducted for retinal, optic nerve, or occipital lobe damage. Baseline visual acuity should be measured because **cataracts, corneal ulcers,** or hemorrhage may occur. The ears should be examined for ruptured tympanic membrane. Vital signs should be assessed, including screening for hypertension. The cervical spine and the entire musculoskeletal system should be evaluated for injury.

TREATMENT

Treatment consists of restoring or maintaining respiratory effort. If the person is apneic, cardiac function ceases in a few minutes. If the person is in cardiac arrest, CPR must be initiated and continued for extended periods. Cardiac monitoring is indicated, along with observation for cerebral edema and respiratory insult. Fractures and lacerations, burns, and other injuries need to be treated according to facility protocol. Tetanus prophylaxis must be confirmed or administered if necessary. Follow-up eye examinations should be

conducted because cataracts may develop in the year after the lightning strike.

EXTREME HEAT (HYPERTHERMIA)

SYMPTOMS AND SIGNS

The person with hyperthermia may be experiencing heat stroke or heat exhaustion as a result of prolonged exposure to extremely hot temperatures. Heat stroke occurs when the person has a body temperature of 105°F or greater. The skin is hot, red, and usually dry. The patient may have a dry mouth, headache, nausea or vomiting, dizziness and weakness, and shortness of breath. The pulse is rapid and strong at the onset, gradually becoming weak, and the blood pressure decreases. The pupils are constricted. Patients exhibit anxiety, mental confusion, irritability, aggression, and even hysterical behavior. In extreme cases, the person collapses, experiences altered levels of consciousness, and may have seizure activity.

Heat exhaustion produces profuse sweating, fatigue, headache, weakness, nausea, dizziness, and possible heat or muscle cramps. The pulse is weak and rapid; the skin is pale, cool, and moist; and the body temperature is normal or subnormal. The pupils are dilated.

ETIOLOGY

Heat stroke results when the body's heat-regulating systems are unable to cope with the exposure to severe external heat sources. As the body overheats, its temperature rises to 105° to 110°F. Approximately one half of patients fail to perspire, whereas the rest do. Because there is no effective cooling mechanism taking place, the body stores the heat, eventually resulting in damage to the brain cells and subsequently permanent brain damage or death. The aged, infants, children, and malnourished and debilitated people are the most susceptible to heat stroke. Others who experience heat stroke are those who work near furnaces and intense sources of heat as well as athletes who are exposed to the combination of high temperatures and high humidity.

Heat exhaustion is the result of salt or water depletion. Generally, the person is involved in strenuous activity in a hot, humid environment. As a result, the person experiences prolonged and profuse sweating, causing the loss of excessive amounts of salt and water. This mimics a mild state of shock.

DIAGNOSIS

Diagnosis of heat stroke is made by symptoms, especially the elevated body temperature. The history of exposure to high temperatures and humidity, along with the altered level of consciousness, aids in the diagnosis.

Diagnosis of heat exhaustion is made from the history and clinical symptoms, specifically the moist, pale skin and normal or below-normal body temperature.

TREATMENT

Treatment of heat stroke, possibly a life-threatening condition, must be aggressive and instituted promptly. It consists of cooling the body down. The first step is to move the person to a cooler environment, to remove what clothing possible, and to cool the body by pouring cool water over it or soaking it with a cool wet cloth. If the person begins to shiver, the cooling process should be slowed. It is imperative to bring the core temperature of the body below 100°F. The person should be transported to an emergency facility where vital signs can be monitored.

Treatment of persons with heat exhaustion consists of moving them to a cool place and applying cool compresses. They should be lying down with the feet elevated. If the person is fully conscious, give 4 ounces of cool water every 10 to 15 minutes.

EXTREME COLD (HYPOTHERMIA)

SYMPTOMS AND SIGNS

Hypothermia, a generalized severe cooling of the body, causes the person to shiver and have a feeling of extreme cold or numbness. Fatigue is followed by loss of coordination, thick speech, and disorientation. The skin is blue and puffy, with the pulse being slow and weak. Core body temperature drops below 95°F. Breathing is slow and shallow, and the pupils are dilated. As the body temperature drops, there is confusion, stupor, and unconsciousness.

ETIOLOGY

Hypothermia can occur when a person is exposed to wind, cold, or cold water for prolonged periods. The elderly, very young, exhausted, and physically debilitated persons have the greatest risk of hypothermia. Sudden immersion in cold water can cause hypothermia. Lack of adequate clothing or wetness can add to the risk.

DIAGNOSIS

Diagnosis is made by the history, the clinical picture, and the finding of below-normal body temperature.

TREATMENT

Treatment of hypothermia, a life-threatening condition, must be aggressive and immediate. Any wet clothing must be removed, and gradual rewarming of the body is begun by wrapping the person in warm blankets while keeping the body dry. If auxiliary sources of heat such as hot packs or warm stones are not available, the warmth from another person's body helps to warm the patient. If the person is conscious, warm liquids should be given orally and in small quantities. The patient should be transported to an emergency facility, where vital signs can be monitored.

FROSTBITE

SYMPTOMS AND SIGNS

Frostbite, usually occurring on the face, fingers, toes, and ears, causes the skin area involved to become white (Fig. 15–10). The person does not realize that the condition is occurring because there is little or no pain as the tissue freezes. As the freezing deepens, the underlying tissue becomes firm, and the skin has a waxy appearance.

ETIOLOGY

Frostbite occurs when tissue is exposed to cold air, water, or objects. Ice crystals form between the cells of the skin. As the freezing continues, fluid that is drawn from the cells subsequently freezes. People who have undergone trauma plus exposure to cold weather, the elderly, newborns, those with wet clothing, and those with tightly laced footwear are at greatest risk when exposed to cold temperatures.

DIAGNOSIS

Diagnosis is made by visual examination and a history of exposure to cold. The depth or degree of the frostbite is determined by the color and appearance of the skin.

TREATMENT

Treatment consists of moving the patient from the cold environment. Superficial frostbite should be warmed with an external source of even heat. The temperature of the heat source should not be above 105°F. The area should *never* be

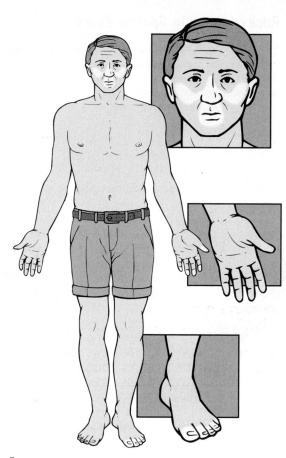

Figure 15–10

Usual sites of frostbite.

rubbed. Patients suffering from frostbite should be treated by a physician if possible. Rewarming of deep frostbite (frozen tissue) should not begin until professional medical care can be provided. The person should be kept warm, vital signs should be monitored, and alcohol should *never* be given.

Bites

Bites can occur at any time and at any place on the body. They range from the annoying insect bite to bites by domestic animals, humans, or reptiles. Insect bites may be insignificant or life threatening. For example, mosquito bites can cause merely itching or can cause **encephalitis,**

and tick bites can cause Rocky Mountain spotted fever, malaria, or Lyme disease. Animal bites range from mere nips that cause no serious disease to life-threatening bites that carry the risk of rabies.

INSECT BITES

SYMPTOMS AND SIGNS

The symptoms and signs of an insect bite or sting vary with the type of insect that has bitten or stung the patient. Usually, there is a sharp, stinging pain, which may be followed by itching, redness, or swelling at the site. If the patient is experiencing a systemic reaction to the bite, he or she has itching on the palms of the hands or soles of the feet, the neck, or the groin, or generalized itching, including a rash over the entire body. As an allergic reaction develops, the patient experiences generalized edema, **dyspnea,** weakness, nausea, shock, and unconsciousness.

ETIOLOGY

The injury occurs when the insect either bites or stings the patient. **Venom** is injected into the tissue, resulting in the body's response to a foreign protein. Some of the more common types of bites or stings are those of mosquitoes, bees, wasps, hornets, spiders, fire ants, ticks, and fleas. Occurring less often are bites by black widow spiders, brown recluse spiders, and scorpions.

DIAGNOSIS

Diagnosis is made by visual examination and history. It is hoped that the patient can identify or give a description of the offending insect. Certain insect bites or stings have characteristic signs.

TREATMENT

The first step in treating an insect sting is to check whether the stinger is still present. If it is present, it must be removed to prevent further damage. The best method of removal is scraping across the area with a plastic card or a fingernail. The use of forceps or tweezers squeezes more venom into the site. The area is cleaned with soap and water. Application of a dry dressing, cold pack, or **anesthetic** sprays affords comfort. The person should be observed for any signs of allergic reaction to the sting or bite. Lyme disease, the result of a tick bite, and encephalitis, the result of a mosquito bite, are discussed in Chapters 7 and 13, respectively.

People with black widow spider, brown re-

469

cluse spider, or scorpion bites should be transported to an emergency facility. Aggressive treatment includes cleansing of the wound, the administration of medication for pain relief, cold applications, the administration of antivenin, and monitoring of vital signs.

Rocky Mountain Spotted Fever

SYMPTOMS AND SIGNS

Rocky Mountain spotted fever, a tick-borne disease, is a severe systemic infection. It is the most commonly reported rickettsial disease in

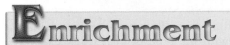

ALTITUDE SICKNESS

Altitude sickness or acute mountain sickness is a disorder associated with the low oxygen content of the atmosphere at high altitudes. It occurs when individuals make a rapid ascent into altitudes usually above 8000 feet. Symptoms include nausea and vomiting, headache, dizziness, difficulty sleeping, and air hunger. Mild symptoms that mimic jet lag or the flu can subside as the body adjusts to the higher altitude. More severe and even life-threatening altitude sickness can cause prostration, cardiac disturbances, and cerebral edema with possible seizures and death. Pulmonary edema is another severe state of altitude sickness. It is possible for those with heart problems to experience angina and subsequent myocardial infarction triggered by the high altitude (Fig. 15–11).

In addition to the high elevation, dehydration is a contributing factor. Those who experience symptoms should descend to a lower altitude and drink plentiful amounts of water. Rest and curtailing stressful activities helps in the relief of symptoms and is a necessary intervention for shortness of breath and increased heart rate.

Prevention includes acclimating one's self to the higher altitudes slowly over a period of a few days, drinking extra fluids, and avoiding alcohol and smoking. It is best not to climb more than 3000 feet a day when at elevations greater than 8000 feet.

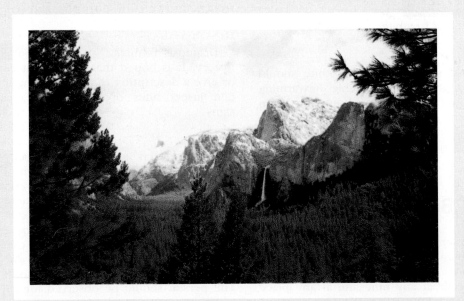

Figure 15–11
Typical site for onset of altitude sickness. (Courtesy of David L. Frazier, 1999.)

the United States. The patient may recall being bitten by a tick, typically during outdoor activity such as camping and hiking. Several days to 2 weeks later, there is a sudden onset of fever, severe headache, vomiting, **malaise,** and **myalgia.** Four days after the onset of fever, a characteristic **maculopapular** rash is noted, which spreads over the body. Small hemorrhages appear under the skin, the characteristic sign that gives the disease its name. Inflammation of blood vessels (vasculitis) affects the skin and other organs, leading to systemic manifestations in the heart, lungs, kidney, and nervous system. After 2 to 3 weeks, the skin begins to peel.

ETIOLOGY

The causative agent, *Rickettsia rickettsii,* is transmitted by the wood tick and is carried in the feces of infected ticks. It is introduced into the bloodstream of a person during a prolonged tick bite (4–6 hours). Once it is in the bloodstream, the organism, an intracellular parasite, reproduces in certain cells and destroys them. The disease cannot be transmitted from person to person.

DIAGNOSIS

Although Rocky Mountain spotted fever is difficult to diagnose, a history of a tick bite or recent outdoor activity in tick-infested areas and the onset of severe systemic symptoms, with the appearance of the characteristic rash, suggest the disease. Laboratory findings include a positive complement fixation reaction, which measures the **antigen–antibody** reaction occurring in the body, and thereby the severity of infection. Changes in blood-clotting components in the blood may be noted. Isolation of the organism in a blood culture confirms the diagnosis.

TREATMENT

The treatment of choice for Rocky Mountain spotted fever is antibiotic therapy with tetracycline and symptomatic relief with the administration of analgesics. Infection confers lifetime immunity.

Preventive measures include wearing protective clothing, with application of insect repellent to clothing and exposed skin. Visual inspection of the skin for the presence of ticks should be made every few hours during and after outdoor activity in infested areas. If found, the tick should be removed carefully with tweezers, without handling the tick.

Malaria

SYMPTOMS AND SIGNS

Malaria is an acute, sometimes chronic, serious, infectious illness. It is characterized by a classic cycle of chills, fever, and sweats, in that order. The patient also may have headache, nausea, fatigue, and myalgia. Although the course and severity of the disease can vary, bouts of malaria usually last from 1 to 4 weeks. Signs include an enlarged spleen, an enlarged liver, and anemia. The symptoms have a tendency to recur and may persist for years.

ETIOLOGY

Malaria is caused by four species of the protozoan genus *Plasmodium,* which is transmitted from infected human to human by the bite of mosquito **vectors** or, less commonly, by blood transfusion or intravenous drug use. After they are introduced into the body, the protozoan parasites feed on hemoglobin and reproduce within red blood cells (RBCs). Malaria is endemic in tropical and subtropical areas such as South and Central America, Asia, and Africa and usually is brought to the United States by travelers returning from these areas.

DIAGNOSIS

Laboratory testing reveals decreased hemoglobin level, decreased platelet count, prolonged **prothrombin time (PT),** and a positive serum antibody test result. Diagnosis is confirmed by identifying the *Plasmodium* organism in a blood smear.

TREATMENT

Malaria is treated with chloroquine, an antimalarial drug, given orally. **Antipyretics** are given for fever. Packed RBCs may be required for anemia. Each new case of malaria must be reported to the local board of health.

A prophylactic course of chloroquine may be given when a person is traveling to known endemic areas.

ANIMAL BITES

SYMPTOMS AND SIGNS

Broken skin with evidence of teeth marks is the usual clinical picture of an animal bite. Puncture wounds are present, with possible tearing of the skin. Bleeding is usually evident, and the flesh actually may be bitten away. A discoloration of the skin occurs, indicating bruising to the area. The patient usually reports pain at the site.

ETIOLOGY

The bite occurs when the animal is agitated, frightened, threatened, or angry. Bites can be from domestic animals, such as cats and dogs; farm animals; or wild animals, such as skunks, bats, raccoons, and foxes. Human bites also have been recorded.

DIAGNOSIS

Diagnosis is made by a history and by physical examination. The pattern of the teeth marks is helpful in determining the type of animal that did the biting.

TREATMENT

Treatment consists of cleaning the wound. If bleeding cannot be controlled, **hemostasis** is achieved by **cautery** or suture. Depending on the site and severity of the wound, plastic surgery may be indicated for repair.

Rabies is transmitted through the saliva of infected animals. If the animal is a domestic pet, it is usually not too difficult to confirm the last rabies inoculation or to quarantine the animal for the time necessary to rule out rabies infection. If it is not possible to determine whether the animal is rabid, the person probably will have to undergo a series of injections to confer immunity to rabies.

As in most invasive trauma, a sterile dressing should be applied. Tetanus prophylaxis is confirmed or administered if necessary, and antibiot-

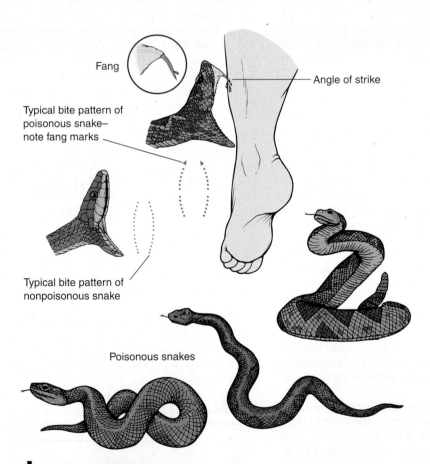

Fang

Angle of strike

Typical bite pattern of poisonous snake— note fang marks

Typical bite pattern of nonpoisonous snake

Poisonous snakes

Figure 15–12

Snakebite. (Redrawn with permission of Patient Care Magazine. Copyright 1976, Patient Care Publications, Inc., Montvale, NJ. All rights reserved.)

ics may be prescribed as an additional prophylactic measure.

SNAKE BITES

SYMPTOMS AND SIGNS

The patient may indicate experiencing a bite or actually seeing the snake or may not be aware of the bite happening. There is a noticeable bite to the skin or possibly only a slight skin discoloration. Burning pain is present, and swelling begins in the area of the bite; however, this may be delayed, developing slowly. The pulse rate becomes rapid, and the patient begins to experience weakness, visual difficulties, and nausea and vomiting. These signs and symptoms of the poisoning may take 30 minutes to several hours to develop. Coral snakes are extremely poisonous and leave chew-type small teeth marks rather than the two distinct fang marks of the other poisonous snakes (Fig. 15–12).

ETIOLOGY

The poisoning from the snake bite usually takes 1 to 2 days to develop unless the person is allergic to the foreign protein of the venom. There are four kinds of poisonous snakes in the United States: rattlesnakes, copperheads, water moccasins, and coral snakes. Rattlesnakes account for the greatest number of poisonous snake bites. Nonpoisonous snakes also account for snakebites, and all snakebites should be treated as poisonous by the first aid provider.

DIAGNOSIS

Diagnosis is made by history and visual examination of the area. Two typical fang marks are indicative of poisonous snakes, other than the coral snake (see Fig. 15–12).

TREATMENT

Treatment consists of removing the person from the area of the snake and keeping her or him calm and quiet. The **emergency medical service (EMS)** system should be activated. The area of the bite should be cleansed with soap and water. Any jewelry, including rings, or constricting objects should be removed from the affected limb. The extremity should be immobilized and, if possible, kept below the level of the heart. Transportation to the nearest emergency facility should be initiated as soon as possible so that aggressive treatment can begin immediately. If it is not possible to reach emergency care within 30 minutes, consideration should be given to suctioning the bite with equipment from a snakebite kit. Antivenin may be given to the patient and vital functions are supported. The protocol for snakebite treatment indicates that cold should *not* be applied, the wound should *not* be cut, tourniquets should *not* be applied, and electrical shock should *not* be applied.

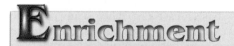

POISONING

Poisons are any substances that, when introduced into the body, cause illness or injury; many cause death. Poisons can be introduced into the body by absorption through the skin, ingestion through the gastrointestinal tract, inhalation through the respiratory system, and injection through a sting, bite, or hypodermic needle. The signs and symptoms vary according to the poison and the method of introduction into the body.

Ingested or swallowed poisons can include foods, alcohol, chemicals, medications, and plants. Inhaled poisons include gases such as carbon monoxide, carbon dioxide, nitrous oxide, chlorine, and fumes from chemicals or drugs. Absorbed poisons include chemicals or oils from certain plants. Injected poisons include venom injected by insects, spiders, ticks, or snakes or drugs given via a hypodermic needle.

Because of the vast number of poisons and methods of introduction into the body, it is impossible to identify symptoms, etiology, diagnosis, and treatment for each toxic substance. General guidelines to follow are identifying the toxic substance and contacting a poison control center or emergency facility for assistance. Of utmost importance is that the rescuer or care provider not compromise his or her own safety, especially when inhalation of toxic fumes could be involved.

Cumulative Trauma (Repetitive Motion Trauma, Overuse Syndrome)

Cumulative trauma disorders, or repetitive motion injuries, are common to numerous occupations. They account for more time lost from work than any other single factor. At risk are those in industry who have repetitive tasks, including those who keyboard on a regular and continuous basis, cashiers who scan products across conveyor belts, those who target practice, those engaging in certain sports, and phlebotomists.

These soft tissue injuries develop over time as a result of repetitive activities that cause continued stress on specific muscles or nerves. They can result from improper posture of the wrist, arm, back, shoulder, or legs. Many occur because of pressure centered on the hand or wrist with

474

frequent repetitive motion for an extended time. In the industrial setting, improper use of hand-held tools, especially with excessive or improper grip, can cause cumulative trauma disorders. Additionally, continuous vibration contributes to increased occurrence of trauma. These disorders include but are not limited to **white finger (Raynaud's phenomenon),** trigger finger, carpal tunnel syndrome, tennis elbow, thoracic outlet syndrome, de Quervain's disease, synovitis, tenosynovitis, and nonspecific **tendinitis.** Cumulative trauma develops over an extended time period, so the onset of symptoms is **insidious.** Much investigation is necessary to pinpoint the repetitive task that has caused this trauma.

CARPAL TUNNEL SYNDROME

SYMPTOMS AND SIGNS

The patient experiences a numbness of hands and fingers with pain in these areas at night. Swelling of the wrist or hand and "fluttering" of the fingers are additional symptoms. The patient

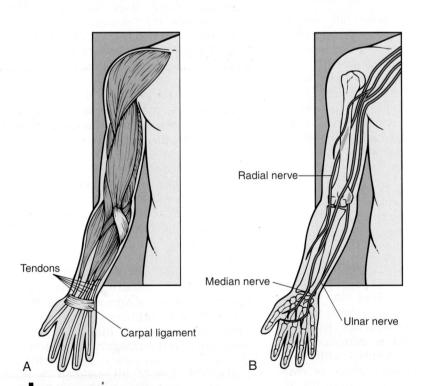

Radial nerve

Tendons

Median nerve

Carpal ligament

Ulnar nerve

A   B

Figure 15–13

Anatomy of arm, wrist, and hand. *A,* Muscles, tendons, and carpal ligament. *B,* Nerves. (Redrawn from Lesson Plan for Ergonomic Seminar Slides. Farmington Hills, MI: Ergonomics, Aro, ARO Tool Products/Ingersoll-Rand Professional Tools, 1994.)

Enrichment

DE QUERVAIN'S DISEASE

de Quervain's disease is an inflammation of the tendons of the thumb. It is caused by irritation of the long abductor and short extensor tendons. Repetitive motion causes edema and tenderness in the thumb and its base.

often is observed cradling the arm or rubbing the hand or arm.

ETIOLOGY

Tendons, blood vessels, and the median nerve pass through a narrow tunnel from the wrist leading to the hand (Fig. 15-13*A* and *B*). Carpal tunnel syndrome results when the tendons become inflamed from repetitive overuse of the hand, wrist, or fingers, causing entrapment of the median nerve as it passes through the wrist, resulting in the pinching of the median nerve (Fig. 15-14).

DIAGNOSIS

The clinical picture, along with the history of the repetitive motion activities, suggests carpal

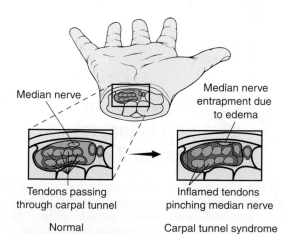

Median nerve

Median nerve entrapment due to edema

Tendons passing through carpal tunnel

Inflamed tendons pinching median nerve

Normal

Carpal tunnel syndrome

Figure 15–14

Entrapment of the median nerve in the carpal tunnel space. (Redrawn from Lesson Plan for Ergonomic Seminar Slides. Farmington Hills, MI: Ergonomics, Aro, ARO Tool Products/Ingersoll-Rand Professional Tools, 1994.)

tunnel syndrome. There are two specific minor tests that aid in the confirmation of the diagnosis. One is the median nerve percussion test, in which the examiner taps his or her fingers along the inside of the affected wrist, eliciting a pins-and-needles sensation in the hand and fingers. The other is the Phalen wrist flexor test, in which the patient presses the backs of the hands together to bend the wrists as much as possible without forcing them together for 60 seconds. The fingers should be kept pointing toward the floor. In a positive test result, the patient experiences numbness and tingling of the hand or fingers. [order a test called EMG.]

TREATMENT

Treatment consists of physical therapy and identification and cessation of the repetitive motion to rest the wrist and hand. Anti-inflammatory drugs are prescribed, and a splint may be applied to maintain the wrist in a neutral position. As a final resort, surgery to divide the carpal ligament is performed to relieve pressure on the nerve.

Prevention is important, so **ergonomic** studies and correction of improper repetitive activities should take place.

TENNIS ELBOW

SYMPTOMS AND SIGNS

The patient has pain in the outer aspect of the elbow and lower arm. Weakness is exhibited in the affected extremity.

ETIOLOGY

The extensor attachment to the lateral humeral condyle becomes inflamed. Repetitive motion in the elbow, usually with stress to the joint, causes this inflammatory condition.

DIAGNOSIS

Diagnosis is made by the clinical picture and physical examination.

TREATMENT

Treatment consists of stopping the repetitive task and resting the affected arm. An elastic brace can be placed distal to the elbow to alter the fulcrum of the activity. Nonsteroidal anti-inflammatory drugs (NSAIDs) are also helpful in decreasing the inflammation. Steroid injections into the joint space may afford relief.

TRIGGER FINGER

SYMPTOMS AND SIGNS

A lump or knot appears on the flexor tendon of the affected index finger.

ETIOLOGY

The cause of trigger finger is excessive use of the index finger resulting from difficult repetitive finger movement or trauma to the tendon sheath.

DIAGNOSIS

Diagnosis is made from the clinical picture, history, and physical examination.

TREATMENT

As with other cumulative trauma, cessation of the repetitive activity and rest of the affected part is the prescribed course of treatment.

THORACIC OUTLET SYNDROME (BRACHIAL PLEXUS INJURY)

SYMPTOMS AND SIGNS

Thoracic outlet syndrome is the compression of the brachial plexus nerves. It causes the patient to experience pain in the arm of the affected side. **Paresthesia** of the fingers also is experienced, along with weakness and diminished grasp in the fingers and thumb. The small muscles of the hand may even begin to waste away.

ETIOLOGY

The performance of repetitive tasks that cause continual hyperabduction of the arm is one of the causative factors of this condition. Other causes include a continual drooping of the shoulder girdle, a cervical rib, or a fibrous band that develops around the nerve plexus.

DIAGNOSIS

Diagnosis is made from the clinical picture, history, and physical examination. **Electromyography (EMG)** aids in confirmation of the diagnosis.

TREATMENT

The cessation of any continued hyperabduction of the arm helps to relieve symptoms. When a cervical rib is the cause, it may be surgically removed. Entrapment of the brachial plexus nerves by the anterior scalene muscle usually ne-cessitates a surgical release of any fibrous band or entrapping tissue.

TENDINITIS

SYMPTOMS AND SIGNS

The patient experiences nonspecific pain anywhere along the route of the tendon or its attachments. The most common symptom is acute pain.

ETIOLOGY

Tendinitis is an inflammation of a tendon. It is caused by an insult to the area from prolonged or improper activity of the affected part. Calcium deposits often are associated with tendinitis, and the bursa around the tendon also may be involved.

DIAGNOSIS

Nonspecific tendinitis is difficult to diagnose. A careful history indicates the event or events that caused the stress to the involved area. If the shoulder is involved, a 50 to 130° **abduction** of the affected arm causes pain.

TREATMENT

Treatment is aimed at reducing pain, decreasing inflammation, and preserving the integrity of the joint involved. Resting the involved area is important, along with administering anti-inflammatory drugs and applying ice. Steroids may be injected into the joint space. If the joint (e.g., the shoulder) becomes fixed, the adhesions that have formed may need to be released surgically to allow full range of motion of the joint.

Physical and Psychological Assault Trauma

Violence by others takes many forms, including child abuse, spouse abuse, abuse against elders, psychological abuse, sexual abuse, and rape. Victimization of individuals has become so prevalent that health-care providers are trained to identify people who have been victimized, to treat their physical and emotional trauma, and to report required incidents or suspicion of abuse.

Violence crosses all areas of society, affecting both sexes, occurring at all socioeconomic levels, and including the entire age spectrum. The number of occurrences continues to increase, even though societal and cultural values in the United States make abusive behavior unacceptable, and health-care providers are encouraged to provide unconditional support for victims.

CHILD ABUSE

SYMPTOMS AND SIGNS

Often, children who are victims of child abuse are identified as such by teachers, day-care providers, or health-care providers. The injuries to the child encompass many forms, including bruises, fractures, burns, bites, and welts and can even be fatal (Fig. 15–15).

Bruising takes on many telltale appearances, such as finger marks, which wrap around with or without evidence of rings; imprints of electrical cords or hangers; and horizontal wraparound effects of belts or straps, with possible buckle marks. These bruises are on soft tissue and not over bony prominences where normal falls

would cause them to be. The bruising often is in areas that normally are covered by clothing and the bruises are in various stages of healing.

Burns from cigarettes appear as small circles (the diameter of a cigarette), often on hands, feet, buttocks, or genitals. These are at various stages of healing. Another form of burn is the scald burn with the pattern of "dipping," straight lines with no splash marks, a result of the child's being held in scalding water (Fig. 15–16A and B).

Other observable injuries include teeth marks, with bruising caused by human bites, and raised areas or welts caused by spankings with sticks, paddles, or belts on the buttocks or legs. There may be a fracture, usually greenstick, of a long bone.

Often, the child is withdrawn, avoids eye contact, and does not respond appropriately to painful stimuli. When asked how the injury happened, the child denies any abuse while protecting the abuser. In other cases, the child exhibits unusually aggressive behavior and has a neglected appearance.

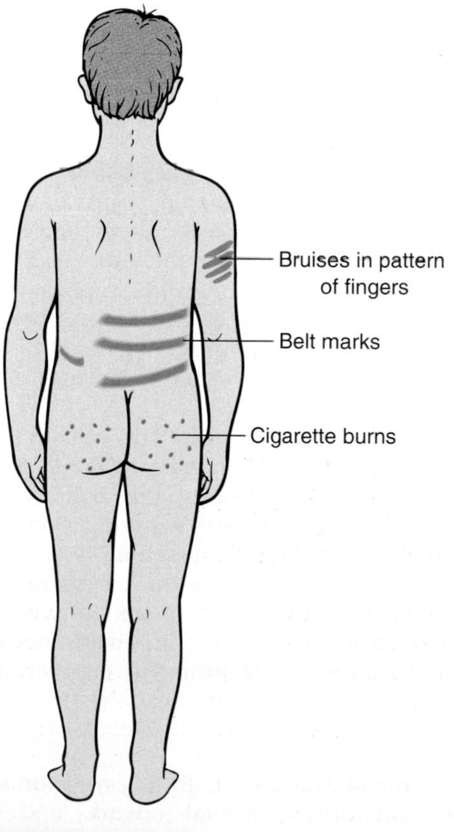

ETIOLOGY

There are many causes of child abuse. These include emotional immaturity of the abuser; stress caused by economic, social, or employment difficulties; poor parenting skills; drug or alcohol abuse; history of being an abused child; unrealistic expectations of the child; and a physically or mentally challenged child.

DIAGNOSIS

Diagnosis is made by history and the clinical picture. Child abuse is not easy to diagnose; nevertheless, health-care providers, teachers, and

Figure 15–15

Typical marks of child abuse.

- Bruises in pattern of fingers
- Belt marks
- Cigarette burns

Enrichment

FAMILY VIOLENCE

The occurrence of family violence is increasing. All members of the family, regardless of age, sex, or place in the family line, are at risk for violence or abuse. The elderly and children are often targets of the aggressive behavior of the stronger member of the family. Many members of dysfunctional families do not realize that abusive and violent behavior is not acceptable in today's society.

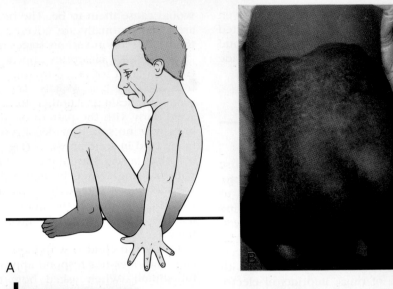

A

Figure 15–16

A, Typical pattern of scald dip burn. B, Scalded child. (B from Slide Set, Behrman RE, Kliegman RM, Arvin AM (eds): Nelson Textbook of Pediatrics, 15/E. Philadelphia, WB Saunders, 1996.)

day-care providers are required by law in most states in the United States to report suspected child abuse to the local or state law enforcement or child protective agency.

TREATMENT

Any injuries must be treated in an appropriate manner. Documentation of the injuries is necessary, and the health-care provider must remain alert for patterns of injuries. Radiographic studies of long bones and of the skull of infants and toddlers should be taken to investigate the extent of abuse. Emotional support for the child should be given unconditionally. Abusive parents and others need help from proper agencies.

Prevention is the best treatment. Parents need to be taught good parenting skills and sources for crisis intervention. They need to be taught alternatives to striking and methods of controlling their reactions (e.g., counting to 10).

SHAKEN BABY SYNDROME

SYMPTOMS AND SIGNS

Shaken baby syndrome (SBS) refers to the injuries incurred by the infant or toddler who has been shaken forcibly enough to cause intracerebral bleeding with resulting closed head injury. The baby may experience altered levels of consciousness to complete loss of consciousness. Irritability, changes in skin color to paleness or

cyanosis, vomiting, lethargy, and convulsions are additional symptoms. Most of the time, there is no outward indication of physical trauma. There may be fractured or dislocated bones and neck or spinal injuries.

ETIOLOGY

The repeated rapid shaking results in the brain continually striking the inside of the cranial vault and then recoiling against the other side of the skull. As a result, tiny vessels rupture causing minor or major bleeds in and around the brain. The swelling and hemorrhage may lead to permanent severe cerebral (brain) damage or even death.

A form of child abuse, SBS usually occurs when the caregiver becomes irritated or upset and loses control, shaking the baby violently. There are incidents of SBS resulting from tossing the baby into the air and catching it or even the jostling in a back pack as the caregiver jogs or runs, bouncing the baby up and down. Young children have large heads and weak neck muscles and therefore are prone to intracerebral injury.

DIAGNOSIS

The manifestation of three symptoms, subdural hematoma, cerebral edema, and retinal hemorrhage, leads to the diagnosis of SBS. However, it is not necessary for all three conditions to be present.

TREATMENT

Immediate and aggressive intervention, including life-sustaining measures, is necessary. Bleeding and cerebral edema must be controlled and intracranial pressure reduced. Nevertheless, damage may be permanent, even fatal. When the child survives, he or she may have visual deficits from retinal insults, including blindness, mental retardation, or cerebral palsy.

SBS may be prevented by educating caregivers about the dangers of shaking a baby in anger and about methods of controlling their outrage. Parents should be made aware of the importance of providing their children with competent caregivers. All caregivers, including parents, should develop a plan for dealing with a crying baby.

ELDER ABUSE

SYMPTOMS AND SIGNS

It is rare for the elderly abuse victim to complain of the abuse. The evidence of the abuse usually is discovered as the result of examination for another purpose. Signs are similar to those of other forms of abuse, are varied, and often are hidden by clothing. Signs include bruising, fractures, malnutrition, poor hygiene, and poor general health status.

ETIOLOGY

As with other forms of abuse, abuse of the elderly is a complex situation. Often, the elderly are dependent on their children for survival, including financial support and physical care. Society presumes that this group of people are protected by love, gentleness, and caring. Some of the elderly requiring care have diminished mental capacity and are confused. The care of the elderly can be a source of stress to the care provider not only because of the physical care demands but also because of the financial and emotional pressures. With the breakdown of the nuclear family structure and the stresses of being a single parent, the additional task of caring for an elderly person can become an overwhelming burden. Additionally, current society puts emphasis on youth. Often, the "sandwiched" generation no longer can cope, and abuse takes place. Other cases of elder abuse have a financial basis, either in being unable to afford the necessities that the elderly person requires or in taking control of the elderly person's finances for the abuser's personal gain.

DIAGNOSIS

Diagnosis is made by an evaluation of the situation and physical examination. Psychological abuse is difficult to diagnose. Many of the victims believe that revealing their child's abusive behavior will suggest that they have failed as parents or will jeopardize their living arrangements.

TREATMENT

Treatment consists of treating any trauma in an appropriate manner. Counseling should be made available to all parties involved. If necessary, the victim should be removed from the abusive environment. Prevention is the best treatment; however, that is not always possible.

PSYCHOLOGICAL OR EMOTIONAL ABUSE

SYMPTOMS AND SIGNS

Symptoms of psychological or emotional abuse, the systematic diminishment of another, take on many forms. Often, the abused person offers no complaints. Although emotional battering transcends age groups, children are the most frequent victims. The guilt that these victims carry often leads to self-destructive behavior, including anorexia, bulimia, obesity, alcoholism, self-mutilation, drug addiction, depression, and suicide. Others manifest the guilt by emotional guarding and turn the anger and rage inward against themselves. These persons display a lack of self-esteem and self-worth and frequently are unable to bond with others.

ETIOLOGY

The cause of this form of abuse is unknown. Often, the parent is the abuser, denying the child love and protection. The abuse can be active, with the parent telling the child, "You're stupid," "I'm ashamed of you," or "You'll never amount to anything." It can be passive in the form of intentional neglect. Often, it is a combination of the two. The abuse can take on the verbal form, or it may be shown by the abuser's actions. The response to the abuse often is buried so deeply that it does not surface until later in life.

DIAGNOSIS

Emotional abuse is difficult to diagnose because no physical contact is required. The comments usually are made to the child in private or in the home environment. The abusive behavior takes place over time, making it difficult to identify at a given time. The victim believes that he or she is responsible for the behavior and does not realize that it is a form of abuse. The victims often defend the abusive behavior, believing that they deserved it.

TREATMENT

The best treatment is prevention. Education of the population as to what constitutes emotional abuse and ways to prevent the many forms is important. A building of self-esteem and self-worth is necessary to begin the healing process. Because of the varied forms of emotional abuse, each individual must believe in himself or herself and address his or her specific guilt, possibly with the help of a therapist.

BATTERED SPOUSE SYNDROME

SYMPTOMS AND SIGNS

The victim, most often female, has evidence of bruising in various stages of healing, usually in an area of the body that is concealed by clothing. She or he has a tendency to avoid eye contact with the examiner.

ETIOLOGY

Battering of spouses is a complex issue. There is no one specific cause. Stress is suggested as an important factor, along with alcohol ingestion and possible intoxication. Cultural and societal values that made wives their husbands' "property" and the mindset according to which women are expected to be submissive to their mates have contributed to spouse abuse. Some women are victimized because they do not have the physical strength that their spouses do. Women can be the abusers also, and some women abuse their spouses even to the point of dismemberment or setting the spouse on fire. It is believed that many of these cases are retaliation for battering that has been received.

DIAGNOSIS

Diagnosis is made from information provided by the victim or others. Physical examination indicates physical injuries. As with child abuse and sexual abuse, the injuries are varied and often occur on areas of the body that normally are covered by clothing. Assessment of the emotional state is difficult but necessary. Often, intervention results from law enforcement involvement; other times, the abusive trauma is discovered by the physician and staff when the victim is seen for another reason in the office or health-care facility.

TREATMENT

Treatment involves normal protocol for physical injuries. Discussing the situation in a nonjudgmental way is imperative. Referral to appropriate agencies for counseling is indicated; nevertheless, the health-care provider must recognize that the victim may not want or seek counseling and may elect to stay in the abusive situation. Listening is of the utmost importance; however, it is inappropriate to impose one's opinion of the situation on the victim.

SEXUAL ABUSE

SYMPTOMS AND SIGNS

Sexual abuse takes on many forms, thus symptoms and signs can be numerous and different. Any form of nonconsensual sexual activity can be considered sexual abuse. Some examples of sexual abuse are fondling of the genitals or breasts, penetration of the vagina or rectum with fingers or other objects, and the forcing of the victim to touch the perpetrator on or around the sex organs. The victim often does not report any unwanted advances or activity and usually appears subdued. If the victim is a young female, she may have itching or burning in the urethral and vaginal areas and exhibit symptoms of a urinary tract infection. Such children have an unusual obsession with the genital region and frequently touch themselves abnormally. They often exhibit aggressive behavior.

ETIOLOGY

As with other forms of abuse, the cause of sexual abuse is a complicated matter. Domination, control, and power issues can be reasons for this unacceptable form of behavior. Many of the perpetrators were sexually abused as children, and they do not regard what they are doing as wrong. Some just have a sociopathic approach to society and its norms. It is important to consider that victimization occurs to both sexes and that the abuser can be of either sex. There are cases of females sexually assaulting any age male.

DIAGNOSIS

Diagnosis is made from a history given by the victim and is confirmed by a physical examination. Often, the sexual abuse is combined with physical abuse and the treatment of that abuse may lead to the confidence from the victim of the unwanted sexual activity. Many times, the removal of the victim from a physically abusive environment allows the victim to feel safe enough to discuss the sexual abuse. Perpetrators of sexual abuse of children have been baby-sitters, relatives, or even a parent.

TREATMENT

Any trauma is treated according to the protocol of the facility. Law enforcement agencies should be notified with the victim's consent or according to local or state policy. If possible, the victim is removed from the situation. Emotional support is provided, and reinforcement is given to the victim that he or she is not responsible

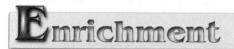

DNA PARENTAGE TESTING

DNA parentage testing is the most reliable and powerful method of providing parentage for legal and medical reasons. It conclusively answers difficult questions, resolves disputes, and helps streamline court proceedings.

Testing is based on a highly accurate analysis of the genetic profiles of the mother, child, and alleged father. Deoxyribonucleic acid (DNA), the unique genetic blueprint within each nucleated cell of a person's body, determines the genetic pattern and individual characteristics. A child inherits half of this DNA pattern from the mother and half from the father. If the mother's and child's patterns are known, the father's can be deduced with virtual certainty.

There are no age restrictions for DNA testing because DNA makeup is set at conception. Testing can be performed before a child is born, and newborns can be tested safely at delivery using umbilical cord blood. In fact, samples can be taken from persons of any age, even postmortem. Only ½ teaspoon of blood is required.

DNA technology is so powerful that the genetic patterns of a deceased father can be reconstructed from grandparents, siblings, or other children to determine paternity.

From DNA Diagnostics Center, Fairfield, Ohio, 1999.

for the sexual abuse. If the victim is receptive to counseling, arrangements are made to assist the victim in dealing with the abuse. If the victim is a child, child protective services may be involved, and if the situation warrants, the child is removed from the environment.

RAPE

SYMPTOMS AND SIGNS

The symptoms and signs of rape vary with the degree of violence incurred by the victim. Many present to an emergency care facility, physician's office, or clinic, or a law enforcement agency stating, "I've been raped." Some report having pain in the pelvic and perineal regions or being choked or restrained in some manner. Others relate the threat of death. Bruising is noted in any area of the body. Signs of rape include torn clothing, dirt and debris ground into clothing or hair, disheveled appearance, withdrawal, anxiousness, avoidance of eye contact, and bruising, tears, or lacerations around or on the genitals, rectum, or mouth. Pelvic and rectal examination often reveals tenderness in those areas and evidence of trauma. If the victim has not bathed or douched, evidence of semen may be present on the inner aspects of the thighs, genital areas, or pubic region. There may be trauma to any part of the body, including the breasts. If the victim is male, bruising or lacerations in the anal region are indicative of sodomy.

ETIOLOGY

Rape is a crime of violence and domination, not a sexual act. It occurs when both parties of the sexual act are not in mutual consent and is a forceful act. Rape can occur to either female or male victims, most frequently being committed on females. Rape can be date rape, occurrence rape, husband against wife, or a violent act by an unknown perpetrator.

DIAGNOSIS

Diagnosis is made by the history, clinical picture, and physical examination, including pelvic examination and sex crime evidence gathering. Samples of debris, clothing, saliva, hair, pubic hair, fingernails, and scrapings from under the nails are collected. A urinalysis is obtained, along with blood tests for sexually transmitted diseases, AIDS, and possible pregnancy. Photographs may be taken for documentation of injury.

481

TREATMENT

Any trauma is treated in an appropriate manner. Counseling at a rape crisis center should be offered. Information concerning the risks of possible pregnancy, sexually transmitted diseases, and AIDS is given, along with follow-up testing protocol. If there is no religious objection, prophylaxis for pregnancy may be considered.

Reinforcement that the victim is a survivor of a violent crime and is not responsible for the incident is necessary. The victim needs to believe that she or he just happened to be in the wrong place at the wrong time. Everyone dealing with the victim and her or his family must be nonjudgmental and never tell the victim that she or he "asked for it."

Summary

Individuals with various injuries from traumatic occurrences present in the medical care setting with minor to life-threatening conditions. These conditions need special consideration because they are common and frequently complicated, requiring special assessment and trained personnel. From the insect bite to severe open trauma, the threats to homeostasis include pain, infection, hemorrhage, respiratory distress, cardiac arrest, and shock. Significant psychological stress and strong emotional responses are consequential in most traumatic events.

- Abrasions, avulsions, and lacerations are soft tissue injuries requiring measures to prevent infection, repair damage, and promote healing without unnecessary scarring.
- Thermal insults give emphasis to the body's vulnerability to excess cold and heat. Burns, frostbite, hypothermia, and hyperthermia are treated after careful assessment of the degree of insult to the body; fluid and electrolyte balance and vital signs are monitored.
- A rapid ascent to high altitudes associated with low oxygen content and dehydration can produce unpleasant and sometimes serious symptoms termed altitude sickness.
- Electrical shock and lightning injuries are classified by severity of injury. Severe burns, respiratory and cardiac arrest, and cerebral edema are grave complications.
- Certain insects such as mosquitoes and ticks and animals such as dogs are vectors of serious diseases, including Rocky Mountain spotted fever, malaria, and rabies.
- Severe allergic reactions and poisoning are life-threatening complications of insect bites that require immediate medical intervention.
- Prevention of certain cumulative trauma is achieved by ergonomic studies in the workplace, with the correction of improper repetitive activities.
- Physical and psychological assault trauma can be difficult to diagnose by obvious injury alone. Sensitivity in obtaining information from the victim, a physical examination, and even criminal evidence gathering can help pinpoint the extent and nature of abuse.
- DNA parentage testing is available to determine paternity.

Review Challenge

REVIEW QUESTIONS

1. What are the major types of trauma?
2. What are some ways in which environmental factors can result in trauma?
3. What is the difference between an abrasion and an avulsion?
4. When is it appropriate to use tetanus toxoid in prophylactic treatment?
5. When is débridement of a wound necessary?
6. How are the depth and extent of burns assessed?
7. What are the possible effects of an electrical shock?
8. What are the types of lightning strikes? Which treatments may be required?
9. How are the signs and symptoms of heat stroke and heat exhaustion different?
10. What is the treatment for heat stroke? For heat exhaustion?
11. What are some precautions in the treatment of frostbite?
12. Which spider bites require emergency care?
13. What is Rocky Mountain spotted fever, and how is it transmitted?
14. Why is an animal quarantined after biting a human?
15. What are the signs and symptoms of a poisonous snake bite?
16. What is the relationship between repetitive activities and carpal tunnel syndrome?
17. Which physical patterns may be observed in child abuse?
18. How may elder abuse, child abuse, sexual abuse, or battered spouse syndrome be noted during the history and physical examination?
19. What testing is available for the rape victim?
20. How can parentage be determined in the laboratory?

Heat Exhaustion

The mother of a 14-year-old girl called the office about her daughter, who had just come home from marching band practice, where she had been for approximately the past 3 hours. The girl was complaining of nausea, weakness, and headache. On questioning, the mother revealed that her daughter's skin appears pale, cool, and moist. The weather has been hot and humid, and the girl told her mother that she had been practicing the marching routines for about 2½ hours before she felt ill. The mother took the girl's temperature, which was 98.2° and said her pulse was faint and fast.

The mother was advised to have her daughter lie down with feet slightly elevated in a cool environment, to loosen her clothing, and to place cool compresses on the girl's face and forehead, neck, chest and abdomen, arms, back, and legs. She also was instructed to give her daughter 4 oz of cool water to drink every 15 minutes. The office advised that they would call back in 1 hour to get a progress report.

The diagnosis was heat exhaustion.

Questions

1. What is the significance of the cool, moist skin?
2. What measures could have been taken to prevent the onset of heat exhaustion?
3. Compare the moist cool skin with sweating of heat exhaustion with the skin condition of heat stroke.
4. What could be the anticipated outcome of treatment, as suggested to the mother?
5. If the girl's condition did not improve in an hour, what would you expect to be the next step in treatment?
6. What is the significance of loosening clothing and applying cool compresses?
7. Why would the mother be instructed to use cool compresses and not ice?
8. Why would the patient with heat stroke require treatment in an emergency facility versus the heat exhaustion victim being treated at home?

REAL-LIFE CHALLENGE

Spousal Abuse

A 36-year-old woman is in the office being treated for pain and reduced hearing in the left ear. She is very vague about any history, only that her left ear is painful, she has noted some blood coming out of the canal, and she has reduced hearing in her left ear. Bruising is noted around the ear on the left cheek, on the left side of the neck, and behind the left ear on the skull. These areas are tender to touch. The patient is very quiet, at times is tearful, and has on a long-sleeved turtleneck shirt and long pants. She is hesitant to remove her shirt for the taking of her blood pressure or for any other examination.

Examination reveals recent trauma to the left ear, blood is visualized in the canal, and otoscopic examination confirms a ruptured tympanic membrane. Audiometry verifies reduced hearing capability in the left ear. Various stages of healing bruises are noted on arms, neck, and chest. Further examination discloses similar bruising to legs. The patient denies any abusive trauma and says she incurred the injuries in a fall. She avoids eye contact, tending to keep eyes downward. Her demeanor is subdued, and her posture also appears subdued with slumping shoulders.

Gentle questioning eventually brings out that her husband, a man of large stature, recently lost his job as a result of drinking and aggressive or near-violent behavior. She also admits that in the past 2 weeks since the loss of his job, her husband has been "slapping her around" and that last night he struck her on the left side of her face and across the ear with his open hand. The patient does not want to file a police report and says she cannot leave the situation.

She is referred to an ear nose and throat specialist for treatment of the ruptured tympanic membrane. An appointment for follow-up is made for 2 days later, at which time additional support for the psychosocial situation will be supplied. She is instructed to call immediately for any recurrence of the abusive behavior. She also is advised to see whether she can get her husband to make an appointment for an examination.

Questions

1. What is typical behavior for a "battered" spouse?
2. What is the significance of the alcohol consumption and the loss of employment in the onset of the abusive relationship?
3. Why didn't the victim want the abuse reported?
4. What are the legal responsibilities of your office in this situation?
5. What might be the reasons the victim feels she cannot leave the abusive situation?
6. Explain the mechanics of the impact of the slapping to cause the ruptured tympanic membrane.
7. Discuss the implications of both the abusive husband and the battered wife being patients in the practice.

RESOURCES

National Clearinghouse on Child Abuse and Neglect and Family Violence Information
1-800-394-3366

National Resource Center on Child Sexual Abuse
1-800-543-7006

National Child Abuse Hotline, Childhelp USA
1-800-4-A-CHILD   1-800-422-4453

Boys Town
1-800-448-3000

Covenant House Nineline
1-800-999-9999

National Domestic Violence Hotline
1-800-799-7233

National Center for Missing and Exploited Children
1-800-843-3678

American Trauma Society (ATS)
8903 Presidential Parkway, Ste 512
Upper Marlboro, MD 20772
1-800-556-7890
(http:www.amtrauma.org)

GLOSSARY

Abduct: move an arm or leg away from the body

Abruptio placentae: detachment of the placenta from the uterus before birth; often results in severe bleeding

Abscess: a localized collection of pus surrounded by swollen tissue

Acidemia: a decreased pH of the blood (increased hydrogen ion concentration)

Acidosis: a pathologic condition resulting from an abnormal increase in hydrogen ion in the body (decrease in pH) from the accumulation of acid or loss of the alkaline reserve

Acute abdomen: an abdominal condition of sudden onset, accompanied by pain from intra-abdominal inflammation or infection

Adenocarcinoma: a cancerous tumor arising from glandular tissue

Adenoma: a benign neoplasm in which cells are derived from glandular epithelium

Adenosarcoma: a cancerous gland-like tumor, such as Wilms' tumor

Agglutination: the clumping of antigens with antibodies, or of the red blood cells from one type of blood to the red blood cells of another type

Aggregation: the coming together of substances, e.g., platelets, blood cells, diseases

Agranulocytosis: a condition of the blood marked by a sudden decrease in the number of granulocytes (a type of white blood cell); occurs in lesions of the throat or other mucous membranes or as a side effect of the administration of certain drugs or radiation

Alkalosis: excessive alkalinity of body fluids

Allergen: an antigenic substance capable of producing an allergic response in the body

Amblyopia: reduced vision in an eye without a detectable organic lesion

Amnesia: a loss of memory; inability to recall past experiences

Amniotic fluid: a transparent albuminous liquid made by the amnion and the fetus; surrounds and protects the fetus during pregnancy

Amyloid: a waxy, starch-like protein that tends to build up in tissues and organs in certain pathologic conditions

Analgesia, analgesic: relief of pain

Anaphylaxis: a severe systemic allergic response characterized by redness, itching, swelling, and water buildup (angioedema); in severe cases, life-threatening respiratory distress occurs and the blood pressure drops rapidly (anaphylactic shock)

Anastomosis (anastomoses): the surgical or pathologic connection between two vessels or tubular structures

Anesthesia, anesthetic: partial or complete loss of sensation caused by injury, diseases, or the administration of an anesthetic agent

Angina pectoris: paroxysmal chest pain, which often radiates to the arms and may be accompanied by a feeling of suffocation and impending death; the most common cause is a shortage of oxygen to the cardiac muscle linked with coronary artery disease

Angioplasty: repair of a narrowed blood vessel through surgery or other angiographic procedures

Angiotensin-converting enzyme (ACE): an enzyme found on the surface of blood vessels in the lungs and other tissues with vasopressor action

Angiotensin-converting enzyme inhibitors: agents that inhibit angiotensin-converting enzyme (a potent vasoconstrictor) and promote relaxation of blood vessels

Ankylosis: immobility of a joint

Anorexia, anorectic: loss of appetite for food

Antibody (antibodies): an immunoglobulin that may combine with a specific antigen to destroy or control it

Anticholinesterase: any enzyme that counteracts the action of the choline esters

Anticoagulant: any substance that delays or prevents blood clotting

Antiemetic: a medication that prevents or relieves nausea and vomiting

Antigen: any substance that stimulates the immune system to produce antibodies

Antimicrobial: a substance that kills microorganisms or suppresses their growth

Antipyretic: a drug or treatment that reduces or relieves fever

Antitrypsin: a substance that inhibits trypsin, an enzyme that hastens the hydrolysis of protein.

Anxiolytic: a substance that diminishes anxiety

Aphasia: a nerve defect that results in loss of speech

Aphonia: inability to produce normal speech sounds or loss of voice

Aphthous ulcers: recurrent painful canker sores in the mouth

Apnea, apneic: the temporary cessation of breathing

Arrhythmia: variation or loss of normal rhythm of the heartbeat

Arthrodesis: the immobilization of a joint accomplished surgically

Arthroplasty: surgical reconstruction or replacement of a diseased joint

Asymptomatic: without symptoms

Asystole: the absence of contractions of the heart; cardiac standstill

Atrophy: a wasting away; a degeneration of a cell, tissue, organ, or muscle because of disease or other influences

Audiogram: the record of a hearing test

Aura: a sensation or phenomenon that signals the onset of an epileptic seizure or a migraine

Auscultation: a diagnostic technique of listening for sounds within the body, particularly the lungs, heart, or abdominal viscera

Autoantibody: an antibody that attacks and destroys the body's own cells

Autoimmunity, autoimmune: an immune response resulting in the presence of self-antigens or autoantigens on the surface of certain body cells; may result in allergy or autoimmune disease

Autosome, autosomal: any of the 22 ordinary paired chromosomes in humans, distinguished from the sex (X and Y) chromosomes

Azoospermia: an absence of spermatozoa in the semen

Azotemia: an excess of urea or other nitrogenous bodies in the blood

Barium: a pale, soft, alkaline metallic element; a radiopaque barium (barium sulfate) compound commonly used in radiographic studies of the gastrointestinal tract

Battle's sign: bogginess of the temporal region of the head that may indicate fracture at the base of the skull

Bifurcate: split into two branches

Bilirubinemia: the presence of bilirubin in the blood

Bilirubinuria: the presence of bilirubin (a yellow- or orange-tinged pigment in the bile) in the urine

Biopsy: the excision of tissue from the living body, followed by microscopic examination, for the purpose of exact diagnosis

Blood gases: the gases present in the blood that are a result of utilization of oxygen and production of carbon dioxide during metabolism; the blood is analyzed for evidence of deviations (acidosis or alkalosis) from normal levels

Blood urea nitrogen (BUN): a measurement of urea nitrogen (a substance formed during protein breakdown) in the serum or plasma; an elevated BUN level may indicate impaired renal function

Breech: buttocks

Bronchoscopy: examination of the bronchial tree with a bronchoscope to obtain a biopsy, remove an obstruction, or diagnose a disease

Bruit: an abnormal sound heard in auscultation

Cachexia: a profound and marked wasting disorder, usually associated with malnutrition and such diseases as cancer and tuberculosis

Calculus (calculi): a stone usually composed of mineral salts (e.g., kidney stones and gallstones); or calcified deposits on the teeth

Carcinogen, carcinogenic: a substance that produces cancer or that causes transformation of a normal cell to a cancerous one

Cardiac sphincter: the circular muscle at the opening of the esophagus into the stomach

Cardiomegaly: enlargement of the heart

Cast: a negative mold or copy formed in a hollow organ or part (e.g., kidney or bronchi); a urinary cast is a small structure formed within the urinary system from mineral or protein matter and extruded from the body in the urine

Cataract: a progressive disease in which the lens of the eye becomes cloudy, impairing vision or causing blindness

Catatonic posturing: a state of not being able to move, with the assumption of a rigid, often bizarre posture

Cautery: an instrument or chemical that destroys tissue, as a therapeutic measure

Cephalalgia: pain in the head; headache

Cephalic: referring to the head; cranial

Cerclage: encircling of the cervix with a metal ring or suture ring to treat cervical incompetence during pregnancy to help prevent spontaneous abortion

Cheilectomy: surgical removal of abnormal bone around a joint, also refers to surgical removal of a lip

Cholangiogram: a diagnostic radiographic study of the gallbladder and bile ducts

Cholecystogram: a diagnostic radiographic study of the gallbladder

Cholinergic: an agent that produces the effect of acetylcholine at the connections of muscles and nerves

Chorea: the ceaseless occurrence of involuntary muscular movements of the limbs or facial muscles

Circadian rhythm: the biologic clock in humans; the rhythmic repetition of certain phenomena, such as hunger, fatigue, and blood pressure, that tend to fluctuate within a 24-hour period

Circumoral cyanosis: a bluish discoloration around the mouth

Clean-catch urine specimen: a urine specimen obtained by cleaning the genitalia and then capturing a midstream urine sample for laboratory analysis

Closed reduction: the nonsurgical manipulative reduction of a dislocation or fracture

Coagulation: the process of clot formation

Cognitive: pertaining to the mental processes of thinking, knowing, remembering, and perceiving

Collateral: a small side branch of a blood vessel or nerve

Colporrhaphy: suturing of the vagina

Comedo (comedones): a blackhead, as seen in acne

Commissurotomy: surgical incision of component parts at the sites of junction between adjacent cusps of the heart valves to increase the size of the opening

Computed tomography (CT): a diagnostic technique using ionizing x-rays passed through a patient around specific sections of the body at multiple angles; useful in the detection of tumors

Contracture: immobility of muscles or a joint caused by shortening or wasting of tissue or muscle fibers

Continuous positive airway pressure (CPAP): a form of respiratory therapy in which ventilation is assisted by a flow of oxygen delivered at a constant pressure throughout the respiratory cycle

Corneal ulcer: ulcerative keratitis

Corticotropin, or adrenocorticotropic hormone (ACTH): a hormone secreted by the anterior lobe of the pituitary

489

Craniotomy: incision into the skull, usually to relieve pressure, to remove a lesion, or to control bleeding

Creatinine: an important nitrogen compound that is a normal constituent of urine and blood; increased levels may indicate renal damage

Cryotherapy: the therapeutic use of cold

Cul-de-sac: an area at the end of the abdominal cavity that is midway between the rectum and the uterus

Cyanosis, cyanotic: bluish appearance of the skin and mucous membrane that usually indicates reduced hemoglobin levels in the blood

Cytology, cytologic: the scientific study of cells

Débride: remove foreign material or dead tissue in a wound

Demise: destruction or death

Demyelination: loss of the myelin sheath of a nerve

Dermatomes: a configured zone of skin innervated by a spinal cord segment

Dialysate: the fluid that passes through a semipermeable membrane during dialysis

Dialysis (dialyses): a procedure that filters out unwanted substances from the blood, usually in cases of renal failure

Diaphoresis, diaphoretic: profuse perspiration

Diplopia: double vision

Discoid: shaped like a disk

Diuresis, diuretic: increased formation and excretion of urine

Doppler: ultrasonographic technique used to evaluate blood flow velocity

Dorsiflexion: to bend a joint toward the posterior aspect of the body; for example, the hand is dorsiflexed when it is extended or bent backward at the wrist

Dyspareunia: pain or discomfort in the pelvis or vagina during or after sexual intercourse

Dysphagia: difficulty in swallowing

Dysphasia: difficulty in speaking, usually caused by a lesion in the central nervous system

Dysphonia: hoarseness; difficulty in speaking

Dyspnea: labored or difficult breathing

Dysrhythmia: an abnormal cardiac rhythm

Echocardiogram, echocardiography, echocardiographic: an ultrasonographic study of the motion of the walls or structures of the heart

Ectopic: out of normal position

Effacement: the thinning or obliteration of the cervix during labor

Electrocardiogram, electrocardiography, electrocardiographic: a record of the electrical activity of the heart

Electromyogram, electromyography, electromyographic: an electrodiagnostic assessment of the activity of skeletal muscles

Embolus (emboli): a mass (e.g., foreign body, blood clot, or a piece of tumor) that breaks off and causes occlusion of an artery

Emergency medical service (EMS): trained services provided on the scene

Encephalitis: inflammation of the brain

Endarterectomy: the surgical excision of the innermost lining of an artery to remove blockage

Endemic: refers to a disease that is prevalent in a particular geographic area or in a population

Endometriosis: a growth of endometrial tissue at various sites outside the uterus

Endometrium: the lining of the uterus that changes with the menstrual cycle; if the ovum is fertilized, the endometrium serves as the place where implantation occurs

Endoscopy: examination of any cavity of the body with an endoscope

Enzyme-linked immunosorbent assay (ELISA): a test used to detect antibodies to the acquired immunodeficiency syndrome (AIDS) virus in blood serum

Epigastric: refers to the upper middle region of the abdomen

Epiphysis (epiphyses), epiphyseal: the long end of a bone where bone growth occurs

Epistaxis: bleeding from the nose

Ergonomics: the science concerned with people and their work; it entails mechanical principles enhancing efficiency and well-being in the work environment

Ergot: a drug obtained from a fungus that grows on rye plants

Erythrocyte sedimentation rate (ESR): a measurable reflection of the acute-phase reaction in inflammation and infection

Esophagoscopy: examination of the esophagus with an esophagoscope

Exacerbation: an increase in the severity of a disease or aggravation of its symptoms

Exotoxin: bacterial toxins excreted outside of the bacterial cell

Exsanguination: excessive loss of blood from a part

Exudate: fluid, cells, or cellular debris that has oozed into tissue because of injury or swelling

Fascia: a fibrous membrane that covers, separates, and supports the muscles

Fasciculation: involuntary contraction or twitching of muscles

Fibrin: a protein material produced by the action of thrombin on fibrinogen

Fibrosis, fibrotic: the abnormal formation of fibrous tissue

Fissure: a crack or groove on a surface

Fistula: an abnormal tube-like passageway

Fluorescein angiography: a procedure in which light-sensitive material is injected into a blood vessel

Foramen (foramina): an opening or hole in a bone, allowing the passage of nerves or blood vessels

Fowler's position: a semisitting position, usually 45°, used to facilitate breathing and drainage

Fulguration: tissue destruction with high-frequency electrical sparks

Fulminant: refers to severe pain with sudden onset

Gamete: male or female sex cell

Gangrene: death of tissue caused by a decrease or absence of blood supply

Gastrectomy: surgical removal of the stomach

Gastroscopy: visual examination of the stomach using a gastroscope

Giemsa stain: a process of staining bacteria for identification

Glenoid: having the semblance of a socket

Glomerulosclerosis: hardening of the renal glomerulus

Glomerulus (glomeruli): a tiny ball of microscopic blood vessels on the end of the renal tubules

Goitrogenic: pertaining to substances causing goiters

Gram stain: a process of staining bacteria for identification

Guthrie test: a test to detect phenylketonuria

H_2-receptor antagonist: chemical agent that blocks the interaction of histamine or acetylcholine with receptors in stomach cells; drugs that inhibit secretion of gastric acid

Hallucination: a false perception of reality; may be visual, auditory, or olfactory

Hallux: the great toe

Hematemesis: vomiting of blood

Hematocrit: the percentage of the total blood volume consisting of erythrocytes

Hematopoiesis, hematopoietic: pertaining to the production and the development of blood cells or a substance that stimulates their production

Hematuria: blood in the urine

Hemiparesis: paralysis affecting one side of the body

Hemoccult: trademark for a guaiac reagent strip test for occult blood

Hemodynamic: refers to forces involved in the circulation of blood within the body

Hemolysis, hemolytic: the destruction of red blood cells with the release of hemoglobin

Hemoptysis: spitting up blood

Hemostasis: the condition of controlled bleeding

491

Hepatomegaly: enlargement of the liver

Histoplasmosis: a systemic respiratory disease caused by a fungus

Homeostasis: a state of equilibrium within the body

Human chorionic gonadotropin (hCG): hormones produced by the placenta and detected in the urine and blood of a pregnant woman

Humoral: refers to body fluids or substances found in them

Hyaline membrane: a membrane that forms in the lung sacs of a developing fetus; a respiratory distress syndrome of the newborn

Hydronephrosis: accumulation of urine in the renal pelvis caused by obstruction, forming a cyst

Hymen: the membrane partially covering the entrance to the vagina

Hyperalimentation: infusion of life-sustaining fluids, electrolytes, and elements of nutrition intravenously or via the gastrointestinal tract

Hypercapnia: increased carbon dioxide levels in the blood

Hypercoagulable: refers to the increased ability of any substance to coagulate, especially blood

Hyperemic: refers to an excessive amount of blood in a part or area

Hyperesthesia: increased sensitivity to pain

Hyperglycemia: an increase in the normal blood glucose level

Hyperlipidemia: an increase of fat levels in the blood

Hyperparathyroidism: a condition caused by overactive parathyroid glands

Hypertrophy, hypertrophic: enlargement of an organ or structure

Hyperuricemia: excessive uric acid levels in the blood

Hypoalbuminemia: low albumin levels in the blood

Hypocalcemia: too little calcium in the blood

Hypokalemia: low potassium levels in the blood

Hypoparathyroidism: a condition caused by greatly reduced function of the parathyroid glands

Hypovolemic shock: a condition that occurs when blood in the circulatory system is decreased (e.g., hemorrhage)

Hypoxia: decreased oxygen levels in the tissues

Idiopathic: refers to a disease without a known or recognizable cause

Immunocompetence: the ability of the immune system to defend the body against disease

Immunocompromised: refers to an immune system incapable of fighting disease

Immunodeficiency: the diminished ability of the immune system to react with appropriate cellular immunity response; often the result of loss of immunoglobulins or aberrance of B or T cell lymphocytes

Immunogen: an antigen (i.e., a substance capable of stimulating an immune response)

Immunoglobulin: a protein that can act as an antibody

Immunoincompetence: immunodeficiency

Immunosuppressive: refers to suppressing the body's immune response to antigens

Infarct, infarction: an area of dead tissue caused by lack of blood supply

Insidious: refers to the onset of a disease without symptoms

Intractable: incurable or resistant to treatment

Intravenous pyelogram, intravenous pyelography: radiographic study of the renal pelvis and ureter using injected dye

Intravenous urogram, intravenous urography: radiographic study of the urinary tract using injected dye

Intrinsic: refers to the essential nature of a substance or structure

Intrinsic factor: a substance normally found in gastric juices; essential for the absorption of vitamin B_{12}

Ischemia, ischemic: holding back or obstructing the flow of blood

Ischemic necrosis: the death or sloughing off of small areas of tissue or bone, caused by insufficient circulation or lack of blood supply

Jaundice: yellowing of the skin

Karyotype: a picture of chromosomes in the nucleus of a cell

Keratin: a hard protein substance found in hair, nails, and skin

Keratoconjunctivitis sicca: dryness of the conjunctiva due to a decrease in lacrimal function

Keratolytic: a substance that causes shedding of the skin

Kernicterus: a form of icterus (bile pigmentation of tissues and membranes) occurring in infants

Laparoscopy: a surgical procedure to examine the abdomen using an endoscope called a laparoscope

Laryngoscopy: visual examination of the larynx using a laryngoscope

Laser photocoagulation: coagulation of the blood vessels in the eye using a laser

Lavage: the cleaning out of a cavity with liquid

Leukocytosis: a slight increase in the numbers of white blood cells

Leukopenia: a decrease in the number of white blood cells

Leukorrhea: a white or yellow mucous discharge from the vagina

Lipase: a fat-splitting enzyme produced by the pancreas

Lithotripsy: crushing of stones (e.g., kidney stones and gallstones)

Lumbar puncture: a surgical procedure to withdraw spinal fluid for analysis or the injection of an anesthetic solution

Lumpectomy: removal of just the tumor from the breast

Lymph: a mostly clear, colorless, transparent, alkaline fluid found within the lymphatic vessels; formed in tissues throughout the body

Lymphadenitis: inflammation of the lymph nodes

Lymphadenopathy: disease of the lymph nodes

Lymphocyte: one of two types (B cells and T cells) of leukocytes (white blood cells) found in blood, lymph, and lymphoid tissue

Lymphocytosis: an excessive number of lymph cells

Macrophage: a monocyte blood cell

Macula: a small spot or a colored area

Maculopapular: pertaining to or consisting of macules and papules

Magnetic resonance imaging (MRI): a procedure similar to computed tomography that does not require x-rays; a large magnetic field is applied and creates an image; useful in visualizing the cardiovascular system, brain, and soft tissues

Malaise: a feeling of discomfort, illness, or uneasiness

Malocclusion: improperly positioned teeth and faulty contact of the teeth

Mastectomy: surgical removal of breast tissue; can be partial or radical

McBurney's point: the point of special tenderness in acute appendicitis; corresponds with the normal position of the base of the appendix

Meconium: the first stool of a newborn, greenish black and a tarry consistency

Mediastinal shift: abnormal movement of the structures within the mediastinum to one side of the chest cavity

Mediastinum: the area in the chest between the lungs

Megakaryocyte: a large bone marrow cell having large or many nuclei

Megaloblastic: pertaining to abnormally large red blood cells found in pernicious anemia

Melanin: the black pigment found in the basal layer of the epidermis

Meningitis: inflammation of the coverings around the brain and spinal cord

Menorrhagia: painful menstruation

Metabolic acidosis: excessive acid in the body fluids caused by dehydration, diarrhea, vomiting, renal disease, or hepatic impairment

Metastasis (metastases), metastatic, metastasize: spreading of a malignant disease or pathogenic microorganisms from one organ or part to another not directly connected with it

Metatarsophalangeal: pertaining to the metatarsus and phalanges of the toes

Monocyte: a phagocytic white blood cell that engulfs and destroys cellular debris

Murmur: a blowing sound heard when listening to the heart or vessels with a stethoscope

Mutation: a variation or change in genetic structure

Mutism: a condition of being unable to speak

Myalgia: muscle pain

Mycoplasma: microscopic organisms that lack a rigid cell wall; some species cause infections in humans

Myelin: the protective fat and protein covering around the axons of many nerves

Myelogram, myelography: radiographic study of the spinal cord after the injection of a dye

Necrosis, necrotic: death of tissue

Neoplasm, neoplasia, neoplastic: abnormal formation of new tissue; can be benign or malignant

Neovascularization: the formation of new blood vessels

Nephron: the functioning unit of the kidney or renal tubule

Neurotransmitter: a chemical released by the terminal end fibers of an axon

Nociceptors: nerves that receive and transmit painful stimuli

Normal flora: the presence of normal bacteria and fungi adapted for living in, and characteristic of, the area considered (e.g., skin, intestine, or vagina)

Nuchal rigidity: neck stiffness

Nullipara: a woman who has never produced viable offspring

Oliguria: scanty urination

Oncogene: a gene in a virus that can prompt a cell to turn malignant

Opacity: the state of being opaque or not transparent

Open reduction: exposure of a fractured or dislocated bone through a surgical incision to realign the bone ends

Ophthalmoscopy, ophthalmoscopic: an examination of the interior of the eye

Opportunistic infection: infection resulting from a defective immune system

Orchitis: inflammation of the testes

Orthodontics: branch of dentistry concerned with correction of dentofacial structures (e.g., teeth)

Orthopnea: a condition in which breathing becomes easier in an upright standing or sitting position

Orthoptic training: eye muscle exercises

Ortolani's sign: an assessment maneuver designed to detect a hip dislocation

Osteophyte: a bony outgrowth, usually branch shaped

Ostomy: a surgical opening of the bowel to the outside of the body

Otitis media: middle ear infection

Otoscopy: visual examination of the ear using an otoscope

Oxygen saturation: refers to the oxygen content in blood, divided by oxygen capacity and expressed in volume percent

Palliative: alleviating symptoms without curing the underlying cause

Panhypopituitarism: a condition in which the entire pituitary gland ceases to function and is not producing any pituitary hormones

Papule: a circular area on the skin that is reddened and elevated

Paresis: partial paralysis

Paresthesia: abnormal, usually increased, sensations

Paronychia: inflammation of soft tissue surrounding the nail

Partial thromboplastin time (PTT): evaluates the coagulation sequence of plasma and screens for platelet abnormalities

Patch test: a screening test in which a small piece of material containing the allergy-causing substance is placed on the skin; redness or edema indicates a positive reaction

Pathogenesis: the development of disease; pathologic mechanisms

Pathologist: one who specializes in the study of disease

Peau d'orange: the skin is dimpled, resembling the skin of an orange

Pelvic inflammatory disease (PID): inflammation of the female pelvic organs, usually caused by bacteria

Perfusion: delivery of oxygen and other nutrients to the tissue by the blood

Pericoronitis: inflammation of the gum around the crown of a tooth

Periosteum: the fibrous covering of long bones

Peritonitis: inflammation of the membrane that lines the abdominal cavity and covers the viscera

Pessary: an object placed in the vagina to support the uterus

Petechia (petechiae): a tiny spider-like hemorrhage under the skin

Phagocyte, phagocytic, phagocytosis: the process by which cells surround and digest certain particles (e.g., bacteria, protozoa, and debris)

Phlebotomy: surgical puncture of a vein to withdraw blood

Photophobia: unusual sensitivity to light

Phototherapy: treatment of disease by exposure to light

Plaque: a deposit of hardened material lining the blood vessel; or a gummy accumulation of microorganisms that clings to teeth and is considered the forerunner of caries and periodontal disease

Plasmapheresis: the process of separating blood into its components by centrifuging

Polyposis: a condition of multiple polyps

Positive end-expiratory pressure (PEEP): mechanical ventilation with pressure maintained, thereby increasing the volume of gas remaining in the lungs at the end of expiration

Positron emission tomography (PET): a non-invasive radiographic study of the blood flow in specific organs and body tissues

Postprandial: after meals

Primipara: a woman who has delivered one child of at least 20 weeks' gestational age

Proctoscopy: visual examination of the rectum with a proctoscope

Prodromal: refers to the initial stage of a disease before the onset of actual symptoms

Prophylaxis, prophylactic: the prevention of disease

Prostate-specific antigen (PSA): an enzyme that is measured in a blood test to detect cancer of the prostate

Proteinuria: the presence of protein in the urine

Prothrombin time (PT): measures the time taken for clot formation

Proton pump inhibitor: a drug that blocks gastric acid secretion; used to treat ulcers of the gastrointestinal tract and gastroesophageal reflux disease (GERD)

Pruritus: itching

Pseudoneurologic: refers to a neurologic symptom that is without clinical basis

Pseudopregnancy: false pregnancy, also known as pseudocyesis

Purpura: a red-purple discoloration of the skin caused by multiple minute hemorrhages in the skin or mucous membrane

Purulent: containing pus

Pustule: a small elevation of the skin containing pus

Putrefaction: decomposition of organic matter

Pyelonephritis: a purulent infection of the kidney tissue and renal pelvis

Pyuria: pus in the urine

Raccoon eyes: dark discoloration (bruising) around the eyes; a sign of possible basilar skull fracture

Radioimmunoassay: a test that measures minute amounts of antibodies or antigens by the use of radioactive substances

Rale: an abnormal crackling sound made by the lungs during inspiration; indicative of fluid in a bronchus

Raynaud's phenomenon: a temporary constriction of arterioles in the skin causing short episodes of numbness and color changes in the fingers and toes. This condition is usually idiopathic

Reflux: a backward flow

Renal calculi: kidney stones

Reticuloendothelial: refers to the system responsible for phagocytosis of cellular debris, pathogens, and foreign substances and for removing them from the circulation

Retrovirus: a family of viruses that contains RNA (ribonucleic acid) and reverse transcriptase; some retroviruses are oncogenic and can induce tumors

Rheumatoid factor: a macroglobulin type of antibody; increased levels are found in the blood of persons with rheumatoid arthritis

Rhonchus: dry rattling in the throat or bronchus caused by partial obstruction

RNA: ribonucleic acid; controls protein synthesis in cells and takes the place of DNA in some viruses

Schick test: an intradermal skin test to detect immunity to diphtheria; a positive result indicates lack of immunity or negative immunity

Sclerosis, sclerosing: hardening of a body part

Sclerotherapy: a sclerosing solution is injected into a vein as a form of treatment for varices

Seborrhea: the excessive secretion of sebum from sebaceous glands

Sebum: oily secretion of sebaceous glands

Semi-Fowler position: patient lying on the back with the head elevated 8 to 10 inches and the knees flexed

Senile: refers to growing old with decreased physical and mental capacity

Septicemia: a disease in which pathogenic microorganisms or toxins are present in the blood

Sequestrum: a segment of dead bone; the result of an abscess from a bacterial infection in a bone and bone marrow

Serology, serologic: a study of blood serum to measure antibody titers

Sigmoidoscopy: visual examination of the sigmoid colon with a sigmoidoscope

Sinopulmonary: pertaining to the paranasal sinuses and lungs

Skeletal traction: a method of immobilization and reduction of a long bone fracture in which traction is applied by means of pins and wires

Somatoform: psychogenic symptoms without an underlying disease process

Splenomegaly: enlarged spleen

Squamous cell: flat and scaly epithelial cell

Status asthmaticus: severe asthmatic episode that does not respond to normal treatment

Steatorrhea: the presence of malabsorbed fat in the feces

Stenosis, stenosed: narrowing of an opening

Stent: a device used to hold tissue in place or provide support

Steri-Strips: trademark for sterile adhesive strips used to approximate and hold together the edges of a wound

Stress incontinence: leakage of urine when stress is placed on the perineum

Stridor: a high-pitched respiratory sound due to air passageway obstruction

Subluxation: partial dislocation

Substernal retraction: the chest wall under the sternum sinks in with each respiration

Sulfonylurea: oral hypoglycemic agent that stimulates the pancreas to produce insulin

Supine: lying on the back

Surfactant: an agent (normally present in the lungs as a phospholipid) that lowers surface tension; abnormal in the lungs of premature infants or in hyaline membrane disease

Symptomatic: concerning the nature of a symptom indicative of a disease

Syncope: fainting, lightheadedness

Synovial: pertaining to fluid around a joint

Synthesize: to produce a substance by combining two or more elements or chemicals

Tachycardia, tachycardic: rapid heartbeat; more than 100 beats per minute

Tachypnea: rapid and shallow respirations

Tamponade: compression of a part by pressure or a collection of fluid

Tendinitis: inflammation of a tendon

Tetany: hyperexcitability of nerves and muscles due to low serum calcium levels; a syndrome characterized by intermittent tonic spasms of the extremities, cramps, and convulsions

Tetralogy of Fallot: a congenital cardiac condition

Thallium scan: a cardiac stress test using intravenous thallium injection to diagnose ischemia and coronary artery disease

Thoracentesis: surgical puncture into the thoracic cavity to remove accumulated air or fluid

Thrill: vibration felt on palpation, especially over the heart

Thrombocytopenia: reduced number of thrombocytes (platelets)

Thyroidectomy: surgical removal of the thyroid gland

Thyrotoxicosis: a toxic condition caused by hyperactivity of the thyroid gland

Tinnitus: ringing in the ears

Tonometry: measurement of intraocular pressure

Toxin, toxic: poisonous substance

Toxoplasmosis: a disease caused by infection with protozoa found in many mammals and birds

Transcutaneous electrical nerve stimulation (TENS): electrical stimulation of nerves for relief of pain

Transferrin: globulin in blood serum that transports iron

Trousseau's phenomenon: when pressure is applied to the upper arm, muscular spasms result, indicating latent tetany

Truss: a device that holds a reduced hernia in place

Turgor: normal tension in a cell that results in normal strength and tension of the skin

Tympanic membrane: eardrum

Tzanck test: diagnostic test that examines the tissue of a lesion to determine the type of cell present

Ulcer, ulceration: a crater-like sore on the skin or mucous membrane

Uremia: toxic condition of excessive waste products, protein, and nitrogen in the blood caused by renal insufficiency

Vaginismus: a spasm of the muscles surrounding the vagina, causing painful contractions of the vagina

Valsalva's maneuver: forced exhalation with the mouth and nose closed, causing increased intrathoracic pressure, slowing of the heart rate, increased venous pressure, and a reduced amount of return blood flow to the heart

Varicocele: a condition in which the veins in the scrotum near the testicles are swollen and enlarged

Vector: carrier of infectious agent of disease from one person to another (usually insects)

Venom: poison secreted by an animal

Ventricular shift: lateral movement of one of the ventricles of the brain to one side caused by pressure on the other side

Vertex: top of the head

Vesicle: a small blister-like elevation of the skin containing clear fluid

Vitrectomy: a surgical procedure that removes the contents of the vitreous chamber

Western blot test: a test to identify and analyze protein antigens

Wheal: a smooth, round elevated area of the skin with red edges and a white center, which is usually accompanied by itching; hives

White blood cell, white blood cell count (WBC) see Appendix 1: Common Laboratory and Diagnostic Tests, under Blood Analysis

Xerostomia: dry mouth; reduced amount of saliva

Zygote: fertilized ovum

COMMON LABORATORY AND DIAGNOSTIC TESTS

Values may vary according to laboratory reference values. These values are for reference only. Results of one test alone usually are not conclusive and should be considered with results of other diagnostic procedures and the symptoms and signs, along with the physical examination, to arrive at a diagnosis.

BLOOD ANALYSIS

Complete Blood Count (CBC). Evaluation of cellular components of the blood. Includes red blood cell count, red blood cell indices, white blood cell count, white blood cell differential, hemoglobin, hematocrit, and platelet count. Sometimes referred to as hemogram. Often the differential must be ordered specifically as CBC with differential.

Red Blood Count (RBC). Count of erythrocytes in a specimen of whole blood.

Normal RBC:

Adult male: 4.5.7–6.1 million/μl
Adult female: 4.0–5.5 million/μl
Infants and children: 3.8–5.5 million/μl
Newborns: 4.8–7.1 million/μl

An elevated RBC is indicative of many disorders, including but not limited to erythremia, polycythemia, erythrocytosis, dehydration, burns, anoxia, diarrhea, cardiovascular disease, poisoning, and pulmonary disease. A decreased RBC also is indicative of many disorders, including but not limited to anemias, bone marrow suppression, hemorrhage, liver diseases, thyroid disorders, cardiovascular disease, vitamin deficiency, and ingestion of certain drugs. When the RBC is abnormal, morphology of the cells should be examined. As with most blood tests, results should

be evaluated with other tests, along with symptoms and signs, to determine a diagnosis.

Hemoglobin (Hgb). Measurement of the oxygen-carrying pigment of the red blood cells.

Normal:

Adult male: 14.0–18.0
Adult female: 12.0–16.0
Infants and children: 11.5–15.5
Newborns: 14.5–22.5

An elevated Hgb is indicative of many disorders, including but not limited to CHF, COPD, dehydration, burns, diarrhea, erythrocytosis, high altitudes, and thrombotic thrombocytopenia. A decreased Hgb also is indicative of many disorders, including but not limited to iron deficiency anemia, hemorrhage, hemolytic reaction to drugs or chemicals, liver diseases, SLE, and pregnancy.

Hematocrit (HCT). Measurement of the percentage of red blood cells in a volume of whole blood.

Normal:

Adult male: 37–52%
Adult female: 36–48%
Infants and children: 28–45%
Newborns: 48–69%

An elevated HCT is indicative of many disorders, including but not limited to dehydration, burns, diarrhea, eclampsia, pancreatitis, shock, and polycythemia. A decreased HCT also is indicative of many disorders including but not limited to anemia, bone marrow hyperplasia, CHF, fluid overload, burns, thyroid disorders, pancreatitis, pregnancy, pneumonia, and ingestion of certain drugs.

White Blood Count (WBC). Count of white blood cells in a whole blood specimen.

Normal:

Adult male: 4500–11,000/μl
Adult female: 4500–11,000/μl
Infants and children: 6000–17,500/μl
Newborns: 9000–30,000/μl

An elevated WBC is indicative of many disorders, including but not limited to acquired hemolytic anemia, anorexia, abscess, appendicitis, bacterial infections, bronchitis, burns, biliary disorders, respiratory disorders, disorders of the GI tract, renal disorders, blood disorders, lactic acidosis, poisoning, pregnancy, sepsis, shock, tonsillitis, trauma, uremia, and ingestion of certain drugs. Similar to an abnormal RBC, a differential should be evaluated, and, as with most blood tests, results should be evaluated with other tests, along with symptoms and signs, to determine a diagnosis. A decreased WBC is indicative of many disorders, including but not limited to AIDS, anemias, chemical toxicity, Hodgkin's disease, influenza, legionnaire's disease, radiation therapy, shock, septicemia, vitamin B12 deficiency, cirrhosis, hepatitis, hypothermia, leukopenia, tuberculosis, and ingestion of certain drugs.

Differential White Blood Cells (Differential Leukocyte Count). An assessment by percentage of leukocyte distribution in a specimen of 100 white cells.

Granulocytes

Normal:

Segmented Neutrophils (SEGs) Adult: 50–62%
Band Neutrophils (Bands) Adult: 3–6%
Eosinophils (EOS) Adult: 0–3%
Basophils (BASOS) Adult: 0–0.75%
Monocytes (MONOS) Adult: 3–7%
Lymphocytes (LYMPHS) Adult: 25–40%

Increased neutrophils are indicative of many disorders, including but not limited to allergies, asthma, acute infections, appendicitis, burns, diabetic acidosis, cardiovascular disorders, disorders of the GI tract, leukemia, respiratory disorders, poisoning, pyelonephritis, septicemia, tonsillitis, and ingestion of certain drugs. A decrease in neutrophils is indicative of many disorders, including but not limited to endocrine disorders, anaphylactic shock, carcinoma, chemotherapy, anemias, pneumonia, septicemia, radiation therapy, and ingestion of certain drugs.

Increased bands are indicative primarily of pharyngitis.

Increased SEGs are indicative primarily of pernicious anemia.

Increased eosinophils are indicative of many disorders including but not limited to allergies, asthma, cancer, dermatitis, diverticulitis, eczema, Hodgkin's disease, leukemia, parasitic infection, pernicious anemia, radiation therapy, sickle cell anemia, tuberculosis, and ingestion of certain drugs. Decreased eosinophils also are indicative of many disorders including but not limited to aplastic anemia, CHF, eclampsia, infections, stress, and ingestion of certain drugs.

Increased basophils are indicative of many disorders, including but not limited to allergic reactions, Hodgkin's disease, hypothyroidism, radiation therapy, sinusitis, urticaria, and ingestion of certain drugs. Decreased basophils also are indicative of many disorders, including but not limited to acute infections, anaphylactic shock, endocrine disorders, pregnancy, radiation therapy, stress, and ingestion of certain drugs.

Increased lymphocytes are indicative of many disorders including but not limited to endocarditis, infectious mononucleosis, leukocytosis, lymphocytic leukemia, syphilis, toxoplasmosis, and ingestion of certain drugs. Decreased lymphocytes also are indicative of many disorders, including but not limited to aplastic anemia, Hodgkin's disease, immunoglobulin deficiencies, leukemia, renal failure, SLE, uremia, and ingestion of certain drugs.

Increased monocytes are indicative of many disorders including but not limited to Epstein-Barr virus, Hodgkin's disease, leukemia, rheumatoid arthritis, syphilis, SLE, tuberculosis, and ingestion of certain drugs. Decreased monocytes are primarily indicative of aplastic anemia and hairy-cell leukemia.

Platelet Count (Thrombocyte Count). Count of platelets in a whole blood specimen.

Normal:

Adults: 150,000–400,000/μl

Increased platelet count is indicative of many disorders including but not limited to anemias, carcinoma, fractures, liver disorders, heart disease, hemorrhage, acute infection, inflammation, leukemia, pancreatitis, pregnancy, rheumatoid arthritis, surgery, and ingestion of certain drugs. A decreased platelet count is indicative of many disorders including but not limited to anemias, bone marrow disorders, autoimmune disorders, severe burns, carcinoma, liver disorders, DIC, hemolytic disease of the newborn, infections, radiation therapy, leukemias, and ingestion of certain drugs.

BLOOD CHEMISTRIES

Chemistries. Normal chemistry profile may contain blood serum levels for albumin, alkaline phosphatase, aspartate aminotransferase, bilirubin, calcium, creatinine, lactate dehydrogenase, phosphorus, total protein, urea nitrogen, and uric acid.

***Albumin* –** Measurement of one of two major protein factions of blood.

Normal:

Adult: 3.5–5.0 g/dl

Increased levels of serum albumin are indicative of many disorders, including but not limited to dehydration, diarrhea, meningitis, carcinoma, myeloma, nephrosis, nephrotic syndrome, peptic ulcers, pneumonia, rheumatic fever, SLE, uremia, vomiting, and ingestion of certain drugs. Below-normal levels of serum albumin are indicative of many disorders, including but not limited to ascites, alcoholism, burns, CHF, Crohn's disease, diabetes mellitus, edema, hypertension, kidney disorders, GI disorders, trauma, stress, and ingestion of certain drugs.

***Alkaline Phosphatase* –** Measurement of enzyme found in bone, liver, intestine, and placenta.

Normal:

Adult: 2–4 U/dl

Elevated alkaline phosphatase levels are indicative of many disorders, including but not limited to alcoholism, liver disorders, diabetes mellitus, fractures, GI disorders, endocrine disorders, hepatitis, Hodgkin's, disease, leukemia, neoplasms, myocardial infarction, bone disorders, disorders of the pancreas, kidney disorders, and ingestion of certain drugs. Below-normal levels of alkaline phosphatase are indicative of many disorders, including but not limited to pernicious anemia, cretinism, hypothyroidism, malnutrition, nephritis, and ingestion of certain drugs.

***Aspartate Aminotransferase (AST)* –** Measurement of enzyme found primarily in heart, liver, and muscle.

Normal adult female: 8–20 U/L
Normal adult male: 8–26 U/L

Elevated AST levels are indicative of many disorders, including but not limited to acute myocardial infarction (MI), alcoholism, liver disorders, insult and injury to tissue including trauma, cerebral and pulmonary infarctions, and ingestion of certain drugs. Decreased AST levels are indicative of many disorders, including but not limited to diabetic ketoacidosis, liver disease, uremia, and ingestion of certain drugs.

***Bilirubin* –** A by-product of hemoglobin breakdown, bilirubin is produced in the liver, spleen, and bone marrow.

Total: Normal adult: < 1.5 mg/dl
Direct: Normal adult: 0.0–0.3 mg/dl
Indirect: Normal adult: 0.1–1.0 mg/dl

Total bilirubin is divided into direct bilirubin, primarily secreted by the intestinal tract, and indirect bilirubin primarily circulating in the bloodstream. Obstructive or hepatic jaundice results in an increased amount of direct bilirubin entering the bloodstream rather than the GI tract and the filtering and elimination of it by the kidneys. Some conditions that cause an increase in direct bilirubin include but are not limited to biliary obstruction, pancreatic cancer (head of pancreas), cirrhosis, hepatitis, and ingestion of certain drugs. Hemolytic jaundice causes the amounts of indirect bilirubin to accumulate in the blood because of the increased breakdown of Hgb. Some conditions that cause an increase in direct bilirubin levels include but are not limited to pernicious and sickle cell anemia, autoimmune hemolysis, cirrhosis, hepatitis, intracavity and soft tissue hemorrhage, MI, septicemia, hemolytic transfusion reaction, and ingestion of certain drugs.

***Calcium* –** Measurement of blood serum calcium levels.

Normal adult:

8.2–10.2 mg/dl

Calcium acts in bone formation, impulse conduction, and myocardial and skeletal muscle contractions, and in the blood-clotting process. Elevated serum calcium levels are indicative of many disorders, including but not limited to endocrine disorders, hepatic disease, respiratory acidosis, leukemia, neoplasms, blood disorders, respiratory disorders, and ingestion of certain drugs. Decreased serum calcium levels are indicative of many disorders, including but not limited to alkalosis, bacteremia, burns, chronic renal disease and other renal disorders, endocrine disorders, osteomalacia, rickets, vitamin D deficiency, and ingestion of certain drugs.

***Creatinine* –** Measurement of an indicator of renal function.

Normal adult female: 0.5–1.1 mg/dl
Normal adult male: 0.6–1.2 mg/dl

Serum creatinine is excreted continually by the renal system, and elevated levels are indicative of a slowing of glomerular filtration. Other conditions that may contribute to elevation of serum creatinine include but are not limited to CHF, diabetes mellitus, kidney disorders, hypovolemia, metal poisoning, endocrine disorders, subacute bacterial endocarditis, SLE, and ingestion of certain drugs. Decreased serum creatinine levels are indicative of diabetic ketoacidosis and muscular dystrophy.

Lactate Dehydrogenase – Measurement of body tissue intracellular enzyme released after tissue damage.

Normal adult:

45–102 U/L

Elevated lactate dehydrogenase levels are indicative of many disorders, including but not limited to alcoholism, anoxia, burns, cardiomyopathy, CVA, cirrhosis, CHF and myocardial infarction, neoplasms, anemias and leukemia, renal disorders, muscle and bone pain, respiratory disorders, shock, trauma, and ingestion of certain drugs. Decreased levels of lactate dehydrogenase develop postradiation and after the ingestion of oxalates.

Total Protein – A reflection of the total amounts of albumin and globulins in blood serum.

Normal adult:

6.0–8.0 g/dl

Increased total protein is indicative of many disorders, including but not limited to Addison's disease, Crohn's disease, dehydration, diarrhea, renal disease, vomiting, protozoal diseases, and ingestion of certain drugs. Decreased total protein is indicative of many disorders, including but not limited to burns, cholecystitis, cirrhosis, CHF, diarrhea, hyperthyroidism, edema, leukemia, peptic ulcer, nephrosis, malnutrition, ulcerative colitis, and ingestion of certain drugs.

Urea Nitrogen/Blood Urea Nitrogen (BUN) – An assessment of the urea content in the blood that gives an indication of the functioning of the renal glomeruli.

Normal adult:

5–20 mg/dl

An elevated urea nitrogen level can be caused by prerenal (inadequate renal circulation or abnormally high levels of blood protein), renal (impaired renal filtration and excretion), or postrenal (lower urinary tract obstruction) etiologies.

Uric Acid – An end-product of the metabolism of purines.

Normal adult female: 2.4–6.0 mg/dl
Normal adult male: 3.4–7.0 mg/dl

Elevated uric acid levels are indicative of many disorders, including but not limited to gout, hyperuricemia, hemolytic, pernicious and sickle cell anemias, arteriosclerosis, arthritis, CHF, dehydration, diabetes mellitus, fasting, exercise, hypothyroidism, intestinal obstruction, acute infections, lead poisoning, leukemia, neoplasms, nephritis, polycystic kidney, renal failure, starvation, stress, uremia, urinary obstruction, and ingestion of certain drugs. Decreased uric acid levels are indicative of many disorders, including but not limited to acromegaly, carcinomas, Hodgkin's disease, pernicious anemia, and ingestion of certain drugs.

Thyroid Function Tests. An evaluation of all three thyroid levels is important in diagnosing thyroid disorders.

Thyroid Thyroxine (T4) – The hormone thyroxine is produced in the thyroid gland from iodide and thyroglobulin in response to stimulation by thyroid-stimulating hormone (TSH) produced by the pituitary gland. T4 stimulates T3 to be produced. It also stimulates the basal metabolism. In the process of negative feedback, circulating levels of T4 influence the levels of TSH.

Normal adult:

5.0–12.0 μg/dl

Increased levels of T4 usually indicate the presence of hyperfunctioning thyroid disorders, including Graves' disease, hyperthyroidism, and thyrotoxicosis, and ingestion of certain drugs. Decreased levels of T4 are indicative of hypothyroid disorders, including acromegaly, cretinism, and goiter, as well as hypothyroidism, liver disease, endocrine disorders, GI tract disorders, pituitary tumor, and ingestion of certain drugs.

Triiodothyronine (T3) – T3 stimulates the basal metabolic rate for metabolism of carbohydrates and lipids, protein synthesis, vitamin metabolism, and bone calcium release.

Normal adult:

80–230 ng/dl

An increase in T3 levels is indicative of but not limited to Graves' disease, hyperthyroidism, thyrotoxicosis, and ingestion of certain drugs. Decreased levels of T3 are indicative of but not limited to iodine and thyroid deficiency disorders, including goiter and myxedema, renal failure, starvation, thyroidectomy, and ingestion of certain drugs.

Thyroid-Stimulating Hormone (TSH) – TSH, produced in the anterior lobe of the pituitary gland, stimulates the production and release of T3 and T4 by the thyroid gland.

Normal adult:

$< 10 \mu U/ml$

An increase in TSH levels may be indicative of but not limited to Addison's disease, goiter, hyperpituitarism, hypothyroidism, thyroiditis, and ingestion of certain drugs. A decrease in TSH may be indicative of but not limited to Hashimoto's thyroiditis and hyper- and hypothyroidism.

Lipid Profile. A lipid profile consists of comparison of results of four serum lipids, total cholesterol, triglycerides, high-density lipoproteins (HDLs), and low-density lipoproteins (LDLs). One consideration is the ratio of HDL:LDL; the recommended ratio is 3.4:5.0.

Total Cholesterol – A widely distributed sterol that facilitates the absorption and transport of fatty acids. Found in foods of animal origin, cholesterol is synthesized continuously in the body.

Normal adult:

< 29 years < 200 mg/dl
30–39 years < 225 mg/dl
40–49 years < 245 mg/dl
> 50 years < 265 mg/dl

Elevated serum cholesterol levels are indicative of many disorders, including but not limited to atherosclerosis, CHD, CHF, biliary disorders, kidney disorders, lipid disorders, and ingestion of certain drugs. Decreased levels of serum cholesterol are indicative of many disorders including but not limited to anemias, carcinoma, cirrhosis, liver disease, hepatitis, endocrine disorders, GI tract disorders, and ingestion of certain drugs.

Triglycerides – Triglycerides, the principal lipids in blood, are simple fat compounds of three molecules of fatty acid, oleic, palmitic, or stearic.

Normal adult female:

20–29 years	10–100 mg/dl
30–39 years	10–110 mg/dl
40–49 years	10–122 mg/dl
50–59 years	10–134 mg/dl
> 59 years	10–147 mg/dl

Normal adult male:

20–29 years	10–157 mg/dl
30–39 years	10–182 mg/dl
40–49 years	10–193 mg/dl
50–59 years	10–197 mg/dl
> 59 years	10–199 mg/dl

Elevated triglyceride levels are indicative of many disorders, including but not limited to arteriosclerosis, MI, aortic aneurysm, hypercholesterolemia, hyperlipoproteinemia, alcoholism, diabetes mellitus, gout, renal disease, starvation, and malnutrition. Decreased triglyceride levels are indicative of many disorders, including but not limited to cirrhosis, malabsorption, hyperalimentation, and ingestion of certain drugs.

HDL Cholesterol – High-density lipoprotein transports cholesterol and other lipids to the liver for excretion. HDL is believed to lower the risk of coronary artery disease.

Normal adult female: 30–85 mg/dl
Normal adult male: 30–70 mg/dl

Increased levels of HDL are indicative of but not limited to alcoholism, hepatic disorders, cirrhosis, and ingestion of certain drugs. Decreased levels of HDL are indicative of many disorders, including but not limited to arteriosclerosis, hypercholesterolemia, hyperlipoproteinemia, CHD, diabetes mellitus, liver disease, kidney disease, bacterial infections, and ingestion of certain drugs.

LDL Cholesterol – Low-density lipoprotein has a high cholesterol content, and it delivers lipids to body tissues.

Normal adult:

80–190 mg/dl

Elevated levels of LDL are indicative of many disorders, including but not limited to diabetes mellitus, anorexia nervosa, renal failure, hepatic disease, and ingestion of certain drugs. Decreased levels of LDL are indicative of but not limited to hyperlipoproteinemia, arteriosclerosis, pulmonary disease, stress, and the ingestion of certain drugs.

Electrolytes (lytes). Blood serum test for chloride, potassium, sodium, and carbon dioxide.

Chloride – An anion found predominately in extracellular spaces.

Normal adult:

97–106 mEq/L

Increased blood serum levels of chloride may be the result of several disorders, including but not limited to metabolic disorders, dehydration, diabetes insipidus, hyperventilation, hyperparathyroidism, acidosis, respiratory alkalosis, CHF, Cushing's disease, nephritis, renal failure, and ingestion of certain drugs. Decreased blood serum levels of chloride may be the result of several disorders, including but not limited to metabolic alkalosis, diabetes, severe vomiting, burns, overhydration, salt-losing diseases, some diuretic therapies, CNS disorders, diaphoresis, fasting, fever, heat exhaustion, acute infections, gastric obstructions, uremia, and ingestion of certain drugs.

Potassium – Potassium is the main cation of intracellular fluid. Potassium is important in nerve conduction, muscle function, osmotic pressure, acid–base balance and myocardial activity.

Normal adult:

3.5–5.3 mEq/L

Increased blood serum levels of potassium may be the result of several disorders, including but not limited to renal failure, dehydration, burns, trauma, chemotherapy, metabolic acidosis, Addison's disease, uncontrolled diabetes, dialysis, hemolysis, intestinal obstruction, sepsis, shock, pneumonia, uremia, and ingestion of certain drugs. Decreased blood serum levels of potassium may be the result of several disorders, including but not limited to alkalosis, anorexia, vomiting, diarrhea, malabsorption, starvation, diuresis, excessive sweating, draining wounds, severe burns, endocrine disorders, pancreatitis, GI stress, and ingestion of certain drugs.

Sodium – Sodium is the major cation of extracellular fluid and the main base in the blood. Its functions include chemical maintenance of osmotic pressure, acid–base balance, and nerve transmission.

Normal adult:

135–145 mEq/L

Increased blood serum levels of sodium may be the result of several disorders, including but not limited to severe burns, CHF, excessive fluid loss caused by vomiting, diarrhea, sweating, Addison's disease, nephrotic syndrome, pyloric obstruction, diabetes insipidus, hypertension, hypovolemia, toxemia, malabsorption syndrome, diuresis, edema, hypothyroidism, and ingestion of certain drugs. Decreased blood serum levels of sodium may be the result of several disorders, including but not limited to bowel obstruction, dehydration, coma, Cushing's disease, diabetes mellitus, glomerulonephritis, hyperthermia, myxedema, certain renal conditions, and ingestion of certain drugs.

Carbon Dioxide – Carbon dioxide in normal blood plasma comes from bicarbonate.

Normal adult:

20–30 mEq/L

Increased blood serum levels of carbon dioxide may be the result of several disorders, including but not limited to emphysema, aldosteronism, mercurial diuretics, severe vomiting, airway obstruction, bradycardia, cardiac disorders, renal disorders, and ingestion of certain drugs. Decreased blood serum levels of carbon dioxide may be the result of several disorders, including but not limited to severe diarrhea, diabetic acidosis, salicylate toxicity, starvation, acute renal failure, alcoholic ketosis, dehydration, high fever, head trauma, malabsorption syndrome, uremia, and ingestion of certain drugs.

Clotting and Coagulation Studies

Partial Thromboplastin Time (PTT). PTT is an evaluation of the functioning of the coagulation sequence. PTT is a screening process used for coagulation disorders and to monitor the effectiveness of heparin therapy.

Normal values or standardized times must be checked with laboratory because of various processes that may be used.

Increased standardized times may be indicative of many disorders, including but not limited to cardiac surgery, DIC, abruptio placentae, factor defects, hemodialysis, obstructive jaundice, vitamin K deficiency, presence of circulating anticoagulants, and ingestion of certain drugs. Decreased standardized times are indicative of acute early hemorrhage and extensive cancer.

Prothrombin Time (PT). Prothrombin time is a measurement of the time taken for clot formation after the addition of reagent tissue thromboplastin and calcium to citrated plasma. In the clotting process, prothrombin converts to thrombin. Adequate vitamin K is necessary for adequate prothrombin production. This test assists in the evaluation of the clotting mechanism and in monitoring oral anticoagulant therapy.

Normal values:

11.0–13.0 sec; may vary according to laboratory

An increase in prothrombin time may be indicative of several disorders, including but not limited to vitamin K deficiency, liver disorders, anticoagulant therapy, prothrombin deficiency, salicylate intoxication, DIC, SLE, clotting disorders, biliary obstruction, CHF, pancreatitis, snakebite, vomiting, toxic shock syndrome, and ingestion of certain drugs. A decreased prothrombin time may be indicative of certain disorders, including but not limited to deep vein thrombosis, MI, peripheral vascular disease, spinal cord injury, pulmonary embolism, and ingestion of certain drugs.

Platelet Count (Thrombocyte Count). Count of platelets in a whole blood specimen.

Normal adults:

150,000–400,000/μl

Increased platelet count is indicative of many disorders, including but not limited to anemias, carcinoma, fractures, liver disorders, heart disease, hemorrhage, acute infection, inflammation, leukemia, pancreatitis, pregnancy, rheumatoid arthritis, surgery, and ingestion of certain drugs. A decreased platelet count is indicative of many disorders including but not limited to anemias, bone marrow disorders, autoimmune disorders, severe burns, carcinoma, liver disorders, DIC, hemolytic disease of the newborn, infections, radiation therapy, leukemias, and ingestion of certain drugs.

Bleeding Times. Bleeding time is a screening test for coagulation disorders, a measurement of the time required for the platelet clot to form.

Normal time at most laboratories is 3–10 minutes.

Increased bleeding times are indicative of several disorders, including but not limited to thrombocytopenia, DIC, aplastic anemia, platelet dysfunction, vascular disease, leukemias, liver disorders, aspirin ingestion, and ingestion of certain drugs. Decreased bleeding time is clinically insignificant.

Erythrocyte Sedimentation Rate (ESR). The rate at which red blood cells (erythrocytes) fall

out of well-mixed whole blood to the bottom of the test tube. An alteration in blood proteins occurs during inflammatory and necrotic processess, causing an aggregation of red cells, therefore making them heavier and thus fall rapidly when placed in a special vertical test tube. A higher ESR is the result of faster settling of the cells. Although not diagnostic of any particular disease process, an elevated ESR provides an indication of an ongoing disease process.

Normal values by Westergren method:

Adult male: 0–15 mm/hr
Adult female: 0–20 mm/hr
Children 0–10 mm/hr

Normal values by Wintrobe method:

Adult male: 0.41–0.51 mm/hr
Adult female 0.36–0.45 mm/hr

Increased ESRs may be indicative of many disease processes, including but not necessarily limited to collagen diseases, infectious processes, inflammatory disorders, cancer, heavy metal poisoning, toxemia, PID, anemia, pain, pregnancy, pulmonary embolism, renal disorders, arthritis, subacute bacterial endocarditis, and ingestion of certain drugs. Decreased levels may be found in CHF and ingestion of certain drugs.

Glucose Monitoring

Glucose Tolerance Test (GTT). GTT is a test that provides an evaluation of patients who have symptoms of diabetes mellitus or diabetic complications as well as a screening test for gestational diabetes. The test measures blood glucose levels at the following intervals: fasting, 30 minutes, 1 hour, 2 hours, and 3 hours after ingestion of dose of glucose. Urine samples also are taken at these intervals.

Normal adult levels:

Fasting 70–110 mg/dl
30 min 110–170 mg/dl
1 hr 120–170 mg/dl
2 hr 70–120 mg/dl
3 hr 70–120 mg/dl

All urine samples should test negative for glucose.

Increased glucose values or decreased glucose tolerance are indicative of certain disorders, including but not limited to diabetes mellitus, excessive glucose ingestion, certain endocrine disorders, hepatic damage, postgastrectomy, CNS lesions, pancreatitis, pheochromocytoma, and ingestion of certain drugs. Decreased glucose values or increased glucose tolerance may be indicative of certain disorders, including but not limited to Addison's disease, hypoglycemia, malabsorption, pancreatic disease, liver disease, hypoparathyroidism, hypopituitarism, and ingestion of certain drugs.

Fasting Blood Glucose (FBS) Levels. The amount of glucose found in the blood after 8 hours of fasting.

Normal adult levels:

Serum—70–110 mg/dl

Increased levels of blood glucose are indicative of several disorders, including but not limited to diabetes mellitus, excessive glucose ingestion, certain endocrine disorders, hepatic damage, postgastrectomy, CNS lesions, pancreatitis, pheochromocytoma, and ingestion of certain drugs. Decreased glucose values may be indicative of certain disorders, including but not limited to Addison's disease, hypoglycemia, malabsorption, pancreatic disease, liver disease, hypoparathyroidism, hypopituitarism, and ingestion of certain drugs.

2-Hour Postprandial. Blood glucose levels 2 hours after ingestion of a normal meal, usually the noon meal.

Normal adult levels:

65–139 mg/dl

Increased postprandial levels of blood glucose are indicative of several disorders, including but not limited to diabetes mellitus, excessive glucose ingestion, certain endocrine disorders, hepatic damage, postgastrectomy, CNS lesions, pancreatitis, pheochromocytoma, and ingestion of certain drugs. Decreased postprandial glucose values may be indicative of certain disorders, including but not limited to Addison's disease, hypoglycemia, malabsorption, pancreatic disease, liver disease, hypoparathyroidism, hypopituitarism, and ingestion of certain drugs.

Glycosylated Hemoglobin/Glycohemoglobin. Glycohemoglobin is a measurement of the blood glucose bound to hemoglobin and provides an overall view of the past 120 days of glucose saturation.

Normal adult levels:

5.5–8.5%

Increased glycohemoglobin levels are indicative of several disorders, including but not limited to poorly controlled diabetes mellitus, iron deficiency anemia, splenectomy, alcohol or lead toxicity, and hyperglycemia. Decreased levels of glycohemoglobin may be indicative of certain diseases, including but not limited to hemolytic anemia, chronic blood loss, chronic renal failure, and pregnancy.

Toxicology Studies, Drug Screens

Drug Levels. Digoxin, digitoxin, theophylline, lidocaine, lithium, and various drugs for therapeutic or toxic levels.

Digoxin – Digoxin is a cardiac glycoside used to treat CHF and cardiac arrhythmias. Blood level studies provide information concerning the therapeutic or toxic levels.

Normal therapeutic level:

0.8–2 ng/ml

Levels above 2 ng/ml indicate a toxicity of the drug. Medical intervention is necessary to return levels to therapeutic. Levels below 0.8 ng/ml indicate that more digoxin is necessary to achieve the expected therapy.

Digitoxin – Digitoxin is a cardiac glycoside used to treat CHF and cardiac arrhythmias. Blood level studies provide information concerning the therapeutic or toxic levels

Normal therapeutic level:

20–35 ng/ml

Levels above 35 ng/ml indicate a toxicity of the drug. Medical intervention is necessary to return levels to therapeutic. Levels below 20 ng/ml indicate that more digitoxin is necessary to achieve the expected therapy.

Theophylline – Theophylline, a bronchodilator, is used to treat asthma and obstructive respiratory disorders. Blood level studies provide information concerning the therapeutic or toxic levels.

Normal therapeutic level:

8–20 μg/ml

Levels above 20 μ/ml indicate a toxicity of the drug. Medical intervention is necessary to return levels to therapeutic. Levels below 8 μg/ml indicate that more theophylline is necessary to achieve the expected therapy.

Lidocaine – Lidocaine is used to treat ventricular arrhythmias. Blood level studies provide information concerning the therapeutic or toxic levels.

Normal therapeutic level:

1.5–6 μg/ml

Levels above 6 μg/ml indicate a toxicity of the drug. Medical intervention is necessary to return levels to therapeutic. Levels below 1.5 μg/ml indicate that more lidocaine is necessary to achieve the expected therapy.

Lithium – Lithium is used to treat bipolar disorders.

Normal therapeutic level:

0.6–1.2 mEq/L

Levels above 1.2 mEq/L indicate a toxicity of the drug. Medical intervention is necessary to return levels to therapeutic. Levels below 0.6 mEq/L indicate that more lithium is necessary to achieve the expected therapy.

CARDIAC ENZYMES/CARDIAC ISOENZYMES

Cardiac enzymes and isoenzymes are released by the myocardium as a result of an MI. Monitoring the levels of these enzymes assists in the evaluation of the extent of the insult to the myocardium and the progress of the healing process.

Creatine Kinase (CK) – Creatine kinase, an enzyme found in certain body tissues, becomes elevated in damage to cardiac and skeletal muscles.

Normal adult levels:

Female: 96–140 U/L
Male: 38–174 U/L

Values may vary according to laboratory.

In MI, levels begin to rise in 2-6 hours, peak at 18–36 hours, and return to baseline 3-6 days after the onset of the MI. The increased levels should be part of the total evaluation to confirm an MI.

CK Isoenzymes – Isoenzymes increase during an MI and are more specific in the diagnosis of an MI.

Normal values:

MM CK3 (muscle): 90–100%
MB CK2 (heart): 0–4%
BB CK1 (brain): 0%

MB CK2 begins to rise within 6-24 hours after the myocardial insult; it usually peaks at 24 hours and then returns to normal within 72 hours.

Lactate Dehydrogenase (LDH) – LDH, an enzyme found in kidney, heart, skeletal muscle, brain, liver, and lung tissue, is released from the cell, increasing serum levels and indicating cellular necrosis.

Normal values:

150–450 U

Values may vary according to laboratory.

Levels of LDH begin to rise at 12 hours postinsult, reach a peak at 24 hours, and return to normal later than CK.

Lactate Dehydrogenase Isoenzymes – Lactate dehydrogenase isoenzymes are found in many body tissues and are released when tissue necrosis occurs. There are five different LDH isoenzymes, and elevation of LDH1 and LDH2 usually point to cardiac involvement and subsequent necrosis of myocardial tissue.

Normal values: % of total

LDH1 17–27%
LDH2 29–39%
LDH3 19–27%
LDH4 8–16%
LDH5 6–16%

LDH1 and LDH2 usually are increased in myocardial insult and necrosis. LDH1 will peak first and then in 48 hours a ratio inversion occurs between LDH1 and LDH2.

Aspartate Aminotransferase (AST, SGOT)– Measurement of enzyme found primarily in heart, liver, and muscle.

Normal adult female: 8–20 U/L
Normal adult male: 8–26 U/L

Elevated AST levels are indicative of many disorders, including but not limited to acute MI, alcoholism, liver disorders, insult and injury to tissue including trauma, cerebral and pulmonary infarctions, and ingestion of certain drugs. Decreased AST levels are indicative of many disorders, including but not limited to diabetic ketoacidosis, liver disease, uremia, and ingestion of certain drugs.

Alanine Aminotransferase (ALT, SGPT) — ALT evaluates liver insult and is a measurement of an enzyme product found in the liver, certain body fluids, and in the liver, heart, kidneys, pancreas, and musculoskeletal tissue.

Normal adult levels:

7–56 μ/L

Elevated ALT levels are indicative of certain disorders, including but not limited to liver insult and liver disease, CHF, muscle injury, MI, pancreatitis, pulmonary embolism, severe burns, trauma, shock, and ingestion of certain drugs. Decreased levels of ALT are not found.

URINE STUDIES

Urinalysis (UA). A screening test, using a urine specimen, that gives a picture of the patient's overall state of health and the state of the urinary tract. Measurements include pH and specific gravity of the urine and presence of ketones, protein, sugars, bilirubin, and urobilinogen. Color and odor are noted, as is the presence of abnormal blood cells, casts, bacteria, other cells, and crystals.

Routine urinalysis—Normal
  Characteristics
    Color and clarity—Pale to darker yellow and clear
    Odor—Aromatic
    Chemical nature—pH is generally slightly acidic, 6.5
    Specific gravity—1.003–1.030, reflects amount of waste, minerals, and solids in urine
    Constituent Compounds
      Protein—None, or small amount
      Glucose—None
      Ketone bodies—None
      Bile and bilirubin—None
      Casts—None, or small amount of hyaline casts
      Nitrogenous wastes—Ammonia, creatinine, urea, and uric acid
      Crystals—None to trace
      Fat droplets—None

Refer to Table 11–1 for abnormal findings and related pathology.

Culture and Sensitivity (C & S) of Urine.
Culture — Sample of urine specimen is placed in/on culture medium to see whether microbial growth occurs. If growth occurs, identification of the pathogenic microbe is determined.

Sensitivity — A portion of the specimen is placed on a sensitivity disk (which has been impregnated with specific antibiotics) to determine to which antibiotic the pathogen is resistant or to which it will be responsive.

Normal—no growth

Growth will indicate pathogens residing in urinary tract. Sensitivity will identify antimicrobials to which pathogens are sensitive.

CARDIOLOGY TESTS

Electrocardiogram (ECG) (12 lead). A recording of electrical activity of the myocardium used to diagnose ischemia, arrhythmias, conduction difficulties, and activity of cardiac medications.

Normal—no dysrhythmias/arrhythmias. A 12-lead electrocardiogram (ECG) consists of three limb leads—I, II, III; three augmented limb leads—AVR, AVL, AVF; and six precordial chest leads—V1, V2, V3, V4, V5, and V6. The conduction of the impulse through the myocardium is traced by three specific areas of the systolic and diastolic complex. The P wave represents atrial depolarization, the conduction of the stimulus from the SA node through the atrium to the AV node. The QRS complex represents ventricular depolarization, the conduction of the stimulus from the upper portion of the ventricle and below the AV node through the bundle of His, the right and left bundle branches, and the Purkinje fibers and relay throughout the ventricular myocardium. The T wave represents the repolarization of the ventricular myocardium. The 12-lead ECG is used to detect conduction abnormalities, dysrhythmias, myocardial ischemia, myocardial damage; to monitor recovery from an MI; and to assist in evaluation of the effectiveness of cardiac medications. Lead II normally is used to evaluate cardiac rhythm. Refer to Table 10–1—Arrhythmias for explanation of cardiac arrhythmias/dysrhythmias.

Echocardiogram. An ultrasound (acoustic imaging) examination of the cardiac structure to define the size, shape, thickness, position, and movements of the cardiac structures, including valves, walls, and chambers.

Normal—shows no abnormalities. This noninvasive procedure assists in diagnosing cardiac diseases and disorders, including structural abnormalities, congenital defects, myocardial damage, and blood flow through all structures of the heart.

Holter Monitor. A miniature electrocardiograph that records the electrical activity of the heart for an extended period of time, usually 24 to 48 hours. The patient records all activities during the time period for the examiner to correlate activity with cardiac abnormalities.

Normal—no dysrhythmias. Refer to ECG.

Thallium Scan. A scan to indicate myocardial profusion and the location and extent of myocardial ischemia or infarction and predict the possible prognosis of the condition.

Normal—no evidence of myocardial ischemia or infarction. Normal tissue absorbs the isotope on injection whereas the ischemic area will not immediately absorb the isotope. As the scan is repeated in 5 minutes, ischemic tissue will absorb the isotope, differentiating it from the infarcted areas, which will never absorb the isotope. This test may be done either under stress or without the stress factor.

MUGA Scan (Multigated Blood Pool Study). A scan that assesses the function of the left ventricle and identifies abnormalities of the myocardial walls.

Normal—55–65% ejection fraction, symmetrical contraction of the left ventricle. A radioactive isotope is injected to show all four chambers and the great vessels simultaneously. A series of images is taken during both systole and diastole, then either shown as a movie or superimposed to relate ventricular function and allowing the ejection fraction to be calculated. This test may be done either under stress or without the stress factor.

Stress Testing, Treadmill, Exercise Tolerance Testing. An assessment of cardiac function during moderate exercise on a treadmill or stationary bicycle after a 12-lead electrocardiogram.

Normal—negative. The stress test measures the effects of exercise on myocardial output and oxygen consumption by the concurrent evaluation of the monitored electrocardiogram and oxygen consumption. This test is done in a safe environment to identify individuals who are prone to myocardial ischemia during activity.

Pulse Oximeter. An instrument (spectrophotometer) that provides a noninvasive measurement of the O_2 saturation of the arterial blood.

Normal—arterial blood oxygen saturation 95% or greater.

Cardiac Catheterization. Fluoroscopic visualization of right or left side of heart by passing a catheter into right or left chambers and injecting dye. Angiograms consist of the catheter being passed into the coronary vessels, where the dye is injected and fluoroscopic images are recorded.

Normal varies with the area being assessed. Normal would indicate normal anatomy and physiology, normal chamber volumes and pressures, normal wall and valve motion, and patent coronary arteries. Normal value for cardiac output is 5–8 L/min.

IMAGING STUDIES

Radiographs. Visualization of internal organs and structures by electromagnetic radiation. Radiographs of bone; the abdomen; the chest; paranasal sinuses; kidneys, ureters, and bladder (KUB); and mammograms do not require contrast medium. Contrast medium is used to distinguish soft tissue and some organs such as the gallbladder, esophagus, stomach, and small and large intestines.

Normal results vary with the area being studied by the imaging process. Interpretation of the imaging is done by the radiologist, with a report being dictated and transcribed for the ordering physician. Often the ordering physician visually inspects the films or images to evaluate the area him/herself.

Magnetic Resonance Imaging (MRI). Uses a magnetic field instead of radiation to visualize internal tissues. It is possible to view tissue and organs in a three-dimensional manner with MRI. It is helpful in determining blood flow to tissues and organs, in studying condition of blood vessels, to detect tumors, to differentiate healthy and diseased tissues, and to detect sites of infection. The patient is not exposed to ionizing radiation during MRI.

Normal results vary with the area being studied during the MRI. Interpretation of the MRI is done by the radiologist, with a report being dictated and transcribed for the ordering physician. Often the ordering physician visually inspects the films or images of the MRI to evaluate the area him/herself.

Computerized Tomography (CT) Scans. A radiographic technique using a scanner system that can provide images of the internal structure of tissue and organs both geographically and characteristically.

Normal results vary with the area being studied during the CT scan. Interpretation of the scan is done by the radiologist, with a report being dictated and transcribed for the ordering physician. Often the ordering physician visually inspects the films or images of the CT scan to evaluate the area him/herself.

Fluoroscopy. A real-time imaging process that provides continuous visualization of the area being imaged. Films are made of the process for more extensive examination. Used in procedures and to study the functioning of tissues and organs.

Normal results vary with the area being studied during fluoroscopy. Interpretation of the procedure is done by the radiologist, with a report being dictated and transcribed for the ordering physician. Often the ordering physician performs a procedure using fluoroscopy as a diagnostic tool and also as a guide for the procedure.

Sonograms, Ultrasound, Echogram. A beam of sound waves is projected into target tissues or organs, resulting in a bouncing back of the wave off the target structure. An outline of the structure is produced and recorded on film for examination. Tissue, organs, and systems that may be studied by ultrasound include but are not limited to abdominal aorta, brain, breast, eye and orbit, gallbladder, pelvis for gynecologic structures, heart, kidney, liver, lymph nodes, pancreas, prostate, spleen, thyroid, urinary bladder, upper GI tract, and pregnant pelvis for obstetric diagnostic examination.

Normal examinations vary with the area being examined. Interpretation of the ultrasound scan is done by the radiologist, with a report being dictated and transcribed for the ordering physician. Often the ordering physician visually inspects the films or images of the ultrasound to evaluate the area him/herself.

Myelogram. An imaging examination of the spinal cord and spinal nerve roots. Contrast medium (dye) or air is injected into the subarachnoid space and recorded on radiographic film. Fluoroscopy generally is used in this procedure.

Normal will reveal no lesions or abnormalities.

It is used to diagnose ruptured or bulging disks, spinal cord lesions and tumors, spinal cord and spinal nerve trauma and edema, and other conditions involving the spinal cord and spinal nerves.

STOOL ANALYSIS

Guaiac Tests. For occult blood. A qualitative detection of red blood cells in the stool.

Normal—negative

Presence of blood in the stool specimen is indicative of trauma, lesion, or other insult to the GI mucosa, producing blood.

Ova, Larva and Parasite Tests. A microscopic examination of stool to detect presence of parasites at various stages of development.

Normal—none detected

A positive examination result indicates parasitic infection of the GI tract.

ENDOSCOPY TESTS

Endoscopy. Visual inspection of internal organs or cavities of the body by a fiberoptic instrument using the appropriate scope. Additionally, during the diagnostic procedure, removal of pathology and repair of insult to the tissue may be accomplished.

Gastroscopy — Visualization of the stomach by a gastroscope.

Normal—Appearance of upper GI tract is within normal limits.

Hemorrhagic areas or erosion of a vessel may be revealed. Additional abnormal findings may include neoplasm, gastric ulcers, hiatal hernia, gastritis, and esophagitis.

Colonoscopy — Visualization of colon with a colonoscope.

Normal—Appearance of large intestinal mucosa is normal.

Inflammation, areas of ulceration, bleeding areas, strictures, polyps, colitis, diverticula, benign or malignant tumors, or foreign bodies may be observed in abnormal findings.

Sigmoidoscopy — Visualization of the sigmoid portion of the colon and the rectum with a sigmoidoscope.

Normal—Normal appearance of mucosa of sigmoid colon.

Inflammatory bowel disease, polyps, benign and cancerous tumors, and foreign bodies may be some of the abnormal findings during a sigmoidoscope examination.

Proctoscopy — Visualization of the rectum with a proctoscope.

Normal—Normal appearance to rectal mucosa and to anal canal.

Rectal prolapse, hemorrhoids, rectal strictures, fissures, abscesses, and fistula are some of the abnormal findings during a proctoscopic examination of the rectum.

Cystoscopy — Visualization of the structures of the urinary tract with a cystoscope.

Normal — The urethra, urethral orifices, urinary bladder interior, and male prostatic urethra appear normal.

Cancer of the bladder, BPH, bladder calculi, prostatitis, ureteral strictures, urinary fistulas, vesicle neck stenosis, ureterocele, polyps, and abnormal bladder capacity are some of the abnormal findings during a cystoscopic examination of the urinary bladder.

Ureteroscopy — Visualization of the ureters and pelvis of the kidney.

Normal — normal appearance of the ureters and pelvis of the kidney and its structures.

Renal or ureteral stones, inflammation or bleeding of the urethral mucosa, and lesions or abnormal structures of the renal pelvis are some of the abnormal findings in a ureteroscopic examination.

Bronchoscopy — Visualization of the trachea and bronchi with a bronchoscope.

Normal — nasopharynx, larynx, trachea, and bronchi are normal in appearance.

Abnormalities revealed in a bronchoscopic examination include but are not limited to bronchitis, carcinoma and other tumors, inflammatory process, tuberculosis, abnormal structures and disorders of the larynx and trachea, foreign bodies, and various pulmonary infections.

ARTERIAL BLOOD GASES

Arterial Blood Gas (ABG) Analysis. A measurement of dissolved oxygen and carbon dioxide in arterial blood. Also a measurement of pH and O_2 saturation of the arterial blood. ABGs are used to assess oxygenation and ventilation, along with acid–base balance. Additionally, they provide information regarding the effectiveness of therapy and the status of critical patients and are used in conjunction with pulmonary function studies.

Normal values are listed; however, these studies are complex and require the interpretation of a physician along with other diagnostic studies and consideration of symptoms and signs to provide a diagnosis or an evaluation.

Normal adult values:

pH: 7.35–7.45
$PaCO_2$: 35–45 mm Hg
PaO_2: 75–100 mmHg
HCO_3: 22–26 mEq/L
O_2 saturation: 96–100%

Increased pH is indicative of several disorders, including but not limited to alkali ingestion, diarrhea, vomiting, hyperventilation, high altitude sickness, metabolic acidosis, fever, and ingestion of certain drugs. Decreased pH is indicative of several disorders, including but not limited to asthma, cardiac disease, MI, renal disorders, Addison's disease, pulmonary disorders, respiratory acidosis, sepsis, shock, and malignant hyperthermia.

Increased $PaCO_2$ is indicative of several disorders, including but not limited to late-stage asthma, brain death, CHF, respiratory disorders, hypoventilation, renal disorders, poisoning, pneumothorax, respiratory acidosis, near drowning, and ingestion of certain drugs. Decreased $PaCO_2$ is indicative of several disorders, including but not limited to early-stage asthma, hyperventilation, dysrhythmias, respiratory alkalosis, metabolic acidosis, and ingestion of certain drugs.

Increased PaO_2 is indicative of but not limited to hyperventilation and hyperbaric oxygen exposure. Decreased PaO_2 is indicative of several disorders, including but not limited to ARDS, asthma, cardiac disorders, head injury, anoxia, hypoventilation, respiratory disorders, pneumothorax, respiratory failure, shock, smoke inhalation, and CVA.

Increased O_2 saturation is indicative of hyperbaric oxygenation. Decreased O_2 saturation is indicative of several disorders, including but not limited to anoxia, cardiac anomalies and disorders, carbon monoxide poisoning, ARDS, CVA, hypoventilation, respiratory disorders, pneumothorax, shock, smoke inhalation, and near drowning.

PULMONARY FUNCTION STUDIES

Pulmonary function studies are complex and include evaluation of several tests' results. Most tests are performed by respiratory therapists and results usually are reported to a pulmonologist for evaluation and correlation with symptoms and signs. Normal values are reported here; however, significance of these values is incomplete without the review and opinion of the pulmonologist, often assisted by the respiratory therapist.

Pulse Oximeter. An instrument (spectrophotometer) that provides a noninvasive measurement of the O_2 saturation of the arterial blood.

Normal — arterial blood oxygen saturation 95% or greater.

Peak Flow. A measurement of inspiratory effort.

Approximately 300 L/min and is based on sex, height, and age.

Spirometry. A measurement of lung capacity, volume, and flow rates used in the evaluation of asthma, bronchitis, COPD, and emphysema.

Methacholine Challenge. A measurement of lung volumes before and after inhalation of methacholine chloride used for diagnosis of asthma.

Normal—negative

Sputum Studies. Sputum studies are analyses and cultures of sputum (material expelled from the respiratory tract) to detect the presence of pathogens.

Normal—negative

Positive results might include respiratory disorders such as fungal infections, mycobacteria, tuberculosis, or carcinoma.

Pulmonary Function. Normal findings are reported in percentages of observed values and by expected values calculated to include allowances for age, sex, weight, and height. Abnormal results are considered to be less than 80% of calculated values. Consult a respiratory therapist for interpretation of values.

Tidal Volume—Normal: 500 ml
Expiratory Reserve Volume—Normal: 1500 ml
Residual Volume—Normal: 1500 ml
Inspiratory Reserve Volume—Normal: 2000 ml

MISCELLANEOUS TESTS

Bone Marrow Studies. Aspiration of bone marrow by needle from the sternum, posterior superior iliac spine, or the anterior iliac crest for diagnosis of neoplasms, metastasis, and blood disorders. Provides a basis for evaluation of hematologic disorders and infectious diseases.

Immune and Immunoglobulin Studies. Studies of the functioning or nonfunctioning of the patient's immune system.

Normal adult:

IgA: 60–400 mg/dl
IgG: 700–1500 mg/dl
IgM: 60–300 mg/dl
IgD: 0–8.0 mg/dl
IgE: 3–42 IU/ml

Increased levels of immunoglobulins are indicative of many disorders and need to be evaluated by a physician. Some disorders include arthritis, cancer, chronic infections, sinusitis, asthma, food and drug allergies, liver disease, SLE, and ingestion of certain drugs. Decreased levels of immunoglobulins are indicative of many disorders, including but not limited to AIDS, bacterial infection, advanced cancer, hypogammaglobulinemia, and ingestion of certain drugs.

Biopsies. The excision of tissue from the living body, followed by microscopic examination, for purpose of exact diagnosis.

Normal—no abnormal cells seen.

Abnormal findings are dependent on cell structure discovered during microscopic examination.

Lumbar Puncture. A surgical procedure to withdraw spinal fluid for analysis. A measurement and analysis of the chemical components of the cerebrospinal fluid used in diagnosis of CNS diseases and disorders.

Normal adult:

Appearance: Clear, colorless
Specific gravity: 1.006–1.008
Pressure: 90–150 mm H_2O
AST: 0–19 U
Bicarbonate: 22.9 mEq/L
WBC: 5 cells
Glucose: 40–70 mg/dl
Total protein: 15–60 mg/dl
Lactic acid: 10–24 mg/dl
VDRL: Negative
Bacteria or viruses: None present

Pressure is dependent on height and also whether patient is positioned in a sitting or horizontal position.

Abnormal findings are indicative of disorders or insults to the CNS.

Electroencephalogram. A recording of the electrical activity of the cerebral cortex of the brain, it helps to identify the locale of insult to cerebral tissue.

Normal—shows symmetrical patterns of electrical brain activity.

Abnormal findings include information to identify CNS or brain insults, hematomas, CVAs, epilepsy, brain tumors, and seizure activity. Lack of any activity is an indication of brain death.

Electromyelogram. An electrodiagnostic assessment and recording of the activity of the skeletal muscles; a nerve conduction study assessing the state of the muscle at rest and during contraction to provide an average picture of local electrical activity of the muscle.

Normal—nerve conduction normal and muscle action potential is normal.

Abnormal findings help to identify the site and cause of muscle disorders and neuronal lesions, particularly of involvement of the anterior horn of the spinal cord.

Gastric Analysis. Used in the diagnosis of pernicious anemia and peptic ulcers. The contents of the stomach are analyzed for acidity, appearance, and volume.

Normal adult:

Bile 0 or minimum
Mucus evenly mixed
Blood 0 or scant
Fasting acidity 2.5 mEq/L
Quantity 62 ml/hr
pH 1.0–2.5

Increased levels of gastric acid are indicative of certain disorders, including but not limited to post–massive small-intestinal resection, gastric or duodenal ulcer, hyperplasia, and hyperfunction of gastric cells. Decreased gastric acid levels are indicative of several disorders, including but not limited to pernicious anemia, postvagotomy, renal failure, rheumatoid arthritis, gastric cancer, atrophic gastritis, and vitiligo.

Pregnancy Tests (Human Chorionic Gonadotropin [hCG/UCG]). Used in diagnosis of pregnancy, abortion, ectopic pregnancy, and uterine pathology.

Normal:

negative

A positive result is indicative of pregnancy, either intrauterine or ectopic.

SCREENING

Tuberculosis (TB) Screening (Mantoux). An intradermal injection of tuberculin is given usually on the inner aspect of the lower arm. Results are read in 48 and 72 hours.

Normal:

negative

Positive—Localized thickening of the skin in the area, along with a redness, indicates the presence of active or dormant tuberculosis.

Positive reaction requires further investigation, usually including a chest radiograph.

Prostate-Specific Antigen (PSA). A serum blood test to determine the level of the prostate-specific antigen. This is a screening test that should be followed by a digital rectal examination (DRE) of the prostate gland to determine any abnormalities. Often additional diagnostic studies are indicated.

PSA blood tests are reported as nanograms per milliliter.

PSA is considered as a marker in the screening for prostatic cancer. Zero to 4 ng/ml usually are considered to be in the normal range; 4 to 10 ng/ml are considered borderline; values greater than 10 ng/ml are considered high. However, increasing age makes slightly higher values acceptable.

Acceptable levels for up to age 40 years 0–2 ng/ml
40–50 years 0–4 ng/ml
50–60 years 0–5 ng/ml
60–70 years 0–6 ng/ml

Any increase of 20% or more in the PSA value in 1 year's time is suspicious and requires further investigation. Above-acceptable levels may be indicative of cancer. Additional investigation, including biopsy, is recommended.

The PSA screening should be completed before the DRE. A constant increase in the PSA leads to suspicion of prostate cancer. PSA levels that fluctuate up and down usually are not indicative of cancer but of an inflammatory process in the prostate or of BPH. PSA is a screening tool and must be combined with a DRE for a more accurate screen. Men older than 50 years of age are encouraged to have prostate screening on an annual basis; however, men older than 70 years of age may or may not be subjected to screening because of the high incidence of prostatic cancer in this group and the treatment protocol of watchful waiting without significant intervention.

Pap Smear (Papanicolaou test). A cytologic examination of cells that have been scraped or aspirated from the cervix and cervical os. A screening test done annually, especially before any female hormones are prescribed.

Results of Pap smears are now reported in two different formats. A system based on classes and the Bethesda System, a system using descriptive diagnostic terms, are the two methods of reporting results to the physician.

Class System:
Class I Negative with no abnormal or unusual cells seen.
Class II Negative smear but with some reservation based on the presence of inflammatory cells or evidence of infection. Additional causes may be regeneration of cervical cells or changes related to trauma, infections, or childbirth. A repeat Pap smear and treatment of the underlying cause may be indicated.
Class III Presence of some abnormal cells that may be considered premalignant. Changes may vary from mild dysplasia to severe dysplasia. Further evaluation, possibly including colposcopy, is indicated.
Class IV Indicative of a high degree of suspicion for malignancy. Prompt and complete evaluation is indicated.
Class V Indication of high probability of more extensive malignancy. Prompt and complete evaluation to determine the extent of disease is indicated.
Bethesda System: The physician may relate the results as normal or abnormal because surface cervical cells may appear abnormal but are not always malignant.
Dysplasia. Although not cancer, dysplasia may develop into very early cancer of the cervix. The cells in dysplasia undergo a series of changes in their appearance, appear abnormal in microscopic examination, and have not invaded nearby healthy tissue. The cells are described as mild, moderate, severe according to their appearance under the microscope.
Squamous intraepithelial lesion (SIL) describes the appearance of abnormal changes on the surface of the cervix. SIL cells are classified further as low grade, having early changes in size, shape, and number, or high grade, containing a large number of precancerous cells with a very different appearance from normal cells.
Cervical intraepithelial neoplasia (CIN) is a description of a new abnormal growth of surface layers of cells. Additional information is provided by using the term CIN and the numbers 1, 2, and 3 to describe how much of the cervix contains abnormal cells.
Carcinoma in situ refers to a preinvasive cancer that has not invaded deeper tissues and contains only surface cells.
Atypical glandular cells of undetermined significance (AGCUS) describes slightly abnormal glandular cells of the cervix.
Atypical squamous cells of undetermined significance (ASCUS) describes slightly abnormal squamous cells of the cervix possibly caused by a vaginal infection or by HPV (human papillomavirus).
Inflammation. Inflammation is present in the cervical cells, and white blood cells also were seen.
Hyperkeratosis. Hyperkeratosis describes dried skin cells on the cervix, often resulting from cervical cap or diaphragm usage or a cervical infection.

Abnormal results range from insignificant to precancerous to invasive cancer of the cervix. Repeat Pap smears in 6 months are often all that is indicated for mild dysplasia and class II Pap smears. Colposcopy and further investigation may be indicated in other abnormal findings. The physician discusses abnormal findings with the patient, and a course of treatment or follow-up is determined.

Mammogram. A radiographic examination of the soft tissues of the breast. A screening test done on an annual basis for women older than 40 years of age to detect the presence of breast disease. This screening also should be accompanied by a manual examination of the breast tissue by a physician. Monthly breast self-examinations are recommended.

Normal:

negative for disease

Identification of abnormal conditions may indicate further investigation. Various benign disorders, including fibrocystic disease of the breast, may be responsible for a positive interpretation. Malignant neoplasms of the breast tissue may be detected, and further investigation, including ultrasound or biopsy of any suspicious area found on the mammogram, is indicated.

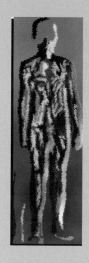

Index

Note: Page numbers in *italics* refer to illustrations; page numbers followed by t refer to tables.

Index